Understanding Medical Terminology

5th edition

Author

Sister Agnes Clare Frenay, S.S.M., R.N., B.S. in Nr., M.S. in Nr. Ed.

Professor Emeritus of Nursing
Saint Louis University School of Nursing and
Allied Health Professions
St. Louis, Mo.

Illustrator

Helen M. Smith, R.N., B.F.A., M.A., F.I.A.L.

Saint Louis University School of Medicine,
St. Louis, Mo.

Published by

The Catholic Hospital Association

St. Louis, Missouri 63104

Contributing Illustrators

Sister Jeanne Derer, S.S.M., B.S., A.D.A.

Sister Susan Scholl, S.S.M., B.S., R.N.

FIFTH EDITION
Copyright © 1973

by THE CATHOLIC HOSPITAL ASSOCIATION
St. Louis, Mo. 63104

Previous editions copyrighted 1958, 1962, 1964 and 1969

Library of Congress Catalog Card No. 72-97662
ISBN 0-87125-006-3

A. M. D. G.

Dedicated to Christ, the Divine Healer,

and to all those in the health professions

who offer Christ-like service

to the patient

Foreword

The Catholic Hospital Association is happy to have the opportunity to publish the Fifth Edition of UNDERSTANDING MEDICAL TERMINOLOGY. Sister Agnes Clare Frenay, SSM has drawn on her twenty years of teaching experience and her close association with the latest medical developments to produce a highly practical, comprehensive text.

The author's contribution to education and to the health field in particular cannot be overestimated. Her dedication to producing the finest available medical terminology text and updating each edition with the latest information to meet the quickening pace of medical progress has benefited both instructors and students in the allied health field.

Previous editions have been translated into a seven-volume Braille edition by the American Printing House for the Blind in Louisville, Kentucky. Similar transcriptions have been produced by the New York Assocation for the Blind. The Library of Congress was given permission to transcribe this text into large type in connection with their program for blind persons.

In 1969, in recognition of the author's noteworthy contribution to literature in the health field, the Board of Trustees of The Catholic Hospital Association awarded Sister Agnes Clare a plaque at their annual convention.

The officers and the Executive Board of The Catholic Hospital Association hope that the Fifth Edition will continue to effectively contribute to the ever-increasing needs of education in the health field.

SISTER MARY MAURITA, RSM
Executive Vice President

June 1973

Preface

Approximately two years of library research have made the fifth edition of UNDERSTANDING MEDICAL TERMINOLOGY a reality. The content and overall plan of the previous work are retained in this new text, since their practical usefulness has received general recognition. It should be reemphasized that the tables which consider conditions amenable to surgery merely offer examples of how certain health problems may be solved by surgical intervention. Their purpose is to put into sharp relief medical terms in a manner conducive to the integration of knowledge and promotion of a better comprehension of the meaning of terms.

Efforts have been extended to update the text by presenting current information related to medical progress in clear, precise definitions. New illustrations for recently developed surgical procedures add clarification to their meaning.

Primary targets of interest are new medical terms related to orthopedic, cardiovascular and blood disorders, immunology, laboratory, radiologic and nuclear procedures. The comprehensive lists of references and bibliography following each chapter provide a rich source of documentation which is further enhanced by the author's consultation with medical experts in various specialties. It is hoped that both factors insure a relatively high degree of reliability of the information presented and that inquisitive minds feel stimulated to explore the professional literature in the health field.

Linguistic improvements of the first chapter are credited to Reverend Marcus A. Haworth, S.J., Ph. D., Professor of Classical Languages at St. Louis University, who gave directives for the changes. This chapter continues to be fundamental to the text and should be the focus of attention in teaching and studying medical terminology.

As in previous editions individual revised chapters of UNDERSTANDING MEDICAL TERMINOLOGY were submitted to faculty members of St. Louis University School of Medicine for preview to insure the correctness of the definitions. Grateful acknowledgement is made to Dr. Vallee L. Willman, Professor of Surgery and Chairman of the Department of Surgery, Dr. Robert M. O'Brien, Clinical Professor Emeritus of Orthopedic Surgery, Dr. Eugene G. Hamilton, Clinical Professor of Gynecology and Obstetrics, Dr. John F. Schweiss, Professor of Surgery and Chairman of the Department of Anesthesiology, Dr. Charles R. Doyle, Clinical Professor of Surgery, Dr. Daniel Sexton, Associate Professor Emeritus of Internal Medicine, Dr. John E. Byrne, Urologist and Dr. Howard J. Aylward, Otolaryngologist.

Recognition and sincere gratitude are extended to Dr. Eugene F. Tucker, Associate Professor of Pathology, St. Louis University and Director of Medical Laboratories, St. Mary's Health Center, and Dr. John A. Gantz, Director of Nuclear Medicine, St. Mary's Health Center, for their unfailing resourcefulness in assisting in the selection and updating of the terms in their specialties.

Sister Mary Imelda Pingel, Chairman and Professor of Physical Therapy, shared her knowledge and experience in editing the chapter of her specialty.

The author's indebtedness to Sister Mary Ernest Freiberger for her gracious willingness and proficiency in typing the manuscript is indeed great. In addition Sister Susan Scholl merits grateful acknowledgement for her contributions to the illustrations of the text. Obviously the kind volunteer, Sister Mary Blanche Kulage, who assisted with the proofreading and index is likewise deserving of heartfelt gratitude.

A very sincere thanks is due to Mr. Art Krings of the Universal Printing Company and Florian W. Beuckman of the Typographic Sales, Inc. for their cooperative efforts in seeing the book through the press.

Mr. George P. Oberst, Vice President and Educational Director of Matthews Book Company, deserves recognition and appreciation for his generosity in making the newest medical texts available to update the terminology.

Gratitude is also expressed to Sister Mary Maurita, RSM, Executive Vice President and Edward J. Pollock, Publisher of the Catholic Hospital Association for publishing the text and to Mrs. Mary Krieger, Director of Publications, for her untiring efforts and support in making the fifth edition a reality.

On previous occasions permissions were granted by Charles Thomas, Publisher and the Harvard University Press to incorporate factual data on laboratory tests in UNDERSTANDING MEDICAL TERMINOLOGY from Dr. Opal E. Hepler's MANUAL FOR CLINICAL LABORATORY METHODS and Drs. Page and Culver's SYLLABUS OF LABORATORY EXAMINATIONS IN DIAGNOSIS.

New copyright permissions were obtained from McGraw-Hill Book Company for including in the text brief statements from the 6th edition of HARRISON'S PRINCIPLES OF INTERNAL MEDICINE, edited by Maxwell M. Wintrobe, M.D. and from the American Psychiatric Association for quoting some definitions of the 3rd edition of A PSYCHIATRIC GLOSSARY.

UNDERSTANDING MEDICAL TERMINOLOGY in its latest revision should provide a basic reference for those who wish to explore the challenges of medical progress.

It is anticipated that the text will undergo further transformations in response to the widening perspectives of the health sciences in the future.

SISTER AGNES CLARE FRENAY, SSM

June 1973

Table of Contents

PART I

TERMS RELATED TO BIOLOGICAL DISORDERS

List of Tables

List of Illustrations

PART I

TERMS RELATED TO BIOLOGICAL DISORDERS

Chapter I
Orientation to Medical Terminology

OBJECTIVES AND VALUES

Medical terminology is the professional language of those who directly or indirectly are engaged in the art of healing. Its strangeness may seem bewildering at first to the average student and its complexity may tax his power of concentration. These difficulties, however, gradually disappear as the student assimilates a working knowledge of the elements of medical terms which enables him to analyze words etymologically and according to their meaning. In the beginning the drudgery of memorizing is somewhat annoying to the novice in the field, but memory work is only a steppingstone to a keener understanding of the professional language. It is obvious that the intellect is constantly engaged in the study of medical terms in various types of mental processes: the analysis of words, their interpretation and, to a moderate degree, the transfer of knowledge, by combining word roots synthetically with prefixes and suffixes.

Since the definitions of terms touch on a number of specialties — medicine, surgery, urology, gynecology, psychiatry, orthopedics, endocrinology, oncology, laboratory diagnosis and others — medical terminology adapts itself easily to the integration and application of knowledge. Professional workers in the health fields, hospital administrators, nurses, medical record librarians and secretaries, medical and radiologic technologists and physical therapists will find in the subject-matter ample material of practical significance for their professional careers.

The terms selected (and a selective process is imperative because of the multiplicity of terms) revolve around the human body in health and disease, the one dynamic power of the biological sciences which never loses its interest value. The time-honored principle to proceed from the normal to the abnormal is realized in the organizational pattern in which anatomic terms form the foundation for diagnostic terms and related operative and symptomatic terms.

Instead of stress on etymological subtleties and Greek and Latin derivations, emphasis is laid on the meaning of word roots and combining forms because this approach facilitates the acquisition and retention of knowledge.

The primary goal of introducing the student to medical terminology is to help him develop the ability to read and understand the language of medicine. Efforts are directed to promote a knowledge of the elements of medical terms, an understanding of standard medical abbreviations, the ability to spell medical terms, and an appreciation of the logical method found in medical terminology.

BASIC CONCEPTS

The majority of medical terms claim Greek and Latin ancestry. Some have been adopted from modern languages, especially from the German and French. Obviously, the process of coining words by usage continues as time goes on and new scientific advances necessitate verbal expression. Theoretically speaking, word formation should safeguard the purity of language by joining Greek roots to Greek prefixes and suffixes and Latin roots to Latin combining forms. In reality, many medical terms are bilingual in their derivation as, for example, teleradiography which combines the Greek prefix "tele" (distant) with the Latin root "radius" (ray) and Greek root "graphein" (to write).

Another peculiarity in medical terminology is the fact that frequently the name of the organ descends from the Latin, while the disease affecting the organ is inherited from the

1

Greek. For instance, "marrow" originates from the Latin **medulla,** but an inflammation of the marrow is termed myelitis from the Greek stem **myelos.**

Concerning the spelling of medical terms, more than one way may be acceptable due to the fact that both the Greek and Latinized spelling of the medical term have been adopted as being correct. Attempts have been made to give both spellings throughout the text.

The scholar of medical terminology may well be filled with awe when he finds in the writings of Hippocrates (460-370 B.C.) a wealth of terms which are still alive after 2000 years although their meaning may have changed. Some refer to human anatomy as acromion, apophysis, olecranon, bronchus, thorax, meninges, peritoneum, symphysis and ureter, others bring to mind obstetrical concepts as bregma, chorion and lochia, still others reflect a knowledge of diseases and deformities as carcinoma, emphysema, ileus, nephritis, phthisis, kyphosis and lordosis. One wonders why Aristotle (384-322 B.C.) mentions alopecia, an abnormal baldness and eye conditions as glaucoma, exophthalmos and leukoma. Was a personal element involved?

It is a worthwhile experience to reach back into antiquity to unravel the intriguing analogies of medical terms. All sorts of creatures from the animal kingdom have found their way into the language of healing. The Greek karkinos, crab means carcinoma and the Latin crab, cancer. Lupus is the Latin word for wolf, coccyx the Greek word for cuckoo. It is obvious why cochlea (G) refers to a snail and cauda equina (L) to a horse's tail. However, one is surprised that muscle from the Latin musculus means little mouse and vermis (L) worm when one considers the potential vigor of the former and the vital significance of the latter as a connecting lobe of the cerebellum.

Startling, too, is our semantic indebtedness to the grapevine. The Greek root staphyle envisions a bunch of grapes and in its combination with cocci reminds of clusters of grapes and berries. Its Latin partner uva is found in uvea and uvula, both referring to grapes.

The search for the origin of terms stirs our academic interest in the culture of the people who have coined the medical words. Thus the warlike spirit of the Hellenistic age is reflected in xiphoid, sword; thyroid, shield and thorax, breastplate. Stapes, stirrup and sella, saddle remind of a horse's trappings, while the ossicles malleus, hammer and incus, anvil depict miniatures of a blacksmith's implements. Even the names of musical instruments take on medical meanings. Salpinx (G), trumpet and tympanum (L), drum are worthy examples of the intuitive perception of ancient minds. The study of medical terminology can become indeed a rewarding experience which unveils the character of genius in the medical language.

The pronunciation of medical terms follows no rigid rules. Flexibility is its outstanding characteristic. Since authorities do not agree upon any special pronunciation, common usage must prevail. Even in the same locality and in the same hospital, there will be discrepancies in pronouncing medical terms. To assist the student in developing the ability to speak the language of medicine, brief discussions of medical subjects have been included in the text for oral reading exercises.

In the process of learning, the cultivation of analyzing medical terms is of primary importance. It simplifies the assimilation of knowledge and promotes the development of a logical mind. To analyze means to unloose, to resolve. The analysis of medical terms is then the systematic breaking up of the term into its component parts — its suffixes, roots and prefixes. This method may convey the meaning in a clear-cut way as, for example:

	Analysis	**Definition**
Appendectomy —	ectomy: removal	Removal of the appendix
	appendec: appendix	

or the meaning may be merely implied requiring a more precise definition as is the case with the term "anemia." A breakup of this word into the prefix "an" and the root "emia" conveys an exaggerated impression since, in reality, anemia does not refer to a total lack of blood which would be incompatible with life, but merely to a condition characterized by a deficiency of red blood cells and hemoglobin. In other words, a definition explains and interprets a medical term, describing its essential properties in contradistinction to an analysis which breaks up the term in its linguistic elements. The introductory chapter seeks to develop an analytic attitude in the student. By making him aware of the structural design of words and helping him to form the habit of analyzing terms, it lays the foundation for the study of medical terminology. Its mastery will render the understanding of the terms offered in the subsequent chapters comparatively easy.[3]

ELEMENTS OF MEDICAL TERMS

I. Suffixes and Compounding Elements

True suffixes refer to a syllable or syllables denoting a preposition or adverb attached to the end of a word, root, or stem to modify its meaning. Many endings are adjectives or nouns added to a root to form compound words. They may be referred to as combining forms or pseudosuffixes. To simplify learning, linguistic distinctions have been disregarded in the following, and modifying endings have been classified according to their meanings into diagnostic, operative and symptomatic suffixes and compounding elements.

In analyzing terms it is advisable to begin with the suffix and proceed to the root or root and prefix. This method of approach may reveal the exact definition of the term, or it may convey its applied meaning.

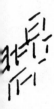

A. Diagnostic Suffixes and Compounding Elements:

Suffix	Term	Analysis	Definition
-cele (G) hernia, tumor, protrusion	cystocele	*kystis:* bladder *kele:* hernia	Hernia of the bladder.
	gastrocele hydrocele	*gaster:* stomach; —; *hydor:* water *kele:* tumor	Hernia of the stomach. Serous tumor as of testis.
	myelocele	*myelos:* marrow *kele:* protrusion	Protrusion of spinal cord through the vertebrae.
-emia (G) blood	hyperglycemia hyperglycosemia	*hyper:* excessive *glykus:* sweet, sugar *haima:* blood	Abnormally high blood sugar.
	polycythemia	*polys:* many, excessive *kytos:* cell —; —;	Abnormal increase of red blood cells and hemoglobin in the blood.
-ectasis (G) expansion, dilatation	angiectasis	*angeion:* vessel *ektasis:* dilatation	Abnormal dilatation of a blood vessel.
	atelectasis —; neonatorum	*ateles:* imperfect; —; —; *neos:* new *natus:* birth, born	An airless, functionless lung. Imperfect expansion of lungs at birth.
	bronchiectasis	*bronchos:* bronchus —;	Abnormal dilatation of a bronchus or bronchi.
-iasis (G) condition, formation of, presence of	lithiasis	*lithos:* stone *iasis:* presence of	Formation of stones.
	cholelithiasis	*chole:* bile; —;	Presence of calculi in the gallbladder.
	nephrolithiasis	*nephros:* kidney; —;	Stones present in the kidney.

NOTE: (G) means that the suffix is a Greek derivative, (L) a Latin. The dash and semicolon refer to the suffix which has already been given. In the analysis the Greek and Latin words are used to show the derivation, but the student needs only to learn the English version.

Suffix	Term	Analysis	Definition
-itis (G) inflammation	carditis iritis poliomyelitis	*kardia:* heart *itis:* inflammation *iris:* rainbow, iris *polios:* gray *myelos:* marrow; —;	Inflammation of the heart. Inflammation of the iris. Inflammation of the gray matter of the spinal cord.
-malacia (G) softening	encephalomalacia osteomalacia splenomalacia	*egkephalos:* brain *malakia:* softening *osteon:* bone; —; *splen:* spleen; —;	Softening of the brain. Softening of the bones. Softening of the spleen.
-megaly (G) enlargement	acromegaly hepatomegaly splenomegaly	*akros:* extreme *megas:* large *hepat:* liver; —; *splen:* spleen; —;	Disease marked by enlargement of bones of head and soft part of extremities and face. Enlargement of the liver. Enlargement of the spleen.
-oma (G) tumor	adenoma carcinoma sarcoma	*aden:* gland *oma:* tumor *karkinos:* cancer; —; *sark:* flesh; —;	Glandular tumor. Malignant tumor of epithelial tissue. Malignant tumor of connective tissue.
-osis (G) condition, disease increase	arteriosclerosis dermatosis neurosis	*arteria;* artery *sklerosis:* hardening *derma:* skin *osis:* condition *neuron:* nerve; —;	Hardening of the arteries. Any skin condition. Functional disorder of the nervous system.
-pathy (G) disease	adenopathy myopathy myelopathy	*aden;* gland *pathos:* disease *mys:* muscle; —; *myelos:* marrow; —;	Any glandular disease. Any disease of a muscle. Any pathological disorder of the spinal cord.
-ptosis (G) falling	blepharoptosis gastroptosis nephroptosis	*blepharon:* eyelid *ptosis:* a falling *gaster:* stomach; —; *nephros:* kidney; —;	Dropping of the eyelid. Downward displacement of the stomach. Downward displacement of the kidney.
-rhexis (G) rupture	angiorrhexis cardiorrhexis hysterorrhexis	*angeion:* vessel *rhexis:* rupture *kardia:* heart; —; *hystera:* uterus; —;	Rupture of a blood vessel or lymphatic. Rupture of the heart. Rupture of the uterus.

B. Operative Suffixes and Compounding Elements:

-centesis (G) puncture	paracentesis abdominal para- centesis thoracentesis	*para:* beside *kentesis:* a puncture *abdomen:* belly; —; *thorax:* chest; —;	Puncture of a cavity. Puncture and aspiration of the peritoneal cavity. Aspiration of the pleural cavity.
-ectomy (G) excision	myomectomy oophorectomy tonsillectomy	*mys:* muscle *oma:* tumor *ektome:* excision *oophor:* ovary; —; *tonsilla:* tonsil; —;	Excision of a tumor of the muscle. Removal of an ovary. Removal of tonsils.

Suffix	Term	Analysis	Definition
-desis (G) binding, fixation	arthrodesis	*arthron:* joint *desis:* fixation	Surgical fixation of a joint.
	spondylosyndesis	*spondylos:* vertebra —;	Surgical fixation of the vertebrae.
	tenodesis	*tenon:* tendon; —;	Fixation of a tendon to a bone.
-lithotomy (G) incision for removal of stones	cholelithotomy	*chole:* bile, gall; —;	Incision into gallbladder for removal of stones.
	nephrolithotomy	*nephros:* kidney; —;	Incision into kidney for removal of stones.
	sialolithotomy	*sialon:* saliva	Incision into salivary gland for removal of stones.
-pexy (G) suspension, fixation	hysteropexy	*hystera:* uterus *pexis:* fixation	Abdominal fixation or suspension of the uterus.
	mastopexy	*mastos:* breast; —;	Fixation of a pendulous breast.
	orchiopexy	*orchis:* testis; —;	Fixation of an undescended testis.
-plasty (G) surgical correction, plastic repair of	arthroplasty	*arthron:* joint *plassein:* to form	Reconstruction operation on joint.
	hernioplasty	*ernos:* a young shoot; —;	Plastic repair of hernia.
	proctoplasty	*proktos:* anus, rectum; —;	Surgical repair of rectum.
-rhaphy (G) suture	perineorrhaphy	*perinaion:* perineum *rhaphe:* suture	Suture of a lacerated perineum.
	staphylorrhaphy	*staphyle:* uvula; —;	Suture of a cleft palate.
	trachelorrhaphy	*trachelos:* neck; —;	Suture of a torn cervix uteri.
-scopy (G) inspection, examination	bronchoscopy	*bronchos:* windpipe *skopein:* to examine	Examination of the bronchi with an endoscope.
	cystoscopy	*kystis:* bladder; —;	Inspection of the bladder with a cystoscope.
	esophagoscopy	*oisophagos:* esophagus —;	Endoscopic examination of the esophagus.
-stomy (G) creation of a more or less permanent opening	colostomy	*kolon:* colon; *stoma:* opening	Creation of an opening into the colon through the abdominal wall.
	cystostomy	*kystis:* bladder —;	Creation of an opening into the urinary bladder through the abdomen.
	gastroduoden- ostomy	*gaster:* stomach *duoden:* duodenum	Creation of an opening between stomach and duodenum.
-tomy (G) incision into	antrotomy	*antron:* antrum *tome:* incision	Incision into the antrum of Highmore to establish drainage.
	neurotomy	*neuron:* nerve; —;	Dissection of a nerve.
	thoracotomy	*thorax:* chest; —;	Opening of the chest.
-tripsy (G) crushing, friction	lithotripsy	*lithos:* stone *tripsis:* crushing	Crushing of a calculus in the bladder or urethra.
	phrenicotripsy	*phren:* diaphragm; —;	Crushing of the phrenic nerve.

C. Symptomatic Suffixes and Compounding Elements:

Suffix	Term	Analysis	Definition
-algia (G) pain	gastralgia	*gaster:* stomach *algos:* pain	Epigastric pain.
	nephralgia	*nephros:* kidney; —;	Renal pain.
	neuralgia	*neuron:* nerve; —;	Lancinating nerve pain.

Suffix	Term	Analysis	Definition
-genic (G) origin	bronchogenic	*bronchos:* windpipe *gennan:* to originate	Originating in the bronchi.
	neurogenic	*neuron:* nerve; —;	Originating in the nerves.
	osteogenic	*osteon:* bone; —;	Originating in the bones.
	pathogenic	*pathos:* disease; —;	Disease producing.
-lysis (G) dissolution, breaking down	hemolysis	*haima:* blood *lysis:* breaking down	A breaking down of red blood cells.
	myolysis	*mys:* muscle; —;	Destruction of muscular tissue.
	neurolysis	*neuron:* nerve; —;	Disintegration of nerve tissue.
-oid (G) like	fibroid	*fibra:* fiber *eidos:* resembling	A tumor of fibrous tissue, resembling fibers.
	lipoid	*lipos:* fat; —;	Fat-like.
	lymphoid	*lympha:* lymph; —;	Resembling lymph.
-osis (G) increase, condition	anisocytosis	*anisos:* unequal *kytos:* cell *osis:* condition	Inequality of size of cells.
	lymphocytosis	*lympha:* lymph; —; —;	Excess of lymph cells.
-penia (G) deficiency, decrease	leukopenia	*leukos:* white *penia:* decrease	Abnormal decrease of leukocytes in the blood.
	neutropenia	*neuter:* neutral; —;	Abnormal decrease of neutrophils in the blood.
-spasm (G) involuntary contractions	chirospasm	*cheir:* hand *spasmos:* spasm or contraction of muscles	A spasm as contraction of the hand. (Writer's cramp)
	dactylospasm	*dactylos:* finger —;	Spasm or cramp in fingers or toes.
	enterospasm	*enteron:* intestine —;	Painful intestinal contractions.

II. Roots

The root stem or main body of a word indicates the organ or part which is modified by a prefix or suffix, or both. Properly, Greek combining forms or roots should be used only with Greek prefixes and suffixes, Latin with Latin. In reality there are many inconsistencies in the word formation of medical terms. A vowel, usually a, i, or o, is often inserted between the combining forms for euphony.

Root	Term	Analysis	Definition
aden- (G) gland	adenectomy	*aden:* gland *ektome:* excision	Excision of a gland.
	adenoma	—; *oma:* tumor	Glandular tumor.
	adenocarcinoma	—; *karkinos:* cancer —;	Malignant tumor of glandular epithelium.
aer- (G) air	aerated	*aer:* air	Filled with air.
	aerobic	*bios:* life	Pertaining to organism which lives only in the presence of air.
	aeroneurosis	—; *neuron:* nerve *osis:* diseased condition	A functional nervous disorder affecting aeroplane flyers.

NOTE: The dash and semicolon refer to the root which has already been given.

Root	Term	Analysis	Definition
angio- (G) vessel	angiotomy	*angeion:* vessel *tome:* a cutting	Dissection of blood vessels.
	angitis or angiitis	—; *itis:* inflammation	Inflammation of the blood vessels or lymphatics.
arth- (G) joint	arthralgia	*arthron:* joint *algos:* pain	Pain in the joints.
	arthritis	—;	Inflammation of the joints.
	arthrology	*itis:* inflammation —; *logos:* study, science	The science of the joints.
blephar- (G) eyelid	blepharedema	*blepharon:* eyelid *oidema:* swelling	Swelling of the eyelids.
	blepharoplasty	—;	Plastic operation upon the eyelid.
	blepharoptosis	*plassein:* to form —; *ptosis:* a falling	Dropping of the upper eyelid.
cardi- (G) heart	cardiac	*kardia:* heart	Pertaining to the heart or esophageal orifice of the stomach.
	phonocardiography	*phono:* sound; —; *graphein:* to write	Graphic recording of heart sounds.
	electrocardiogram	*elektron:* amber; —; *gramma:* writing	A graphic record of the heart beat by an electrometer.
cerebro- (L) brain	cerebral	*cerebrum:* brain	Pertaining to the brain.
	cerebromalacia	—; *malakia:* softening	Softening of the brain.
	cerebrospinal	—; *spina:* a thorn, the backbone	Referring to brain and spinal cord.
cephal- (G) head	cephalad	*kephale:* head *ad:* toward	Toward the head.
	cephalic	—; *ic:* pertaining to	Pertaining to the head.
	cephalitis	—; *itis:* inflammation	Inflammation of the brain.
cerv- (L) neck	cervical	*cervix:* neck *al:* pertaining to	Pertaining to the neck.
	cervicectomy	—; *ektome:* excision	Excision of the neck of the uterus.
	cervicovesical	—; *vesica:* bladder —;	Relating to the cervix uteri and bladder.
cheil, chil- (G) lip	cheilitis	*cheilos:* lip *itis:* inflammation	Inflammation of the lip.
	cheiloplasty	—; *plassein:* to form	Plastic operation of the lip.
	cheilosis	—; *osis:* diseased condition	Morbid condition of the lips due to vitamin B deficiency.
chir- (G) hand	chiromegaly	*cheir:* hand *megas:* large	Abnormal size of the hands, wrists and ankles.
	chiroplasty	—; *plassein:* to form	Plastic surgery on the hand.
	chiropody	—; *pous:* foot	Treatment of conditions of the hands and feet.
chol- (G) bile	cholangitis	*chole:* bile *angeion:* vessel *itis:* inflammation	Inflammation of the bile duct.
	cholecyst	—; *kystis:* bladder, sac	Gallbladder.
	cholecystogram	—; —; *gramma:* mark	A radiogram of the gallbladder.

Root	Term	Analysis	Definition
chondr- (G) cartilage	chondrectomy	*chondros:* cartilage *ektome:* excision	Excision of a cartilage.
	chondrofibroma	—; *fibra:* fiber *oma:* tumor	A mixed tumor composed of fibrous tissue and cartilage.
	chondroma	—; —;	A cartilaginous tumor.
cost- (L) rib	costochondral	*costa:* rib *chondros:* cartilage	Pertaining to a rib and its cartilage.
	costophrenic angle	—; *phren:* diaphragm *angle:* corner	The angle formed by the ribs and diaphragm.
	costosternal	—; *sternon:* breast	Referring to the ribs and breast bone.
crani- (G, L) skull	cranial	*kranion:* skull *al:* pertaining to	Pertaining to the skull.
	craniotabes	—; *tabes:* a wasting	A thinning or atrophy of the skull bones.
	craniotomy	—; *tome:* incision	Surgical opening of skull.
cysto- (G) bladder, sac	cyst	*kystis:* bladder, sac	A bladder; any sac containing a liquid.
	cystography	—; *graphein:* to write	Radiographic examination of the urinary bladder following the introduction of air or opaque solution.
	cystoscope	—; *skopein:* to examine	Instrument for interior examination of the bladder.
cyt- (G) cell	cytology	*kytos:* cell *logos:* study	The study of cell life.
	erythrocyte	*erythros:* red *kytos:* cell	Red blood cell.
	lymphocyte	*lympha:* lymph; —;	Lymph cell, a nongranular leukocyte.
dacry- (G) tear	dacryadenitis	*dakry:* tear *aden:* gland *itis:* inflammation	Inflammation of the lacrimal (tear) gland.
	dacryocele	—; *kele:* hernia	Protrusion of the lacrimal sac.
	dacryocyst	—; *kystis:* sac	The lacrimal sac.
dactyl- (G) finger, toe	dactylitis	*dactylos:* finger *itis:* inflammation	Chronic disease of bones of fingers or toes in young children.
	dactylogram	—; *gramma:* a mark	A fingerprint.
	dactylomegaly	—; *megas:* large	Abnormal size of fingers and toes.
derm- (G) skin	dermatitis	*derma:* skin *itis:* inflammation	Inflammation of the skin.
	dermal	—; *al:* relating to	Relating to the skin.
	dermopathy	—; *pathos:* disease	Any skin disease.
encephal- (G) brain	encephalitis	*egkephalos:* brain *itis:* inflammation	Inflammation of the brain.
	encephaloma	—; *oma:* tumor	Brain tumor.
	encephalography	—; *graphein:* to write	Radiographic examination of head after withdrawal of fluid and replacing it with air.
enter- (G) intestine	enteritis	*enteron:* intestine *itis:* inflammation	Inflammation of the intestines.
	enterocele	—; *kele:* hernia	A hernia of the intestines.
	enterocolitis	—; *kolon:* colon; —;	Inflammation of intestines and colon.

Root	Term	Analysis	Definition
psycho- (G) soul, mind	psychiatry	*psyche:* mind *iatreia:* healing	Medical specialty treating mental and neurotic disorders.
	psychoneurosis	—; *neuron:* nerve *osis:* disease or condition	A functional disorder of mental origin without demonstrable lesion.
	psychopathy	—; *pathos:* disease	Any mental disease usually related to defective character and personality.
pyel- (G) pelvis	pyelitis	*pyelos:* pelvis *itis:* inflammation	Inflammation of the pelvis of the kidney.
	pyelogram	—; *gramma:* a mark	Radiogram of the ureter and renal pelvis.
	pyelography	—; *graphein:* to write	Radiography of a renal pelvis and ureter.
pyloro- (G) pylorus, gatekeeper	pylorus	*pyloros:* gatekeeper	Orifice between stomach and duodenum.
	pylorostenosis	—; *stenosis:* narrowing	Constriction of pylorus.
	pyloromyotomy	—; *mys:* muscle *tome:* a cutting	Incision of the pyloric sphincter to relieve pyloric stenosis.
pyo- (G) pus	pyogenic	*pyon:* pus *genesis:* formation	Pus forming.
	pyometritis	—; *metra:* uterus *itis:* inflammation	Purulent inflammation of the uterus.
	pyonephrosis	—; *nephros:* kidney	Pus in the renal pelvis.
radi- (L) ray	radioactivity	*radius:* ray *activus:* acting	The ability to emit rays which can penetrate various substances.
	radiosensitive	—; *sensitivus:* feeling	Capable of being destroyed by radioactive substances.
	radiotherapy	—; *therapeia:* treatment	The use of radiation of any type in treating diseases.
spondyl- (G) vertebra	spondylitis	*spondylos:* vertebra *itis:* inflammation	Inflammation of vertebrae.
	spondylolisthesis	—; *olisthesis:* a slipping	Forward dislocation of lumbar vertebrae with pelvic deformity.
	spondylosyndesis	—; *syndesis:* a binding together	Surgical formation of an ankylosis between vertebrae.
trachel- (G) neck	trachelitis	*trachelos:* neck *itis:* inflammation	Inflammation of the cervix uteri.
	tracheloplasty	—; *plassein:* to form	Plastic operation of the cervix uteri.
	trachelorrhaphy	—; *rhaphe:* suture	Suturing of a torn cervix uteri.
tubercul- (L) tubercle	tubercle	*tuberculum:* a little swelling	The lesion of tuberculosis: also, a nodular bony prominence.
	tubercle bacillus	—; *bacillus:* rod	Microorganism causing tuberculosis.
	tubercular	—; *aris:* akin to	Relating to a bony prominence.
	tuberculous	—; *ous:* full of	Affected with tuberculosis.
	tuberculoma	—; *oma:* tumor	A tuberculous abscess or tumor.
	tuberculosis	—; *osis:* process	An infectious disease marked by the formation of tubercles in any tissue.
viscer- (L) organ	visceral	*viscus:* organ *al:* pertaining to	Pertaining to the internal organs.
	viscus	—;	Organ.
	viscera	—;	Organs.
	visceroptosis	—; *ptosis:* a dropping	Prolapse of the viscera. Glenard's disease.

III. Prefixes

Among the most frequently used elements in the formation of medical terms are prefixes. A prefix consists of one or two syllables placed before a word to modify its meaning. These syllables are often prepositions or adverbs. Some common prefixes are:

Prefix	Term	Analysis	Definition

ab-
(L)
from,
away from
	abductor
	
	abnormal
	abruptio
	   placentae
		ab: away from
		ductor: that which
		   draws
		—; *norma:* rule
		—;
		ruptere: break
		placenta: a flat cake
			That which draws away from a common center, as a muscle.
			
			Away from or not correponding to rule.
			A tearing away from or the premature detachment of a normally situated placenta.

a, an (G) without, not	anesthesia apnea asthenia atresia	*an:* without *aesthesis:* sensation *a:* without *pnoe:* breath —; *sthenos:* strength —; *tresis:* a perforation	Loss of sensation. Temporary absence of respiration. Debility, loss of strength. Absence or closure of a normal opening or passage.
ad- (L) adherence, increase, near, toward	adductor adrenal adhesion adnexa	*ad:* toward *ductor:* that which draws *ad:* near *ren:* kidney *ad:* to *haerere:* to stick —; *nectere:* to tie, to bind	That which draws toward a common center. A ductless gland above the kidney. Abnormal joining of surfaces to each other. Accessory parts; for example, adnexa uteri.
ante- (L) before	anteflexion antenatal antepartum	*ante:* forward *flectere:* to bend —; *natus:* birth —; *partum:* labor	Forward displacement of an organ; for example, the uterus. Before birth. Before the onset of labor.
anti- (G) against	antisepsis antitoxin antipyretic	*anti:* against *sepsis:* putrefaction —; *toxikon:* poison —; *pyretos:* fever	The exclusion of putrefactive germs. A protein that defends the body against a toxin. A drug that reduces fever.
bi- (L) two, both, double	biceps —; brachii —; femoris biconvex bilateral bifurcation	*bis:* two *caput:* head —; *brachii:* arm —; *femoris:* thigh —; *convexus:* rounded surface —; *latus:* side —; *furca:* fork	Two-headed. Muscle of the upper arm having two heads. Muscle of the thigh. Having two convex surfaces as in a lens. affecting both sides. A separation into two branches.
co- con- (L) together, with	congenital defect conjunctiva connective tissue	*con:* with *genitus:* born *defectus:* imperfection —; *jungere:* to join *con:* together *nectere:* to bind	Born with a defect, hereditary. Mucous membrane which lines eyelids. Tissue which connects or binds together.

NOTE: The dash and semicolon refer to the prefix which has already been given.

Prefix	Term	Analysis	Definition
contra- (L) against, opposite	contraception	*contra:* against *concipere:* to conceive	The prevention of conception.
	contraindication	—; *indicare:* to point out	A condition antagonistic to line of treatment.
	contralateral	*contra:* opposite *latus:* side	Affecting the opposite side of the body.
dys (G) bad, difficult, painful	dysentery	*dys:* painful *enteron:* intestine	Inflammation of intestinal mucous membrane accompanied by pain.
	dysmenorrhea	—; *men:* month *rein:* flow	Painful menstruation.
	dyspepsia	*dys:* bad *peptein:* to digest	Imperfect digestion.
	dysphagia	*dys:* difficult *phagein:* to eat	Difficulty in swallowing.
	dysphasia	—; *phasis:* speech	Impairment of speech.
	dyspnea	—; *pnoe:* breathing	Labored or difficult breathing.
	dystocia	—; *tokos:* birth	Difficult labor.
	dysuria	*dys:* painful *ouron:* urine	Painful or difficult urination.
ec- (G) out	ectropion of eyelid cervix uteri	*ek:* out *trepein:* to turn *cervix:* neck *uteri:* of womb	Eversion as the edge of the eyelid or the turning out of the cervical canal of the uterus.
ecto- (G) outside	ectopic pregnancy	*ecto:* outside *topos:* place *prae:* before *natus:* birth	Gestation outside the uterine cavity.
em, en- (G) in	empyema	*em:* in *pyon:* pus	Pus in a body cavity, especially in the pleural cavity.
	encephalopathy	*en;* in *kephale:* head *pathos:* disease	Any disease of the brain.
endo- (G) within	endocardium	*endon:* within *kardia:* heart	Lining membrane of inner surface of the heart.
	endocarditis	—; —; *itis:* inflammation	Inflammation of the endocardium.
	endocrine gland	—; *krinein:* to secrete *glans:* gland	A ductless gland in which forms an internal secretion.
	endocrinology	—; *logos:* science	The science of the endocrines, or ductless glands.
	endometrium	—; *metra:* uterus	The mucous membrane lining the inner surface of the uterus.
	endometritis	—; —; *itis:* inflammation	Inflammation of the endometrium.
	endoscope	—; *skopein:* to examine	Tubular instrument for examining cavities through natural openings.
	endoscopy	—; —;	Inspection of cavities by use of the endoscope.
	endosteum	—; *osteon:* bone	Membrane lining the medullary cavity of long bones.
	endostitis	—; —; *itis:* inflammation	Inflammation of the endosteum.

Prefix	Term	Analysis	Definition
epi- (G) upon, at, in addition to	epidermis epigastrium epiphysis	*epi:* upon *derma:* skin —; *gaster:* stomach *epi:* at *physis:* a growing upon	Cuticle or outer layer of the skin. Region over the pit of the stomach. A center of ossification at both extremities of long bones.
ex- (L, G) out, away from, over	exacerbation exeresis exophthalmia exophthalmic goiter expectoration exudate	*ex:* over *acerbus:* harsh *ex:* out *eiresis:* taking —; *ophthalmos:* eye —; —; *guttur:* throat —; *pector:* chest —; *sudare:* to sweat	Aggravation of symptoms. Excision of any part. Abnormal protrusion of the eyeballs. A goiter marked by protrusion of the eyeballs. Expulsion of mucus from the lungs. Accumulation of fluid due to inflam- matory condition.
hemi- (G) half	hemiglossectomy hemigastrectomy hemiplegia	*hemi:* half *glossa:* tongue *ektome:* excision —; *gaster:* stomach —; —; *plege:* a stroke	Removal of half a tongue. Removal of one-half of the stomach. Paralysis of one-half of the body.
hyper- (G) above, excessive, beyond	hyperacidity hyperadrenalism hypercalcemia hyperemesis gravidarum hyperemia hyperpyrexia hypertension hypertrophy	*hyper:* excessive *acidus:* sour —; *ad:* near *ren:* kidney *ismos:* state of —; *calx:* lime *haima:* blood —; *emesis:* vomiting *gravida:* a pregnant woman —; *haima:* blood *hyper:* above *pyrexia:* fever —; *tensio:* tension *hyper:* increased *trophe:* nourishment	An excess of acid in the stomach. Excess of adrenal secretion. Excess of calcium in the blood. Excessive vomiting during early pregnancy. Congestion. Fever above 106° F. High blood pressure. Increased size of an organ not due to tumor formation.
hypo- (G) beneath, below, deficient	hypochondriac region hypodermic injection hypoglycemia	*hypo:* beneath *chondros:* cartilage *regio:* area —; *derma:* skin *injectus:* to throw in *hypo:* deficient *glycus:* sugar *haima:* blood	Part of abdomen beneath the ribs. Injection under the skin. Low blood sugar.
para, par- (G) beside, around, near, abnormal	paracentesis parametrium parametritis paranephritis paranoia	*para:* beside *kentesis:* a puncture *para:* around *metra:* uterus —; —; *itis:* inflammation *para:* beside *nephros:* kidney, —; *para:* abnormal *nous:* mind	Puncture of a cavity with tapping. Fat and connective tissue around the uterus. Inflammation of the parametrium. Inflammation of suprarenal capsules; of connective tissue about the kidney. Mental disease marked by systematized delusions of persecution.

Prefix	Term	Analysis	Definition
(Cont'd)	parathyroid	*para:* beside *thyreos:* shield *eidos:* form	Ductless gland near the thyroid gland.
	parotitis	*par:* near *ot:* ear *itis:* inflammation	Inflammation of the parotid gland.
peri- (G) around, about	pericardium	*peri:* around *kardia:* heart	The double membranous sac enclosing the heart.
	pericarditis	—; —; *itis:* inflammation	Inflammation of the pericardium.
	perimetrium	—; *metra:* womb	Peritoneum covering uterus.
	perimetritis	—; —; *itis:* inflammation	Inflammation of the peritoneum covering of the uterus.
	periosteum	—; *osteon:* bone	The membrane that invests and nourishes the bone.
	periostitis	—; —; *itis:* inflammation	Inflammation of the periosteum.
pre- (L) before, in front of	precancerous	*prae:* before *cancer:* crab	Before the development of carcinoma.
	precordium	—; *cor:* heart	Region over the heart.
	preeclampsia	—; *ek:* out *lampein:* to flash	Eclampsia before delivery. (Eclampsia is a major toxemia during pregnancy.)
	prepatellar bursitis	*prae:* in front of *patella:* kneecap *bursa:* sac *itis:* inflammation	Inflammation of the bursa in front of the patella. (Housemaid's knee.)
	presentation	*praesentatio:* a placing before	Manner of the fetus presenting itself at the cervix.
pro- (L, G) in front of, before, forward	procidentia	*procidentia:* a falling forward	A complete prolapse especially of the uterus.
	prognosis	*pro:* before *gnosis:* a knowing	Prediction of end of disease.
	prolapse	*pro:* forward *lapsus:* slide	A downward displacement of an organ, as the rectum or the uterus.
retro- (L) backward, behind, back of	retroflexion	*retro:* backward *flexio:* a bending	A bending or flexing backward; for example, of the uterus.
	retrogasserian neurotomy	*retro:* back of *gasserian:* pertaining to a ganglion *neuron:* nerve *tome:* incision into	Transection of the posterior root of the retrogasserian ganglion.
	retroperitoneal	*retro:* behind *peritonaion:* peritoneum	Located behind the peritoneum.
	retroversion	*retro:* backward *versio:* a turning	A state of being turned back; for example, of the uterus.
semi- (L) half	semicircular canal	*semi:* half *circulus:* a ring *canal:* a channel	One of the three canals in the labyrinth of the ear.
	semicoma	—; *koma:* lethargy	Mild degree of coma.
	semilunar valves	—; *luna:* moon *valva:* one leaf of a double door	Half-moon shaped valves of the aorta and pulmonary arteries.

Prefix	Term	Analysis	Definition
sub- (L) under, beneath, below	subclavicular	*sub:* beneath *clavicular:* a little key	Beneath the clavicle (collar bone).
	subcostal	—; *costa:* rib	Beneath the ribs.
	subcutaneous	—; *cutis:* skin	Beneath the skin.
	subinvolution	—; *involutio:* a turning into	Failure of the uterus to reduce to normal size after childbirth.
	suppuration	*sub:* under; *pur:* pus *tion:* state of	The process of pus formation.
super, supra- (L) above, beyond, superior	supernatant	*super:* above *natare:* to float	Floating on surface.
	supraoccipital	—; *occiput:* back part of the skull	Situated above the occiput.
	suprapubic cystotomy	—; *pubis:* bone of pelvis *kystis:* bladder *tome:* incision	Surgical opening into the bladder from above the symphysis pubis.
	suprarenal	—; *ren:* kidney *al:* pertaining to	Adrenal gland above the kidney.
sym, syn- (G) with, along, together, beside	symphysis of pubis	*sym:* together *physis:* a growing	Fusion of pubic bones on midline anteriorly.
	synarthrosis	*syn:* together *arthron:* joint *osis:* condition	An immovable joint.
	syndactylism	*daktylos:* digit, finger *ismos:* condition	A fusion of two or more fingers or toes; webbing.
trans- (L) across, over	transection	*trans:* across *sectio:* cutting	Incision across the long axis; cross section.
	transfusion	—; *fusio:* a pouring	Injection of the blood of one person into the blood vessels of another.
	transurethral prostatectomy	—; *ourethra:* urethra *prostates:* prostate *ektome:* excision	Excision of the prostate gland through the urethra.
tri- (G) three	tricuspid	*tres, tria:* three *cuspis:* a point	Having three cusps or points; tricuspid valve.
	trifacial	—; *facialis:* facial	Fifth cranial nerve.
	trigone	*trigonon:* a three-cornered figure	A triangular space, especially that of the lower part of the urinary bladder.

Terms Pertaining to the Body as a Whole

A. Anatomical Division of the Abdomen:

1. hypochondriac regions (upper lateral regions beneath the ribs)..............(1) and (3)
2. epigastric region (region of the pit of the stomach).......................(2)
3. lumbar regions (middle lateral regions)..................................(4) and (6)
4. umbilical region (region of navel).......................................(5)
5. inguinal regions (lower lateral regions).................................(7) and (9)
6. hypogastric region (region below the umbilicus).........................(8)

B. Clinical Division of the Abdomen:

1. upper right quadrant..URQ
2. upper left quadrant...ULQ
3. lower right quadrant..LRQ
4. lower left quadrant...LLQ

C. Anatomical Division of the Back:

1. cervical region ....neck
2. thoracic region ....chest
3. lumbar region ....loin
4. sacral region ....sacrum

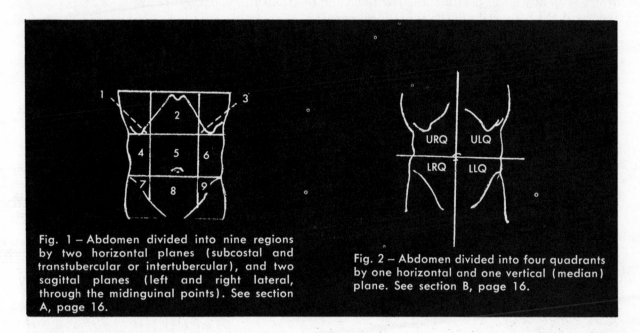

Fig. 1 – Abdomen divided into nine regions by two horizontal planes (subcostal and transtubercular or intertubercular), and two sagittal planes (left and right lateral, through the midinguinal points). See section A, page 16.

Fig. 2 – Abdomen divided into four quadrants by one horizontal and one vertical (median) plane. See section B, page 16.

D. Position and Direction:

1. afferent — conducting toward a structure.
2. anterior or ventral — front of the body (not synonymous in lower limb).
3. central — toward the center.
4. deep — away from the surface.
5. distal or peripheral — away from the beginning of a structure; away from the center.
6. efferent — conducting away from a structure.
7. inferior or caudal — away from the head, situated below another structure.*
8. intermediate — between median and lateral.
9. lateral — toward the side.*
10. medial — toward the median plane.*
11. median — in the middle of a structure.
12. posterior or dorsal — back of the body (not synonymous in lower limb).
13. proximal — toward the beginning of a structure.
14. superficial — near the surface.
15. superior or cephalic — toward the head, situated above another structure.*

E. Planes of the Body:

1. frontal or coronal — vertical plane parallel to the coronal suture of the skull. It divides the body or structure into anterior and posterior portions.
2. horizontal — plane parallel to the horizon.
3. longitudinal — plane parallel to the long axis of the structure.
4. median — lengthwise plane which divides the body or structure into right and left halves.
5. sagittal — any vertical plane parallel to the sagittal suture of the skull and the median plane.
6. transverse — plane at a right angle to the long axis of a structure.

---

* Refer to F. Anatomical Position.

F. Anatomical Position:

Anatomists all over the world apply anatomical terms to the body as though it were in what is known as the **anatomical position.** In this position, the body is erect, the eyes look straight to the front, the upper limbs hang at the sides with the palms facing forward, and the lower limbs are parallel with the toes pointing forward. Whether the body lies face upward or downward, or in any other position, the positions and relationships of structure are always described as if the body were in the anatomical position.

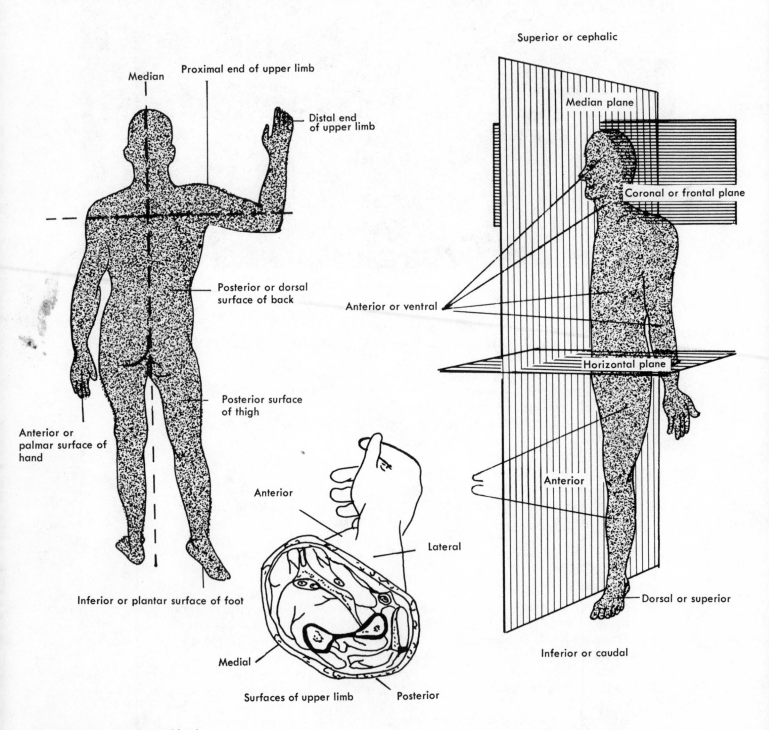

Fig. 3 – Posterior view of body.

Fig. 4 – Directional planes of the body.

REFERENCES AND BIBLIOGRAPHY

1. *Blakiston's Gould Medical Dictionary*, 3rd ed. New York: McGraw-Hill Book Co., 1972.

2. Gordon, Burgess L. (ed.). *Current Medical Information and Terminology*, 4th ed. Chicago: American Medical Association, 1971.

3. *Stedman's Medical Dictionary*, 22nd ed. Baltimore: The Williams and Wilkins Co., 1972.

4. *Taber's Cyclopedic Medical Dictionary*, 12th ed. Philadelphia: F. A. Davis Co., 1973.

Chapter II
Disorders of the Skin and Breast

SKIN

A. Origin of Terms:

1. cutis (L) — skin
2. derma (G) — skin
3. erythema (G) — flush
4. kelis (G) — stain
5. kerato (G) — horny
6. macula (L) — spot
7. onyx, onych (G) — nail
8. papula (L) — pimple
9. pilus, pili (L) — hair
10. pemphix (G) — blister
11. pigmentum (L) — paint
12. psora (G) — itch
13. sebum (L) — tallow
14. squama (L) — scale
15. sudor (L) — sweat
16. tegmen (L) — covering
17. vesic, vesica (L) — blister, bladder

B. Anatomical Terms:[6]

1. corium — the true skin or deeper layer containing blood vessels, lymphatics, hair follicles, nerve endings, connective tissue fibers, sweat and sebaceous glands.
2. derma, dermis — synonymous with corium.
3. epidermis — cuticle or outer layer of the skin.
4. epithelium — the layers of cells covering the surfaces of the body, external as well as internal.
5. integument — the skin, composed of the corium and epidermis.
6. pigment — a coloring substance.
7. sebaceous glands — oil glands of the skin.
8. sebum — oily substance secreted by sebaceous glands.
9. subcutaneous tissue — a layer of loose, connective tissue containing fat.
10. sudoriferous glands — sweat glands.

C. Diagnostic Terms:*

1. acne — any inflammatory condition of the sebaceous glands. The more common forms are:
    a. acne albida — white nodules or milia on face.
    b. acne papulosa — papular lesions.
    c. acne rosacea, simple rosacea — condition characterized by thickened skin especially on the nose, due to hypertrophy of sebaceous glands.
    d. acne vulgaris — a common form of acne, marked by papules, pustules and blackheads.
2. albinism — a congenital lack of normal skin pigment.
3. alopecia — loss of hair, baldness.
4. angioedema, angioneurotic edema, Quincke's edema — diffuse swelling of the loose tissues of the face, eyelids, lips, tongue, larynx, gastrointestinal tract, others.
5. atopic skin disorders — allergic skin conditions such as angioedema, urticaria, atopic drug reactions and food allergy in atopic dermatitis. Atopy or allergy tends to be of the familial type.[5, 31]
6. burn — the effect of exposure to heat, chemicals, electricity or sunshine.
    a. first degree burn — redness or hyperemia involving superficial layers of skin.
    b. second degree — blisters or vesication involving deeper layers of skin.
    c. third degree burn — destruction involving any tissue below the skin.[36]

---

*For additional terms consult Antony N. Domonkos. *Andrews' Diseases of the Skin — Clinical Dermatology*, 6th ed. Philadelphia: W. B. Saunders Co., 1971.

7. callositas, keratosis — a circumscribed thickening and hypertrophy of the horny cells of the epidermis.
8. carbuncle — a circumscribed inflammation of the skin and deeper tissues causing necrosis and suppuration.
9. cellulitis — inflammation of skin and subcutaneous tissue with or without formation of pus.
10. decubitus ulcer — a bedsore.
11. dermatitis — inflammation of the skin.   Some common forms are:
    a. contact dermatitis, dermatitis venenata — inflammatory reaction to an irritant or a sensitizer; for example, poison ivy, ragweeds, metals, chemicals, rubber, others.[26, 9, 13]
    b. exfoliative dermatitis — exfoliation or scaling off of dead skin associated with crust formation, generalized redness and edema.
    c. dermatitis medicamentosa — drug eruption.   Macular, urticarial, vesicular, bullous, pustular or hemorrhagic lesions may occur.[34]
12. eczema — cutaneous, inflammatory condition producing red, papular and vesicular lesions, crusts and scales.
13. epidermophytosis, athlete's foot — parasitic or fungus infection, chiefly affecting the skin between the toes, associated with intense itching, sogginess and scaling of skin.
14. gangrene — a form of necrosis or putrefaction of tissue.
    a. diabetic gangrene — associated with diabetes mellitus.
    b. embolic gangrene — caused by circulatory obstruction due to embolus.
    c. gas gangrene — due to infection with bacillus Welchii, an anaerobic microorganism.
15. impetigo contagiosa — infectious, inflammatory skin disease, characterized by discrete vesicles which change to pustules and crusts.   They appear in crops.
16. leukoderma — white patches of skin due to local absence of pigment.
17. lichen planus — inflammatory condition of skin and mucous membrane characterized by small, flat papules that appear shiny, dry and violet in color.   Linear, anular and irregular patches are found on neck, wrists and thighs.[7]
18. lupus vulgaris — a type of cutaneous tuberculosis, marked by reddish-brown patches in which tiny nodules are embedded.
19. melanoderma — abnormal brown or black pigmentation of the skin.
20. onychia — inflammation of the nail bed.
21. paronychia — infected skin around the nail.
22. pediculosis — infestation with lice.
23. pemphigus — skin disease characterized by the appearance of crops of bullae of various sizes.
24. psoriasis — eruption appearing in circular patches of various sizes, showing a definite line of demarcation.   Remissions and exacerbations are common.
25. pyoderma faciale — cyanotic or reddish erythema associated with deep or superficial cystic lesions or abscesses.[7]
26. rhinophyma — red, large, nodular hypertrophic masses around the tip and wings of the nose; seen in men past 40 years of age.[7]
27. scabies — skin lesion due to animal parasite, associated with the formation of vesicles and pustules and intense itching.
28. steatoma — sebaceous cyst.
29. tinea — any fungus skin disease, frequently due to ringworms.
30. tumors of skin — new growths.   (See Part II — Chapter on Oncology.)
    a. basal cell carcinoma — malignant skin ulcer usually on face.[35]
    b. keloid — new growth of scar tissue.
    c. nevus, mole, birthmark — congenital pigmentation of a circumscribed area of the skin.
    d. squamous cell epithelioma — malignant skin ulcer which affects areas of chronic irritation; for example, scars from burns, or leukoplakic lesions.[25]
31. ulcer — a break in the skin or mucous membrane resulting from varicose veins, trauma or other causes.
32. urticaria, hives, nettle rash — skin eruption of pale or reddish wheals, usually associated

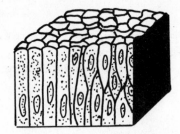

A. Simple, columnar epithelium
(three-dimensional view)

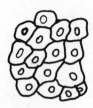

B. Simple, columnar epithelium
(surface view)

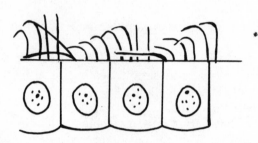

C. Ciliated epithelium

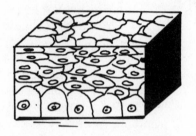

D. Stratified squamous epithelium

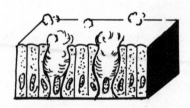

E. Goblet cells

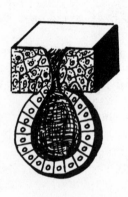

F. Simple alveolar glands

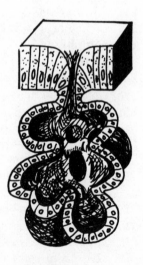

G. Compound alveolar glands

Fig. 5 — Various types of simple epithelium (A, B, C, D) and various types of glands (E, F, G).

with intense itching. May occur as an acute self-limited episode due to food allergy, drug reaction or emotional stress or in chronic form as a characteristic feature of rheumatic and connective tissue disorders.[3]

D. Operative Terms:

1. cryosurgery of skin — freezing the skin with liquid nitrogen or solid carbon dioxide in order to destroy the lesion.[37]
2. curettage of skin — removal of superficial lesions with a skin curette.[30]
3. dermabrasion — surgical removal of nevi or scars using sandpaper or other abrasives.
4. electrodesiccation — the use of short, high frequency electric sparks for drying cells and tissue.
5. fulguration of skin — the use of long, high frequency electric sparks for destroying tissue.
6. incision and drainage of infected skin lesion.
7. Linton flap procedure — operation for stasis dermatitis and ulceration refractory to simpler method. All incompetent communicating veins are ligated and divided to relieve ambulatory venous hypertension in superficial veins. This prevents progression of dermatitis, ulceration and pigmentation of overlying skin in the lower limb.[11]
8. local excision of skin lesion.
9. plastic operation on skin — surgical correction of defect.
10. skin grafting — transfer of skin from a normal area to cover denuded areas. A dermatome may be used to obtain these skin transplants.

E. Symptomatic Terms:

1. anular, formerly annular — ring-shaped.
2. café au lait spots — light brown flat spots, variable in shape and size, seen in neurofibromatosis (von Recklinghausen's disease).[24]
3. chloasma — patches of brown or yellowish pigmentation on a skin otherwise normal.
4. cicatrix of skin — a scar left by a healed wound.
5. cicatrization — healing by scar formation.
6. comedo (pl. comedones), excretory duct of skin plugged by discolored sebum.
7. confluent — lesions joined or run together.
8. depigmentation — partial or complete loss of pigment; occurs in albinism, atrophic skin and scars.
9. dermatographism, dermographia — skin writing. Urticarial wheals appear where skin was marked by pencil or blunt instrument.[3]
10. discoid — shaped like a disc.
11. discrete — lesions are disconnected, separate from one another.
12. ecchymosis (pl. ecchymoses) — purple spot or bruise due to seepage of blood into the skin.
13. eczematoid, eczematous — eczema-like inflammatory lesion which tends to thicken, to become scaly, vesicular, crusty, or weeping.
14. eruption — a rash or skin lesion.
15. erythema — diffuse redness of skin.
16. excoriation — linear break of skin or scratch mark due to surface trauma.
17. granulation — a method of repair or healing following loss of tissue or pyogenic infection.
18. guttate — droplike.
19. kerototic — pertaining to a horny thickening.
20. hyperpigmentation — the presence of an abnormal amount of pigment in the skin seen in a considerable number of systemic diseases such as adrenal insufficiency, acromegaly, and others. In the familial progressive type of hyperpigmentation patches of excessive pigmentation enlarge in size with increasing age.[4]
21. intertriginous — between two folds of skin.
22. macule — discolored patch or spot on the skin.
23. milia (sing. milium) — tiny white nodules appearing on skin, frequently below the eyes.
24. moniloform — beaded.

25. multiform — several forms of the skin lesions.
26. papule — a pimple.
27. petechiae — pin size hemorrhagic spots in the skin.
28. proliferation — process of rapid reproduction of similar cells.
29. pustule — a small elevation of the skin containing pus or lymph.
30. seborrheal, seborrheic — pertaining to seborrhea, an oversecretion of sebaceous glands.
31. serpiginous — creeping in a snakelike manner.
32. vesication, vesiculation — formation of blisters.

BREASTS

A. Origin of Terms:

1. areola (L) — a small area or space
2. lac (L) — milk
3. mamma (L) — breast
4. mastos (G) — breast
5. thele (G) — nipple

B. Anatomical Terms:

1. areola — area of pigmented skin surrounding the nipple. It becomes dark during pregnancy and remains so thereafter.
2. mammary gland — glandular tissue of the breast composed of 15 to 20 compound alveolar lobes, each connected with the nipple by a lactiferous duct.
3. papilla mammae — the nipple.

C. Diagnostic Terms:

1. abscess of breast, mammary abscess — a localized collection of pus of mammary tissue.
2. amastia — absence of a breast.
3. athelia — absence of a breast nipple.
4. breast cancer — malignant mammary tumor, a painless or painful mass which may be associated with skin and muscle attachment, discharge, crusting and retraction of nipple, changes in contour of affected breast and metastases to regional lymph nodes.
   a. carcinoma of breast — malignant tumor usually arising from ductal epithelium of mammary gland.
   b. sarcoma of breast — rare, nonepithelial, malignant mammary tumor, e.g., cystosarcoma and fibrosarcoma.
5. cystic disease of breast — the most common breast lesion composed of gross cysts that may be accompanied by microscopic cysts. Haagensen distinguishes 4 types:
   a. galactoceles, cysts containing inspissated milk.
   b. cysts formed in duct ectasia (dilated duct).
   c. cysts due to fat necrosis caused by trauma.
   d. cysts related to intraductal papilloma.[21]
6. fissure of nipple — a deep furrow in nipple.
7. hyperplasia of breast, hypermastia — abnormally large breast, usually pendulous and sagging.
8. hypoplasia of breast, hypomastia — abnormally small breast.
   a. unilateral hypomastia — one breast underdeveloped the other normal or overdeveloped. This results in mammary asymmetry and disfigurement.[29]
   b. bilateral hypomastia — both breasts are abnormally small.
9. occlusion of lactiferous ducts — blockage of lumen of milk-conveying ducts.
10. Paget's disease of nipple — cancer directly beneath the nipple, seen in elderly women. Areola, nipple and surrounding skin may be weeping and eczematoid.[19]
12. thelitis — inflammation of the nipple.

D. Operative Terms:

1. biopsy of breast — excision of small piece of mammary tissue for diagnostic evaluation.
   a. biopsy of apex of axilla — method of detecting axillary lymph node metastasis.
   b. biopsy of internal mammary node — method of detecting internal mammary node metastasis.[17]
2. mammaplasty, mammoplasty, mastoplasty — surgical reconstruction of the breast.[18]
   a. augmentation mammaplasty — implantation of a retromammary prosthesis for an underdeveloped breast.
   b. reduction mammaplasty — repair of an overdeveloped, pendulous breast by partial removal of the mammary gland and fixation of the breast to its normal position.[23]
3. mastectomy, mammectomy — removal of a breast.
   a. radical mastectomy — removal of an entire breast including axillary dissection and surgical division of pectoralis major and minor muscles.
   b. simple mastectomy — removal of a breast without dissection of axillary lymph nodes.
4. mastopexy — surgical fixation of a pendulous breast.
5. mastotomy — incision and drainage of a breast abscess.

E. Symptomatic Terms:

1. mastalgia, mastodynia — breast pain occurring in premenstrual period, mastitis, mammary cancer and other disorders.
2. peau d'orange — skin simulating orange peel; seen in inflammatory breast cancer.
3. skin retraction — dimpling and puckering of skin due to benign or malignant lesions underneath.

RADIOLOGY

A. General Terms:

1. fluorescence — the property of becoming luminous through the influence of x-rays or other agents.
2. fluoroscopy — direct x-ray examination using a fluoroscopic screen in a darkened room.[3]
3. laminograms, planigrams, tomograms — body section radiograms; x-ray films of a thin layer of body tissue of varying depths without interference with the intervening structures.
4. radiogram, roentgenogram, skiagram (skia (G) shadow) — picture made on a photographic film by means of x-rays.
5. radiography, roentgenography, skiagraphy, — the making of x-ray photographs.
6. radiologist — a physician who uses roentgen, radium and other forms of radiant energy for diagnostic and therapeutic purposes.
7. radiology — the study or science concerned with the use of various forms of radiant energy in the diagnosis and treatment of disease.
8. radium — a radioactive substance used in treating certain diseases.
9. radon — a heavy radioactive gas which is given off in the disintegration of radium.
10. roentgenography — the use of x-rays in the production of an image on a photographic film.
11. roentgenologist — a physician who uses x-rays in the diagnosis and treatment of disease.
12. roentgen rays, x-rays — a form of radiant energy capable of penetrating solid and opaque objects.

B. Terms Related to the Diagnosis of Breast Lesions:

1. mammography, Egan technique — soft tissue mammary radiography based on varying degrees of absorption of the x-ray beam by fatty, fibroglandular and cancerous tissue in the breast in decreasing order of translucency.

2. mammograms, Egan technique — three radiographic views of the breast which outline:
   a. benign lesions, nodules or cysts well circumscribed usually surrounded by a thin halo of radiolucent fat.
   b. malignant lesions, spicular, ragged irregular in shape and poorly circumscribed, frequently associated with thickening and retraction of skin, nipple deformity, axillary lymph node involvement, microcalcifications and venous congestion. Since the presence of fat serves to identify lesions no radiopaque substance is injected into the lactiferous ducts. As a result the breast is not distorted and pathological conditions are clearly delineated. Mammography may also be used in screening studies of asymptomatic women and in postmastectomy follow-up examinations.[14]
3. xerography of breast — an x-ray method of obtaining images of breast structures on selenium-coated metal plates.[14]

C. Terms Related to Therapy of Skin and Breast:

1. laser radiation — an intensely strong, narrow beam of light that may be used to destroy selected skin lesions. Laser means light amplification by the stimulated emission of radiation.[8, 16]
2. radiation therapy in carcinoma of the breast — treatment of value:
   a. in selected inoperable cases for palliation.
   b. as an adjunct to surgery; particularly as postoperative therapy following radical mastectomy.
   c. for postoperative recurrence of lesion.
   d. in the management of metastatic bone involvement
      Radical surgery is the treatment of choice for carcinoma of the breast, since it is not possible to eradicate the disease by radiation therapy. However, there is sufficient clinical evidence that irradiation has brought about five year cures in patients treated for inoperable lesions.[22, 37]
3. radium therapy — treatment of pathological conditions with radium which continually emits radiation at a constant rate regardless of enviromental conditions.
4. superficial x-ray therapy — radiation therapy used for surface lesions; for example, selected skin conditions and tumors.[10]

CLINICAL LABORATORY

A. General Terms:

1. allergen, allergin — substance which produces various allergic manifestations; for example, skin reactions.
2. allergy — hypersensitivity to a particular substance. Eczema, urticaria, dermatitis due to drugs or roentgen-rays are forms of allergic conditions.
3. eosinophilia — abnormal increase of eosinophils in differential white count present in skin diseases such as pemphigus or certain forms of dermatitis.
4. desensitization — process of abating allergic manifestations and making a person susceptible to a substance of therapeutic value by repeatedly giving him small doses of it.

B. Terms Related to Laboratory Diagnosis:

1. frozen section — microscopic study of slides made from fresh tissue of lesion. It is valuable for rapid diagnosis while patient is on operating room table to determine the need for conservative surgery, should the tissue section show a benign lesion, or for radical surgery, should a malignant lesion be found.
2. incisional biopsy — tissue of lesion obtained for pathological verification. This procedure is indicated when the tumor mass is very large. Otherwise excisional biopsy is the method of choice.
3. skin tests for hypersensitivity — small amount of specific protein is scratched or injected into skin to determine the protein causing food allergy or other morbid conditions.

ABBREVIATIONS

A. General:

CC — chief complaint
cc — cubic centimeter
Derm. — dermatology
Dx — diagnosis
FH — family history
FS — frozen section
H — hypodermic
IC — International Classification

MH — marital history
PH — past history
PI — present illness
Rx — take
STD — skin test dose
Subcu. — subcutaneous
TPR — temperature, pulse and respiration
ung. — ointment

B. Coding Systems, Nomenclature, Classification of Books:

H-ICDA — *Hospital Adaptation of ICDA*

ICDA — *International Classification of Diseases Adapted (official)*

NLM — *National Library of Medicine*

SNDO — *Standard Nomenclature of Diseases and Operations*

C. Organizations:[27]

AAMRL — American Association of Medical Record Librarians
ACS — American Cancer Society
AHA — American Hospital Association
AMA — American Medical Association
ANA — American Nurses Association
ANC — US Army Nurse Corps
ANF — American Nurses' Foundation
APHA — American Public Health Association
ARC — American National Red Cross
FNC — Future Nurses' Clubs
ICN — International Council of Nurses

NIH — US National Institutes of Health
NLN — National League for Nursing
NNC — US Navy Nurse Corps
NSC — National Safety Council
OCDM — US Office of Civil and Defense Mobilization
PAHO — Pan American Health Organization
USPC — US Peace Corps
USPHS — US Public Health Service
VA — US Veteran Administration
VNA — Visiting Nurses Association
WHO — World Health Organization

ORAL READING PRACTICE

Pemphigus

There are several forms of **dermatitis** in which a **bullous eruption** develops but they are distinguished from true bullous diseases by a short duration and good **prognosis.**[28]

The term **pemphigus,** derived from the Greek **pemphix,** "blister", points up the chief characteristic of **pemphigus vulgaris,** namely, the formation of blisters. These **blebs** arise suddenly on apparently normal or slightly **erythematous** skin and form oval-shaped or round blisters containing clear **serum.** The blisters tend to be **flaccid** and to break easily. The **epidermis** becomes detached leaving increasingly larger areas of **denudation.** The Nicholsky sign is always positive. It is obtained by pressing on the skin with the finger tip. The epidermis then slides off and a raw surface remains. The **denuded** areas are slow in healing and constitute a continuous threat of infection.

Pemphigus has been compared with a serious burn, but, in reality, the trauma of a burn is a single occasion and the lesion is frequently localized. On the other hand, the injury inflicted upon the skin by numerous crops of **bullae** followed by widespread denudation presents a still graver problem than that of many a burn. The blisters vary in size from a few **millimeters** in diameter to ten **centimeters.** New lesions develop while old ones disappear. Since the crops arise rapidly, often overnight, and old lesions heal slowly, the areas of denudation are extensive.

Eventually, crusts form over the raw surface. If **pyogenic bacteria** get beneath these crusts, foul-smelling pus collects and increases the patient's physical distress. There is no **scarring;** only a **hyperpigmented** lesion remains after healing. The formation of bullae in the **oral cavity** is particularly painful. Blebs about 5 millimeters in diameter are scattered over the **buccal mucosa.** They appear spontaneously, rupture and leave raw **ulcers** which inflict much pain. Blebs may also occur on other **orificial mucous** membranes.

The **etiology** of pemphigus is still unknown. Some authorities believe that it is **metabolic** in nature or caused by **bacterial** or **viral** infections; however, no theory has yielded convincing evidence.

The common type of pemphigus is a chronic, recurrent disease, afflicting only adults. Acute **exacerbations** may be followed by brief or prolonged periods of remission. As a rule, pemphigus vulgaris lasts from several months to years. Untreated, it is a fatal disease, but with the judicious use of **Cortisone** the **prognosis** is favorable.[15, 2, 12]

Table 1

SOME CONDITIONS OF THE SKIN AND BREAST AMENABLE TO SURGERY

Organs Involved	Diagnoses	Operations	Operative Procedures
Skin	Seborrheic keratoses	Epidermal curettage[a]	Lesions frozen with ethyl chloride and curetted
	Basal cell carcinoma — small lesion	Curettage Electrodesiccation[b]	Lesion and all extensions removed with skin curette Remaining cells destroyed by surgical diathermy
Skin Sebaceous glands Hair follicles Nail bed Nail fold	Infected steatoma Furuncle or carbuncle of hair follicles Onychia, paronychia Infected ingrowing toe nail	Incision and drainage of glands of skin; of hair follicles; of nail bed or fold	Surgical opening of infected sebaceous glands, etc. to induce drainage
Subcutaneous areolar tissue	Cellulitis of forearm	Incision and drainage of subcutaneous areolar tissue	Surgical opening of infected area and insertion of drain
Skin, subcutaneous tissue	Dermoid of skin Lipoma of subcutaneous tissue	Local excision of dermoid or lipoma	Removal of benign neoplasm
Skin	Second degree burn	Skin graft	Removal of small sections of skin and implanting them on a raw, clean, granulating surface

Organs Involved	Diagnoses	Operations	Operative Procedures
Skin	Cicatrix of skin due to burn (Structures beneath skin undamaged)	Excision of cicatricial skin lesion Use of split-thickness or full thickness skin graft	Removal of excess scar tissue and replacement by covering area with either half or full thickness of the skin removed by a knife or dermatome
Skin of neck, chin or cheek	Contracture from scar of old burns or injuries	Reconstruction operation *First stage:* Preparation of pedicle or Gillies' tube flap *Second stage:* Excision of scar Coverage of denuded area with pedicle *Third stage:* Removal of pedicle	Skin and subcutaneous tissue from donor area raised and pedicle tubed Removal of deep scar, distal end of pedicle severed and sutured into defect with pedicle still attached Pedicle opened and returned to donor area
Skin of axilla	Cicatricial contracture of axilla	Z-plasty	Defect corrected by using sliding flaps of skin
Breast	Abscess of breast due to Staphylococcus aureus or other infectious agents	Mastotomy with drainage	Surgical opening and evacuation of abscess Insertion of drain
Breast	Carcinoma of breast	Radical mastectomy	Removal of breast, pectoral muscles and lymph nodes
Breast	Overdevelopment of breast (pendulous breast)	Mastopexy	Fixation of a pendulous breast
Breast	Unilateral hypomastia Hypermastia of contralateral breast	Augmentation mammaplasty of underdeveloped breast Reduction mammaplasty of overdeveloped breast	Implantation of a Cronin silicone prosthesis in a retromammary pocket Partial excision of mammary tissue High fixation of breast

aA. N. Domonkos. *Andrews' Diseases of the Skin — Clinical Dermatology*, 6th ed. Philadelphia: W. B. Saunders Co., 1971, p. 967.
bJ. M. Knox *et al.* Curettage and electrodesiccation in the treatment of skin cancer. *Archives of Dermatology*, 82: 197-204, 1960.

REFERENCES AND BIBLIOGRAPHY

1. Baughman, R. and Sobel, R. Psoriasis, stress and strain. *Archives of Dermatology*, 103: 599, June, 1971.
2. Berger, R. S. and Lynch, P. J. Familial benign chronic pemphigus. *Archives of Dermatology*, 104: 380-384, October, 1971.
3. Braverman, Irwin M. Hypersensitivity syndromes. In *Skin Signs of Systemic Disease*. Philadelphia: W. B. Saunders Co., 1970, pp. 239-241 and 245-246.
4. Chernosky, M. E. Familial progressive hyperpigmentation. *Archives of Dermatology*, 103: 581-597, June, 1971.
5. Criep, Leo H. Diagnosis of atopy. In *Dermatologic Allergy: Immunology, Diagnosis, Management.* Philadelphia: W. B. Saunders Co., 1967, pp. 260-265.
6. Cummins, H. The skin and breasts. In Anson, B. J. (ed.) *Morris' Human Anatomy*, 12th ed. New

York: McGraw-Hill Book Co., 1966, pp. 109-130.

7. Domonkos, A. N. Lichen planus — pyoderma, rhinophyma. In *Andrew's Diseases of the Skin — Clinical Dermatology*, 6th ed. Philadelphia: W. B. Saunders Co., 1971, pp. 239-240 and 266-267.

8. _____. Laser radiation. In *Andrews' Diseases of the Skin — Clinical Dermatology*. Philadelphia: W. B. Saunders Co., 1971, pp. 967-968.

9. Elgart, M. L. and Higdon, R. S. Allergic contact dermatitis to gold. *Archives of Dermatology*, 103: 649-653, June, 1971.

10. Epstein, E. Dermatologic radiotherapy. *Archives of Dermatology*, 92: 307-314, September, 1965.

11. Field, Paul. The role of the Linton flap procedure in the management of stasis dermatitis and ulceration in the lower limb. *Surgery*, 70: 920-926, December, 1971.

12. Fincher, D. F. *et al.* Bullous pemphigoid in childhood. *Archives of Dermatology*, 103: 88-90, January, 1971.

13. Fisher, Alexander A. *Contact Dermatitis*. Philadelphia: Lea & Febiger, 1967.

14. Gershon-Cohon, J. Mammography, thermography and xerography. *Ca — A Cancer Journal for Clinicians*, 17: 108-112, May-June, 1967.

15. Goldman, H. M. Dermatologic diseases affecting the oral mucosa. *Postgraduate Medicine*, 49: 125-130, January, 1971.

16. Goldman, L. *et al.* Laser surgery in dermatology. *Cutis*, 5: 571-583, May, 1969.

17. Goldman, W. P. Triple biopsy for carcinoma of the breast: A clinical study of 200 cases. *Surgery*, 70: 628-634, October, 1971.

18. Grant, D. A. Treatment of asymmetry of the breasts. *Southern Medical Journal*, 64: 1097-1105, September, 1971.

19. Greenwood, S. M. Paget's disease in metastatic breast carcinoma. *Archives of Dermatology*, 104: 312-315, September, 1971.

20. Guerra-Rodrigo, F. *et al.* Pemphigus vegetans. *Archives of Dermatology*, 104: 412-419, October, 1971.

21. Haagensen, C. D. Cystic disease of the breast. In *Diseases of the Breast*, 2d ed. Philadelphia: W. B. Saunders Co., 1971, pp. 155-156.

22. _____. The radiotherapy of breast carcinoma. In *Diseases of the Breast*, 2d ed. Philadelphia: W. B. Saunders Co., 1971, pp. 734-753.

23. Hoffman, G. W. *et al.* Reduction mammoplasty. *Southern Medical Journal*, 64: 1106-1111, September, 1971.

24. Lewis, M. and Wheeler, C. E. *Practical Dermatology*, 3rd ed. Philadelphia: W. B. Saunders Co., 1967, pp. 528 and 85.

25. Menn H. *et al.* The recurrent basal cell epithelioma. *Archives of Dermatology*, 103: 628, June, 1971.

26. Mitchell, J. C. *et al.* Allergic contact dermatitis from ragweeds. *Archives of Dermatology*, 104: 73-76, July, 1971.

27. *Nursing Outlook*, 14: 83, December, 1966.

28. Peck, S. M. Studies in bullous diseases. *Archives of Dermatology*, 103: 141-147, February, 1971.

29. Rees, T. D. and Dupuis, C. C. Unilateral hypomastia. *Plastic and Reconstructive Surgery*, 41: 307-310, April, 1968.

30. Reymann, F. Treatment of basal cell carcinoma of the skin with curettage. *Archives of Dermatology*, 103: 623-627, June, 1971.

31. Roane, Jack. Atopic dermatitis, *Southern Medical Journal*, 64: 1395-1397, November, 1971.

32. Ryan, J. G. Pemphigus. *Archives of Dermatology*, 104: 14-20, July, 1971.

33. Sante, L. R. *Manual of Roentgenological Technique*, 18th ed. Ann Arbor, Michigan: Edwards Brothers, Inc. 1956, p. 461.

34. Sherman, W. B. Drug allergy. *Southern Medical Journal*, 64: 22-26, January, 1971.

35. Stellmach, R. K. *et al.* Malignant degeneration of basal cell carcinoma of the face; Basal squamous carcinoma. *Plastic and Reconstructive Surgery*, 48: 471-473, November, 1971.

36. Vistnes, Lars M. and Hogg, G. R. The burn eschar. *Plastic and Reconstructive Surgery*, 48: 56-60, July, 1971.

37. Walter, J. *Cancer and Radiotherapy*. London: The Whitefriars Press Ltd., 1971.

38. Zacarian, S. A. *Cryosurgery of Skin Cancer*. Springfield, Illinois: Charles C. Thomas, Publisher, 1969.

Chapter III
Musculoskeletal Disorders

BONES

A. Origin of Terms:

1. calcaneus (L) — heel bone
2. cancellus (L) — lattice
3. coxa (L) — hip bone
4. diploë (G) — fold
5. femur (L) — thigh
6. genu (L) — knee
7. ischion (G) — hip
8. lacuna (L) — lake
9. medulla (L) — marrow
10. myelos (G) — marrow
11. os (pl. ossa) (L) — bone
12. osteon (G) — bone
13. pes, ped (L) — foot
14. physis (G) — growth
15. pelvis (L) — basin
16. planta (L) — sole
17. pod, podo (G) — foot
18. sternon (G) — breast bone
19. trochanter (G) — runner
20. xiphoid (G) — sword

B. Anatomical Terms:

1. bone, osseous tissue — the hardest type of connective tissue which provides a supporting framework for the body.
2. bone marrow, medulla — soft, central part of bone.
    a. red marrow — fills cancellous bone and manufactures red blood cells and hemoglobin.
    b. yellow marrow — fills the medullary cavity and contains fat cells.
3. cancellous bone — spongy bone composed of a loose latticework of bony trabeculae and bone marrow within the interspace.[77]
4. compact bone, cortex of bone — solid bone rich in calcium.
5. diaphysis — shaft of long bone.
6. diploë — spongy bone between the two tables of the skull.
7. endosteum — membrane lining the walls of the medullary cavity.
8. epiphysis (pl. epiphyses) — extremity of long bones and center of ossification for growing bone.
9. matrix of bone — collagenous fibers and a ground substance in which calcium is deposited.[33]
10. medullary cavity — marrow-filled cavity within the shaft of long bones.
11. ossification — bone formation.
12. osteoblasts — bone forming cells.
13. osteoclasts — bone absorbing cells.
14. osteocytes — bone cells lying in lacunae within intercellular substance.
15. osteoid — calcifiable osseous tissue, yet uncalcified.[77]
16. periosteum — outer covering of bone.
17. trabeculae — slender spicules or anastomosing bars of spongy bone.
18. trochanter — bony prominence of the upper extremity of the femur below the femoral neck.
    a. major or greater trochanter — large bony projection located externally and laterally between femoral neck and shaft.
    b. minor or lesser trochanter — conical bony prominence located medially and laterally at the junction of the femoral neck and shaft.

C. Diagnostic Terms:

1. avascular necrosis of bone — death of bone resulting from deprivation of blood supply due to fracture, extensive removal of periosteum in surgery, exposure to radioactive substances and other causes.[32]
2. cervical rib — a supernumerary rib attached to a cervical vertebra.

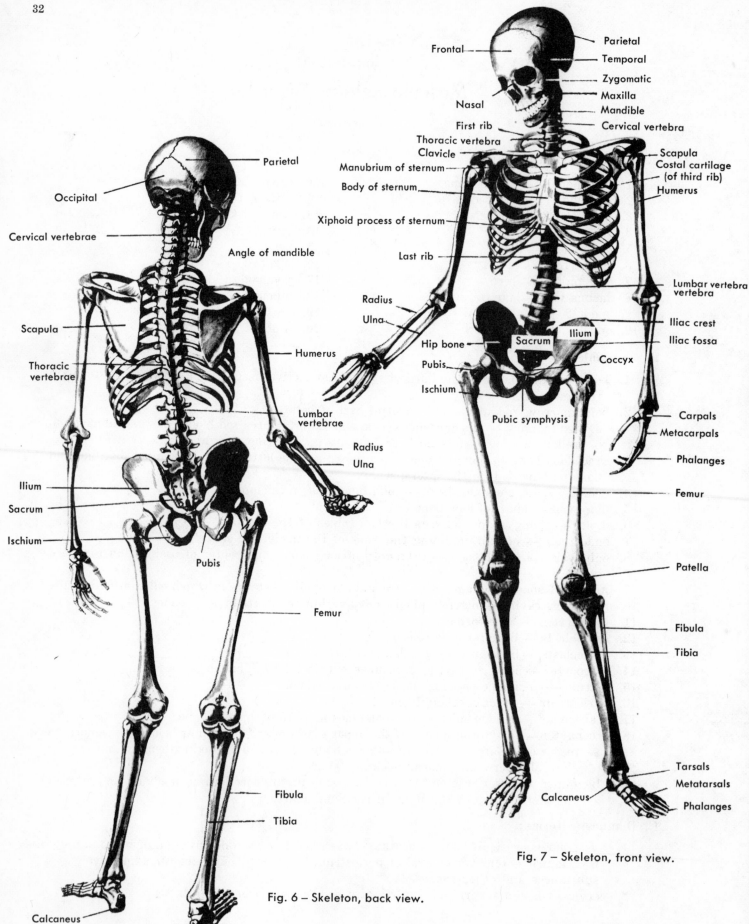

Parietal

Occipital

Cervical vertebrae

Angle of mandible

Scapula

Thoracic
vertebrae

Humerus

Lumbar
vertebrae

Radius

Ulna

Ilium

Sacrum

Ischium

Pubis

Femur

Fibula

Tibia

Calcaneus

Fig. 6 – Skeleton, back view.

Frontal

Parietal

Temporal

Zygomatic

Maxilla

Mandible

Nasal

Cervical vertebra

First rib

Thoracic vertebra

Clavicle

Scapula

Manubrium of sternum

Costal cartilage
(of third rib)

Body of sternum

Humerus

Xiphoid process of sternum

Last rib

Radius

Lumbar vertebra
vertebra

Ulna

Iliac crest

Hip bone

Sacrum

Ilium

Iliac fossa

Pubis

Coccyx

Ischium

Pubic symphysis

Carpals

Metacarpals

Phalanges

Femur

Patella

Fibula

Tibia

Tarsals

Metatarsals

Calcaneus

Phalanges

Fig. 7 – Skeleton, front view.

3. coxa plana — flattening of head of femur.

4. coxa valga — widening of angle between the shaft and neck of femur.

5. coxa vara — diminishing of angle between the shaft and neck of femur.

6. deformity of bone — congenital or acquired abnormality of bone resulting in disfigurement.

7. epiphysitis, acute — inflammatory process of the epiphyseal region of a long bone, marked by tenderness and pain of the joint.

8. epiphysiolysis, slipped epiphysis — a loosening or separation of the epiphysis from the shaft, usually a slipping of the upper femoral epiphysis. There is eversion of the limb resulting in displacement and limping.[63]

9. epulis — a fibrous tumor arising from the gum.

10. Ewing's sarcoma — malignant new growth originating in the shaft of long bones and spreading through the periosteum into soft tissues. Metastases occur early. Femur, tibia, humerus, fibula and pelvic bones are frequently involved.[31]

11. exostosis (pl. exostoses) — bone tumor, osteoma, a benign osseous growth.

12. fibrous dysplasia of bone, Albright's syndrome — metabolic bone disease characterized by rapid resorption of bone and fibrous replacement of marrow, distortion of one or several bones, brownish pigmentation of the skin, and precocious puberty in girls.[57]

13. fracture — a broken bone. Long bone fractures are frequently associated with nerve injury.
    a. nonpenetrating or closed fracture — no external wound present.
    b. penetrating or open fracture — an external wound communicating with the fracture.
       Fractures may be:
       (1) capillary — hairlike line of break.
       (2) comminuted — bone splintered into small fragments.
       (3) complicated — broken bone injuring adjacent structure, e.g. fractured rib piercing the lung.
       (4) compound — an open wound leading down to the fracture.
       (5) depressed — broken bone inwards as in certain skull fractures.
       (6) greenstick — incomplete break which may be associated with bowing of shaft.
       (7) impacted — broken fragment wedged into other bony fragment.
       (8) pathological — a spontaneous fracture due to bone destruction in certain diseases: cancer, syphilis, osteomalacia, osteoporosis, others.
       (9) simple — uncomplicated fracture, no open wound.
       (10) transverse — break across the bone. For example: Colles fracture — transverse fracture of radius above the wrist with displacement of the hand.

14. fracture of hip — a break in upper end of femur. The two main types are:
    a. femoral neck fracture — bone broken through the neck of the femur.
    b. trochanteric fracture — bone broken below, around or between the greater or lesser trochanters.[60, 45, 19]

15. genu valgum — knock knees.[40]

16. genu varum — bowlegs; deformity involving either tibia alone, or femur, tibia and fibula; seen in rickets and corrected by high doses of vitamin D.

17. giant cell tumor, osteoclastoma, benign — osteolytic tumor containing numerous giant cells. It arises at the epiphysis and does not interfere with joint motion until late. It may undergo malignant transformation or recur after removal.[67]

18. myeloma, plasmacytoma — malignant neoplasm derived from plasma cells and usually associated with abnormal protein metabolism. It may occur as
    (1) multiple myeloma — a malignant type of widespread bone destruction with gradual replacement of cancellous bone by neoplasm seen in age groups above 50 years old and as
    (2) solitary myeloma — single lesion found in any location but most frequently in vertebral column. Backpain is severe.[57]

19. osteitis — inflammation of bone.

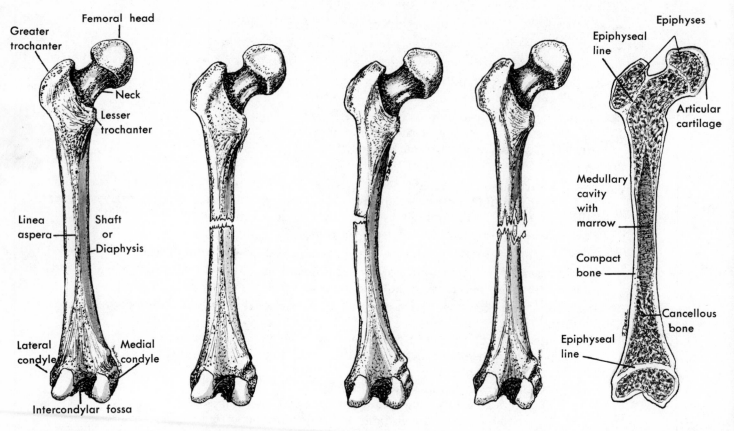

Greater trochanter
Femoral head
Neck
Lesser trochanter
Linea aspera
Shaft or Diaphysis
Lateral condyle
Medial condyle
Intercondylar fossa

Epiphyses
Epiphyseal line
Articular cartilage
Medullary cavity with marrow
Compact bone
Cancellous bone
Epiphyseal line

Fig. 8 – Mature femur-posterior view.

Fig. 9 – Transverse diaphyseal fracture.

Fig. 10 – Greenstick fracture.

Fig. 11 – Comminuted fracture.

Fig. 12 – Immature femur – longitudinal section.

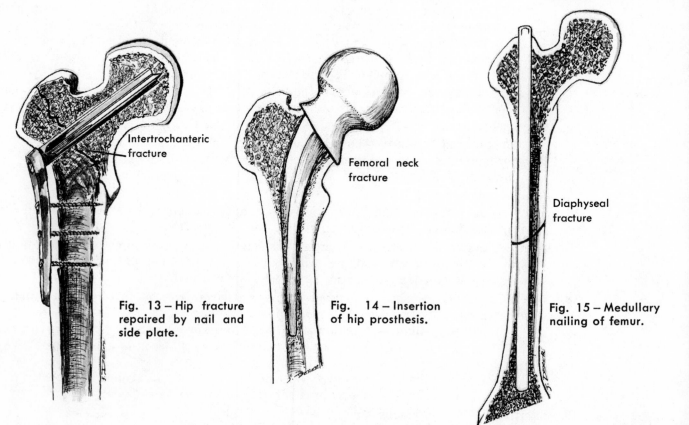

Intertrochanteric fracture

Femoral neck fracture

Diaphyseal fracture

Fig. 13 – Hip fracture repaired by nail and side plate.

Fig. 14 – Insertion of hip prosthesis.

Fig. 15 – Medullary nailing of femur.

20. osteitis deformans, Paget's disease of bone — chronic disorder characterized by bone destruction associated with increase in vascularity and fibrosis, skeletal deformities and pathological fractures; seen in the aged.[62]

21. osteoblastoma, giant osteoid osteoma — benign highly vascular, bone forming tumor, typically found in the spine, where it may cause cord compression and paraplegia.

22. osteochondritis deformans juvenile, coxa plana, Legg-Calvé-Perthes disease — self-limited disease in children, age 4-10; characterized by flattening of the femoral head resulting in limping and restricted motion.[44]

23. osteolysis, osteoclasia — resorption and destruction of osseous tissue.

24. osteogenic sarcoma — rapidly growing, vascular, malignant tumor producing bony tissue.[43]

25. osteoma — benign osseous tumor usually of facial and frontal bones. Headache and seizures may be due to intracranial osteomas.

26. osteomalacia — softening of bone caused by calcium and vitamin D deficiency.

27. osteomyelitis — inflammation of the bone and bone marrow.[3, 36]

28. osteoporosis, porous bone — disorder of protein metabolism characterized by diffuse decrease of bone density and marked increase in porosity which are most pronounced in the spine and pelvis.[54]

29. renal (azotemic) osteodystrophy — bone disorder due to defective mineralization complicating chronic renal failure.[8]

30. rickets, rachitis — calcium and vitamin D deficiency of early childhood which leads to demineralization of bones and deformities.

31. sequestration — process of bone necrosis resulting in dead bone.

32. sequestrum — dead bone separated from surrounding tissue.

33. supernumerary bone — extra bone.

34. whiplash injury of neck — compression of cervical spine involving the bones, joints and intervertebral disks. It is due to a sudden throwing forward and then backward of the head, usually caused by car accident when the collision is from the rear.

D. Operative Terms:

1. amputation — partial or complete removal of limb for crushing injury, intractable pain, gangrene, vascular obstruction or uncontrollable infection.[75, 30, 1, 49]

2. bone grafting, transplantation of bone — insertion of a bone graft.[10, 11]
    a. autografting or autotransplantation of bone — removal of bone from one site and implanting it at another site to promote bone union, replace destroyed bone or immobilize joint in surgical fusion.
    b. homografting or homotransplantation of bone — surgical use of bone from bone bank obtained from amputations, ostectomies or rib resections of nonmalignant, noninfectious cases.

3. epiphyseal arrest — surgical procedure for retarding growth at the epiphysis by equalizing length of lower extremities.

4. epiphyseal stapling — temporary arrest of epiphyseal growth by stapling the epiphysis to control leg length discrepancy.[42]

5. epiphysiodesis — implanting bone grafts across the epiphyseal plate to secure immobilization of epiphysis. Operation is done for slipped femoral epiphysis following insertion of metal pins.

6. exostectomy — removal of a benign bone tumor (exostosis), e.g. a bunion (hallux valgus).

7. ostectomy — excision of a bone.

8. osteoclasis — surgical refracture of a bone in case of malunion of broken parts.

9. osteoplasty — reconstruction or repair of a bone.

10. osteotomy — surgical division or section of a bone.[53, 14]

11. replantation of an extremity — restorative surgery of an accidentally amputated limb to its functional capacity including
    a. restoration of circulation by anastomoses of blood vessels.
    b. internal fixation of diaphyseal fracture of bone by intramedullary nail.
    c. repair of nerves and tendons.
    d. debridement of devitalized tissue.
    e. closure by suturing undamaged soft tissue of dismembered limb to stump.
    f. split-thickness grafts for denuded skin areas.[50, 56]
12. sequestrectomy — surgical removal of a piece of dead bone.
13. surgical correction of fracture — this may be achieved by
    a. closed reduction — manipulation and application of cast, or application of splint or traction apparatus in selected cases when the fractured ends are not in alignment.
    b. open reduction and internal fixation — manipulation and
       (1) insertion of plate and screws.
       (2) insertion of medullary nail for diaphyseal fractures (shaft of long bones); extraction of nail after bone union.
       (3) insertion of a nail with a side plate such as a Jewett nail for intertrochanteric fractures of the femur.
       (4) insertion of a hip prosthesis, Fred Thompson or Austin Moore type, in selected femoral neck fractures. Occasionally prostheses are used for severe fractures of the upper or lower end of the humerus.[5]
    c. simple immobilization — application of a cast or splint when the fractured ends are in apposition.
14. surgical correction of facial defects:
    a. bone grafting of hemimandibular defects.
    b. bone graft reconstruction following hemimandibulectomies.
    c. craniofacial osteotomies for correction of facial anomalies.[80]

E. Symptomatic Terms:

1. callus — substance growing between ends of fractured bone and converted into osseous tissue in the process of repair.
2. crepitation — grating sound made by movement of fractured bones.
3. decalcification — the removal of lime salts, especially from bone.
4. ostealgia, osteodynia — bone pain.
5. phantom limb pain — painful sensation felt by amputee as if the limb were still intact, probably of central origin.

JOINTS, BURSAE, CARTILAGES, LIGAMENTS

A. Origin of Terms:

1. ankyle (G) — stiff joint
2. arthron (G) — joint
3. bursa (L) — purse, sac
4. cartilage (L) — gristle
5. cavus (L) — hollow
6. chondros (G) — gristle
7. condylos (G) — knuckle
8. cubitus (L) — elbow
9. hallux (L) — great toe
10. kyphos (G) — hump
11. ligament (L) — that which ties
12. lordosis (G) — bending backbone
13. luxatio (L) — to dislocate
14. malleus (L) — hammer
15. mandibulum (L) — lower jaw bone
16. meniskos (G) — crescent
17. pes, pedes (L) — foot, feet
18. planus (L) — flat
19. scolios (G) — curved
20. spondylos (G) — vertebra
21. talus (L) — heel, ankle
22. taliped (L) — club footed

B. Anatomical Terms:

1. acetabulum — cup-shaped socket on the external surface of the innominate bone in which the head of the femur lies.
2. articulation — joint.
   a. cartilaginous joint — bones united by fibrocartilage or hyaline cartilage.
   b. fibrous joint — bones united by fibrous tissue.
   c. synovial joint, diarthrodial joint — bones united by a joint capsule and ligaments. Cartilage covers the articular surface of the bones. The joint capsule is composed of a fibrous layer lined by synovial membrane.
3. bursa (pl. bursae) — connective tissue sac containing lubricating fluid, sometimes synovia.
4. intervertebral disc — fibrocartilage between the bodies of the vertebrae composed of
   a. anulus* fibrosus — an outer fibrous ring encircling the nucleus pulposus.
   b. nucleus pulposus — an inner gelatinous mass.
5. ligaments — fibrous, connective tissue bands uniting articular ends of bones.
6. meniscus — fibrocartilage found in certain joints.
7. synovial membrane — inner lining of a joint capsule secreting synovia.

C. Diagnostic Terms:

1. ankylosis — stiff joint.
2. arthritis — inflammation of joints.
   a. atrophic or rheumatoid arthritis which produces constitutional symptoms in addition to painful, inflammatory, multiple joint involvement.[13, 17, 9]
   b. gouty arthritis — metabolic disorder, usually involving one joint (monarticular). Urate crystals are highly increased and found in various tissues. Pain is relieved by colchicine.
   c. infectious arthritis, pyogenic arthritis, septic arthritis —
      (1) acute infectious arthritis — acute inflammatory process affecting synovial and subchondrial tissues and causing articular destruction. It is usually due to pyogenic cocci such as gonococci, meningococci, pneumococci, staphylococci and streptococci.
      (2) chronic infectious arthritis — persistent infection of joint causing pain, swelling, restricted joint motion and deformity.[27, 70]
   d. hypertrophic arthritis, osteoarthritis — a degenerative condition of cartilage and enlargement of bone at the joint margins, occurring particularly in older persons. It often affects the terminal phalanges, knees, hips and spine and results in contractures, deformities and stiffness of affected joints.[27]
   e. Marie Strümpell arthritis, ankylosing spondylitis — painful inflammatory joint disease characterized by progressive stiffening of the spine caused by fusion of vertebral bodies.[27, 68]
   f. traumatic arthritis — a group of disorders resulting from single or repetitive trauma to joints:
      (1) acute synovitis, traumatic synovitis — this may be due to a single episode of articular trauma to the synovial membrane of a joint and may be associated with hemarthrosis and sprains. The articular cartilage is intact.
      (2) disruptive trauma of joint — the major supporting structures have ruptured and the articular cartilage is damaged. Meniscal tears, intraarticular fractures and severe sprains may be present.
      (3) posttraumatic osteoarthritis — residual damage from disruptive trauma may lead to restricted mobility, deformity and articular instability.
      (4) repetitive articular trauma — a chronic arthritis of the affected joints may develop due to occupational hazards or sports.

---

* Spelling of anulus according to *Nomina Anatomica*, 1964, p. 67.

(5) other types of trauma — arthropathy may develop following decompression, radiation, frostbite or the like.[57]

Medicolegal problems may arise when there is an aggravation of pre-existing arthritis and the causal relationship between the traumatic episode and joint affections is veiled.

3. arthropathy — any disease of the joints.

4. bursitis — inflammation of a bursa.

5. chondritis — inflammation of a cartilage.

6. chondroblastoma — benign, vascular, cartilaginous tumor arising from the epiphysis of a long bone.

7. chondrocalcinosis, pseudogout — acute, recurrent joint disease affecting the cartilaginous structures of large joints especially the knee. Synovial fluid contains calcium pyrophosphates.[27]

8. chondroma — benign neoplasm arising from cartilage.[73, 60]

9. chondrosarcoma — malignant tumor derived from cartilage.

10. coxarthrosis — a hip joint; trophic degeneration of hip joint.

11. destructive coxopathy — painful disability of hip joint associated with nocturnal distress of inflammatory type. Joint motion is moderately impaired.

12. dislocation — displacement of a bone from its natural position in a joint.

13. fibrositis, muscular rheumatism, periarthritis, periarticular fibrositis — rheumatoid condition affecting the muscles and tissues around the joints.

14. hallux malleus — hammer toe.

15. hallux valgus — deflection of great toe to outer side of foot and subsequent development of bony prominence.[25]

16. hallux varus — deflection of great toe to inner side of foot.

17. hemarthrosis — bloody effusion in a joint cavity. It is prone to occur in hemophiliacs.[51]

18. herniated intervertebral disc, herniated nucleus pulposus — tear of anulus fibrosus followed by protrusion of the nucleus pulposus, compression of nerve root, back pain with or without sciatic radiation and paresthesias (pricking or numbness) of calf or foot. The rupture usually occurs in the lumbar, sacral and cervical regions of the spine.[74, 41]

19. internal derangement of knee joint — term refers to various joint lesions which interfere with motion (locking, snapping, buckling) due to atrophy of thigh muscles, tenderness or pain and joint swelling. Some leading causes are tears of menisci, ligaments, patellar or quadriceps tendons, loose bodies, fracture or chondromalacia of patellae.[83]

20. kyphosis — hunchback; abnormal posterior curvature of thoracic spine.

21. lordosis — hollow-back; anterior convexity of lower spine.

22. painful shoulder, nonarticular — disorder characterized by tenderness, moderate to agonizing pain and limitation of motion. These symptoms are present in

a. adhesive capsulitis, adhesive bursitis, frozen shoulder — adhesions within the bursa causing stiffness and later atrophic changes.

b. hand-shoulder syndrome — peculiar clinical entity in which pain radiates from shoulder to finger tips. The patient spontaneously immobilizes the affected extremity which leads to atrophy and edema of the hand. Later overactivity of sympathetic nerves results in a sweaty, cold, painful hand followed by stiffness and fibrosis of joints. Syndrome may occur following myocardial infarction.

c. supraspinatus syndrome — disorder caused by adhesions, calcium deposits or tears in rotator cuff resulting in a painful shoulder, limited motion, muscle atrophy and spasm.[12, 4]

23. scoliosis — lateral spinal curvature.

24. spondylitis — inflammation of one or several vertebrae.

25. spondylolisthesis — forward slipping of a lumbar vertebra on the adjacent vertebra below, usually associated with pelvic deformity.[38, 78]

26. spondylosis — ankylosis of vertebrae; also any degenerative lesion of the spine.

27. sprain — injury to joint with tearing of tendons and ligaments.
28. Still's disease — painful rheumatoid arthritis in children associated with retarded growth, glandular and splenic enlargement.[13]
29. subluxation — incomplete dislocation.
30. talipes — clubfoot:
    a. equinus — forefoot touches ground; walking on toes.
    b. planus — arch broken; entire sole rests on ground.
    c. valgus — foot everted; inner side of sole touches ground.
    d. varus — foot inverted; outer side of sole rests on ground.

D. Operative Terms:

1. arthroclasia — surgical breaking of a stiff joint.
2. arthrodesis, artificial ankylosis — surgical fixation of a joint to immobilize the joint.[20, 24, 15]
3. arthrolysis — freeing the joint from fibrous bands or excess cartilage to restore its mobility.
4. arthroplasty — surgical repair of a joint. The hip, knee, elbow and temporomandibular joints are best suited for reconstruction.
    a. arthroplasties of the hip joint.
        (1) Charnley low-friction arthroplasty — a total hip arthroplasty or total hip replacement for rheumatoid arthritis or any type of destructive hip disease. The prosthesis has two components: (1) an acetabular cup or socket of high density polyethylene and (2) a femoral component of Vitallium or stainless steel consisting of a small femoral head for low friction which lodges in the socket and a prosthetic stem embedded in the intramedullary canal of the femur. Acrylic cement is used to seat the acetabular cup and prosthetic stem. The cement provides rigid fixation and stability.[7, 16, 55, 28, 46]

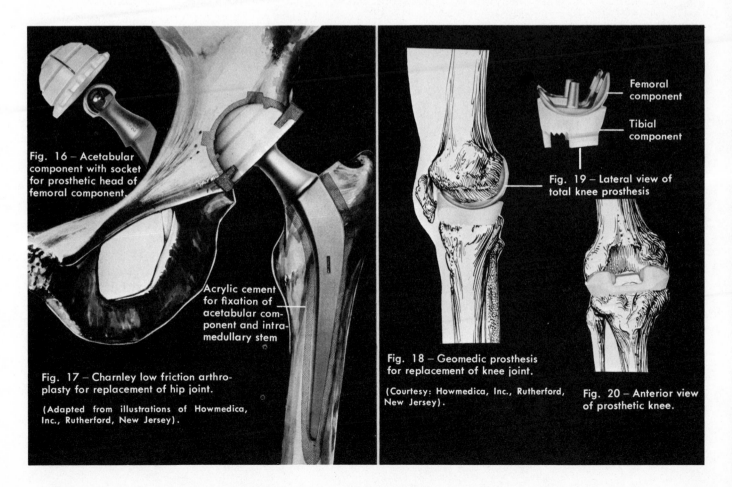

Fig. 16 – Acetabular component with socket for prosthetic head of femoral component.

Acrylic cement for fixation of acetabular component and intramedullary stem

Fig. 17 – Charnley low friction arthroplasty for replacement of hip joint.

(Adapted from illustrations of Howmedica, Inc., Rutherford, New Jersey).

Fig. 18 – Geomedic prosthesis for replacement of knee joint.

(Courtesy: Howmedica, Inc., Rutherford, New Jersey).

Femoral component

Tibial component

Fig. 19 – Lateral view of total knee prosthesis

Fig. 20 – Anterior view of prosthetic knee.

(2) Colonna capsular arthroplasty — operation for congenital dislocation of the hip. This procedure retains the gliding mechanism between the displaced head of the femur and its capsule. The acetabulum is usually deepened and enlarged.[18]

(3) Moore or Thompson prosthetic arthroplasty — surgical repair of arthritic hip including amputation of head and neck of femur, acetabular remodeling and reconstruction and seating of prosthesis in femoral shaft and acetabulum.[66, 76, 52]

(4) Vitallium mold arthroplasty — molding a joint and interposing a nonirritating substance between bony surfaces to improve joint function and lessen pain in rheumatoid arthritis and bony or fibrous ankylosis. Interposition of material between joint surfaces such as autogenous fascia or inert metal (Vitallium) also prevents recurrence of ankylosis.[79]

b. arthroplasties of the knee.

(1) Geomedic total knee arthroplasty — removal of sufficient bone and insertion of femoral and tibial components of the geomedic prosthesis for total knee replacement. See Figs. 18, 19 and 20.

(2) MacIntosh arthroplasty — removal of hypertrophic synovium and menisci and placement of one or both hemispheric discs on articular surface of tibia. The McKeever arthroplasty is a similar operative procedure for relief of pain and restoration of a functional knee joint.[55, 58, 23]

(3) MGH (Massachusetts General Hospital) prosthesis — a stainless steel model of the articular surface of the femoral condyles attached to lower end of femur by an intramedullary stem.[55]

c. arthroplasty of temporomandibular joint — surgical breaking of a stiff joint to relieve disabling ankylosis caused by rheumatic, degenerative, infectious or traumatic arthritis. The mandibular condyle is resected and remodeled.[79]

5. arthrotomy — surgical opening of a joint.

6. bunionectomy, surgical correction of valgus deformity — removal of bony prominence (bunion) from medial aspect of first metatarsal head.[71, 47]

7. chondrectomy — removal of a cartilage.

8. chondroplasty — plastic repair of a cartilage.

9. Harrington instrumentation and fusion — operation for correcting scoliosis. Metal rods and hooks are directly implanted on the spine. Articular fusion is achieved by inserting bone grafts from the ilium.[22, 35]

10. synovectomy — partial or total removal of a synovial membrane lining of a joint capsule.[26]

E. Symptomatic Terms:

1. arthralgia, arthrodynia — joint pain.

2. capsular laceration — tear of a joint capsule.

3. crepitus, articular — the grating of joints.

4. detachment of cartilage — separation of cartilaginous material from a joint. Loose bodies limit motion.

5. effusion, hemorrhagic — bleeding into synovial sac.

6. effusion, synovial — an overproduction of joint fluid.

7. Heberden's nodes — hard nodules at the distal phalangeal joints of the fingers in osteoarthritis.

8. lipping — liplike bony growths at the joints in osteoarthritis; for example: the marginal lipping of the acetabular rim and head of the femur in degenerative hip disease.

9. lumbago — dull, aching pain in the lumbar region of back.

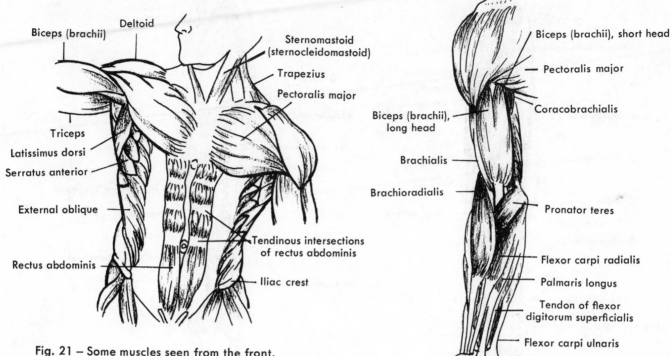

Fig. 21 – Some muscles seen from the front.

Biceps (brachii)
Deltoid
Sternomastoid (sternocleidomastoid)
Trapezius
Pectoralis major
Triceps
Latissimus dorsi
Serratus anterior
External oblique
Tendinous intersections of rectus abdominis
Rectus abdominis
Iliac crest

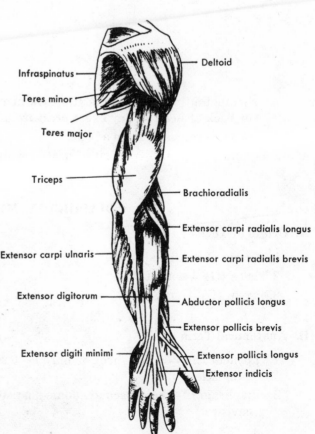

Biceps (brachii), short head
Pectoralis major
Coracobrachialis
Biceps (brachii), long head
Brachialis
Brachioradialis
Pronator teres
Flexor carpi radialis
Palmaris longus
Tendon of flexor digitorum superficialis
Flexor carpi ulnaris

Fig. 23 – Muscles of the front of the upper limb.

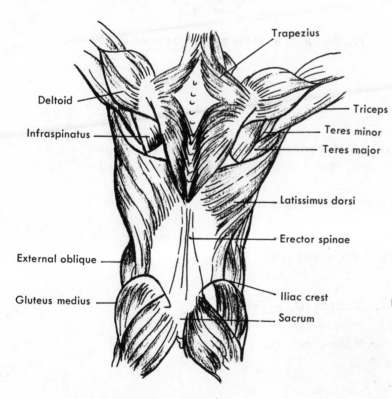

Trapezius
Deltoid
Infraspinatus
Triceps
Teres minor
Teres major
Latissimus dorsi
Erector spinae
External oblique
Gluteus medius
Iliac crest
Sacrum

Fig. 22 – Some muscles seen from the back.

Infraspinatus
Teres minor
Teres major
Deltoid
Triceps
Brachioradialis
Extensor carpi radialis longus
Extensor carpi radialis brevis
Extensor carpi ulnaris
Extensor digitorum
Abductor pollicis longus
Extensor pollicis brevis
Extensor digiti minimi
Extensor pollicis longus
Extensor indicis

Fig. 24 – Muscles of the back of the upper limb.

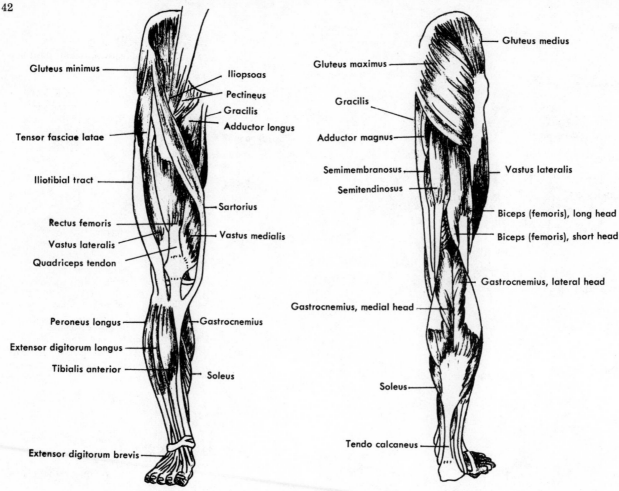

Fig. 25 – Muscles of the front of the lower limb.

Fig. 26 – Muscles of the back of the lower limb.

10. rheumatoid nodules — subcutaneous nodules located over bony prominences, e.g. elbow or back of heel. They exert pressure and are present in advanced rheumatoid arthritis.
11. spur — projection from a bone.
12. tophus, pl. tophi — deposit of urate crystals in subcutaneous tissue near a joint.

DIAPHRAGM, MUSCLES, TENDONS

A. Origin of Terms:

1. fascia (L) — band
2. leios (G) — smooth
3. myo- (G) — muscle
4. phragm (G) — fence, wall
5. rhabdo- (G) — rod, striated
6. tendo-, teno- (G) — tendon

B. Anatomical Terms:

1. aponeurosis — a flat sheet of fibrous tissue which usually serves as an attachment for a muscle.
2. diaphragm — the muscular, dome-shaped septum between the thoracic and abdominal cavities.

3. fascia — a sheet of connective tissue which covers, supports and separates muscles.
4. insertion of muscle — end attached to the bone or cartilage which moves when the muscle contracts (or shortens).
5. muscle — contractile tissue composed of units that have the power to contract when stimulated by a nerve impulse.
6. origin of a muscle — end attached to the bone or cartilage which does **not** move when the muscle contracts (or shortens).
7. tendons — bands of fibrous tissue which attach muscles to bones.

C. Diagnostic Terms:

1. carpoptosia — wrist drop.
2. claudication — limping, intermittent type due to ischemia of leg muscles.
3. contracture — permanent shortening of one or more muscles caused by paralysis, spasm or scar formation.
   a. Dupuytren's contracture — shrinkage of palmar fascia resulting in flexion deformity of one or more fingers.[39]
   b. Volkmann's contracture — flexion deformity of wrist and fingers which may be due to circulatory interference by a tight cast.[34]
4. disuse atrophy — muscle wasting caused by immobilization.
5. fascitis — inflammation of the fascia.
6. graphospasm — writer's cramp.
7. hiatus hernia, diaphragmatic hernia — protrusion of an abdominal organ, usually a portion of the stomach through the esophageal opening of the diaphragm.
8. leiomyoma — benign, smooth muscle tumor.[21]
9. muscular dystrophy — progressive disease of unknown etiology, marked in infants by enlarged calves, waddling gait, sway back and winged shoulders. As the disease advances there is extensive wasting of muscles and development of bizarre deformities.
10. myasthenia gravis — chronic neuromuscular disorder, characterized by weakness, usually first manifested in ocular muscles resulting in bilateral ptosis of eye lids and sleepy appearance. The myasthenic facies is apathetic and expressionless. There may be involvement of the muscles of speech, mastication and swallowing. When the chest muscles are affected, dyspnea may develop. Infrequently weakness of the legs interferes with walking. Symptoms fluctuate in severity ranging from exacerbations to remissions.[48, 29]
11. myoma — benign muscular tumor.
12. myosarcoma — malignant muscular tumor.
13. myositis — inflammatory process of muscles.
14. paralysis — loss of sensation and voluntary movements, either temporary or permanent.
    a. flaccid — lower motor neuron involvement.
    b. spastic — upper motor neuron involvement.[61]
15. polymyositis — a primary myopathy characterized by muscle weakness in pelvic and shoulder girdles, distal lower and upper extremities, muscle pain or tenderness. It may be associated with connective tissue disease.
16. rhabdomyoma — a striated muscle tumor.
17. tenosynovitis, tendosynovitis — inflammation of a tendon and its synovial sheath.
18. torticollis, wryneck — contraction of a sternocleidomastoid muscle, drawing the head to one side and causing asymmetry of face; may be congenital or acquired.

D. Operative Terms:

1. myoplasty — surgical repair of a muscle; for example, by free muscle graft or pedicle graft.
2. myorrhaphy — suture of a muscle.
3. myotasis — stretching of a muscle.

44

4. tenodesis — suture of end of tendon to skeletal attachment (tendon torn at point of insertion).
5. tenoplasty, tendoplasty — surgical repair of a tendon.
6. tenosynovectomy — removal of a tendon and its sheath.

E. Symptomatic Terms:

1. clonic spasm — rapid, repeated, muscular contractions.
2. cramp — prolonged, intense spasm of one muscle.
3. hyperkinesia — purposeless, excessive, involuntary movements.
4. hypotonia — reduced muscle tension associated with muscular atrophy.
5. rigidity, rigor — stiffness, muscular hardness.
6. tonic spasm — excessive, prolonged, muscular contractions.
7. tremors — oscillating, rhythmic movements of muscle groups.[82]

RADIOLOGY

A. Terms Related to Diagnosis:

1. air arthrogram, pneumoarthrogram — air injection into a joint for radiographic evaluation. For example it is possible to outline the menisci of the knee and visualize major tears and displacements of large tears.
2. arthrography — injection of a contrast medium into a joint and making arthrograms.[64, 6]
3. scanogram — a radiogram of a structure of the body using special technique for accurate measurements of its length. Scanograms are made to determine the length of the medullary canal before medullary fixation is attempted. The selection of the medullary nail depends on scanographic findings.
4. scanography — a method of x-ray examination for accurate measurement of the length of structures of the body usually of the long bones.[65] It is used to determine leg length discrepancy.
5. stereoradiography, stereoroentgenography, stereoskiagraphy (stereo (G) - solid) — obtaining an x-ray picture from two similar positions to give the object seen an appearance of relief, depth and solidity.
6. xeroradiography (xeros (G) - dry) — the taking of a radiogram by using a selenium coated plate and developing it without liquid chemicals.[55]

B. Terms Related to Therapy:

1. radiation necrosis of bone — bone destruction by ionizing radiation or radioactive substances.
2. radiotherapy — radiant energy used in the treatment of disease.
3. radiosensitive — capable of responding to irradiation.
4. radioresistant — incapable of receiving benefit from irradiation.
Radiotherapy is the treatment of choice for giant cell tumors and Ewing's sarcoma. According to Ackerman[14] myelomas tend to be radiosensitive and locally radiocurable. Attempts have been made to use radioisotopes in the treatment of myelomas. Osteosarcomas previously thought to be radioresistant have shown radiosensitivity in specific instances.[2]

CLINICAL LABORATORY

A. Terms Related to Blood Chemistry:

1. serum calcium determination — a function test of the parathyroids which produce parathormone. This hormone is concerned with the regulation of the calcium content of the blood. Calcium is important in bone production.
2. serum phosphorus determination — a test designed to obtain the concentration of phosphorus in blood serum. Calcium phosphate is found in the bones and teeth.

B. Terms Related to Urine Studies:

1. Bence-Jones protein — a peculiar type of protein molecule which is excreted in the urine in the majority of cases of multiple myeloma and in certain bone tumors.
2. determination of calcium in urine and feces — these tests are concerned with the calcium balance in the body.
3. normal calcium balance — in health the calcium intake exceeds the calcium excretion of urine and feces together.

C. Terms Related to the Specific Diagnosis of Joint Disease.

1. F-II latex fixation test — serologic test for the detection of the rheumatoid factor (RF).
2. serum uric acid determination — abnormal increase in serum uric acid usually indicative of gouty arthritis or gout.
3. synovial fluid studies — examination of joint fluid to aid in the diagnostic and prognostic evaluation of joint disease by demonstrating the severity of the inflammatory process of synovial tissue. In most cases the synovial fluid is obtained by aspirating the suprapatellar space of the knee joint. The examination includes:
   a. appearance and consistency of joint fluid.
   b. culture of synovial fluid to detect the presence or absence of infective agent.
   c. cytology of joint fluid: red and white cell counts, differential count, identification of crystals such as urate crystals.[27]

Table 2

SERUM CALCIUM AND SERUM PHOSPHORUS IN BONE DISEASES

Serum	Normal Values[a]	Increased Values	Decreased Values
Calcium Adults Children Infants	Method of Clark - Collip 9.5-11.0 mg/100 ml or 4.7-5.5 mEq/L 10.0-11.5 mg/100 ml or 5.0-5.8 mEq/L 10.5-12.0 mg/100 ml or 5.2-6.0 mEq/L	Multiple myeloma Metastases to bone	Renal osteodystrophy Osteomalacia
Phosphorus Adults Children Infants	Colorimeter Method of Bodansky 2.5- 4.0 mg/100 ml 4.5- 5.5 mg/100 ml 5.5- 6.5 mg/100 ml	Renal osteodystrophy	Rickets Osteomalacia

a Cf. Opal E. Hepler. *Manual of Clinical Laboratory Methods*, 4th ed. Springfield, Illinois: Charles C. Thomas, 1955, pp. 305-309. The abbreviation mEq/L refers to milliequivalents per liter.

Table 3

CALCIUM IN URINE AND FECES IN BONE DISEASES

Calcium	Normal Values[a] Method of Wang	Increased Values	Decreased Values
Urine	50-300 mg per 24 hour specimen (Range of 0.2 to 4.6 mg per kg)	Metastases to bone Multiple myeloma Paget's disease	Osteomalacia Renal osteodystrophy Rickets
Feces	0.4-0.8 Gm in 24 hrs. depending on Ca intake Average of 70% of total Ca excreted by body		Osteomalacia

a *Ibid.*, pp. 305-307.

ABBREVIATIONS

A. General:

ASS — anterior superior spine
AP — anteroposterior
Ca — calcium, cancer
C_1 — first cervical vertebra
C_2 — second cervical vertebra
D_1 — first dorsal vertebra
D_2 — second dorsal vertebra
IDK — internal derangement
    of the knee

IM — intramuscular
IS — intercostal space
LIF — left iliac fossa
L_1 — first lumbar vertebra
L_2 — second lumbar vertebra
MSL — midsternal line
Orth. — orthopedics
RIF — right iliac fossa
S — sacral vertebra

B. Amputations and Prostheses:

AE — above the elbow
AK — above the knee
BE — below the elbow
BK — below the knee
HD — hip disarticulation
HP — hemipelvectomy
KB — knee bearing
KD — knee disarticulation

PTB — patellar tendon bearing
    (prosthesis)
SACH — solid ankle cushion heel
    (foot prosthesis)
SD — shoulder disarticulation
THR — total hip replacement
UHMWPE — ultra high molecular
    weight polyethylene
    (cup or socket)

C. Organizations:

MDAA — Muscular Dystrophy
    Association of America, Inc.

NSCCA — National Society for
    Crippled Children and Adults

ORAL READING PRACTICE

Paget's Disease of Bone

When in 1877 Sir James Paget described the disease which now bears his name, he erroneously called it osteitis deformans considering it a form of chronic **inflammatory** affection of osseous tissue. Paget's disease is a peculiar bone disorder with an insidious onset, **asymptomatic** early phase, a plateau of apparent stationary involvement, perhaps lasting years, followed by progressive disease and complications which may terminate life. Its **etiolgoy** is unknown. It is not a metabolic disturbance since it primarily attacks bones under pressure of weight bearing, leaving those of the upper body relatively untouched. An exception is the skull which shows radiologic evidence of **osteoporosis circumscripta,** so termed because **osteoporotic** changes are limited to a circumscribed area.

The incidence of Paget's disease of bone is highest in advancing years and greater in males than in females. It is a rather common affliction amounting to three percent in the age group past forty.

The pathological characteristics comprise concurrent processes of **osteoclastic** and **osteoblastic** activity resulting in marked bone destruction and rapid bone repair, architectural abnormality of new bone, increased **vascularity** and **fibrosis.** Instead of normal resorption and replacement of bone, metabolic processes are disorganized and irregular. New bone may undergo osteolysis as soon as it is formed. Osteoblasts produce coarse, disorted **trabeculae** which **anastomose** in a peculiar fashion exhibiting a mosaic design.

In the skull **osteolytic** (osteoclastic) activity predominates. A lesion of **decalcification** forms, particularly in the outer **cranial** table. It is termed **osteoporosis circumscripta.** Gradually dense areas resembling tufts of cotton appear in the **rarefied** lesion and the **demarcation** between **diploe,** the two cranial tables, becomes indistinct.

The patient's **contour** portrays the influence of pathological, skeletal changes in advanced Paget's disease. His spine is **kyphotic**, stature shortened, position crouched and abdomen pendulous. The **anterolateral** bowing of his legs results in a waddling, slow gait. The face appears small compared to the protruding skull, which characteristically shows **bitemporal** enlargement.

Pain develops with progressive bone involvement and varies from a mild dull ache to intermittent or persistent **ostealgia**. Fractures occur frequently, heal readily and are the most common complication of Paget's disease. They may be occasioned by trivial incidents such as tripping on stairs or turning in bed.

The patient with Paget disease, immobilized because of fracture or intercurrent disease, is likely to develop **hypercalciuria, renal calculi** and **hypercalcemia**. Since bone repair is markedly decreased during immobilization, **osteoporosis** of disuse becomes a problematic issue.[37] Bone destruction persists unabated, thus liberating an excessive amount of calcium which is spilled into urine instead of being **deposited** in bone. This may lead to **nephrolithiasis** and serious **sequelae**. If the kidneys are unable to handle the high surplus of calcium, hypercalcemia is prone to develop. It is signalled by dryness of mouth and nose, nausea and vomiting. Untreated, the **prognosis** may be fatal.

Malignant degeneration of diseased bone is a constant threat. Whenever **osteogenic sarcoma, fibrosarcoma** or malignant **osteoclastoma** develop, the patient has probably reached the terminal phase of his life. **Palliative** measures must be instituted to bring relief of ostealgia and other distressing symptoms.[81, 72]

Table 4

SOME ORTHOPEDIC CONDITIONS AMENABLE TO SURGERY

Organs Involved	Diagnoses	Operations	Procedures
Rib	Supernumerary rib	Costectomy	Removal of rib
Shoulder	Chronic tendinitis	Partial acromionectomy	Removal of outer edge of acromion
Shoulder	Calcified deposits in rotator cuff	Curettment of rotator cuff	Split deltoid approach and scraping of cuff to remove deposits
Humerus	Osteomyelitis of humerus	Osteotomy with curettage and drainage	Surgical opening of bone, scraping of medullary canal and insertion of drain
Humerus	Sequestrum	Sequestrectomy and saucerization	Excision of dead bone and removal of infected or foreign matter, scar and granulation tissue
Ulna Radius	Crushing injury with loss of blood supply to hand and wrist	Amputation of forearm	Removal of forearm below elbow
		Biceps cineplasty for operating prosthetic device	Construction of skin tunnel through biceps muscle; tunneled muscle to move artificial hand
Hand Wrist joint	Traumatic severence of hand Disarticulation at wrist joint	Replantation of hand Internal fixation with Kirschner wires	First wire passed through carpus and up the medullary cavity of radius Second wire crossed from base of 5th metacarpal through cortex of radius Repair of vessels and tendons
Spine	Scoliosis	Harrington's operation instrumentation and fusion for correction of scoliosis	Implantation of metal rods and hooks directly on the spine followed by fusion to provide distractive and compressive forces of spinal curve

Organs Involved	Diagnoses	Operations	Procedures
Spine	Spondylolisthesis	Modified Hibbs arthrodesis of spine	Excision of cartilage from articular facets, packing bone chips into joint spaces; iliac bone grafting
Hip joint	Early degenerative arthritis	High femoral osteotomy	Incision through upper end of femur usually in subtrochanteric region Medial displacement of distal femur resulting in change in weight bearing position of femoral head[a]
Hip joint	Degenerative arthritis	Vitallium mold arthroplasty	Reconstruction of femoral head and placement of deep cup over head
		Austin Moore or Fred Thompson arthroplasty	Replacement of femoral head with hip prosthesis
Hip joint	Advanced rheumatoid arthritis and ankylosing spondylitis of hip — or Advanced osteoarthritis	Charnley low-friction arthroplasty for total hip replacement	Lateral approach with osteotomy of greater trochanter Dislocation of hip and removal of femoral head and neck and of destructive joint lesions Insertion of small femoral head and stem in shaft Cement used for seating the acetabular cup and prosthetic stem to provide rigid fixation[a, b]
Hip joint	Congenital dislocation of hip	Colonna capsular arthroplasty	*Fist stage* Hamstring stretching and surgical division of adductor tendon *Second stage* Reconstruction of acetabulum Placement of capsule-covered femoral head into reconstructed acetabulum
Femur	Slipped femoral epiphysis	Trochanteric osteotomy	Section of femur, abduction and internal rotation of distal fragment, blade-plate fixation
Femur	Fracture of femoral neck	Excision of femoral head and insertion of hip prosthesis Fred Thompson or Austin Moore type Internal fixation by insertion of Smith-Petersen nail	Removal of femoral head and most of neck — replacement by metal prosthesis Three flanged nail driven over guide wire through femoral neck and head, guide wire removed
Femur	Intertrochanteric fracture of femur	Internal fixation by insertion of hip nail Jewett type or Neufeld type of Key type or Holt type	Nail driven over guide wire through femoral neck and into head of femur, side plate fixed to shaft with screws

Organs Involved	Diagnoses	Operations	Procedures
Femur	Transverse diaphyseal fracture of femur	Internal fixation by insertion of intramedullary nail Küntscher type or Lottes type	Medullary nail driven over guide wire into medullary cavity occupying the entire canal
Knee	Recurrent dislocation of patella	Hauser operation	Medial and distal transplantation of tibial tubercle and its patellar tendon[c]
Knee	Chondromalacia of patella	Patelloplasty Complete patellectomy	Partial resection and plastic repair of patella Removal of patella
Knees	Genu valgum	Stapling operation	Oblique skin incision Stapling the medial femoral condyles
Tibia Fibula Foot	Crushing injury and uncontrollable infection of distal portion of lower extremity	Below-knee amputation	Incision of skin flaps Division of anterolateral muscles Ligation of blood vessels Removal of leg and stump closure Application of rigid elastic plaster dressing and prosthetic unit
Foot	Hallus valgus deformity	Keller operation	Resection of proximal half of first phalanx of great toe Excision of bony prominence
Anterior cruciate ligament	Tear of anterior cruciate ligament, separation of anterior attachment	Reconstruction of torn anterior cruciate ligament	Repair of ligament by restoring the anterior attachment
Quadriceps tendon	Old rupture of quadriceps tendon	Repair of old rupture of quadriceps tendon-application of cast	Approximation of tendon ends with heavy braided silk sutures; cast applied with knee extension
Tendon Achilles or Tendon calcaneus	Abnormal shortening of tendon calcaneus	Tenoplasty with lengthening of tendon calcaneus	Surgical repair of tendon
Tendon supraspinatus	Complete rupture of tendon	Tenorrhaphy	Suture of tendon
Sternocleido-mastoid muscle	Torticollis, congenital	Brown and McDowell excision of sternocleidomastoid muscle Tenotomy of upper and lower end of sternocleidomastoid muscle or both ends	Abnormal muscle freed from underlying structures and excised Muscle lengthened by division of one or both ends allowing shortened muscle to retract
Flexor muscles of hip	Hip flexion contracture in spastic cerebral palsy	Myotomies for release of spastic hip flexor muscles	Surgical division of all taut flexor muscles of hip

[a] Robert M. O'Brien, M.D. Personal communications.

[b] R. B. Welch and C. Charnley. Low-friction arthroplasty of the hip in rheumatoid arthritis and ankylosing spondylitis. *Clinical Orthopaedics and Related Research.* 72: 22-27, September-October, 1970.

[c] M. Stewart. Dislocations. In Crenshaw, A. H. (ed.). *Campbell's Operative Orthopaedics*, 5th ed. St. Louis: The C. V. Mosby Company, 1971, p. 451.

REFERENCES AND BIBLIOGRAPHY

1. Ackerman, Lauren V. and del Regato, Juan A. Malignant tumors of bone. In *Cancer, Diagnosis, Treatment and Prognosis*, 4th ed. St. Louis: The C. V. Mosby Co., 1970, pp. 896-924.

2. —————. Radiotherapy of malignant tumors of bone. *Ibid.*, pp. 924-926.

3. Alho, A. *et al.* Osteomyelitis in nonoperative and operative fracture treatment. *Clinical Orthopaedics and Related Research*, 82: 123-133, January-February, 1972.

4. Allman, F. L. Shoulder injuries. *Lawyer's Medical Journal*, 6: 41-62, May, 1970.

5. Anderson, L. D. Fractures. In Crenshaw, A. H. (ed.). *Campbell's Operative Orthopaedics*, 5th ed. St. Louis: The C. V. Mosby Co., 1971, pp. 574-608.

6. Angell, F. L. Fluoroscopic techniques of double contrast arthrography of the knee. *Radiologic Clinics of North America*, 9: 85-98, April, 1971.

7. Beber, C. A. and Convery, F. R. Management of patients with total hip replacement. *Physical Therapy*, 52: 823-828, August, 1972.

8. Black, D. A. K. (ed.). *Renal Disease*, 2d ed. Philadelphia: F. A. Davis Co., 1967, p. 666.

9. Bluhm, G. B. and Barnhart, M. I. Pathophysiology of rheumatoid joint disease. *Clinical Orthopaedics and Related Research*, 74: 34-42, January-February, 1971.

10. Boyd, H. B. Grafting operations. In Crenshaw, A. H. (ed.). *Campbell's Operative Orthopaedics*, 5th ed. St. Louis: The C. V. Mosby Co., 1971, pp. 814-816.

11. Boyne, P. J. Autogenous cancellous bone and marrow transplants. *Clinical Orthopaedics and Related Research*, 73: 199-209, November-December, 1970.

12. Braun, R. M. *et al.* Surgical treatment of the painful shoulder contracture in the stroke patient. *Journal of Bone and Joint Surgery*, 53A: 1307-1312, October, 1971.

13. Calabro, J. J. Rheumatoid arthritis. *Clinical Symposia*, 23: 2-32, 1971.

14. Canale, S. T. *et al.* Innominate osteotomy in Legg-Calvé-Perthes disease. *Journal of Bone and Joint Surgery*, 54A: 25-40, January, 1972.

15. Carroll, R. E. and Dick, H. M. Arthrodesis of the wrist for rheumatoid arthritis. *Journal of Bone and Joint Surgery*, 53A: 1365-1369, October, 1971.

16. Charnley, J. The long-term results of low-friction arthroplasty of the hip performed as a primary intervention. *Journal of Bone and Joint Surgery*, 54B: 61-76, February, 1972.

17. Christian, C. L. Rheumatoid arthritis. In Samter, M. (ed.). *Immunological Diseases*. 2d ed. Boston: Little, Brown and Co., 1971, pp. 1014-1028.

18. Chung, S. M. K. *et al.* The Colonna capsular arthroplasty. A long-term follow-up of fifty-six patients. *Journal of Bone and Joint Surgery*. 53A: 1511-1527, December, 1971.

19. Cozen, L. Does diabetes delay fracture healing? *Clinical Orthopaedics and Related Research*, 82: 134-140, January-February, 1972.

20. Crenshaw, A. H. Arthrodesis. In *Campbell's Operative Orthopaedics*, 5th ed. St. Louis: The C. V. Mosby Co., 1971, pp. 1125-1205.

21. DasGupta, T. K. and Brasfield, R. D. Tumors of muscles and synovial tissues. *Ca — A Cancer Journal for Clinicians*, 21: 379-385, November-December, 1971.

22. Dolan, J. and MacEwen, D. Surgical treatment of scoliosis. *Clinical Orthopaedics and Related Research*, 76: 125-137, May, 1971.

23. Drain, C. B. The athletic knee injury. *American Journal of Nursing*, 71: 536-537, March, 1971.

24. Drennan, D. B. *et al.* Important factors in achieving arthrodesis of the Charkot knee. *Journal of Bone and Joint Surgery*, 53A: 1180-1193, September, 1971.

25. Edmonson, A. S. Postural deformities. In Crenshaw, A. H. (ed.). *Campbell's Operative Orthopaedics*, 5th ed. St. Louis: The C. V. Mosby Co., 1971, pp. 1795-1891.

26. Ellison, M. R. *et al.* The results of surgical synovectomy of the digital joints in rheumatoid arthritis. *Journal of Bone and Joint Surgery*, 53A: 1041-1060, September, 1971.

27. Engleman, E. P. *et al.* Arthritis and allied rheumatic disorders. In Krupp, Marcus A. and Chatton, Milton J. *Current Diagnosis and Treatment*, 11th ed. LosAltos, California: Lange Medical Publications, 1972, pp. 435-455.

28. Eyre, M. K. Total hip replacement. *American Journal of Nursing*, 71: 1384-1387, July, 1971.

29. Farlin, D. E. Myasthenia gravis. In Samter, Max (ed.). *Immunological Diseases*, 2d ed. Boston: Little, Brown and Co., 1971, pp. 1150-1166.

30. Francis, K. C. The role of amputation in the treatment of metastatic bone cancer. *Clinical Orthopaedics and Related Research*, 73: 61-63, November-December, 1970.

31. Friedman, B. *et al.* Round-cell sarcoma of bone. *Journal of Bone and Joint Surgery*, 53A: 1118-1136, September, 1971.

32. Garden, R. S. Malreduction and avascular necrosis in subcapital fractures. *Journal of Bone and Joint Surgery*, 53B: 183-197, May, 1971.

33. Gardner, E. Skeleton. In Gardner, Ernest, Gray, Donald J. and O'Rahilly, Ronan. *Anatomy — A Regional Study of Human Structure*, 3rd ed. Philadelphia: W. B. Saunders Co., 1969, p. 14.

34. Gardner, R. C. Impending Volkmann's contracture following minor trauma to the palm of the hand. *Clinical Orthopaedics and Related Research*, 72: 261-264, September-October, 1970.

35. Goldstein, L. A. The surgical management of scoliosis. *Clinical Orthopaedics and Related Research*, 77: 32-56, June, 1971.

36. Gordon, S. L. *et al.* Recurrent osteomyelitis. *Journal of Bone and Joint Surgery*, 53A: 1150-1156, September, 1971.

37. Hardt, A. B. *et al.* Early metabolic responses of bone to immobilization. *Journal of Bone and Joint Surgery*, 54A: 119-124, January, 1972.

38. Harrington, P. R. and Tullos, H. S. Spondylolisthesis in children — observations and surgical treatment. *Clinical Orthopaedics and Related Research*, 79: 75-84, September, 1971.

39. Honner, R. Dupuytren's contracture. *Journal of Bone and Joint Surgery*, 53B: 240-246, May, 1971.

40. Howorth, B. Knock knees with special reference to the stapling operation. *Clinical Orthopaedics and Related Research*, 77: 233-246, June, 1971.

41. Hutchins, W. C. Miscellaneous affections of joints. In Crenshaw, A. H. (ed.). *Campbell's Operative Orthopaedics*, 5th ed. St. Louis: The C. V. Mosby Co., 1971, pp. 987-1087.

42. Ingram, A. J. Anterior poliomyelitis. In Crenshaw, A. H. (ed.). *Campbell's Operative Orthopaedics*, 5th ed. St. Louis: The C. V. Mosby Co., pp. 1517-1684.

43. Johnson, R. J. *et al.* Osteosarcoma. *Clinical Orthopaedics and Related Research*, 78: 314-321, July-August, 1971.

44. Katz, J. F. Legg-Calvé-Perthes disease: The role of distortion of normal growth mechanism in the production of deformity. *Clinical Orthopaedics and Related Research*, 71: 193-198, July-August, 1970.

45. Lam, S. F. Fractures of the neck of the femur in children. *Journal of Bone and Joint Surgery*, 53A: 1165-1179, September, 1971.

46. Lazansky, M. Complications in total hip replacement with the Charnley technic. *Clinical Orthopaedics and Related Research*, 72: 40-45, September-October, 1970.

47. Le Lievre, J. Current concepts and correction in the valgus foot. *Clinical Orthopaedics and Related Research*, 70: 43-55, May-June, 1970.

48. Liverani, L. and Osserman, R. S. Myasthenia gravis: a nursing care plan. *Nursing Clinics of North America*, 7: 185-195, March, 1972.

49. Maginn, R. and Kaiser, G. C. Profound hypothermia and delayed amputation. *Surgery, Gynecology and Obstetrics*, 126: 1081-1082, May, 1968.

50. Malt, R. A. and McKhann, C. F. Replantation of severed arms. *Journal of American Medical Association*, 189: 716-722, September, 7, 1964.

51. Miller, E. H. The management of deep soft tissue bleeding and hemarthrosis in hemophilia. *Clinical Orthopaedics and Related Research*, 82: 92-107, January-February, 1972.

52. Moore, A. T. and Bohlman, H. R. The classic: metal hip joint. *Clinical Orthopaedics and Related Research*, 72: 3-6, September-October, 1970.

53. Mueller, K. H. Osteotomies of the hip. *Clinical Orthopaedics and Related Research*, 77: 117-127, June, 1971.

54. Newton-John, H. F. The loss of bone with age — osteoporosis and fractures. *Clinical Orthopaedics and Related Research*, 71: 229-252, July-August, 1970.

55. O'Brien, Robert, M., M.D. Personal communications.

56. Paletta, F. K. Replantation of the amputated extremity. *Annals of Surgery*, 168: 720-727, October, 1968.

57. Pinals, R. S. Traumatic arthritis and allied conditions. In Hollander, Joseph L. and Mc Carty, Daniel J. *Arthritis and Allied Conditions*, 8th ed. Philadelphia: Lea & Febiger, 1972, pp. 1391-1410.

58. Potter, T. A. *et al.* Arthroplasty of the knee in rheumatoid arthritis and osteoarthritis — a follow-up study after implantation of the McKeever and Mac Intosh prostheses. *Journal of Bone and Joint Surgery*, 54A: 1-24, January, 1972.

59. Reckling, F. W. *et al.* Acute knee dislocations and their complications. *Lawyer's Medical Journal*, 6: 25-40, May, 1970.

60. Rockwell, M. A. *et al.* Periosteal chondroma. *Journal of Bone and Joint Surgery*, 54A: 102-108, January, 1972.

61. Rooth, H. P. Flexion deformity of the hip and knee in spastic cerebral palsy: Treatment by early release of spastic hip flexor muscles. *Journal of Bone and Joint Surgery*, 53A: 1489-1510, December, 1971.

62. Roper, B. A. Paget's disease involving the hip joint. *Clinical Orthopaedics and Related Research*, 80: 33-38, October, 1971.

63. Russe, O. A. Acute and chronic slipped femoral epiphysis. *Clinical Orthopaedics and Related Research*, 77: 144-148, June, 1971.

64. Sage, F. P. Congenital anomalies. In Crenshaw, A. H. (ed.). *Campbell's Operative Orthopaedics*, 5th ed. St. Louis: The C. V. Mosby Co., 1971, pp. 1892-2044.

65. Sante, L. R. *Manual of Roentgenological Technique*, 18th ed. Ann Arbor, Michigan: Edwards Brothers, Inc., 1956, p. 473.

66. Sarmiento, A. Austin Moore prosthesis in the arthritic hip. *Clinical Orthopaedics and Related Research*, 82: 14-23, January-February, 1972.

67. Shifrin, L. Z. Giant cell tumor of bone. *Clinical Orthopaedics and Related Research*, 82: 59-66, January-February, 1972.

68. Sigler, J. W. *et al.* Clinical features of ankylosing spondylitis. *Clinical Orthopaedics and Related Research*. 74: 14-19, January-February, 1971.

69. Simon, W. H. and Wyman, E. T. Femoral neck fractures. *Clinical Orthopaedics and Related Research*, 70: 152-160, May-June, 1970.

70. Smith, C. B. and Ward, J. R. Chronic infectious arthritis — role of Mycoplasmas. *Journal of Infectious Diseases*, 123: 313-315, March, 1971.

71. Soren, A. Surgical correction of hallux valgus. *Surgery*, 71: 44-50, January, 1972.

72. Steinbach, H. L. and Dodds, W. J. Clinical radiology of Paget's disease. *Clinical Orthopaedics and Related Research*, 57: 277-297, March-April, 1968.

73. Takigawa, K. Chondroma of the bones of the hand. A review of 110 cases. *Journal of Bone and Joint Surgery*, 53A: 1591-1600, December, 1971.

74. Taylor, T. K. Lumbar disc prolapse. *Lawyer's Medical Journal*, 3: 219-255, November, 1967.

75. Tooms, R. E. Amputations. In Crenshaw, A. H. *Campbell's Operative Orthopaedics*. St. Louis: The C. V. Mosby Co., 1971, pp. 885-889.

76. Torgerson, W. R. and Hammond, G. Prosthetic arthroplasty in the treatment of degenerative arthritis of the hip. *Clinical Orthopaedics and Related Research*, 72: 224-232, September-October, 1970.

77. Turek, Samuel L. *Orthopaedics — Principles and Their Application*, 2d ed. Philadelphia: J. B. Lippincott Co., 1967, pp. 11-16.

78. Turner, R. H. and Bianco, A. J. Spondylolysis

52

and spondylolisthesis in children and teenagers. *Journal of Bone and Joint Surgery*, 53A: 1298-1306, October, 1971.

79. Waring, T. L. Arthroplasty. In Crenshaw, A. H. (ed.). *Campbell's Operative Orthopaedics*, 5th ed. St. Louis: The C. V. Mosby Co., 1971, pp. 1235-1297.

80. White, W. L. Plastic surgery and burns. *Surgery, Gynecology & Obstetrics*, 134: 274-276, February, 1972.

81. Wilner, D. and Sherman, R. S. Bone sarcoma associated with Paget's disease. *Ca — A Cancer Journal for Clinicians*, 16: 238-244. November-December, 1966.

82. Wilson, P. D. and Levine, D. B. Internal derangement of the knee joint. In Hollander, Joseph L. and McCarthy, Daniel J. *Arthritis and Allied Conditions*, 8th ed. Philadelphia: Lea & Febiger, 1972, pp. 1411-1421.

83. Yahr, M. D. Essential tremor — senile tremor. In Beeson, Paul B. and McDermott, Walsh (eds.). *Cecil-Loeb Textbook of Medicine*. Philadelphia: W. B. Saunders Co., 1971, pp. 182-183.

Chapter IV

Neurological and Psychiatric Disorders
NERVES

A. Origin of Terms:

1. axon (G) — axis
2. dendron (G) — tree
3. ganglion (G) — knot
4. lemma (G) — sheath
5. nucleus (L) — little kernel
6. plexus (L) — braid
7. radicle (L) — root
8. synapse (G) — clasp

B. Anatomical Terms:

1. nerve — a collection of many nerve fibers.
   a. cranial nerves — 12 pairs of nerves made up of either motor or sensory fibers or both.
   b. spinal nerves — 31 pairs of mixed nerves.
2. nerve cell, neuron — basic component of nerve tissue consisting of a cell body or neuron body and one or more processes. The neuron is the anatomical unit of the central nervous system.
   a. structure of neurons[100]
      (1) axon, axone — slender process of a neuron body arising from specialized protoplasm known as axon hill. It contains many neurofibrils but **no** Nissl bodies.
      (2) cell body — neuron body composed of a nucleus embedded in cytoplasm which contains neurofibrils, Nissl bodies, mitochondria and others. The cell body maintains the nutrition of the whole neuron.
      (3) dendrite, dendron — a protoplasmic extension from the cell body forming an irregular knobby process, which is wide at the base and narrows down rapidly. Dendrites greatly increase the cell body's receptive surface.
      (4) effector — organ of response which reacts to the impulse, for example, a muscle or a gland.
      (5) ganglion (pl. ganglia) — a collection of neural cell bodies lying outside the central nervous system.
      (6) myelin sheath — protective covering of axons, composed of lipids and protein and interrupted by constrictions, the nodes of Ranvier.
      (7) neurilemma, neurolemma, sheath of Schwann — a thin, cellular membrane covering the axis cylinder of a non-medullated nerve fiber or enclosing the myelin sheath of a medullated nerve fiber of **peripheral nerves.**
      (8) neurofibrils — delicate threads found in the cell bodies and processes of neurons.
      (9) Nissl bodies — RNA (ribose nucleic acid) granules present in the cell bodies of neurons.
      (10) receptor — end organ which responds to various stimuli (pain, touch, and others) and converts them into nervous impulses.[100]
   b. classification according to function
      (1) afferent neurons — conduct impulses from receptor to central nervous system.
      (2) association, intercalated or internuncial neurons — located within the central nervous system; transmit impulses between neurons.
      (3) efferent neurons — conduct impulses away from the central nervous system to the effector organ.[100]
3. nerve fiber — the axon with its sheaths.
4. plexus (pl. plexuses) of spinal nerves — a network of nerve fibers. For example:
   a. brachial plexus — an intermingling of the 5th through 8th cervical and the 1st thoracic nerves which supply the upper limb.
   b. sacral plexus — an intermingling of the 4th and 5th lumbar and first four sacral nerves which help to supply the lower limb.

54

5. roots of spinal nerves — they attach the nerves to the spinal cord.
    a. ventral (anterior) root — composed of efferent fibers and has no ganglion.
    b. dorsal (posterior) root — composed of afferent fibers and has a small ganglion.
6. synapse — the point of contact between the axon of one neuron and a dendrite or cell body of another neuron.

C. Diagnostic Terms:

1. Bell's palsy — a functional disorder of the seventh cranial nerve which may result in a unilateral paralysis of facial muscles, and distortion of taste perception. Etiology is unknown.
2. causalgia — posttraumatic paroxysms of unbearable peripheral nerve pain of a burning quality aggravated by heat, slight friction, anxiety and emotion. It appears to be stimulated by efferent sympathetic nerve impulses.[86, 47]
3. Guillain-Barré syndrome, acute idiopathic polyneuropathy — widespread disorder of the peripheral motor nerves, characterized by progressive flaccid paralysis of an ascending type associated with sensory disturbances. When the chest muscles and diaphragm become affected, respiratory difficulties arise. Cranial nerve involvement, particularly that of the facial nerve, may develop last in the course of the disease, or it may be the initial pathology followed by motor impairment of a descending type.[59]
4. herniated nucleus pulposus, herniated intervertebral disc — tear in posterior joint capsule and bulging of portions of intervertebral disc resulting in nerve root irritation and compression followed by sciatic pain and paresthesias and occasionally by paresis or paralysis.[91]
5. neurilemoma, neurilemmoma* — usually a benign, encapsulated, solitary tumor, produced by the proliferation of Schwann cells. It may originate from a sympathetic, peripheral or cranial nerve.[57]
6. neuroma — a tumor of tissue found in nervous system; obsolete term, a more specific designation is preferable, e.g.:
    a. ganglioneuroma — true neuroma.
    b. pseudoneuroma, amputation neuroma — false neuroma or traumatic neuroma.
7. polyneuritis, polyneuropathy — widespread neural lesions due to nutritional deficiencies especially of vitamin B complex. The chief symptoms are pain and paresthesia.
8. radiculitis — and involvement of the spinal nerve roots due to either infection, toxins, trauma, protrusion of intervertebral disk or degenerative diseases.
9. sciatic neuritis, sciatica — a very painful involvement of the sciatic nerve.
10. trigeminal neuralgia, trifacial neuralgia, tic douloureux — paroxysms of lancinating pain of one or more areas innervated by the fifth cranial nerve.
11. trigeminal neurinoma — rare, benign tumor of the trigeminal nerve characterized by mild pain or paresthesia, diminished corneal reflex and weakness of muscles of mastication.[68]

D. Operative Terms:

1. ganglionectomy — excision of a ganglion
2. neuroanastomosis — surgical communication between nerve fibers.
3. neurectomy — excision of a nerve or lesion of a nerve, for example, a solitary neuroma.
4. neurolysis — freeing a nerve from adhesions. In peripheral nerve surgery, dissection is best achieved by use of the Zeiss microscope with 6 to 10 times magnification.[38]
5. neuroplasty — plastic repair of a nerve.
6. neurorrhaphy — suture of an injured nerve.
7. neurotomy — transection of a nerve.
8. supraorbital and supratrochlear neurectomy — surgical procedure for tic douloureux when the first division of the trigeminal nerve causes pain in the area above the eye socket (orbit).[39]

---

* Also — neurolemoma, neurolemmoma.

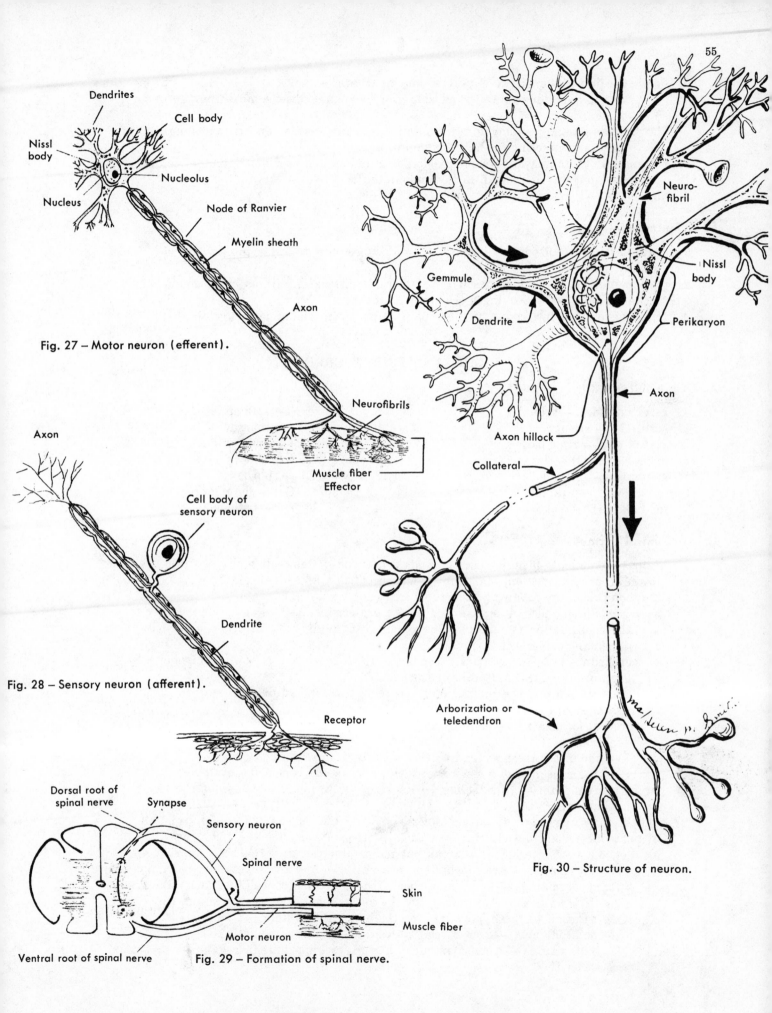

Dendrites

Cell body

Nissl body

Nucleolus

Nucleus

Node of Ranvier

Myelin sheath

Axon

Fig. 27 – Motor neuron (efferent).

Neurofibrils

Muscle fiber Effector

Axon

Cell body of sensory neuron

Dendrite

Fig. 28 – Sensory neuron (afferent).

Receptor

Neuro-fibril

Gemmule

Nissl body

Dendrite

Perikaryon

Axon

Axon hillock

Collateral

Arborization or teledendron

Fig. 30 – Structure of neuron.

Dorsal root of spinal nerve

Synapse

Sensory neuron

Spinal nerve

Skin

Muscle fiber

Motor neuron

Ventral root of spinal nerve

Fig. 29 – Formation of spinal nerve.

9. sympathectomy — excision of part of a sympathetic nerve.
   a. thoracic ganglionectomy for causalgia or Raynaud's disease affecting the upper extremities.
   b. lumbar ganglionectomy for causalgia, Raynaud's disease and thromboangiitis obliterans affecting the lower extremities.
10. trigeminal decompression — compression of ganglion and root of trigeminal complex with dry cottonoid to relieve pain in tic douloureux.[40]
11. vagotomy — transection of a vagus nerve.

E. Symptomatic Terms:

1. aural vertigo — episodic attacks of severe dizziness due to lesion in ear (labyrinthine lesion).
2. paroxysmal pain — sudden, recurrent or periodic attack of pain as in tic douloureux.
3. tactile stimulation — evoking a response by touch.
4. trigger area — point from which the pain starts as in trigeminal neuralgia.

BRAIN AND SPINAL CORD

A. Origin of Terms:

1. cerebrum (L) — brain
2. cord (G) — string
3. cortex (L) — rind, bark
4. encephalon (G) — brain
5. gyrus (L) — convolution
6. lamina (L) — thin plate
7. medulla (L) — marrow
8. meninges (G) — membranes
9. myelo- (G) — marrow
10. occiput (L) — back of head
11. pons (L) — bridge
12. spina (L) — thorn
13. thalamo- (G) — chamber
14. ventricle (L) — little belly or cavity

B. Anatomical Terms:

1. brain, encephalon[16] — major part of central nervous system. It is divided into the forebrain or prosencephalon, midbrain or mesencephalon and hindbrain or rhombencephalon and comprises the following structural and functional components.
   a. cerebellum — second largest part of the brain which serves as a reflex center for the coordination of muscular movements. It is divisible into two hemispheres and a median portion, the vermis.
   b. cerebrum — the largest part of the brain which is divided into two hemispheres by a deep groove, the longitudinal fissure.
   c. cerebral cortex — the surface of the cerebrum composed of gray matter and arranged in folds known as convolutions or gyri.
   d. cerebral localization — definite regions of the cerebral cortex performing special functions:
      (1) the motor areas which influence voluntary muscular activity.
      (2) the sensory areas where sensations reach the conscious level.
   e. corpus callosum — a bridgelike structure of white fibers which joins the two hemispheres.[16]
2. brain stem — upward continuation of cervical cord which consists of numerous bundles of nerve fibers and nuclei. Its structural components include the following:
   a. diencephalon, interbrain[4] — small but important part of forebrain comprising
      (1) epithalamus — area including several nuclei and the pineal body or epiphysis.
      (2) hypothalamus — small mass below the thalamus containing nuclei and fibers. It is an integrating center for the autonomic nervous system and through its relation to the hypophysis for the endocrine system.
      (3) metathalamus — area of the lateral and medial geniculate bodies.
      (4) subthalamus — a mass of nuclei and fibers important in regulating muscular activities.

(5) thalamus — a mass of nuclei situated on either side of the third ventricle. It is the great sensory relay station.[16]

 b. medulla oblongata, myelencephalon, marrow brain — extends from upper cervical cord to pons; contains vital centers regulating heart action, vasomotor activity, respiration, deglutition and vomiting.

 c. mesencephalon, midbrain — extends from pons below to forebrain above and is composed of nuclei and bundles of fibers.

 d. pons — part of metencephalon (afterbrain) composed of bundles of fibers and nuclei which are located between the medulla and midbrain.

3. meninges — covering membranes of the brain and the spinal cord.

 a. dura mater — serves as outer protective coat and is composed of strong fibrous tissue.

 b. arachnoid — is the middle layer and consists of thin meshwork. The subarachnoid space contains cerebrospinal fluid.[16]

 c. pia mater — dips down between the convolutions and adheres closely to the brain.

4. nucleus (pl. nuclei) — a group of nerve cells within the central nervous system.

 a. basal nuclei, formerly basal ganglia — masses of nerve cells deeply embedded in the white matter of the forebrain, for example, the lentiform nucleus.

5. ventricles and aqueduct

 a. lateral ventricles — fluid-filled spaces, one in each cerebral hemisphere.

 b. third ventricle — a fluid-filled space beneath the corpus callosum.

 c. cerebral aqueduct — a narrow canal which connects the third and fourth ventricles.

 d. fourth ventricle — an expansion of the central canal of the medulla oblongata.

 The ventricles contain cerebrospinal fluid which is formed by the capillaries of the choroid plexuses. The fluid seeps from the third ventricle into the cerebral aqueduct and fourth ventricle and from there into the central canal. It reaches the subarachnoid space through openings in the roof of the fourth ventricle and circulates around the cord and brain in this space, thus providing a water-cushion and shock absorber for the delicate nerve tissue.[24]

6. spinal cord — portion of central nervous system located in the vertebral canal and giving rise to 31 pairs of spinal nerves. It extends from the foramen magnum to the second lumbar vertebra and is composed of white substance which surrounds the inner gray matter of the cord. Several lengthwise grooves demarcate the white matter into long columns. The deepest groove is the anterior median fissure which, together with the posterior median septum, almost separates the cord into two equal halves.

The **white matter** consists of myelinated fibers arranged in longitudinal bundles and grouped into 3 columns, the anterior, lateral and posterior funiculi. Afferent white fibers form the ascending nerve tracts which carry impulses from the cord to the brain. Efferent white fibers represent descending nerve tracts which bring messages from the brain to the cord.

The **gray matter** is H-shaped in cross-section and consists mainly of cell bodies. The anterior horn contains motor cells from which the motor fibers of the peripheral neurons arise. Sensory relay neurons are located in the posterior horn.[16]

C. Diagnostic Terms:

1. amyotrophic lateral sclerosis — degenerative disease of the lateral motor tracts of the spinal cord causing widespread muscle wasting, weakness, fasciculations and usually a mild degree of spastic paralysis of lower extremities.

2. anencephalia, anencephalus — absence of brain.

3. brain abscess — localized lesion of suppuration within the brain, generally secondary to ear infection, sinusitis or other infections.

4. brain tumor, intracranial tumor — benign or malignant space-occupying brain lesion.[29, 80]

 a. adnexal tumor — derived from pineal body or choroid plexus. It may compress the aqueduct and cause obstructive hydrocephalus or exert pressure on the hypothalamus and be associated with diabetes insipidus or precocious puberty.

58

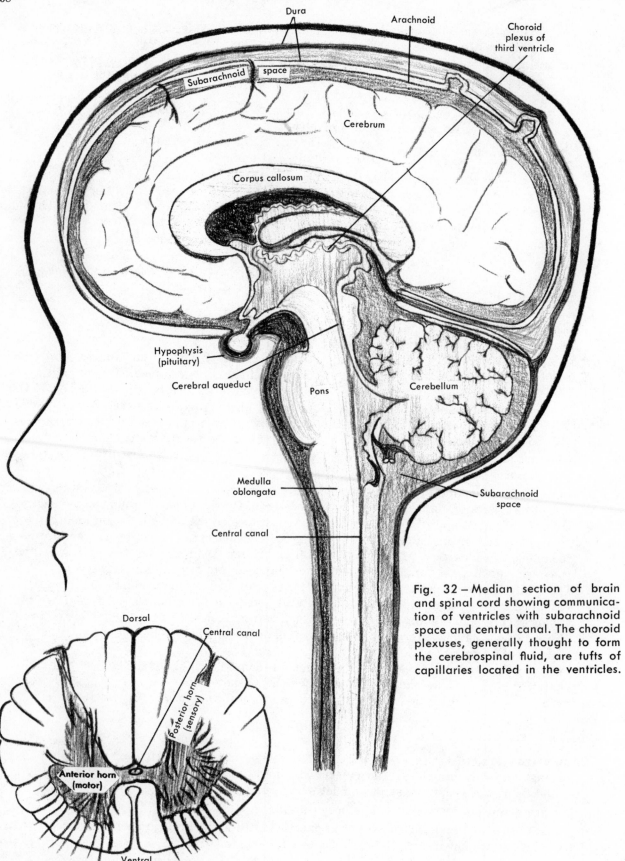

Dura

Arachnoid

Choroid
plexus of
third ventricle

Subarachnoid space

Cerebrum

Corpus callosum

Hypophysis
(pituitary)

Cerebral aqueduct

Pons

Cerebellum

Medulla
oblongata

Subarachnoid
space

Central canal

Fig. 32 – Median section of brain
and spinal cord showing communication of ventricles with subarachnoid
space and central canal. The choroid
plexuses, generally thought to form
the cerebrospinal fluid, are tufts of
capillaries located in the ventricles.

Dorsal

Central canal

Posterior horn
(sensory)

Anterior horn
(motor)

Ventral

Fig. 31 – Transverse section of spinal
cord at level of origin of third lumbar
nerve.

b. congenital tumor — a slowly growing, highly invasive tumor; e.g., a dermoid or teratoma.

c. medulloblastoma — a highly malignant cerebellar tumor which metastasizes freely to the subarachnoid space, cerebrum and cord.

d. meningeal tumor — neoplasm arising from the covering membranes of the brain or cord. The meningioma may cause compression and distortion of the brain.[80, 96]

e. metastatic tumor — most primary tumors may metastasize to the brain, especially breast and lung tumors.

f. pituitary tumor — arises from anterior pituitary (adenohypophysis) and may compress the normal portion of the pituitary, the hypothalamus and optic chiasm.

g. primary brain tumors — comprise a large number of intracranial tumors, especially, the gliomas which contain malignant glial cells. Some neoplasms of the glioma group are presented:[50, 61]

    (1) astrocytoma — a slowly growing tumor containing astrocytes that infiltrate widely into neighboring brain tissue and may undergo cystic degeneration.

    (2) ependymoma — tumor arises from the lining of the ventricular wall, is highly malignant and invasive.

    (3) glioblastoma multiforme — the most malignant glioma, rapidly growing, causing edema and necrosis of brain tissue.

    (4) oligodendroglioma — similar to astrocytoma in behavior, different in histologic structure.[29, 80]

5. cerebral concussion — transient state of unconsciousness following head injury immediately as a result of damage to the brain stem.[41, 87, 50]

6. cerebral palsy — condition characterized by paralysis, incoordination and other aberrations of motor or sensory functions due to pathology of the brain.[60]

7. cerebrovascular disease — any disorder in which one or more of the cerebral blood vessels have undergone pathological changes.[63]

a. cerebral aneurysm, intracranial aneurysm — dilation of an artery of the brain resulting in a thinning and weakening of the arterial wall. Common locations are the internal carotid and middle cerebral arteries. Rupture and hemorrhage may occur and cause serious brain damage.[17]

b. cerebral arteriovenous malformation — structural vascular defect, generally found in young patients with recurrent subarachnoid hemorrhage and epilepsy.

c. cerebral atherosclerosis — a primary degeneration of the intima by atheromatous plaques (lipid deposits) usually located in the basilar artery, the middle and posterior cerebral arteries, and at the branching of the internal carotids. The subsequent narrowing of the vessels may lead to inadequate oxygenation and nutrition of the brain by the reduced cerebral circulation. Brain softening, neural atrophy, and senile plaques add further damage and predispose to physical and mental deterioration.[8]

d. cerebral embolism — sudden occlusion of a cerebral blood vessel by a circulatory embolus composed of air bubble, blood clot, fat cells or bacteria.

e. cerebral infarction — local necrosis of brain tissue due to loss of blood supply in the part by an obstructed endartery.

f. cerebral ischemia — anemia of the brain resulting from diminished cerebral blood flow. Some important causes are circulatory obstruction of the intra- or extracranial arteries by atheroma, thrombus or embolus, severe hypotension, arteritis or stenosis of an artery. Recurrent ischemic episodes are thought to signal impending stroke.[17]

g. cerebral thrombosis — formation of a thrombus within an intracranial artery leading to its occlusion and subsequent necrosis of the area supplied by the thrombosed vessel.

h. cerebrovascular accident, stroke, apoplexy — neurologic disorder caused by pathological changes in the blood vessels of the brain, primarily by arteriosclerosis, thrombosis, embolism, hemorrhage or by arterial hypertension. A softening of brain tissue may occur in the affected lesion. The neurologic deficit is characterized by coma, paralysis of one side of the body, aphasia and convulsions.[17, 8, 51, 23]

i. internal carotid artery occlusion — condition usually due to an atheromatous plaque obstructing the vessel near the bifurcation of the common carotid. It may cause hemiplegia, unilateral blindness and aphasia.[62]

j. intracranial hematoma — local mass of extravased blood which formed subsequent to intracranial hemorrhage. Chronic lesions may become encapsulated. Epidural and subdural hematomas, located above or below the dura mater, are usually due to head injury.[101]

k. intracranial hemorrhage — rupture of a vessel beneath the skull with seepage of blood into the brain coverings or substance. It may be caused by head injury, stroke or ruptured aneurysm. Brain damage depends on the location and extent of the lesion involved.[101]

l. subarachnoid hemorrhage — bleeding into the subarachnoid space which in some cases is associated with excruciating headache, convulsions and coma. It is due to head injury or ruptured intracranial aneurysm.

8. chorea — nervous disorder characterized by bizarre, abrupt, involuntary movements.
   a. Huntington's chorea, adult chorea — hereditary form with onset in adult life, involvement of basal ganglia and cortex, choreaform movements and mental decline.[14]
   b. Sydenham's chorea, juvenile chorea — disorder of childhood and adolescence with insidious onset of jerky movements usually occurring during rheumatic fever.[9]

9. encephalitis lethargica — inflammation of the brain marked by somnolence and ocular paralysis. It is caused by a filtrable virus.[56, 93]

10. encephalocele — protrusion of some brain substance through a fissure of the skull.

11. epilepsy — convulsive disorder consisting of recurrent seizures and impaired consciousness.[35, 36]

12. Friedreich's ataxia — familial disease, seen in the young. Involvement of cerebellum, pyramidal tracts and peripheral nerves result in sensory impairment, unsteady gait, contractures and deformities such as lordosis and high arching feet with toes cocking up. Optic atrophy and myocardial disease may occur.[1]

13. head injury, craniocerebral trauma — injury to the head, usually associated with a fractured skull and affecting directly or indirectly and at varying degree one or more cerebral centers. The severity and extent of brain damage is usually, but not exclusively indicated by
    a. state of consciousness
    b. intracranial pressure
    c. respiratory exchange
    d. circulatory ability to supply the brain with oxygen and nutrients
    e. prevention or control of cerebral hemorrhage, edema and infection.[84, 69, 95, 74, 94, 104]

14. hydrocephalus — a pathologic condition characterized by a dilatation of the ventricles of the brain and an abnormal accumulation of intraventricular cerebrospinal fluid. It may be
    a. obstructive or noncommunicating due to an interference with the circulation of the cerebrospinal fluid through the ventricular system
    b. nonobstructive or communicating due to an interference in absorption of cerebrospinal fluid.
    Some other distinctions comprise:
    a. adult hydrocephalus, hydrocephalus *ex vacuo* — a rare type in which the increased volume of cerebrospinal fluid develops as a compensatory response to brain atrophy in degenerative cerebral disease.[92, 13]
    b. infantile hydrocephalus — relatively common form which occurs before closure of fontanelles and is characterized by increasing cranial enlargement and prominent forehead. Occasionally the process is arrested.[102, 20]

c. posttraumatic hydrocephalus — type due to head injury which may result in ventricular hemorrhage or subarachnoid bleeding and blockage of the aqueduct and fourth ventricle by blood clot.[4]

15. hypertensive encephalopathy — cerebral vasoconstriction and edema. The cerebral arteries are greatly constricted. The swollen, pale and anemic brain is compressed against the skull and ventricles causing increased intracranial pressure.

16. meningitis — inflammation of the meninges resulting from infectious agents such as bacteria, fungi, viruses or other causes.[103]

17. meningocele — protrusion of the meninges through a cranial fissure.

18. microcephalus — abnormally small head sometimes associated with idiocy.

19. multiple sclerosis, disseminated sclerosis — slowly progressive disease, striking the 20-40 age group. Areas of demyelination and scar tissue plaques are scattered throughout the nervous system disrupting nerve transmission. Numbness, fatigability, clumsiness, difficulty in walking and blurring vision may be followed by severe incoordination, spasticity, paralysis, incontinence, scanning speech, intention tremor, nystagmus and blindness.[82, 70]

20. myelitis — inflammation of the spinal cord.

21. neurofibromatosis, von Recklinghausen's disease — hereditary disorder of the nervous system in which multiple neurofibromas and café-au-lait spots are found on the skin. The tumors are usually asymptomatic and rarely cause compression of the spinal cord or sensory nerve damage.[48, 57]

22. paralysis agitans, Parkinson's disease — slowly progressive neurological disorder of middle life, primarily affecting the nuclei of the brain stem. Rigidity, slow movements, tremors, masklike facies and a monotonous voice are clinical findings. Characteristically festination is present. The patient's body is stooped forward; his steps are short, shuffling along with increasing pace, once locomotion has started. His gait is propulsive or retropulsive.[9, 76, 106]

23. poliomyelitis — viral disease with lesions in the central nervous system and varying symptomology.
    forms:
    a. asymptomatic, nonparalytic poliomyelitis — abortive type devoid of symptoms referable to the central nervous system.
    b. paralytic poliomyelitis.
       (1) bulbar poliomyelitis — involvement of cranial nerve nuclei; particularly the respiratory center in the medulla. It is the most serious type of poliomyelitis causing respiratory paralysis.
       (2) spinal paralytic poliomyelitis — usually an involvement of anterior horn cells of the spinal cord resulting in characteristic stiffness of the neck and spine, tightness of the hamstring muscles followed by paralysis of lower extremities. It presents the classical form of poliomyelitis.

24. spina bifida — congenital defect consisting in the absence of a vertebral arch of the spinal column. It may cause a
    a. meningocele — protrusion of the meninges through the defect in the spinal column.
    b. meningomyelocele — herniation of the cord and meninges through the defect of the vertebral column.
    c. syringomyelocele — protrusion of cord and meninges through defect in spine. Cord tissue is a thin-walled sac filled with fluid from the central canal.

25. spinal cord injury — trauma to cord produced by fracture or dislocation of spine may cause irreversible damage and disability.
    a. compression of cervical cord — complete transverse compression of cervical cord may cause lifelong quadriplegia (paralysis of arms and legs) and loss of sphincter control or be fatal due to phrenic nerve injury and subsequent respiratory paralysis.
    b. compression of thoracic or lumbar cord — pressure on this area may cause paraplegia (paralysis below the waist) and sphincter disturbances.[85]
    Compression of spinal cord may also be due to cord tumor and herniated intervertebral disc affecting the spinal nerve root of the lesion.

26. subacute sclerosing panencephalitis (SSPE), Dawson's encephalitis — uncommon form of inflammation of the brain occurring between 4 to 20 years of age. Three stages are recognized:
    a. behavioral disorders at the onset
    b. mental deterioration, myoclonic jerkings and convulsive seizures as the disease progresses
    c. stupor, dementia, rigidity, blindness and coma in the terminal phase.[49, 33, 11]
27. tabes dorsalis, locomotor ataxia — syphilis of the central nervous system clinically recognized by peculiar gait.

D. Operative Terms:

1. carotid artery ligation — tying a carotid artery in its cervical portion (neck) or using a Silverstone or Crutchfield clamp to gradually occlude the blood flow in the extracranial portions of the common or internal carotid artery.[88, 42]
2. carotid endarterectomy — removal of plaques or the intimal lining of a carotid artery in occlusive cerebrovascular disease. This removal may be carried out at the carotid bifurcation and followed by a reconstruction of an internal carotid artery with a Teflor graft.[88, 42]
3. carotid reconstruction operation — repair of carotid artery with a graft or bypass.[88, 42]
4. cingulumotomy — cingulum destruction by stereotaxic surgery with positioning of electrodes in target area. Operation is done under radiographic guidance for relief of psychogenic pain, manic depressive reactions and other disorders.[77]
5. cordectomy — removal of portion of the spinal cord to convert a spastic paraplegia to a flaccid paraplegia. This enhances rehabilitation.
6. cordotomy, chordotomy — section of a nerve fiber tract (usually the spinothalamic tract) within the cord for relief of pain.
    a. percutaneous cordotomy — surgical interruption of the pain fibers in the high cervical cord by means of percutaneous electrical needle. This is done under biplane radiographic control.[88]
    b. selective cordotomy — palliative surgery for obtaining sensory loss in local pain region, as in arm, leg or trunk.
7. craniectomy — removal of part of skull bone; a method of approach to the brain.
8. craniotomy — opening of skull. Burr or trephine openings into the skull are made in order to prepare a bone flap. This osteoplastic flap is separated from the skull during brain surgery and replaced when the skull is closed. Osteoplastic craniotomy is a common method of approach to the brain.[88]
9. cryoneurosurgery — the operative use of cold in the destruction of neurosurgical lesions.
10. decompression of
    a. brain — removal of a piece of skull bone, usually in the subtemporal region with opening of the dura mater to relieve intracranial pressure.
    b. spinal cord — removal of bone fragments, hematoma or lesion to relieve pressure on cord.[88]
11. drainage of meninges for abscess or hematoma — evacuation of subarachnoid or subdural space.
12. excision of brain lesion — complete removal if lesion does not encroach on vital centers.
13. laminectomy — excision of one or more laminae of vertebrae; method of approach to spinal cord.
14. microneurosurgery — use of the surgical binocular microscope which provides a powerful light source, up to 25 times magnification and a clear stereoscopic view of the brain. Microsurgical techniques and dissection are employed for
    a. acoustic tumors
    b. cerebral aneurysms
    c. pituitary tumors
    d. spinal cord tumors and other neurosurgical procedures.[75]

15. operations for parkinsonism — surgical procedures directed toward the destruction of areas of basal nuclei presumably affected by the disease.

    a. pallidotomy, formerly pallidectomy — surgical interruption of nerve pathways coming from globus pallidus to relieve intractable tremor and rigidity. Division of nerve fibers is usually achieved by use of electrocautery or chemical solution. Cryogenic agents, ultrasonic waves and stereotaxic techniques may be employed.

    b. thalamotomy formerly thalamectomy — partial destruction of thalamus for relief of tremors and rigidity. The stereotaxic instrument is applied to the skull. By means of radiographic visualization the target area is located and lesions are created by electrolytic, chemical, ultrasonic or cryogenic methods.[88]

16. stereotaxic neurosurgery — operative procedure that uses three dimensional measurement for precisely locating the neurosurgical target area in

    a. acromegaly

    b. cerebral aneurysm

    c. diabetic retinopathy

    d. manic depressive reactions[77]

    e. Parkinson's disease

    f. psychogenic pain[77]

    g. temporal lobe epilepsy.[43]

17. stereotaxy — the use of stereotaxic instrument fixed onto the skull with screws like a scaffold. From this a probe, containing either a chemical, electrical or cryogenic agent, is introduced through a burr opening into the target area of the brain.[88]

18. surgical shunts for hydrocephalus — detour channels, surgically created to relieve an accumulation of cerebrospinal fluid in the brain.

    a. ventriculoatrial or ventriculocaval shunt — insertion of Holter or Pudenz valve to channel the cerebrospinal fluid from the lateral ventricle to either an atrium or the superior vena cava via the jugular vein. This operation is performed for communicating hydrocephalus.[28, 44]

    b. ventriculocisternostomy, Torkildsen operation — surgical procedure for obstructive hydrocephalus. A catheter is used to shunt the fluid from a ventricle to the cisterna magna.[88, 43]

19. tractotomy — section of a nerve fiber tract within the brain stem for relief of intractable pain.

20. trephination — cutting a circular opening or boring a hole into skull; a method of approach to the brain.

21. ultrasonotomy — a neurosurgical procedure in the treatment of certain severe psychiatric disorders in which discrete brain lesions are produced (usually in the prefrontal lobes) by the use of ultrasound (high frequency sound waves).[3]

E. Symptomatic Terms:

1. analgesia — loss of normal sense of pain.

2. anesthesia — loss of sensation; may be associated with unconsciousness.

3. aphasia — difficulty with the use or understanding of words due to lesions in association areas.

    a. motor aphasia — verbal comprehension intact, but patient unable to use the muscles which coordinate speech.

    b. sensory aphasia — inability to comprehend the spoken word if auditory word center is affected and the written word if the visual word center is involved. The patient will not understand the spoken or written word if there is an involvement of both centers.

4. ataxia — motor incoordination.

5. aura — patient's awareness of pending epileptic seizure.

6. cerebrospinal otorrhea — escape of cerebrospinal fluid from the ear following craniocerebral trauma. It is due to a fistulous communication between the ventricular system or subarachnoid space and the ear.[84]

7. cerebrospinal rhinorrhea — escape of cerebrospinal fluid from the nose following craniocerebral trauma. It is due to a fistulous passage leading from the ventricular system or subarachnoid space to the nose.[84]
8. coma — state of unconsciousness or deep stupor.
9. convulsion — paroxysms of involuntary muscular contractions and relaxations.
10. diplegia — paralysis on both sides of body.
11. dysarthria — incoordination of speech muscles affecting articulation.
12. dyskinesia — abnormal involuntary movement and body posture due to brain lesion.
    a. athetosis — slow, wormlike, writhing movement especially in hands and fingers.
    b. ballism — violent, flinging, shaking or jerking movements of extremities.
    c. chorea — quick, explosive, purposeless movements.
    d. dystonia — abnormal posture from twisting movements usually of limbs and trunk.
13. euphoria — a sense of well-being associated with mild elation.
14. fasciculation — involuntary twitchings of groups of muscle fibers.
15. festination — quick, shuffling steps; accelerated gait seen in Parkinson disease.
16. hemiparesis — slight degree of paralysis of one side of body.
17. hemiplegia — paralysis affecting one side of body.
18. hyperesthesia — increased sensibility to sensory stimuli.
19. intention tremor — trembling when attempting voluntary movement.
20. nystagmus — constant movements of the eyeballs as seen in the brain damage and disorders of vestibular apparatus.
21. paraparesis — slight paralysis of lower limbs.
22. paraplegia — paralysis of lower limbs and at varying degrees of lower trunk.
23. paresis — partial paralysis.
24. paresthesia — abnormal sensation, heightened sensory response to stimuli.
25. scanning speech — hesitant, slow speech, pronouncing words in syllables.
26. syncope — fainting.
27. tic — involuntary, purposeless contractions of muscle groups as twitching of facial muscles, eye blinking or shrugging of shoulder.

PSYCHIATRIC DISORDERS

A. Origin of Terms:

1. analysis (G) — dissolving
2. catatonia (G) — stupor
3. dement (L) — unsound mind
4. dynamo (G) — power
5. hallucinate (L) — to wander in mind
6. mania (G) — madness
7. ment (L) — mind
8. phren (G) — mind
9. psyche (G) — soul, mind
10. psychedelic (G) — mind-manifesting
11. schizo (G) — split
12. soma (G) — body

B. General Terms:

1. commitment — legal consignment of a mentally unsound or defective individual to an institution.
2. descriptive psychiatry — system of psychiatry which implies the study of clinical patterns, symptoms and classification.
3. dynamic psychiatry — the study of emotional processes, their origins, and the mental mechanisms. Implies the study of the active, energy-laden, and changing factors in human behavior and its motivation, as opposed to the older, more static and descriptive study of clinical patterns, symptoms, and classification. Dynamic principles convey the concepts of change, of evolution, and progression or regression.[3]
4. ego — in psychoanalytic theory, one of the three major divisions in the model of the psychic apparatus, the others being the id and superego. The ego represents the sum of certain mental mechanisms, such as perception and memory, and specific defensive mechanisms. The ego serves to mediate between the demands of primitive instinctual

drives (the id), of internalized parental and social prohibitions (the superego), and of reality. The compromises between these forces achieved by the ego tend to resolve intrapsychic conflict and serve an adaptive and executive function. As used in psychiatry, the term should not be confused with its common usage in the sense of "self-love" or "selfishness."[3]

5. mental health — a state of being which is relative rather than absolute, in which a person has effected a reasonably satisfactory integration of his instinctual drives. His integration is acceptable to himself and to his social milieu as reflected in his interpersonal relationships, his level of satisfaction in living, his actual achievement, his flexibility, and the level of maturity he has attained.[3]

6. orthopsychiatry — an approach to the study and treatment of human behavior that involves the collaborative effort of psychiatry, psychology, psychiatric social work, and other behavioral, medical and social sciences in the study and treatment of human behavior in the clinical setting. Emphasis is placed on preventive techniques to promote healthy emotional growth and development, particularly of children.[3]

7. psychiatry — the medical science which deals with the origin, diagnosis, prevention, and treatment of mental and emotional disorders. It also includes such special fields as mental retardation, and the emotional components of physical disorders, mental hospital administration, and the legal aspects of psychiatric disorders.[3]

8. psychodynamics — a predictive science which recognizes unconscious drives in human behavior.

9. psychometry — psychological testing; for example, Binet-Simon's intelligence test.

C. Diagnostic Terms:

1. mental retardation, mental deficiency — abnormally low intellectual functioning from birth or childhood associated with impairment of maturation, social adjustment and learning ability. There are five degrees of retardation:
   a. borderline mental retardation ....IQ 68-83
   b. mild mental retardation ....IQ 52-67
   c. moderate mental retardation ....IQ 36-51
   d. severe mental retardation .... IQ 20-35
   e. profound mental retardation ....IQ under 20
   Clinical subcategories of mental retardation include those related to
   a. maternal infection, intoxication and trauma.
   b. disorders of metabolism, growth and nutrition
   c. chromosomal abnormality
   d. psychosocial environmental deprivation and others.[18]

2. neurosis, pl. neuroses — disorder in which the dominant trait is anxiety. It may be expressed directly or controlled unconsciously by psychological mechanisms. There is no distortion of reality or personality disorganization. Some neuroses are presented:
   a. anxiety neurosis — overconcern bordering on panic usually associated with somatic manifestations.
   b. hysterical neurosis — involuntary functional disorder or psychogenic loss, initiated by emotionally charged situation relevant of underlying conflict.
   c. hysterical neurosis, conversion type — disorder of special senses or voluntary nervous system characterized by loss of sight, hearing, smell, feeling of pain, and associated with ataxia (muscular incoordination) and paralysis. The patient seems indifferent about his symptoms which bring relief from unpleasant obligations.
   d. neurasthenic neurosis, neurasthenia — chronic fatigability, weakness and exhaustion causing genuine distress. No secondary gain is sought by patient.[18]
   e. traumatic neurosis — any functional nervous condition which follows an accidental injury.[6]

---

* Note: The *Diagnostic and Statistical Manual of Mental Disorders*, 1968, gives many other conditions not mentioned here.

3. organic brain syndrome — syndrome characterized by impairment of orientation, memory, mental functioning related to comprehension, learning and acquisition of knowledge, defective judgment, shallowness of affect and emotional instability. Functional brain tissue is impaired at varying degree. The syndrome may be acute or chronic, reversible or irreversible, and related to the patient's basic personality pattern, interpersonal relations and conflicts, as well as environmental factors.[18]

4. personality disorder — condition marked by maladaptive behavior pattern that is deeply ingrained and nonpsychotic. Some examples are:
   a. alcohol addiction — dependence on alcohol as evidenced by appearance of withdrawal symptoms when alcohol is withheld.
   b. drug dependence — addiction to or dependence on opiates, synthetic analgesics, barbiturates, psychostimulants, hallucinogens and others. Habitual use is necessary for diagnosis. Withdrawal symptoms may be absent.[15]
   Other personality disorders are:
   c. cyclothymic personality — individual manifesting mood swings from elation to depression.
   d. inadequate personality — individual unable to respond to intellectual, emotional, social and physical demands in a satisfactory manner.
   e. schizoid personality — individual being oversensitive, shy, seclusive, unsociable, eccentric and autistic; apparently detached in conflict situation.[18]

5. psychophysiologic disorder — any disorder representing the visceral expression of or functional response to emotion, for example: irritable colon, mucous colitis, heartburn, hyperventilation.[31]

6. psychosis, pl. psychoses — a major mental illness in which the patient's intellectual functioning is impaired to a degree that he cannot meet the ordinary demands of life and exhibits abnormal patterns of thought, feeling and action.[18]

7. psychoses associated with organic brain syndrome:
   a. acute alcoholic intoxication — disorder comprises a variety of acute brain syndromes caused by alcohol such as delirium tremens, alcoholic hallucinosis, others.
   b. Korsakov's psychosis — a chronic brain syndrome associated with a prolonged use of alcohol. Clinical features are peripheral neuropathy, disorientation, impaired memory and confabulation.[97, 22]
   c. presenile dementia — cortical brain syndrome in age group below sixty.
   d. psychosis with brain trauma — psychosis developing after head injury. If it occurs in childhood, mental retardation is a common sequel.
   e. psychosis with cerebral arteriosclerosis — condition similar to presenile and senile psychosis. Arterial occlusion of brain vessels may result in physical and mental deterioration.
   f. psychosis with cerebrovascular disturbance — common circulatory disorder usually associated with cerebral thrombosis, embolism or hemorrhage.
   g. senile dementia — a chronic organic brain syndrome due to brain atrophy in the aging process resulting in physical and mental deterioration at various degrees.[72]

8. psychoses not attributed to physical conditions:
   a. manic-depressive illness — disorder characterized by unusual mood swings from normal to depression or elation or alternating high or low spirits with intervening remissions.[25, 34, 89]
   b. schizophrenia — severe mental disorder of psychotic depth marked by disturbances in behavior, mood, and ability to think. Altered concept formation may lead to a distortion of reality, delusions and hallucinations which tend to be self-protective. Emotional disharmony and bizarre regressive behavior are frequently present.[81, 5] The American Psychiatric Association distinguishes 11 types, some of which are given here:
      (1) catatonic type — marked disturbance in activity with either generalized inhibition (mutism, stupor, negativism, waxy appearance) or by excessive

motor activity and excitement. Gross personality disorganization is a prominent feature.[45]

(2) hebephrenic type — shallow inappropriate emotions, disorganized thinking, unpredictable childish behavior and mannerisms, indicative of gross personality disorganization.

(3) latent type — prepsychotic or borderline schizophrenia with definite symptoms but no schizophrenic episode.

(4) paranoid type — schizophrenia in which grandiose or persecutory delusions are dominant characteristics. They are usually associated with hostility, aggressiveness and hallucinations.[18]

D. Terms Related to Shock Therapy:

Several types of shock therapy are employed in psychiatric treatment:
1. carbon dioxide therapy — the use of carbon dioxide inhalations to alter favorably the course of mental illness.
2. electroconvulsive or electroshock treatment — the use of electric current to cause unconsciousness and/or initiate convulsions.
3. electronarcosis — narcoticlike state produced as therapeutic measure.
4. electrostimulation — avoidance of convulsive seizures when using electric current.
5. insulin coma therapy — inducing hypoglycemic reaction by the administration of large doses of insulin.
6. subcoma insulin therapy — producing drowsiness or somnolence by insulin injection, but no coma.

E. Terms Related to Psychotherapy:

Psychotherapy may be defined as treatment of emotional and personality problems by psychological means. The following terms refer to psychotherapeutic techniques.
1. abreaction — an expressive form of psychotherapy which encourages a reliving of repressed emotional stress situations in a therapeutic setting. It releases painful emotions and increases insight.[7]
2. activity therapy — program of activities prescribed for patients on the basis of psychological understanding of their specific needs. Types of therapy are:
   a. bibliotherapy   c. music therapy   e. recreational therapy
   b. educational therapy d. occupational therapy
3. group psychotherapy — a method of psychotherapy applied to a group. Group leaders help patients to gain insight into their emotional difficulties and conflicts, to understand their causes and to translate their defensive reactions into acceptable behavior.
4. hypnosis — a state of semiconscious suggestibility. Through verbal suggestion the patient's attention is withdrawn from other stimuli and focused on the therapist's procedure. Under hypnosis symptoms are made to disappear. Posthypnotic suggestion is important.[78]
5. milieu therapy — the utilization of a modified and controlled environment in the treatment of mental disease.[90]
6. narcoanalysis — psychotherapy is offered under the influence of drugs.
7. persuasion — a form of psychotherapy which utilizes reasoning and moralizing discussions to change faulty attitudes.
8. play therapy — psychotherapeutic approach to children who tend to reveal their hidden resentments, feelings and frustrations in play. An analytic therapist uses his interpretations of play as a guide to treatment.
9. psychoanalysis — system of psychotherapy developed by Sigmund Freud. Psychoanalytic treatment seeks to influence behavior by bringing into awareness unconscious emotional conflicts in an effort to overcome them.[37]

10. supportive psychotherapy — therapeutic efforts directed toward a strengthening of the patient's ego in order to reduce anxiety. The real problem remains unsolved and may become acute again at a crucial moment.[37]

11. transference — a patient's unconscious reaction to a psychiatrist which is a repetition of an early childhood relationship to a parent, sibling or other. The psychiatrist utilizes the transfer situation to gain insight into the patient's disturbing emotional conflicts and to plan his psychotherapy accordingly.

F. Terms Related to Psychopharmacology:

1. antianxiety agents — drugs which exhibit a central calming effect. They are used in the treatment of mild to moderate anxiety.

2. antidepressants — psychic energizers which relieve despondency, tension, fatigue and mental depression.

3. antipsychotic agents — drugs used in treating psychoses and controlling excitation of central nervous system.

4. ataractics — tranquilizing agents widely used in psychiatric disorders such as agitation, aggressive outbursts, psychomotor overactivity and the like. They are the same as antianxiety agents.

5. hallucinogens — chemical agents producing hallucinations, disturbed thought processes and depersonalization in normal persons.

6. psychedelics — drugs which apparently expand consciousness and enlarge vision.

7. psychopharmacology — science dealing with drugs that affect the emotions.

8. psychotogens — drugs producing psychotic behavior.

G. Symptomatic Terms:

1. aggression — forceful, self-assertive, attacking action, verbal, physical or symbolic.

2. agitation — chronic restlessness, important psychomotor reaction of emotional stress.

3. ambivalence — opposing drives or emotions; for example, love and hatred for the same person.

4. amnesia — a loss of memory, pathological in nature.

5. anaclitic — leaning on; refers to dependence of infant on mother, abnormal later in life.

6. autism — a form of thinking which seeks to satisfy unfulfilled desires but completely disregards reality factors.

7. blocking — a sudden interruption in the stream of thought.

8. body image — the conscious and unconscious picture a person has of his own body at any moment. The conscious and unconscious images may differ from each other.[3, 65]

9. catalepsy — diminished responsiveness usually characterized by trance-like states. May occur in organic or psychological disorders or under hypnosis.[3]

10. catharsis — a wholesome emotional release by talking about one's problems or repressed feelings.

11. circumstantiality — the inclusion of numerous details in conversation before the essential idea is expressed.

12. confabulation — the more or less unconscious defensive filling in of actual memory gaps by imaginary experiences, often complex, that are recounted in a detailed and plausible way; seen principally in organic psychotic disorders.[3]

13. cyclothymic — refers to mood swings out of proportion to stimuli.

14. delirium — syndrome characterized by clouding of consciousness, incoherence of ideas, mental confusion, bewilderment, hallucinations and illusions.

15. delusions — false beliefs resulting from unconscious needs and maintained irrespective of contrary evidence.
    a. delusions of grandeur — exaggerated ideas about one's position and importance.
    b. delusions of persecution — false ideas that one is the target of persecution.
    c. delusions of reference — erroneous assumption that casual, unrelated remarks are directed to oneself.

16. dementia — an irreversible impairment of intellectual capacities.
17. depersonalization — loss of sense of one's own identity.
18. dyssocial behavior — the term refers to individuals who are not classifiable as antisocial personalities but who follow more or less criminal pursuits, such as racketeers, dishonest gamblers, prostitutes and dope peddlers; formerly called sociopathic personalities.[3, 18]
19. empathy — an objective insight into the feelings of another person in contrast to sympathy which is subjective and emotional.
20. hallucinations — false sensory perceptions without actual external stimulation.
21. illusions — falsely interpreted sensory perceptions.
22. incoherence in speech — illogical flow of ideas which is difficult to comprehend by the hearer.
23. libido — a psychoanalytic term denoting the psychic drive that energizes living.
24. malingering — a conscious simulation of illness used to avoid an unpleasant situation or for personal gain.[3]
25. mental mechanism — term refers to a number of intrapsychic processes primarily functioning on an unconscious level such as most of the defense mechanisms. Thinking, memory and perception are included.[32, 3]
    a. compensation — an individual's striving to make up for deficiencies.
    b. conversion — emotional conflict expressed in somatic symptoms.
    c. denial — reality factors denied in an effort to resolve emotional conflict.
    d. displacement — tension reducing mechanism in which an emotional response is transferred from its real source to a more acceptable substitute.
    e. dissociation — a group of ideas, memories and feelings which have escaped from normal consciousness and the control of the individual.
    f. identification — unconscious imitation of another.
    g. projection — mental mechanism by which unacceptable desires are disowned and attributed to another.
    h. regression — an anxiety evading mechanism, a readoption of immature patterns of thought, behavior and emotional responses.
    i. repression — a common mechanism which excludes unacceptable desires, impulses and thoughts from conscious awareness.
    k. sublimation — the channelling of undesirable impulses and drives away from their primitive objectives into activities of a higher order. This defense mechanism is nonpathogenic.[32, 3]
26. phobia — any morbid fear.
27. sensory deprivation — experience of being cut off from usual external stimuli and the opportunity for perception. May occur in various ways such as through loss of hearing or eyesight, by solitary confinement, by travelling in space. May lead to disorganized thinking, depression, panic, delusions and hallucinations.[3]

RADIOLOGY

A. Terms Related to Radiographic Diagnosis:

1. cerebral angiography — a method of demonstrating the cerebral blood vessels by taking a series of radiograms during the injection of a contrast medium. The carotid artery is generally the vessel of choice for the injection.[71]
Angiography is a valuable diagnostic aid in the detection of aneurysms, space-occupying lesions, and brain tumors with specific vascular patterns. It, likewise, helps to determine the presence of collateral circulation.
2. encephalography, pneumoencephalography — the intrathecal introduction of air followed by x-ray examination of the brain. The air rises in the subarachnoid space and demonstrates the ventricular system. Since this procedure may cause a severe reaction, a fractional method of pneumoencephalography has been developed and has yielded excellent radiographic studies. It consists of injecting a small amount of air into the lumbar subarachnoid space.[58, 67, 79]

3. discography — a valuable diagnostic aid in the detection of herniated lumbar intervertebral discs. A contrast medium is directly injected into the disc and followed by radiograms of the spine.
4. myelography — the injection of a radiopaque substance into the subarachnoid space either by lumbar or cisternal puncture. This permits the observation of its rise and fall in the spinal canal with the fluoroscope when the position of the patient is changed.[71, 83]
5. ventriculography — the introduction of air into the ventricular system following the removal of cerebral fluid. This procedure permits radiographic examination of the brain.[60]
6. vertebral angiography — a diagnostic tool in neurology primarily used in the detection of subarachnoid hemorrhage. Two methods are employed: (1) the direct percutaneous anterior approach and (2) the indirect filling of the vertebral artery with a radiopaque substance followed by radiographic examination.

B. Terms Related to Therapy:

radioresistant neoplasms — tumors composed of cells which cannot be destroyed by radiotherapy; for example, many brain tumors are radioresistant.

CLINICAL LABORATORY

A. Terms Related to Cerebrospinal Fluid Studies:

1. collection of cerebrospinal fluid —
   a. cisternal puncture — removal of cerebrospinal fluid from the cisterna magna, for example, in case of blocking of central canal of spinal cord.
   b. lumbar puncture — needle puncture of subarachnoid space of the lumbar cord used in determining cerebrospinal fluid (CSF) pressure and removing CSF for diagnostic evaluation or other purposes.
   c. ventricular puncture — removal of ventricular fluid, rarely done on adults except for ventriculography, but a common procedure for infants with open fontanels.
2. examination of cerebrospinal fluid (CSF)
   a. chemical analysis of CSF: chloride, protein, glucose, bilirubin, others.
   b. cytology of spinal fluid — cell count and differential leukocyte count of spinal fluid.
   c. Lange colloidal gold test — test for cerebrospinal fluid. The curve obtained aids in the differential diagnosis of disorders of the nervous system.
   d. Queckenstedt test — diagnostic maneuver consisting in compression of one or both jugular veins which normally results in a quick, brief rise of pressure of the cerebrospinal fluid. In blockage of vertebral canal, the rise in CSF is minimal or absent.
   e. turbidity of spinal fluid — cloudy appearance due to the presence of microorganisms, granules or flaky material in spinal fluid.
   f. VDRL of spinal fluid — qualitative and quantitative tests for neurosyphilis.
   g. xantochromic — canary yellow. Xantochromic spinal fluid may occur in cerebral hematoma, subarachnoid hemorrhage, toxoplasmosis, abscesses and tumors.[46, 55]

B. Terms Related to Echoencephalography and Electroencephalography:

1. echoencephalography — rapid determination of intracranial midline displacements using ultrasonic pulse echo techniques. As soon as the density is altered, a pulse beam of high frequency sound, emitted by the transmitter, will echo back and be recorded on an oscillographic screen. The procedure aids in the detection of pressure-producing and space-occupying brain lesions.[83]
2. electroencephalogram — a device for measuring and recording delicate electrical impulses generated in the brain. The aparatus is an aid to medical diagnosis and treatments and directly increases the chance of success in brain surgery.[83]

3. electroencephalography — a tracing or recording of brain waves. Marked irregularities indicate pathological conditions such as epilepsy, brain tumors, scars and other disorders.
4. electronystagmography — electrical stimulation of the eyeball to induce nystagmus for the recording of eye movements in nystagmus.[99]
5. rheoencephalography — graphic registration of the changes in conductivity of nerve tissue caused by vascular factors.[92, 64]

C. Terms Related to Psychometric Tests:[73]

1. intelligence tests — devices set up to determine an individual's native intellectual ability including the level of his functioning in various areas. The following tests have been widely accepted.
   a. Stanford-Binet — shows range of mental ability by age. It is assumed that mental growth stops at the age of fifteen.
   b. Wechsler Adult Intelligence Scale — a verbal and a performance test designed to measure the intellectual capacity of adults at different age levels.
   c. Wechsler Intelligence Scale for Children — test devised primarily to classify children according to their intellectual abilities.
2. projective tests — methods employed to uncover a subject's unconscious attitudes, needs and relationships to others. When taking a test, the subject projects the pattern of his own psychological life and thus reveals the underlying dynamics of his personality structure. Of value are the following:
   a. Minnesota Multiphasic Personality Inventory — affords insight into various phases of the patient's personality.
   b. Rorschach Personality Test — attempts to detect conscious or unconscious personality traits and conflicts through eliciting the individual's associations to a set of ink blots.
   c. Thematic Apperception Test — uses twenty pictures to stimulate projective expression of personality traits.

D. Terms Related to Neurological Examination:[83, 60, 54, 21]

1. Babinski reflex — extension of the great toe with or without plantar flexion of other toes when examiner strokes the sole. A positive Babinski suggests organic disease of the pyramidal tracts.
2. Brudzinski sign — when head is passively flexed on chest, the patient draws up legs reflexly. This occurs in meningeal irritation and meningitis.
3. carotid compression test — evaluation of cerebral blood flow by compressing the carotid arteries digitally. This may lead to the detection of cerebrovascular insufficiency. An irritable carotid sinus reflex is evoked by unilateral compression.[25]
4. Kernig sign — when the patient is supine and his thigh is flexed upon the abdomen, he is unable to extend the leg. This sign is present in meningeal irritation and meningitis.
5. Romberg sign — inability of ataxics to stand steady with their eyes closed and feet together.

E. Terms Related to Miscellaneous Tests:[105]

1. barbiturate serum concentration — Method of Schreiner
   Potentially fatal level of intoxication with
   a. most short acting barbiturates .... 3.5 mg/100 ml
   b. phenobarbital approximately ...... 8.0 mg/100 ml
2. ethanol blood concentration
   Marked intoxication .... 0.3 - 0.4%
   Alcoholic stupor .... 0.4 - 0.5%
   Coma .... over 0.5%

ABBREVIATIONS

A. General:

ANS — autonomic nervous system
CA — chronological age
CBF — cerebral blood flow
CBS — chronic brain syndrome
CNS — central nervous system
CP — cerebral palsy
CR — conditioned reflex
CS — conditioned stimulus
CSF — cerebrospinal fluid
CVA — cerebrovascular accident
DCR — direct cortical response
DSM — **Diagnostic and Statistical Manual of Mental Disorders**
DT — delirium tremens
ECT — electroconvulsive therapy
EEG — electroencephalogram
Ej — elbow jerk
EST — electric shock therapy

ICT — insulin coma therapy
IQ — intelligence quotient
Kj — knee jerk
LP — lumbar puncture
LSD — lysergic acid diethylamide
MAO — monoamine oxidase
MS — multiple sclerosis
NREM — no rapid eye movements (sleep)
OBS — organic brain syndrome
PEG — pneumoencephalogram
PNS — peripheral nervous system
REM — rapid eye movements (deep sleep)
SLE — St. Louis encephalitis
SNS — sympathetic nervous system
SR — stimulus response
UCR — unconditioned reflex

B. Tests:

IMP — Inpatient Multidimensional Psychiatric (Scale)
IPAT — Cattle's Institute for Personality and Ability Testing Anxiety Scale
MAS — Taylor Manifest Anxiety Scale
MMPI — Minnesota Mulitphasic Personality Inventory
MSRPP — Multidimensional Scale for Rating Psychiatric Patients

PMA — Primary Mental Abilities Test
SAT — School Ability Test
SB — Stanfort-Binet Test
TAT — Thematic Apperception Test
WAIS — Wechsler Adult Intelligence Scale
WISC — Wechsler Intelligence Scale for Children

C. Organizations:

AA — Alcoholics Anonymous
ABPN — American Board of Psychiatry and Neurology
APA — American Psychiatric Association
BDAC — Bureau of Drug Abuse Control
GAP — Group for Advancement of Psychiatry

NAMH — National Association of Mental Health
NARC — National Association for Retarded Children
NIMH — US National Institute for Mental Health

ORAL READING PRACTICE

Drug Addiction, a Psychiatric Disorder

The problem of **addiction** in the United States remains unsolved, although the passage of the Harrison Narcotic Act (1914) has brought about a decline in the incidence of narcotic addicts. Unfortunately, this decrease has been counterbalanced by an increasing occurrence of barbiturate addicts.

The drugs which most commonly cause addiction in this country are opium, morphine, heroin, demerol, marihuana, cocaine, benzedrine, and the barbiturates. Since 1950 the problem of heroin addiction among adolescents and young adults has become acute in the large metropolitan areas. Males become more easily addicted than females. Ready availability makes doctors and nurses prone to develop addiction. Then there are the emotionally unstable, borderline psychotic, psychoneurotic, and psychopathic individuals who fall prey to the allurements of opiates. Perhaps the largest number of the unfortunate members of the human society belong to those engaged in underworld activities, a world filled with misery, crime and moral defeats.

Among the habit producing agents narcotics merit first attention. Narcotic addiction is a psychiatric disorder in which the use of opiates, because of the intense feeling of well-being it produces, has become a compulsive act. There are three phases recognizable in the addiction to opiates and synthetic analgesic drugs: tolerance, physical dependence and habituation.

Tolerance refers to the diminishing effect of the drug after continuous use. Consequently, the addict will take increasingly larger doses to attain the desired pleasurable effect and comfort provided by the drug.

Physical dependence reveals an altered physiological state resulting from the frequent administration of the drug.

Psychological dependence or **habituation** manifests an emotional response compelling the addict to use the drug as an escape measure from unpleasant situations and a psychological crutch for a new lease on life.[26, 52, 30, 27, 19]

Table 5

SOME CONDITIONS AMENABLE TO NEUROSURGERY

Organs Involved	Diagnoses	Operations	Operative Procedures
Brain	Rupture of middle meningeal artery Epidural hemorrhage Epidural hematoma	Surgical exploration of subtemporal region Removal of epidural hematoma	Drilling exploratory burr holes Burr hole enlarged for exposure of hematoma Removal of epidural hematoma by suction
Brain Subarachnoid space	Subarachnoid hemorrhage from ruptured aneurysm of internal carotid artery	Ligation of carotid artery[a] Intracranial clipping or ligation of aneurysm	Tying the carotid artery in the neck Applying a clip or ligature to the aneurysmal sac
Brain Subdural space	Subdural hematoma of the brain	Drainage of subdural space Craniotomy and excision of hematoma	Evacuation of the clot through trephine opening in the skull Surgical opening of the skull and removal of subdural hematoma
Brain Dura mater	Craniocerebral injury: open depressed fracture with dural laceration	Decompression, suture of dura mater	Elevation of depressed fracture and repair of dural laceration
Brain Meninges	Meningioma, benign	Craniotomy with excision of meningioma	Opening into skull, osteoplastic flap, removal of tumor
Brain Glial tissue	Primary malignant glioma	Craniotomy with resection of tumor	Opening into skull, osteoplastic flap, removal of tumor

Organs Involved	Diagnoses	Operations	Operative Procedures
Brain Choroid plexus Ventricles	Obstructive, non-communicating hydrocephalus Nonobstructive, communicating hydrocephalus	Ventriculocisternostomy, Torkildsen procedure Ventriculocaval shunt Insertion of Holter or Pudenz valve[a]	Shunting cerebrospinal fluid from third ventricle to the cisterna magna by means of plastic catheter Shunting the cerebrospinal fluid from the lateral ventricle to the superior vena cava via the jugular vein by the insertion of a one-way valve
Brain Hypophysis	Pituitary tumor Hyperpituitarism	Stereotaxic cryo-hypophysectomy	Diamond drill dissection of anterior wall of sella turcica using the surgical microscope Accurate placement of cryoprobes for destruction of hypophysis and tumor
Brain Basal nuclei	Paralysis agitans or Parkinson's disease	Stereotaxic thalamotomy[a]	Introduction of radiofrequency electrode through burr hole Electrode carried to the surgical target by stereotaxic instrument Destruction of ventrolateral nucleus of thalamus[a]
Brain Trigeminal nerve	Trigeminal neuralgia (Tic douloureux)	Retrogasserian neurotomy	Transection of sensory root of trigeminal nerve
Brain Vestibulocochlear nerve	Acoustic neurilemmoma	Suboccipital craniectomy Microneurosurgical excision of acoustic tumor[b]	Excision of portion of skull, transmeatal approach Removal of acoustic tumor from internal auditory canal by microdissection[b]
Spinal cord	Intractable pain due to any cause	Cordotomy Percutaneous high cervical cordo-tomy[a]	Transection of pain tracts in spinal cord Stereotaxic method used for locating and interrupting the spinothalamic tract in the cervical cord[a]
Spinal cord Ganglia	Intractable pain in extremity due to Causalgia Raynaud's disease Buerger's disease	Sympathectomy	Removal of sympathetic chain and ganglia
Spinal cord Subarachnoid space	Intractable pain in malignant disease	Alcohol injection as nerve block	Injection of alcohol into sub-arachnoid space
Lumbar spinal cord Sensory nerve roots	Intractable pain of posterior spinal nerve roots at lumbar level	Posterior lumbar rhizotomy	Section of posterior spinal nerve roots in lumbar region
Spinal cord Sensory nerve roots	Intractable pain due to herniated nucleus pulposus	Laminectomy Excision of herniated nucleus pulposus[a]	Removal of laminae of vertebrae concerned and lesion[a]

[a] Edmund A. Smolik, M.D. Personal communications.

[b] Robert A. Rand. Acoustic tumor microsurgery. *Journal of Neurosurgery,* 28: 159-161, February, 1968.

REFERENCES AND BIBLIOGRAPHY

1. Adams, R. D. Diseases of the spinal cord. In Wintrobe, Maxwell M. (ed.). *Harrison's Principles of Internal Medicine*, 6th ed. New York: McGraw Hill Book Co., 1970, pp. 1724-1727.

2. Appleton, F. J. Psychiatric drugs: A usage guide. *Diseases of the Nervous System*, 32: 607-616, September, 1971.

3. *A Psychiatric Glossary*, 3rd ed. Washington, D.C.: American Psychiatric Association, 1969, *verbatim*, with permission.

4. Aström, K. E. *et al.* Traumatic diseases of the brain. In Wintrobe, Maxwell M. (ed.). *Harrison's Principles of Internal Medicine*, 6th ed. New York: McGraw Hill Book Co., 1970, pp. 1764-1774.

5. Ayd, F. J. Neuroleptic therapy for chronic schizophrenia. *Diseases of the Nervous System*, 33: 35-39, January, 1972.

6. Barahal, H. S. Traumatic neurosis. *Lawyer's Medical Journal*, 6: 63-78, May, 1970.

7. Batchelor, Ivor R. C. (ed.). *Henderson and Gillespie's Textbook of Psychiatry*, 10th ed. London: Oxford University Press, 1969, p. 179.

8. Brain, Lord and Walton, John N. Disorders of the cerebral circulation. In *Brain's Diseases of the Nervous System*, 7th ed. London: Oxford University Press, 1969, pp. 279-335.

9. —————. Extrapyramidal syndromes. *Ibid.*, pp. 513-555.

10. Buchtel, B. C. *et al.* Radiographic diagnosis of meningioma. *Southern Medical Journal*, 64; 973-977, August, 1971.

11. Canady, M. E. SSPE-Helping the family cope. *Amercian Journal of Nursing*, 72: 94-96, January, 1972.

12. Carey, M. E. *et al.* Experience with brain abscesses. *Journal of Neurosurgery*, 36: 1-9, January, 1972.

13. Cassidy, F. M. Adult hydrocephalus. *American Journal of Nursing*, 72: 494-497, March, 1972.

14. Chase, T. N. *et al.* Huntington's chorea. *Archives of Neurology*, 26: 282-284, March, 1972.

15. Cheatham, J. S. A profile of the drug dependent patient. *Southern Medical Journal*, 64: 1354-1357, November, 1971.

16. Chusid, Joseph G. Central nervous system: In *Correlative Neuroanatomy & Functional Neurology*, 14th ed. Los Altos, California: Lange Medical Publications, 1970, pp. 1-70.

17. —————. Disorders due to vascular disease. *Ibid.*, pp. 304-319.

18. Committee on Nomenclature and Statistics of the American Psychiatric Association. *Diagnostic and Statistical Manual of Mental Illness*, 2d ed. Washington, D.C.; American Psychiatric Association, 1968.

19. Condon, Alice and Roland, Arlene. Drug abuse jargon. *American Journal of Nursing*, 71: 1738-1739, September, 1971.

20. Conquist, S. *et al.* Hydrocephalus and congestive heart failure caused by intracranial arteriovenous malformations in infants. *Journal of Neurosurgery*, 36: 249-254, March, 1972.

21. Cunningham, R. D. The eye as a mirror to neurologic disease. *Modern Treatment*, 8: 717-741, August, 1971.

22. Curran, J. R. *et al.* Alcoholic myopathy. *Diseases of the Nervous System*, 33: 19-22, January, 1972.

23. DeVivo, D. C. *et al.* Vertebrobasilar occlusive disease in children. *Archives of Neurology*, 26: 278-281, March, 1972.

24. Dodge, P. R. and Fishman, M. A. The choroid plexus — two-way traffic? *New England Journal of Medicine*, 283; 316-317, August 6, 1970.

25. Dorzah, Joe *et al.* Depressive disease: Clinical cause. *Diseases of the Nervous System*, 32: 269-273, April, 1971.

26. DuPont, R. L. and Katon, R. N. Development of a Heroin-Addiction Treatment Program. *Journal of American Medical Association*, 216: 1320-1324, May 24, 1971.

27. Fink, M., Freedman, A. M., Zaks, A. M., Resnick, R. B. Narcotic antagonists: Another approach to addiction therapy. *American Journal of Nursing*, 71: 1359-1363, July, 1971.

28. Fischer, E. G. Ventriculo-direct atrial shunts. *Journal of Neurosurgery*, 36: 438-440, April, 1972.

29. Fishman, R. A. Intracranial tumors and states causing increased intracranial pressure. In Beeson, Paul B. and McDermott, Walsh (eds.). *Cecil-Loeb Textbook of Medicine*, 13th ed. Philadelphia: W. B. Saunders Co., 1971, pp. 273-288.

30. Foreman, N. J. and Zerwekh, J. V. Drug crisis intervention. *American Journal of Nursing*, 71: 1736-1739, September, 1971.

31. Freedman, Alfred M., Kaplan, Harold I. and Sadock, Benjamin J. Psychophysiological disorders. In *Modern Synopsis of Comprehensive Textbook of Psychiatry*. Baltimore: The Williams & Wilkins Co., 1972, pp. 431-478.

32. —————. Theories of personality and psychopathology: I Freudian School. *Ibid.*, pp. 97-118.

33. Furr, S. C. Subacute sclerosing panencephalitis. *American Journal of Nursing*, 72: 93-95, January, 1972.

34. Gallemore, J. *et al.* Precipitating factors in affective disorders. *Southern Medical Journal*, 64: 1248-1252, October, 1971.

35. Glaser, G. H. The epilepsies. In Beeson, Paul B. and McDermott, Walsh (eds.). *Cecil-Loeb Textbook of Medicine*, 13th ed. Philadelphia: W. B. Saunders Co., 1971, pp. 260-271.

36. Goldring, S. The role of prefrontal cortex in grand mal convulsion. *Archives of Neurology*, 26: 109-119, February, 1972.

37. Gregory, Ian. *Fundamentals of Psychiatry*, 2nd ed. Philadelphia: W. B. Saunders Co., 1968, pp. 3-4 and pp. 233-234.

38. Gurdjian, E. Stephens and Thomas, L. Murray. Use of microsurgery in neurolysis. In *Operative Neurosurgery*, 3rd ed. Baltimore: The Williams and Wilkins Co., 1970, p. 582.

39. —————. Supraorbital and supratrochlear neurectomy and avulsion. *Ibid.*, pp. 188-189.

40. —————. Trigeminal decompression. *Ibid.*, pp. 192-194.

41. _____. Head injury, skull fracture, concussion, others. *Ibid.*, pp. 235-289.

42. _____. Endarterectomy of carotid bifurcation. Teflon graft reconstruction of internal carotid artery. *Ibid.*, pp. 306-309.

43. _____. Stereotaxis. Cingulotomy, fornicotomy, thalamotomy, amygdalotomy. *Ibid.*, pp. 216-219.

44. _____. Surgical treatment of hydrocephalus — Ventriculocisternal intubation — Ventriculocaval shunt. Insertion of Holter valve. *Ibid.*, pp. 199-210.

45. Hearst, E. D. *et al.* Catatonia: Its diagnostic validity. *Diseases of the Nervous System*, 32: 453-456, July, 1971.

46. Hepler, Opal E. *Manual of Clinical Laboratory Method*, 4th ed. Springfield, Illinois: Charles C. Thomas, Publisher, 1955, pp. 150-157.

47. Ingram, A. J. Miscellaneous affections of the nervous system. In Crenshaw, A. H. (ed.). *Campbell's Operative Orthopaedics*, 5th ed. St. Louis: The C. V. Mosby Co., 1971, pp. 1685-1738.

48. Izumi, A. K. *et al.* Von Recklinghausen's disease associated with multiple neurolemomas. *Archives of Dermatology*, 104: 172-176, August, 1971.

49. Johnson, R. T. Subacute sclerosing panencephalitis. In Beeson, Paul B. and McDermott, Walsh (eds.). *Cecil-Loeb Textbook of Medicine*, 13th ed. Philadelphia: W. B. Saunders Co., 1971, pp. 241-242.

50. Kahn, E. A. and Crosby, E. D. Gliomas of the cerebral hemispheres. In Kahn, Edgar A. *et al. Correlative Neurosurgery*, 2d ed. Springfield, Illinois: Charles C. Thomas, Publisher, 1969, pp. 44-67.

51. Kent, H. Postpartum hemiplegia. *Southern Medical Journal*, 64: 1456-1459, December, 1971.

52. Kilcoyne, M. *et al.* Nephrotic syndrome in heroin addicts. *The Lancet*, 1: 17-20, January 1, 1972.

53. Kimmel, M. E. Antabuse in a clinic program. *American Journal of Nursing*, 71: 1173-1175, June, 1971.

54 Klawanas, H. L. *et al.* Neurologic examination in an elderly population. *Diseases of the Nervous System*, 32: 274-279, April, 1971.

55. Krentz, M. J. and Dyken, P. R. Cerebrospinal fluid cytomorphology — sedimentation vs. filtration. *Archives of Neurology*, 26: 253-257, March, 1972.

56. Kriel, R. L. Diagnosis and management of viral encephalitis. *Postgraduate Medicine*, 50: 99-103, July, 1971.

57. Larmon, W. A. Infections and neoplasms of bone. Tumors of nerve origin. In Sabiston, David C. (ed.). *Davis-Christopher Textbook of Surgery*, 10th ed. Philadelphia: W. B. Saunders Co., 1972, pp. 1381-1398.

58. LeMay, M. J. and New, P. E. Pneumoencephalography and isotope cisternography in the diagnosis of occult normal-pressure hydrocephalus. *Radiology*, 96: 347-358, August, 1970.

59. Lichtenfield, P. Autonomic dysfunction in the Guillain-Barre syndrome. *American Journal of Medicine*, 50: 772-780, June, 1971.

60. Low, Neils L. Cerebral palsy. *Medical Clinics of North America*, 56: 1273-1280, November, 1972.

61. Margolis, M. T. *et al.* Choroidal arteries in the diagnosis of thalamic tumors. *Journal of Neurosurgery*, 36: 287-298, March, 1972.

62. McDowell, F. H. Cerebrovascular diseases. In Beeson, Paul B. and McDermott, Walsh, *Cecil-Loeb Textbook of Medicine*, 13th ed. Philadelphia: W. B. Saunders Co., 1971, pp. 189-216.

63. Miller Fischer, C. *et al.* Cerebrovascular diseases. In Wintrobe, Maxwell M. (ed.). *Harrison's Principles of Internal Medicine*, 6th ed. New York: McGraw-Hill Book Co., 1970, pp. 1727-1764.

64. Mintz, A. Y. *et al.* Changes in the nervous system during cerebral atherosclerosis. *Geriatrics*, 26: 134-144, September, 1971.

65. Murray, R. The concept of body image. *Nursing Clinics of North America*, 7: 593-595, December, 1972.

66. New, R. F. and Weiner, M. A. Radiological investigation of hydrocephalus. *Radiologic Clinics of North America*, 9: 117-140, April, 1971.

67. Newton, T. H. and Potts, D. G. (eds.). *Radiology of the Skull and Brain*. St. Louis: The C. V. Mosby Co., 1971.

68. Palacios, E. and MacGee, E. E. The radiographic diagnosis of trigeminal neurinomas. *Journal of Neurosurgery*, 36: 153-156, February, 1972.

69. Parsons, L. C. Respiratory changes in head injury. *American Journal of Nursing*, 71: 2187-2191, November, 1971.

70. Paterson, P. Y. The demyelinating diseases: clinical and experimental correlates. In Samter, Max (ed.). *Immunological Diseases*, 2d ed. Boston: Little, Brown and Co., 1971, pp. 1269-2199.

71. Peterson, H. O. and Kieffer, S. A. *Introduction to Neuroradiology*, Hagerstown, Maryland: Medical Department Harper & Row, Publishers, 1972.

72. Pfeiffer, E. Psychotherapy with elderly patients. *Postgraduate Medicine*, 50: 254-258, November, 1971.

73. Piotrowski, Z. A. Psychological testing of intelligence and personality. In Freedman, Alfred M. and Kaplan, Harold I. (eds.). *Comprehensive Textbook of Psychiatry*, Baltimore: The Williams and Wilkins Co., 1967, pp. 509-530.

74. Potts, D. G. Increased intracranial pressure: causes and associated skull changes. In Newton, T. H. *et al. Radiology of the Skull and Brain*. St. Louis: The C. V. Mosby Co., 1971, pp. 819-822.

75. Rand, R. W. Microneurosurgery for aneurysm of the vertebral-basilar artery system. *Journal of Neurosurgery*, 27: 330-332, October, 1967.

76. Richardson, E. P. *et al.* Degenerative diseases of the nervous system. In Wintrobe, Maxwell M. (ed.). *Harrison's Principles of Internal Medicine*, 6th ed. New York: McGraw Hill Book Co., 1970, pp. 1817-1833.

77. Richardson, D. E. Stereotaxic cingulumotomy and prefrontal lobotomy in mental disease. *Southern Medical Journal*, 65: 1221-1223, October, 1972.

78. Rodger, B. P. Therapeutic conversation and posthypnotic suggestion. *American Journal of Nursing*, 72: 714-717, April, 1972.

79. Rovit, R. L. Progressive ventricular dilatation following pneumoencephalography. A radiological sign of occult hydrocephalus. *Journal of Neurosurgery*, 36: 50-59, January, 1972.

80. Russell, D. S. and Rubinstein, L. J. *Pathology of Tumors of the Nervous System*, 3rd ed. Baltimore: The Williams and Wilkins Co., 1971, pp. 5-358.

81. Sankar, D. V. (ed.). *Schizophrenia — Current Concepts and Research*. Hicksville, New York: PJD Publications LTD., 1969, pp.76-79.

82. Scheinberg, L. C. The demyelinating diseases. In Beeson, Paul B. and McDermott, Walsh (eds.). *Cecil-Loeb Textbook of Medicine*, 13th ed. Philadelphia: W. B. Saunders Co., 1971, pp. 251-260.

83. Schmidt, R. P. Neurologic diagnostic procedures. In Beeson, Paul B. and McDermott, Walsh (eds.). *Cecil-Loeb Textbook of Medicine*, 13th ed. Philadelphia: W. B. Saunders Co., 1971, pp. 174-176.

84. Schneider, R. C. Craniocerebral trauma. In Kahn, Edgar A. *Correlative Neurosurgery*, 2d ed. Springfield, Illinois: Charles C. Thomas, Publisher, 1969, pp. 533-596.

85. _____. Trauma to the spine and spinal cord. *Ibid.* pp. 597-648.

86. Simmons, J. C. H. Peripheral nerve injuries. In Crenshaw, A. H. (ed.). *Campbell's Operative Orthopaedics*, 5th ed. St. Louis: The C. V. Mosby Co., 1971, pp. 1739-1794.

87. Smith, H. B. Cerebral concussion: Diagnosis and evaluation. *Lawyer's Medical Journal*, 3: 339-368, February, 1968.

88. Smolik, Edmund, A., M.D. Personal communications.

89. Spalt, L. *et al.* Suicide: an epidemiologic study. *Diseases of the Nervous System*. 33: 23-29, January, 1972.

90. Stainbrook, E. Milieu therapy. In Freedman, Alfred M. and Kaplan, Harold I. (eds.). *Comprehensive Textbook of Psychiatry*. Baltimore: The Williams and Wilkins Co., 1967, pp. 1296-1304.

91. Stauffer, N. *et al.* The lumbar disk syndrome and its operative treatment. *Postgraduate Medicine*, 49: 87-93, February, 1971.

92. *Stedman's Medical Dictionary*, 22d ed. Baltimore: The Williams and Wilkins Co., 1972, p. 1098.

93. Steinman, A. J. Influence of age on infection with St. Louis encephalitis virus. *Journal of Infectious Diseases*, 123, 316, March, 1971.

94. Sugar, Oscar. Nontraumatic neurosurgical emergencies. *Surgical Clinics of North America*, 52: 171-182, February, 1972.

95. Suwanwela, C. *et al.* Intracranial arterial narrowing and spasm in acute head injury. *Journal of Neurosurgery*, 36: 314-323, March, 1972.

96. Taren, J. A. Meningiomas. In Kahn Edgar A. *et al. Correlative Neurosurgery*, 2d ed. Springfield, Illinois: Charles C. Thomas, Publisher, 1969, pp. 68-86.

97. Tartar, R. E. and Jones, B. M. Motor impairment in chronic alcoholics. *Diseases of the Nervous System*, 32: 632-636, September, 1971.

98. Thomashefsky, A. J. Acute autonomic neuropathy. *Neurology*, 22: 251-255, March, 1972.

99. Toglia, J. U. and Morena, S. Labyrinthine versus central nystagmus: Electronystagmographic observation. *Diseases of the Nervous System*, 32: 623-626, September, 1971.

100. Truex, Raymond C. and Carpenter, Malcolm B. *Strong and Elwyn's Human Neuroanatomy*, 6th ed. Baltimore: The Williams and Wilkins Co., 1969, pp. 117-202.

101. Tucker, Eugene, F., M.D. Personal communications.

102. Weller, R. O. and Shulman, K. S. Infantile hydrocephalus: clinical histological and ultrastructional study of brain damage. *Journal of Neurosurgery*, 36: 255-265, March, 1972.

103. Wiebe, R. A. *et al.* Clinical factors relating to prognosis of bacterial meningitis. *Southern Medical Journal*, 65: 257-264, March, 1972.

104. Wilson, C. B. Complications of head injuries in childhood. *Postgraduate Medicine*, 51: 130-134, March, 1972.

105. Wintrobe, Maxwell M. (ed.). *Harrison's Principles of Internal Medicine*, 6th ed. New York: McGraw-Hill Book Co., 1970, pp. 2010-2011.

106. Yahr, M. D. The treatment of parkinsonism: current concepts. *Medical Clinics of North America*, 56: 1377-1392, November, 1972.

Chapter V

Cardiovascular Disorders

HEART AND CORONARY ARTERIES

A. Origin of Terms:

1. cardia (G) — heart
2. cardium (L) — heart
3. cor (L) — heart

4. corona (G) — crown
5. cuspid (L) — point, cusp
6. luna (L) — moon

B. Anatomical Terms:

1. cavities of the heart — the four heart chambers
   a. atria (sing. atrium) — the two chambers which form the base of the heart and receive the venous blood.
   b. ventricles — the two chambers which lie anteriorly to the atria and propel blood into arteries.
2. conduction system of the heart — specialized neuromuscular tissue for the conduction of impulses.[56]
   a. atrioventricular bundle, bundle of His — a bundle of modified muscle fibers within the interventricular septum and walls of the ventricles.
   b. atrioventricular node (AV node) — found in interatrial septum. It relays impulses to the atrioventricular bundle which in turn causes the contraction of the ventricles.
   c. Purkinje fibers — cardiac muscle fibers of the conduction system which ramify beneath the endocardium.
   d. sinoatrial node, sinus node (SA node) — node situated in the wall of the right atrium. It is the pacemaker of the heart since it transmits impulses to both atria stimulating them to contract simultaneously.
3. heart wall and covering
   a. endocardium — interior lining of the heart wall.
   b. myocardium — the heart muscle.
   c. myocardial sinusoids — endothelium-lined spaces lying between the myocardial muscle fibers and enabling the ventricular myocardium to absorb blood in a sponge-like manner.
   d. pericardium — covering of the heart, composed of a fibrous and serous pericardium. The former fits loosely around the heart. The latter consists of a visceral layer or epicardium which adheres closely to the myocardium and a parietal layer which lines the inner surface of the fibrous pericardium. The pericardial cavity is a narrow space between the parietal and visceral layers. It contains a minimal amount of serum that serves as a lubricant.
4. orifices and valves of the heart and great vessels.[56]
   a. atrioventricular orifices and valves — openings and cuspid valves between atria and ventricles.
      (1) mitral valve, bicuspid valve — valve between left atrium and left ventricle. It contains two endothelial folds or cusps which come together when the ventricle contracts.
      (2) tricuspid valve — three endothelial folds or cusps which guard the right atrioventricular orifice.
   b. foramen ovale — opening between the two atria in fetal life. It normally closes after birth.
   c. semilunar valves — half moon-shaped flaps within the aorta and pulmonary trunk which prevent the blood from flowing back into the ventricles.

5. sinuses, arteries and nerves:[56]
   a. aortic sinuses, sinuses of Valsalva — 3 dilated spaces of the root of the aorta, related to the 3 cusps of the aortic valve.
   b. coronary arteries — branches of the ascending aorta arising from the right and left aortic sinuses. These blood vessels with their branches supply the heart muscle and form numerous anastomoses of small arteries and precapillaries. In the event of a sudden occlusion of a major coronary artery these anastomotic channels may not be able to provide adequate collateral circulation. But if a major coronary artery is slowly occluded, these channels may enlarge and maintain a sufficient blood supply to the heart muscle.[56]
   c. coronary sinus — a short trunk into which most of the veins of the heart empty.
   d. internal thoracic arteries, internal mammary arteries — blood vessels, usually arising from the subclavian arteries and passing downward on either side of the sternum. They are approximately the same caliber as the coronary arteries. They can be surgically relocated from the chest wall to the myocardium or to a coronary artery distal to an obstructing lesion to revascularize the heart muscle.[167]
   e. parasympathetic fibers — preganglionic fibers which reach the heart via the vagus nerves. Ganglia in the heart have postganglionic fibers distributed to both the atria and ventricles. Impulses slow the heart and depress contractions.
   f. sympathetic fibers carried by the cervical and thoracic cardiac nerves to the heart muscle — fibers involved in control of the heart rate and the force of its contraction. Afferent fibers join the vagus nerve to aid in regulation of blood volume and heart rate.[167]

C. Diagnostic Terms:

1. aneurysm — a dilatation or bulging out of the wall of the heart, aorta or any other artery. Thrombi may form in the sac, break off and lead to embolism. Aneurysm may rupture.[32, 21]
2. anomalies, congenital — gross structural defects of the heart or great intrathoracic vessels arising during fetal development.[167, 116, 147, 175, 72, 2]
   a. atrial septal defect — abnormality resulting in a shunting of oxygenated blood from the left into the right atrium. There are wide variations of atrial septal defects in size, position and shape. Shunting is minimal when the defect is small. A persistent foramen ovale is one of the septal defects which may be encountered.
   b. isolated pulmonic stenosis, pure pulmonary stenosis — a narrowing of the pulmonary valve or of the infundibulum associated with an intact ventricular septum. The stenotic defect causes pulmonary outflow tract obstruction. (Infundibulum is the cone-shaped area of the right ventricle from which the pulmonary artery begins.)
   c. patent ductus arteriosus — persistence of communication between pulmonary artery and aorta after birth. In normal infants the closure of the ductus takes place during the first six weeks of life.
   d. tetralogy of Fallot — a complex of congenital defects usually considered as having four parts:
      (1) ventricular septal defect — a malformation of the septum of the ventricles.
      (2) pulmonic stenosis — same as isolated type except that involvement is associated with other defects.
      (3) dextroposition of the aorta — a transposition of the aorta to the right.
      (4) hypertrophy of the right ventricle — increased size of the ventricle, nature's way of compensating for the added work load imposed by the defects. The first two are essential parts of the complex.
   e. ventricular septal defect — anomaly existing in various forms, for example:
      (1) isolated absence of the ventricular septum, partial or total — occasionally multiple.
      (2) defect associated with other anomalies.

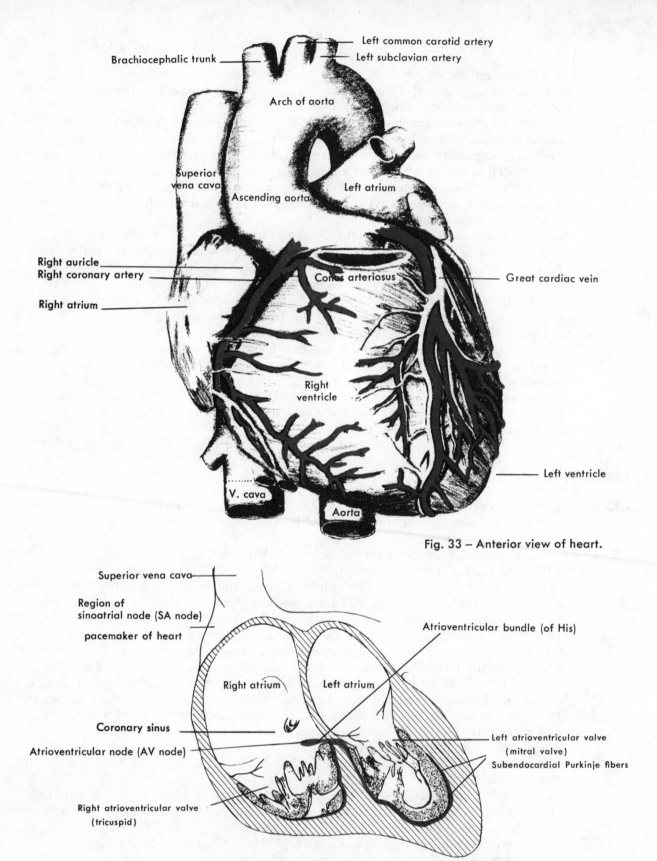

Left common carotid artery

Left subclavian artery

Brachiocephalic trunk

Arch of aorta

Superior vena cava

Left atrium

Ascending aorta

Right auricle

Conus arteriosus

Great cardiac vein

Right coronary artery

Right atrium

Right ventricle

Left ventricle

V. cava

Aorta

Fig. 33 – Anterior view of heart.

Superior vena cava

Region of sinoatrial node (SA node)

pacemaker of heart

Atrioventricular bundle (of His)

Right atrium

Left atrium

Coronary sinus

Atrioventricular node (AV node)

Left atrioventricular valve (mitral valve)

Subendocardial Purkinje fibers

Right atrioventricular valve (tricuspid)

Fig. 34 – Schematic diagram of conduction system of heart. Impulses pass from sinoatrial node through both atria stimulating them to contract. The atrioventricular node is thereby activated, and transmits impulses to the atrioventricular bundle and its right and left limbs, resulting in the contraction of both ventricles.

3. cardiac arrest — cessation of effective heart action, usually caused by asystole or ventricular fibrillation.

4. cardiac arrhythmias — irregularities of heart action including disturbances of rate, rhythm and conduction, either related or unrelated to other cardiac disease. Some major arrhythmias which seriously interfere with cardiac and circulatory efficiency are presented.[11, 88, 98, 20, 70]

    a. atrial arrhythmias — disorders of rhythm caused by abnormal foci in the atrial wall which discharge impulses more frequently than those from the sinoatrial node. These ectopic foci usually originate in myocardial irritability provoked by ischemia and drug toxicity. They readily take over the pacemaker function of the sinoatrial node. If uncontrolled, atrial arrhythmias may become life-threatening.[112]

        (1) atrial fibrillation — extremely rapid, vermicular, ineffectual contractions of the atria resulting in irregularity of rhythm in the ventricles. The atrial rate is 350 per minute or more.[139, 136]

        (2) atrial flutter — rapid, regular cardiac action of 250-350 beats per minute usually occurring in paroxysms, which are more prolonged than atrial tachycardia. The atrial impulse may produce a rapid ventricular rate or result in an atrioventricular block of varying degree (e.g. 2:1, 3:1 or 4:1)

        (3) paroxysmal atrial tachycardia (PAT) — small, rapid, regular contractions of the atria initiated by an irritable center within the atrium outside the sinoatrial node. Rate is about 160-220. Ventricular contractions are in 1:1 ratio with atrial contractions. This arrhythmia (PAT) is practically indistinguishable from nodal paroxysmal tachycardia. The patient may encounter a sudden forceful thump and subsequent attack of palpitation.

    b. atrioventricular nodal arrhythmias — disorders arising in the atrioventricular node.[112]

        (1) atrioventricular nodal rhythm — pacemaker function assumed by AV node in response to sustained failure of sinoatrial node to send impulses to the atrioventricular node.

        (2) premature atrioventricular nodal contractions (PNC) — arrhythmia due to irritation of the atrioventricular node which produces an ectopic stimulus and subsequent premature nodal contractions.[112]
        Frequent recurrence of PNC's may signal progressive myocardial infarction.

    c. ventricular arrhythmias — disorders of rhythm arising within the ventricles.[148, 41, 44]

        (1) premature ventricular contractions (PVC) — the most common disturbance of rhythm, frequently an index of myocardial damage and anoxia. If more than 6 PVC's per minute occur, ventricular efficiency may be seriously impaired.

        (2) ventricular fibrillation — extremely rapid contractions, irregularity in rhythm and force resulting in no ejection of blood from the fibrillating ventricles. It may terminate in ventricular standstill.

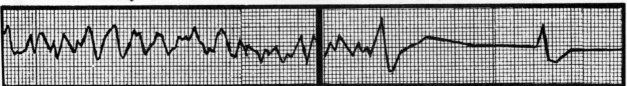

Fig. 35 – Ventricular fibrillation: life-threatening arrhythmia.

Fig. 36 – Terminal ventricular fibrillation and ventricular standstill – the dying heart.

        (3) ventricular tachycardia — disorder heralding a high degree of irritability frequently associated with myocardial infarction. The irritable center within the ventricular wall produces a rapid ventricular rate which may change to ventricular fibrillation or ventricular standstill. The rate is 150-250 or more and the rhythm slightly irregular. Sudden dizziness, precordial pain, dyspnea and weakness are common complaints.

d. conduction disturbances — abnormalities in the cardiac conduction system.[88, 149, 120, 67, 137]

    (1) atrioventricular block — delay or obstruction of impulses arising above or within the atrioventricular node.[88]

        (a) first degree heart block — prolongation of atrioventricular conduction time, delay of impulses on their ventricular pathway. Possible causes: increased vagal tone, myocardial ischemia, drug toxicity.

        (b) second degree or partial heart block — **type one,** benign form — blockage of one atrial beat after 6 to 8 conducted beats and dropping of respective ventricular beat (Wenckebach pause); **type two,** serious form — not all impulses are transmitted to the bundle of His by the atrioventricular node resulting in various ratios (2:1, 3:1, 4:1, other) of atrial contractions to ventricular contractions.[88] Wrist pulse is 40-50 beats per minute.

        (c) third degree or complete block — no atrial impulses are transmitted to the bundle of His by the atrioventricular node. Wrist pulse is 30 to 40 beats per minute.

    (2) bundle branch block — obstruction of the wave of excitation in either branch of the atrioventricular bundle.

    (3) Stokes-Adams syndrome — cardiac standstill which occurs with certain forms of heart block, causes syncope and possible fatal convulsions.

    (4) Wolff-Parkinson-White syndrome — a congenital disorder of atrioventricular conduction which may be associated with recurrent paroxysmal tachycardia, atrial flutter or other ectopic rhythms.[11, 107, 102, 161]

5. cardiac tamponade, pericardial tamponade — compression of the heart by effusion or hemorrhage in the pericardium which may seriously obstruct the venous inflow to the heart, raise the venous pressure, reduce the cardiac output, cause hypotension, distention of the neck veins and orthopnea.

6. cardiopulmonary arrest — heart-lung arrest due to sudden and unexpected cessation of respirations and functional circulation.

7. congestive heart failure — condition in which the heart is unable to pump adequate amounts of blood to tissues and organs. This is generally due to diseases of the heart causing low cardiac output. It can result from other conditions (anemia, hyperthyroidism) in which the demand for blood is greater than normal and the heart fails despite high cardiac output.[167, 171, 58, 59, 106]

8. coronary atherosclerosis — chronic disorder characterized by the presence of lipid deposits which form fibrous fatty plaques within the intima and inner media of the coronary arteries.[131]

9. coronary atherosclerotic heart disease — the most common heart condition. Progressive thickening of the intima of the coronary arteries leads to occlusion, caused by narrowing of the lumen and intravascular clotting.[31, 109, 18, 16, 124, 95]

10. cor pulmonale — heart-lung disease characterized by right ventricular hypertrophy due to pulmonary disorders which seriously impair ventilatory function and result in pulmonary hypertension.
    a. acute form — caused by massive pulmonary embolism occurring within hours.
    b. chronic form — caused by diffuse pulmonary fibrosis, obstructive emphysema or obstructive vascular disease developing within months.

11. cytomegalovirus-induced perfusion syndrome — a systemic disorder characterized by enlarged liver and spleen, fever, atypical lymphocytosis, viruria, immunologic aberrations and hematologic abnormalities. The cytomegalovirus (CMV) is undergoing further investigational studies in relation to virus-induced autoimmunity in man. CMV infections may develop following cardiopulmonary bypass.[83, 84]

12. endocarditis, bacterial — acute or subacute disease of the lining of the heart and especially valve leaflets. It is caused by infective organisms which enter the blood stream and

initiate a bacteremia clinically recognized by fever, fatigue, heart murmurs, splenomegaly, embolic episodes and areas of infarction.

13. Libman-Sacks endocarditis — condition characterized by verrucose lesions found in the endocardium of patients with terminal disseminated lupus erythematosus.[35]

14. ischemic heart disease — cardiac disease in which the prominent feature is a markedly reduced blood supply to the heart muscle, generally due to coronary atherosclerosis. The resultant myocardial ischemia may produce myocardial infarction, heart failure or angina pectoris.[167, 133, 17, 25]

15. myocardial disease, primary:
    a. myocarditis — inflammation of the heart muscle which may result in myocardial fibrosis, followed by cardiac enlargement and congestive heart failure.
    b. myocardosis — condition characterized by cardiac dilatation, congestive failure and embolization.[168]

16. myocardial disease, secondary:
    heart disease associated with noninfectious systemic diseases such as
    a. amyloidosis
    b. carcinoidosis
    c. collagen diseases
    d. endocrinopathy
    e. sarcoidosis
    f. systemic muscular and neurological disorders.

17. myocardial infarction, acute — clinical syndrome manifested by persistent, usually intense cardiac pain, unrelated to exertion and often constrictive in nature followed by diaphoresis, pallor, hypotension, dyspnea, faintness, nausea and vomiting. The underlying disease is usually coronary atherosclerosis which progressed to coronary thrombosis and occlusion and resulted in a sudden curtailment of blood supply to the heart muscle and myocardial ischemia.[29, 17, 133]

18. pericarditis — inflammation of the covering membranes of the heart. Its distinctive feature is pericardial friction rub, a transitory, scratchy or leathery sound elicited on ausculation.
    a. constrictive pericarditis, chronic — disorder characterized by a rigid, thickened pericardium which prevents adequate filling of the ventricles and may lead to congestive heart failure.
    b. purulent pericarditis — disease caused by pyogenic bacteria which may be associated with purulent, pericardial effusion.[49, 42]

19. rheumatic heart disease — involvement of the heart occurring in the course of rheumatic fever and attacking the myocardium, pericardium and endocardium with the valvular endocardium as the site of predilection.[150]

20. valvar heart disease, chronic — disorder referring to any permanent organic deformity of one or more valves.[69] Stenosis of the valve tends to increase the cardiac work load and precipitate cardiac failure.[150]
    a. aortic stenosis — reduction in the valve orifice interfering with the emptying of the left ventricle.
    b. mitral stenosis — a very common sequela of rheumatic fever, marked by the development of minute vegetations and thrombi which narrow the orifice of the valve leaflets. Calcifications form as the disease progresses.[140]
    c. tricuspid stenosis — defect associated with mitral stenosis. It reduces the valve to a small triangular opening which causes resistance in the flow of blood from the right atrium to the right ventricle and leads to congestion of the lungs and liver.

D. Operative Terms:

1. biopsy of pericardium — excision of a small piece of pericardial tissue for microscopic study.

2. cardiac biopsy — excision of tissue from the heart for the purpose of diagnosing various disease states. This can be done at the time of the operation or by means of a biotome adapted to an intracardiac catheter.[167] Under fluoroscopic control the biotome is passed through the right saphenous vein to the right atrium and right ventricle for biopsy. Tissue studies aid in the evaluation of the patient's condition prior to cardiovascular surgery.[93]

3. cardiac massage, open — emergency thoracotomy and manual compression of the heart, 40-60 times a minute, in an attempt to force blood from the ventricles into the aorta and pulmonary artery.

4. cardiac transplantation, heart transplantation — removal of a human cadaver heart for implantation into a recipient who is in irreversible cardiac failure. The procedure includes a median sternotomy, cannulation of vena cavae, cardiopulmonary bypass, surgical division of the ascending aorta, main pulmonary artery and atria, the excision of donor and recipient hearts and implantation of donor heart by atrial and vascular anastomoses to recipient.[26, 65, 66, 174, 167, 144]

5. correction of aortic coarctation — excision of contracted lesion of aorta and joining cut ends by suture or inserting a graft.

6. correction of congenital septal defects:[175]
   a. atrial septal defect — closure of defect under direct vision using cardiopulmonary bypass with or without hypothermia.
   b. ventricular septal defect — repair of defect by
      (1) direct suture or
      (2) use of ventricular patch such as an Ivalon pledget.
         Extracorporeal circulation with or without hypothermia is employed.

7. correction of patent ductus arteriosus —
   a. catheter closure of ductus — under fluoroscopic control a catheter is percutaneously placed into the femoral artery and advanced across the ductus through the right heart. A closure plug is rammed into the ductus. No thoracotomy is needed.[125] This method has been employed infrequently.[167]
   b. complete division of patent ductus — the ductus is divided and the pulmonic and aortic ends are closed separately by suture.[167]

8. correction of transposition of the great vessels.
   a. Blalock-Hanlon operation — surgical creation of an atrial septal defect as a palliative method which provides increased intracardiac mixing of the oxygenated and unoxygenated blood.[167]
   b. Mustard operation — surgical revision of the atrial septum transposing the venous return to match the transposed outflow tracts.[167, 159, 175]
   c. Rashkind operation, atrioseptostomy by balloon catheter — surgical creation of an atrial septal defect for palliation.[127]

9. mitral commissurotomy — separation of the stenotic valve at points of fusion.

10. myocardial revascularization — operative procedure which supplies the ischemic heart muscle with systemic arterial blood. Various techniques are used, for example:
    a. aortocoronary artery bypass — direct revascularization by placing autogenous grafts of a saphenous vein from the ascending aorta to the coronary arteries distal to the occlusions. Vascular obstructions are thus bypassed and adequate blood flow to the heart is immediately restored. Since single grafts become frequently occluded in the early postoperative period, multiple grafts are advocated to safeguard permanent circulatory efficiency.[122, 43, 1, 142, 10, 164, 130, 86]
    b. Vineberg-Sewell bilateral implants — indirect revascularization by implanting both internal thoracic (internal mammary) arteries in the left ventricle to promote the growth of collaterals to the interventricular branches of the coronary arteries. Weeks or months may elapse before the collateral circulation will be established.[103, 38, 39, 128, 13, 121]

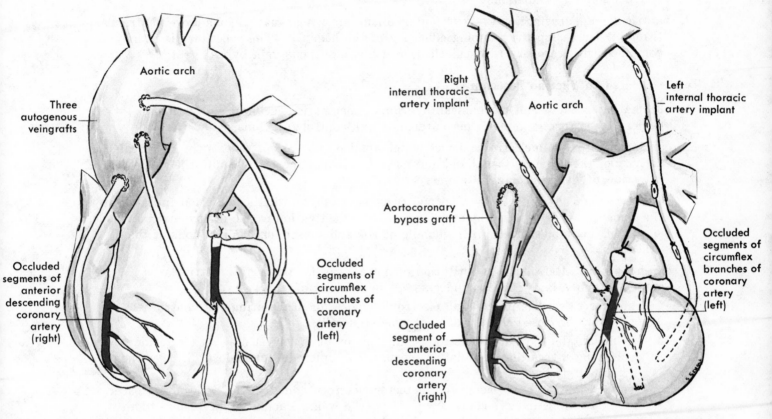

Fig. 37 – Direct myocardial revascularization by triple aortocoronary artery bypass.

Fig. 38 – A combination of direct and indirect myocardial revascularization.

12. pericardiectomy — incision and partial dissection of the pericardium to relieve the heart from constricting fibrous adhesions.

13. pulmonary banding — operation performed on infants who are unable to withstand a complete correction of an interventricular septal defect. The pulmonary artery is partially tied off to diminish the amount of blood to the lung.[92, 74]

14. tetralogy of Fallot — the following operations may be performed:
    a. shunting procedures, anastomoses of left subclavian and pulmonary artery and aorta.
    b. correction of pulmonary stenosis by valvotomy or valvoplasty.
    c. direct vision cardiac surgery, removal of pulmonic obstruction and repair of interventricular defect using hypothermia and heart-lung machine, or machine alone.[167, 23]

15. valve replacement surgery — removal of incompetent or stenotic valve and its replacement with a prosthetic valve graft.[115, 68]
    a. aortic valve replacement with frozen irradiated homograft; tendency to develop valve leakage.[5]
    b. excision of aortic valve and fresh viable homograft cusp replacement.[154]
    c. excision of calcified aortic valve and seating of Starr-Edwards aortic prosthesis; tendency to form thromboemboli.[135]
    d. excision of incompetent or stenotic mitral valve and seating of Starr-Edwards mitral prosthesis.[170]
    e. mitral valve replacement using unstended fresh semilunar valve homografts.[172]

16. valvotomy — incision into a valve.

   a. mitral valvotomy — splitting the two commissures (areas of fusion) of the mitral valve to widen its opening.

   b. pulmonary valvotomy — incising the valve of the pulmonary artery to improve the pulmonary circulation.

17. ventricular aneurysmectomy — excision of aneurysm which may harbor large ventricular thrombi, decreasing the pumping efficiency of the heart.[167]   The procedure is usually combined with coronary revascularization using saphenous vein bypass grafts.[104]

E. Terms Related to Specific Procedures:

1. automation — the use of mechanical, hydraulic, pneumatic, electrical and electronic devices to perform automatic measurements and control functions.

2. cardiac monitor — an electronic device which applied to a patient reveals the electrical activity of the heart by visual and auditory signals and thereby permits the immediate detection of dangerous arrhythmias.

3. cardiac pacing, physiological — a normal response to myocardial stimulation initiated at the sinoatrial node followed by atrial contractions, activation of the atrioventricular node, spread of the impulse through the bundle of His and subsequent contractions of the ventricles.

4. cardiac pacing, electronic — substitution of normal cardiac pacing in ventricular standstill and Adams-Stokes syndrome[60, 28] by the use of

   a. an external cardiac pacer — an electronic device for stimulating the ventricles through the closed chest wall in cardiac standstill.

   b. an implantable cardiac pacer, for permanent or temporary use — an electronic device achieving myocardial stimulation by means of epicardial or endocardial electrodes. Types of pacing are:

      (1) atrial-triggered pacing — a detector electrode added to the endocardial pacer. Its tip is in close contact with the atrial wall.   Pacing is in response to an atrial myocardial pickup rather than at a fixed rate.[33]

      (2) demand pacing — impulse is fired by pacemaker, if QRS complex fails to occur within a given period; pacing impulse is withheld if QRS complex develops within a certain interval.[113, 89, 132]

      (3) epicardial pacing, fixed rate — two electrodes attached to the epicardium with braided or coiled leads.   Through a subcutaneous tunnel the leads are connected to a battery operated pacer embedded in the abdominal or chest wall.   The electric battery is effective for about 3 years.   A thoracotomy is needed.[24]

      (4) transthoracic pacing — ventricular stimulation achieved by a thin wire electrode which is inserted through the chestwall into the myocardium by means of a transthoracic needle.   A battery powered pacer serves as a power source. Since pacing can be quickly initiated, transthoracic pacing is an effective emergency measure for resuscitating patients in cardaic arrest.[113]

      (5) transvenous endocardial pacing — an electrode catheter introduced into the heart through the jugular vein, its tip lodged in the right ventricular apex and the battery case located in a subcutaneous pouch below the clavicle.   The rate is fixed, usually 75 impulses per minute.   No thoracotomy is required. Transvenous pacing may be used temporarily for myocardial stimulation to control bradycardia and prevent ventricular standstill.[113, 24, 3, 73, 157]

      (6) ventricular-triggered pacing — on intracardiac electrode introduced transvenously into the right ventricular apex.   Method is similar to endocardial pacing.[117]

5. cardiac resuscitation — restoration of the heart beat by drugs, electrical myocardial stimulation, closed or open chest cardiac compression.

6. cardiopulmonary bypass — a mechanism for diverting the blood around the heart and lungs for the purpose of providing inflow occlusion to the heart. This enables the surgeon to operate on a bloodless heart muscle under direct vision.

7. cardiopulmonary resuscitation — heart-lung revival achieved by establishing a patent airway and restoring respiratory and circulatory functions.

8. cardioversion — direct current (DC) countershock applied to the chest to convert abnormal rhythms to normal sinus rhythm.[167]

9. coronary artery perfusion — introduction of blood into the coronary arteries by catheters during procedures in which the root of the aorta is opened.[167]

10. countershock — use of an external electronic defibrillator to terminate the disorderly electrical activity within the heart that provokes the arrhythmia. In ventricular fibrillation a brief high voltage shock abruptly stops the chaotic twitching of the ventricular muscle fibers. If effective the natural cardiac pacemaker regains control and restores normal contractions.

11. defibrillator — mechanical device for applying electric shock to the closed chest or to the open heart to terminate abnormal cardiac rhythms.

12. diastolic augmentation procedure — a circulatory assistive technique in which a balloon, placed in the aorta, is inflated during diastole and collapsed during systole (phase-shift). This reduces the pressure against which the heart pumps yet increases diastolic pressure and thus favorably influences coronary flow.[167, 94]

13. direct current defibrillation — countershock by a capacitor discharge defibrillator (DC type) instead of alternating current of the old type defibrillator (AC type).

14. elective cardiac arrest, cold anoxic arrest — standstill of the heart induced by cross-clamping the aorta and cardiac cooling. The temperature may be lowered by perfusing the coronary arteries with a cold solution, instilling a coolant into the pericardial sac or applying ice to the myocardium. Cold anoxic arrest provides a motionless, dry operative field conducive to aortic valve surgery and repair of congenital defects.[167]

15. exhaled-air ventilation — artificial respiration using the mouth-to-mouth, mouth to nose or mouth-to-tracheal stoma method to restore ventilatory lung function.

16. external arteriovenous (AV) shunt — procedure used to facilitate access to the patient's circulation by cannulation of blood vessels for prolonged hemodialysis. One piece of Silestic tubing is inserted into an artery, the other into an adjacent vein. They are then brought on top of the skin and connected with each other by a removable Teflon connector.[129]

17. external cardiac compression — the application of rhythmic pressure (60 times per minute) over the lower sternum to compress the heart and produce artificial circulation.

18. extracorporeal circulation — blood circulating outside of the body, a form of cardiopulmonary bypass. It may be achieved by using a heart-lung machine.

19. flowmetry of blood (in man) — measurement of blood flow.
    a. Doppler ultrasonic flowmetry — technique for obtaining phasic, continuous and instantaneous measurement of velocity (speed) of blood flow in various cardiovascular disorders, especially in aortic valvar disease, and venous thrombosis.[6, 145, 173]
    b. electromagnetic flowmetry — quantitation of blood flow by electromagnetic technique; useful as a diagnostic adjunct to cardiac catheterization and vascular surgery especially by measuring flow in shunts, bypass grafts and anastomoses.[152]

20. heart-lung machine — apparatus used to substitute for cardiopulmonary function. It permits a direct vision approach to cardiac lesions requiring corrective surgery. Venous blood returning to the heart is not allowed to enter the right atrium, but is sucked away by two tubes, one in each of the main veins. It is then pumped into an artificial lung. After this the oxygen laden blood enters a reservoir, passes through filters and is pumped to the patient's arterial system. Many different types of heart-lung machines are now in use.

21. hyperbaric oxygenation, hyperbaroxia — the clinical use of elevated atmospheric pressure produced in a hyperbaric chamber. Its principal effects are increased oxygenation and oxygen tension. Hyperbaroxia is thought to be of value in cardiac surgery and the treatment of cardiogenic shock due to acute myocardial infarction.[57]

22. induced hypothermia — artificial reduction of the body temperature in an effort to lower the metabolic requirements of the patient. He is then better able to tolerate the interruption of cardiac inflow.

23. medical electronics — the use of electronics in medical areas. Electronics refers to the action of charged electrical particles in any medium: solid, liquid or gas.

24. normothermia — environmental temperature that maintains body temperature and metabolic requirements at normal levels. In current cardiovascular surgery, normothermia is usually preferred to induced hypothermia.[25]

25. oscillation — a movement to and fro.

26. oscillometer — instrument for measuring any kind of oscillations; for example, those related to blood pressure.

27. oxymetry — measuring the amount of oxygen in a series of blood samples either chemically or by reading cuvette oxymeters of the samples obtained through a catheter from each heart chamber or vessel.[105]

28. perfusion in intracardiac surgery — method of providing oxygenated blood to the body by a heart-lung machine while interrupting the circulation through the heart.

29. precordial shock — electrical treatment of arrhythmias.
    a. elective procedure for converting certain tachyarrhythmias to normal rhythm. It is known as cardioversion.
    b. emergency procedure for controlling ventricular fibrillation. It is usually referred to as defibrillation.[113]

30. sphygmomanometer — instrument measuring blood pressure.

31. stethoscope — instrument for listening to sounds within the body.

32. synchronized direct current (DC) countershock — electric shock producing cardioversion by the use of a synchronized capacitator. The synchronizer is contraindicated in ventricular fibrillation.

33. transducer, medical use — a transforming device which transmits energy from a patient to a monitoring machine.

34. treadmill exercise tolerance — stress test for evaluating the ability of the coronary circulation to meet the metabolic demands of an increasing exercise load. The patient is subjected to graded exercise on the treadmill or bicycle ergometer until his electrocardiogram shows ischemic changes.[133, 8, 111]

35. two-step exercise test, Master's test — exercise test of coronary reserve. Within 1½ minutes the patient goes up and down 15 to 25 times 2 steps, each 9 inches high. A postexercise electrocardiogram is taken at once. If it is negative a 3 minute double two-step test is performed. As soon as the patient experiences pain the exercise is discontinued.[108, 22]

36. Valsalva maneuver — effective treatment for paroxysmal atrial tachycardia and similar disorders. The patient is instructed to inhale deeply, hold his breath and then strain down forcefully while slowly counting for 10 seconds. The Valsalva maneuver is also used as a test for cardiac reserve.[75]

F. Symptomatic Terms:

1. anasarca — massive edema with serous effusion especially in the right pleural and peritoneal cavities. It occurs in right heart failure and systemic congestion.

2. anginal syndrome, angina pectoris — syndrome characterized by short attacks of substernal, precordial pain which radiates to the shoulder and arm. It is provoked by exertion and relieved by rest.

3. Aschoff bodies — nodular lesions of the myocardium, pathognomonic (characteristic) of rheumatic disease.

4. asystole — cardiac standstill, no contractions of the heart.

5. bradycardia — slow heart action.

6. cardiac edema — retention of water and sodium in congestive heart failure due to circulatory impairment.

7. cardiac syncope — fainting associated with marked sudden decrease in cardiac output.

8. cardiogenic shock — syndrome related to cardiovascular disease, primarily to myocardial infarction, cardiac tamponade, massive pulmonary embolism or others. It is clinically characterized by mental torpor, reduction of blood pressure and pulse pressure, tachycardia, pallor, cold, clammy skin and signs of congestive heart faliure.[94]

9. carotid sinus syncope, vasopressor type — fainting or clouded consciousness without change in heart rate. It is due to hyperirritability of the carotid sinus or local disease.

10. ischemia — reduced blood supply to an organ usually due to arterial narrowing or occlusion in advanced atherosclerosis.
   a. cerebral ischemia — local anemia in the brain.
   b. myocardial ischemia — inadequate blood supply to the heart muscle.

11. murmur — blowing sound heard on auscultation.

12. palpitation — subjective awareness of skipping, pounding or racing heart beats.

13. postinfarction (Dressler's) syndrome — syndrome developing within the first week or weeks after myocardial infarction. It exhibits the clinical features of a benign form of pericarditis with or without effusion.

14. sinus rhythm — normal cardiac rhythm initiated at the sinoatrial node.

15. systole — rhythmical contractions of the heart particularly of those of the ventricles which pump the blood through the body.

16. tachycardia — rapid heart action.

ARTERIES, CAPILLARIES, VEINS

A. Origin of Terms:

1. angio (G) — vessel
2. artery (G) — air duct
3. diastole (G) — expansion
4. hemangio- (G) — blood vessel
5. phleb- (G) — vein
6. pulsus (L) — stroke, beat
7. systole (G) — contraction
8. thrombos (G) — clot
9. varix (L) — swollen vein
10. vena (L) — vein

B. Anatomical Terms:

1. aorta — the main artery of the trunk.

2. blood pressure
   a. systolic — the force exerted by the blood against the arterial walls at the end of the contraction of the left ventricle.
   b. diastolic — the force exerted by the blood against the arterial walls at the end of the relaxation of the left ventricle.

3. coats of arteries:
   a. tunica externa, adventitia — outer coat.
   b. tunica media — middle coat.
   c. tunica intima — inner coat.

C. Diagnostic Terms:

1. **acute limb ischemia** — a sudden catastrophic interruption of the blood flow to an extremity demanding emergency surgery to save the limb and the life of the patient, particularly if he is debilitated and advanced in years. Vascular disorders such as acute arterial embolization and the deposition of atheromatous plaques associated with bleeding and a relatively rapid thrombus formation precipitate the occlusive event. The limb is waxy pale, cold, painful or insensitive to touch and exhibits rigidity or deep muscle tenderness.[96]

2. **aneurysm of aorta** — dilatation of a weakened part of the wall of the vessel.
   a. **dissecting type** — progressive splitting of middle coat which may involve the entire circumference of the aorta. When pulsating blood is driven between the media and intima, the tear may rapidly extend the whole length of the aorta causing excruciating, ripping pain. A cystic medial necrosis with excess mucoid material is a frequent pathological finding.
   b. **fusiform type** — tubular swelling of the walls of the aorta involving the three coats and circumference.
   c. **sacculated type** — saclike bulging of a weakened part of the aorta formed by the middle and outer coats.

3. **aortic arch syndrome, pulseless disease** — group of disorders characterized by occlusion of vessels of the arch of the aorta.[76]

4. **aortic atresia** — congenital absence of normal valvar opening into aorta. Heart failure develops within days.[76]

5. **aortic stenosis** — congenital or acquired narrowing of valvar opening into aorta.

6. **aortoiliac disease, Leriche's syndrome** — gradual thrombosis of terminal aorta near the bifurcation and extending to the iliac arteries. Claudication and trophic changes may be present.[76]

7. **arteriosclerosis** — degenerative, vascular disorder characterized by a thickening and loss of elasticity of arterial walls. It assumes 3 distinctive morphologic forms.
   a. **atherosclerosis** — the most common form in which an intimal plaque or atheroma is produced by focal lipid deposits. In the beginning the atheroma is soft and pasty. With time the plaque may undergo fibrosis and calcification or it may ulcerate into the arterial lumen. Ulcerated plaques are prone to cause mural thrombosis and eventually arterial occlusion. Arteriosclerosis and atherosclerosis are frequently used as synonyms.
   b. **arteriolosclerosis** — a vascular disorder which affects the small arteries and arterioles and seems to be secondary to hypertension.
   c. **Mönckeberg's medial calcific sclerosis, medial calcinosis** — a vascular disorder in which ring-like calcifications occur in the media of muscular arteries. It is clinically of little importance since the medial lesions fail to encroach on the arterial lumen.[131]

8. **arteriosclerosis obliterans** — arterial obstruction of extremities, particularly affecting the lower limbs and causing ischemia.[76]

9. **carotid occlusive disease** — extracranial cerebrovascular disorder characterized by atheromatous lesions which obstruct the internal carotids and if progressive and severe may lead to reduced blood flow to the brain, transient ischemic attacks, cerebrovascular insufficiency and stroke.[166]

10. **coarctation of aorta** — constriction of a segment of the aorta.[76]

11. **dilatation of aorta** — abnormal enlargement of the aorta.

12. **embolism** — a "throwing in"; blocking of a blood vessel by a clot or other substance brought to its place by the circulating blood.[47, 118]

13. **hypertension** — a pathological elevation of the blood pressure.[114, 61, 153]

14. **hypertensive vascular disease** — sustained high blood pressure associated with cardiovascular, renal and retinal changes.[46, 143, 14]

15. **peripheral arterial insufficiency of extremities** — impaired circulation to the extremities, particularly to the lower limbs. It is characterized by claudication, coldness, pallor, trophic changes, ulceration and gangrene in the involved extremity.[7]

16. peripheral vascular disease — any disorder directly affecting the arteries, veins and lymphatics except those of the heart.[77]
17. phlebitis — inflammation of the veins.
18. phlebosclerosis — a hardening of the walls of the veins.
19. Raynaud's disease — painful vascular disorder characterized by peripheral spasms of the digital arterioles of the fingers and toes which may result in gangrene.
20. rupture of an aneurysm — a break in the weakened vascular wall of an aneurysm associated with hemorrhage.
21. subclavian steal syndrome — symptom complex of cerebrovascular insufficiency, usually due to segmental atheromatous occlusion of the subclavian artery proximal to the vertebral artery. Since the circulation through the vertebral artery is reversed, the subclavian is said "to steal" cerebral blood. A delay in the arrival time of the radial pulse on the affected side is diagnostic of reversed vertebral artery flow. A localized murmur and a difference in brachial blood pressure are common manifestations. The patient may experience dizziness, vertigo, light headedness, tinnitus, blurred vision, headache and ataxia.[158, 90]
22. thoracic outlet syndromes — neurovascular compression syndromes affecting the structures of the thoracic outlet. Offending lesions are detected by angiography. Included are:
    a. cervical rib and scalenus anticus syndrome — a cutoff or torsion of subclavian artery may be present.
    b. scalenus anticus and pectoralis minor syndrome — a cutoff or torsion of subclavian artery and a compression or thrombosis of axillary veins may be demonstrated by angiography.
    c. scalenus anticus syndrome and tightness of costoclavicular space — a ridge-like compression of subclavian artery and venous compression or thrombosis may produce the syndrome.[97, 81]
23. thromboangiitis obliterans, Buerger's disease — inflammatory, obstructive disease involving primarily the peripheral blood vessels of the lower extremities.
24. thrombophlebitis — inflammatory reaction of the walls of veins to infection, associated with intravascular clotting.[34]
25. thrombosis — formation of blood clots in a blood vessel, leading to circulatory obstruction.[110]
26. varicose veins, varicosity — condition of having distended and tortuous veins, most commonly present in lower extremities.[30]

D. Operative Terms:

1. anastomosis of blood vessels — end-to-end union of two different blood vessels or two segments of same blood vessel after excision of lesion.
2. anastomosis for aortic coarctation — joining the aortic segments end-to-end after removal of constricted region or joining the left subclavian to the descending aorta if former method is not feasible.
3. aneurysmectomy — removal of an aneurysm.
4. aneurysm, resection of — excision of aneurysm and repair of arterial defect by insertion of homograft or prosthesis.
5. arterial homograft — arteries obtained at autopsies under aseptic technic and preserved by freezing, dry freezing or chemicals in a blood vessel bank. They are used for replacing the excised segments of an artery.
6. bypass graft, autogenous — implantation of an autograft, usually a segment of a saphenous vein to bypass a vascular obstruction such as occlusive lesions of the coronary, femoropopliteal or carotid-subclavian arteries. The occluded vascular segment is left in place. Circulatory efficiency is usually restored.
7. embolectomy — emboli may be excised directly or removed by retrograde method via femoral arteries by balloon catheter. With balloon deflated Fogarty catheter is inserted into a vein where embolus is located. When in proper position, the balloon is inflated. By withdrawing the catheter the clot is pulled through the incision to the body surface.[50, 87]

8. endarterectomy — removal of the inner coat (intima) of an artery for occlusive vascular disease.
9. femoropopliteal arterial reconstruction — bypass surgery for restoring the circulation in femoral artery occlusion. The saphenous vein is removed from the knee to the saphenofemoral junction and the obstruction is bypassed by an autogenous graft of the saphenous vein.
10. femorotibial bypass grafting — autogenous graft of reversed saphenous vein or reversed cephalic vein placed from common femoral artery to posterior or anterior tibial artery to bypass the obstructed arterial segment.[82, 160]
11. phleborrhaphy — suture of a vein.
12. phlebotomy — opening of a vein; for example, to reduce high red count in polycythemia vera by bloodletting.
13. shunt for portal hypertension — method of diverting a large volume of blood from the hypertensive portal system into the normal systemic venous circulation. This operation prevents hemorrhages from esophageal varices which result from portal hypertension. Procedures used at present are:
    a. an anastomosis of the portal vein and the inferior vena cava, known as portacaval shunt.
    b. an anastomosis of the splenic vein with the left renal vein.
14. subclavian steal syndrome operations:
    a. carotid-subclavian anastomosis — joining the carotid and subclavian arteries to improve cerebral blood flow.
    b. carotid-subclavian bypass graft — implanting an autograft in carotid and subclavian arteries to bypass the occluded segment of the subclavian artery.[4, 27]
    c. subclavian-subclavian bypass — inserting a knitted preclotted Dacron graft and anastomosing one end of the graft with the right and the other end with the left subclavian artery thus creating a crossover bypass of the occluded arterial segment.[45]
15. thrombectomy — removal of a thrombus; for example, from an occluded portal vein.
16. vein stripping — surgical procedure to relieve varicosity.
17. venesection — incision into a vein.

E. Symptomatic Terms:

1. acrocyanosis — bluish discoloration of finger tips and toes.
2. angiospasm, vasospasm — involuntary contractions of the muscular coats of blood vessels; spasm of blood vessels.
3. claudication — limping.
    a. lower extremity claudication — inadequate blood supply associated with cramping pains in the calf muscles. It is usually relieved by rest, thus being intermittent.[167]
    b. upper extremity claudication, brachial claudication — inadequate blood supply to an arm causing intermittent or persistent cramping pain.
4. extravasation — escape of fluid; serum, lymph or blood into the adjacent tissues.
5. digital — referring to fingers and toes.
6. digital blanching — fingers and toes becoming pallid due to vasospasm of digital arterioles; seen in Raynaud's disease.
7. ischemia — local anemia of an organ or part resulting from circulatory obstruction or vasospasm.
8. paroxysmal digital cyanosis — attacks of cyanosis caused by the interruption of blood flow in palmar and plantar arteries.
9. pedal circulation — circulation in the foot.
10. pulse — contractions of an artery which can be felt by a finger.
    a. bigeminal pulse — coupled beats.
    b. Corrigan or water hammer pulse — strong, jerky beat followed by a sharp decline and collapse of beat.
    c. dicrotic pulse — arterial beat with weak secondary wave which may be mistaken for two beats.

11. pulse deficit — difference between apical heart rate and radial pulse rate, found in cardiac disease.
12. vasoconstriction — a narrowing of the vascular lumen, resulting in decreased blood supply.
13. vasodepression — collapse due to vasomotor depression.
14. vasodilatation — a widening of the vascular lumen, increasing the blood supply to a part.
15. vasomotor — referring to nerves which control the muscular contractions of blood vessels.

RADIOLOGY

A. Terms Related to the Radiographic Examination of the Blood Vessels:

1. aortography — injection of opaque solution for x-ray examination of the aorta.[9, 164]
   a. abdominal — direct injection of contrast medium into the aorta for examining the abdominal arteries.
   b. thoracic — retrograde injection of contrast medium through a catheter introduced through the ulnar or radial artery or the carotid artery into the aorta.
2. arteriography — radiographic examination of arteries following the injection of a contrast medium.
3. femoral arteriogram — radiographic examination of the femoral and popliteal arteries after the injection of a contrast medium. A few seconds later serial films are made to detect the presence and extent of occlusive vascular disease.[162]
4. percutaneous splenoportography — radiological study of directional blood flow patterns in portal hypertension. After the injection of 40 ml of 50% Hypaque into the spleen, radiograms are taken at intervals to visualize the splenic and portal veins. The demonstration of collateral blood flow, an opaque coronary vein and short gastric veins are predictive of bleeding, especially from gastroesophageal varices. The procedure is combined with taking spleen pressures. Their elevation adds further evidence of pending hemorrhage.[79]
5. splenoportogram — a radiological image of the portal circulation obtained by injecting radiopaque material into the spleen.
6. venography — radiographic examination of veins following the injection of an opaque solution.[155, 156, 126]

B. Terms Related to the Radiographic Examinations of the Heart:

1. angiocardiography — the injection of opaque material into the basilic or cephalic veins of the arm for examining the chambers of the heart and pulmonary circulation.
   a. rapid biplane angiocardiography — the technic of simultaneously obtaining angiograms in two planes, at right angles to each other, with a speed of 10 to 12 exposures per second. It is then possible to study the atria and ventricles in the state of contraction (systole) and dilatation (diastole).[12, 72]
   b. selective angiocardiography — technic employed to concentrate an opaque solution in the specific area of the heart or blood vessel selected for study.
   c. selective coronary arteriography, **Sones technique** — injection of contrast medium into right and left coronary orifices through a tapered catheter that is manipulated under fluoroscopic or television guidance. High speed cineradiograms record the spread of the radiopaque dye through the coronary arteries. The degree of coronary opacification can be determined by direct viewing of the fluoroscopic or television screen. If there is a marked narrowing of the coronary arteries, surgery is recommended.[100]
   d. selective internal mammary arteriography, **Sones technique** — injection of a contrast medium into the internal mammary artery implants of patients who had undergone a Vineberg operation. It is an effective method for postoperative evaluation since it demonstrates how the radiopaque dye enters the myocardial tunnel and to what extent revascularization has been accomplished.[100, 24]

e. selective retrograde aortography and left ventriculography — retrograde aortic catheterization for passing a radiopaque catheter across the aortic valve into the left ventricle. The correct position of the catheter is ascertained either by fluoroscopic or television guidance or a radiograph. This method discloses ventricular septal defects, aneurysms, mitral and aortic regurgitation and other pathology.[48]

f. selective right ventricular angiography — visualization of the anatomical structures involved in tetralogy of Fallot, transposition of the great vessels, patent ductus arteriosus and similar conditions.

g. successive angiocardiograms — serial films taken at accurately recorded intervals. They reveal the time and sequence of filling of the great vessels and chambers of the heart as well as their position, size and configuration.

2. barium swallow in cardiovascular disorders — the patient drinks a barium solution while fluoroscopic and radiographic examinations are performed to reveal abnormalities of the cardiac outline and esophageal displacement.

3. cardiac tomography — sectional radiography of the heart.

4. cardiovascular spot-filming, intercalative angiography — electronically controlled spot-filming of an opacified portion of the cardiovascular system.[5]

5. cineangiocardiography — radiography of the heart and great blood vessels in motion. This complex procedure combines cardiac catheterization and selective angiocardiography. Under fluoroscopic guidance the cardiac catheter is maneuvered through the heart chambers and pulmonary artery. An image amplifier visualizes the cardiovascular structures. A motion picture camera takes from 16 to 128 pictures per second during the injection of a contrast medium. The amplified image can be seen on a television screen for group visualization. The motion pictures are projected on a screen for slow motion study of the route of the contrast medium. Cineangiocardiography offers another valuable diagnostic aid in congenital heart disease.[52]

6. radiokymography — the use of roentgen rays for recording the pulsations of the cardiac borders.[52]

CLINICAL LABORATORY

A. Terms Related to Selected Tests in Cardiovascular Conditions:

1. antistreptolysin-O titer — a diagnostic aid for rheumatic fever which may be used as screening test in statewide programs.
   Normal values — low titers of 50 Todd units or less; normal range up to 200 units.
   Increase — high titers in most cases of active rheumatic fever and streptococcal infections.[141]

2. blood culture — method of isolating the causative microorganisms in specific infectious diseases by placing blood withdrawn from a vein on or in suitable culture media. It is of value in establishing the diagnosis of bacterial endocarditis.

3. central venous pressure (CVP) — measurement of pressure within the superior vena cava reflecting the pressure of the right atrium and expressed in centimeters of water pressure. CVP provides some index of the adequacy of the pumping action of the heart and of the blood volume in the vessels.
   Normal values — usually CVP .... 5 - 8 cm of water
   Increase indicative of overload of right heart in congestive heart failure.
   Decrease suggestive of reduced blood volume and need of fluid replacement.[19]

4. circulation time — time needed for a particle of blood to pass through the entire systemic and pulmonary circulation. Ether with normal saline, calcium gluconate and other substances may be used as tracers.
   Normal values — (ether) right circuit time (arm to lung) 3.5 - 9 seconds
   Increase in cardiac failure and hypertension
   Decrease in anemia and hyperthyroidism.

5. C-reactive protein antiserum — nonspecific test for tissue breakdown and disseminated inflammatory conditions. It is often used to follow the clinical course of the disease. Results are usually positive in rheumatic fever and carditis, rheumatoid arthritis, arteriosclerotic heart disease with myocardial infarction, Hodgkin's disease, widespread invasive malignancies and infections.[141]

6. erythrocyte sedimentation rate — speed with which red blood cells settle when mixed with anticoagulant.

   Normal values — Wintrobe and Landsberg's method
   Men .... 0 - 9 mm
   Women and girls .... 0 - 20 mm

   Increase in coronary thrombosis, rheumatic fever, rheumatoid arthritis, pericarditis, tuberculosis and others.

7. serum enzymes of the heart muscle:
   a. creatine phosphokinase (CPK) — enzyme released into the blood following injury to the heart muscle or skeletal muscles.
   b. glutamic oxalacetic transaminase (GOT) — enzyme widely distributed in body tissues but found in its highest concentration in the heart muscle and liver.
   c. lactic dehydrogenase (LDH) — enzyme primarily found in the heart muscle, skeletal muscles and kidneys, also in cerebrospinal fluid, serum and serous effusion.

8. serum enzyme tests of diagnostic value in acute myocardial infarction:
   a. serum creatine phosphokinase (SCPK) — determination of serum CPK valuable in the early diagnosis of acute myocardial infarction with or without congestive heart failure. The serum enzyme is elevated 6 hours after the first occurrence of symptoms and CPK drops to a normal level within 72 hours.

   Normal values
   serum creatine phosphokinase .... males.... 0 - 20 international units
   females.... 0 - 14 international units

   Increase in early myocardial infarction.[146, 53]

   b. serum glutamic oxalacetic transaminase (SGOT) — valuable test in the detection of myocardial infarction. It aids in differentiating acute myocardial infarction from pericarditis, aortic aneurysm and acute pulmonary embolism. The release of transaminase into the blood is highly increased after a myocardial infarct.

   Normal values
   transaminase (SGOT) .... 0 - 28 Sigma-Frankel units
   .... 5 - 17 international units

   Increase in acute myocardial
   infarction .... 70 - 600 Sigma-Frankel units
   or over.

   This rise occurs within 12-24 hours after the onset of manifestations and SGOT returns to normal within 3-5 days.[146, 53]

   c. serum lactic acid dehydrogenase (SLDH) — determination of LDH activity in serum. A peak level of 3500 units of SLDH signals a grave prognosis in myocardial infarction.

   Normal values
   serum lactic acid dehydrogenase .... 100-350 Berger-Broida units
   .... 60-250 international units

   Increase in acute myocardial infarction within 48 hours after the onset of myocardial infarction lasting 5-10 days.[146, 53]

9. thrombotest — Owren's method — a capillary blood test designed as a guide to anticoagulant dosage control for quick determination at bedside and in office.
   Normal values .... 10 - 20%.

B. Terms Related to Cardiac Catheterization and Coronary Artery Catheterization:

1. cardiac catheterization, **right side** — a procedure of diagnostic value in detecting various cardiac defects and diseases. A radiopaque cardiac catheter is inserted into an accessible vein and passed into the heart and pulmonary artery.
   Various technics may be employed. If the basilic or the cephalic vein is used as a starting point, the catheter passes through the innominate vein and superior vena cava into the right atrium, right ventricle and pulmonary artery. If the saphenous vein is used, the catheter enters the heart through the inferior vena cava and traces its course through the cardiac chambers and pulmonary artery. Oxygen saturation of the blood in the chambers and the pressure recorded therein determine the defect within the heart, if present. Although this procedure is of great diagnostic value in congenital heart lesions it is incomplete if cineangiography does not accompany the hemodynamic data.[119]
   In **atrial septal defect** the catheter findings usually demonstrate a left to right shunt in the right atrium and the catheter may pass readily into the left atrium.
   In **patent ductus arteriosus** the catheter moves from the right atrium to the right ventricle and pulmonary artery. It may pass through the open ductus and enter the descending aorta if it is large. A left to right shunt of fully saturated blood will be found.[119, 54]

2. cardiac catheterization, **left side** — there are several ways of accomplishing the objective of obtaining pressures and blood samples in the left side of the heart.
   a. The **suprasternal** or **Radner method** may be done by inserting a needle behind the suprasternal notch and directing it downward into the left atrium. The pulmonary artery, aorta and left ventricle can be entered by the same method.
   b. The **transseptal** or **Ross method** consists of inserting a long needle through a catheter up to the right atrium and then pushing the needle out the catheter and puncturing the atrial septum at the foramen ovale.[119, 54]

3. cardiac pressures — pressures created by the force of the contraction within the heart chambers upon the circulating blood.

Normal values — resting individual	Intracardiac and Intravascular Pressures[119]
right atrium	2 - 4/ mm Hg
right ventricle	25 - 30/ 0 mm Hg
pulmonary artery	25 - 30/10 mm Hg
left atrium	4 - 6 mm Hg
left ventricle	120/ 4 mm Hg
aorta	120/80 mm Hg

Increase in some cardiac defects.

4. hemodynamics — a study of blood circulation and blood pressure.

5. oscilloscope — an instrument for recording electric vibrations as those made by blood pressure or heart sounds upon a television monitoring screen.

6. percutaneous transfemoral catheterization of **coronary arteries**, Judkins technique — a method of choice for rapid selective catheterization of both coronary arteries using preshaped right and left catheters with coronary-seeking tip configurations and positive control feature.[80]
   Under fluoroscopic or television guidance a catheter is introduced percutaneously into the common femoral artery and advanced via aortic arch to the coronary orifice.
   Catheter manipulation differs for selective left and right coronary artery catheterization.
   Following contrast injection rapid direct serial radiography and cinephotofluorography provide coronary visualization thereby revealing the presence and extent of occlusive arterial heart disease.[119]

C. Terms Related to Special Recordings of Heart Action:

1. ballistocardiography — electrographic recording of bodily movements during the cardiac cycle.[37, 55]

2. echocardiography — graphic recording of ultrasound waves reflected from the heart for the purpose of
   a. studying the development of mitral stenosis from the onset of rheumatic heart disease
   b. determining the severity of mitral stenosis and
   c. appraising the leaflet motion after mitral valvotomy.[165, 63, 64]

3. electrocardiography — graphic recording of the electrical waves of the cardiac cycle or spread of excitation throughout the heart. It is an invaluable diagnostic aid in the detection of arrhythmias and myocardial damage. The meaning of the waves is:[53, 151]
   a. P wave — wave reflects the contraction of the atria.
   b. PR interval — period in which the impulse passes through the atria and AV node, normally 0.16 - 0.20 seconds.

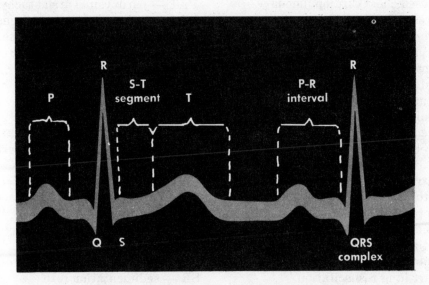

Fig. 39 – Normal electrocardiographic cycle.

   c. QRS complex — waves represent ventricular excitation or depolarization of the ventricular myocardium, normally 0.12 seconds.[163, 112]
   d. Q wave — downward deflection and beginning of the complex.
   e. R wave — large upward wave.
   f. S wave — second large downward deflection and end of the QRS complex.
   g. ST segment — the interval between the completion of depolarization and recovery of ventricular muscle fibers. The segment may be depressed or elevated in myocardial injury.
   h. T wave — recovery phase following the contraction. Inversion of the T wave usually reflects injury or ischemia of the heart muscle.[112]

4. electrokymography — recording of the movements of the heart and great vessels by an electrokymograph.

5. kinetocardiography, precordial cardiography — a method of recording vibrations of the chest wall produced by heart action.[55]

6. phonocardiography — graphic recording of heart sounds, usually on an oscilloscope for quick scanning or upon a tape recorder for a permanent record.[55]

7. phonocardiography, intracardiac — sound tracing recorded from within the cardiac chambers through a phonocatheter which has a microphone at the tip. Method seeks to detect minor defects not revealed by cardiac catheterization.

8. plethysmography — instrumental recording of variations in size of a part or organ caused by fluctuations in the size of the vascular bed.

9. ultrasound cardiography — same as echocardiography.[91, 71, 62, 169]

10. vectorcardiography — graphic recording of the direction and magnitude of the electrical forces of the heart.[101]

ABBREVIATIONS

ACG — angiocardiography
AHA — American Heart Association
ASD — atrial septal defect
ASHD — arteriosclerotic heart disease
ASO — arteriosclerosis obliterans
AV — atrioventricular, atriovenous
BBB — bundle branch block
BP — blood pressure
CCCR — closed chest cardiopulmonary resuscitation
CCU — coronary care unit
CHD — coronary heart disease
CHF — congestive heart failure
CPB — cardiopulmonary bypass
CPK — creatine phosphokinase
CPR — cardiopulmonary resuscitation
CRP — C-reactive protein
CVA — cerebrovascular accident
CVD — cardiovascular disease
CVP — central venous pressure
DM — diastolic murmur
ECG — electrocardiogram
EKG — electrocardiogram
ESR — erythrocyte sedimentation rate
Hg — mercury
HLR — heart-lung resuscitation
HVD — hypertensive vascular disease
IASD — interatrial septal defect
IVC — inferior vena cava
IVSD — interventricular septal defect
LA — left atrium
LD — lactic dehydrogenase
LHF — left heart failure

LV — left ventricle
LVH — left ventricular hypertrophy
M — murmurs
MI — myocardial infarction
mm Hg — millimeters of mercury
MS — mitral stenosis
PA — pulmonary artery
PAC — premature atrial contractions
PAT — paroxysmal atrial tachycardia
PDA — patent ductus arteriosus
PPS — postperfusion syndrome
PVC — premature ventricular contractions
RA — right atrium
RCA — right coronary artery
RF — rheumatic fever
RHF — right heart failure
RV — right ventricle
RVH — right ventricular hypertrophy
SA — sinoatrial (node)
SBE — subacute bacterial endocarditis
SGOT — serum glutamic oxalacetic transaminase
SGPT — serum glutamic pyruvic transaminase
SLD — serum lactic acid dehydrogenase
SR — sedimentation rate
SVC — superior vena cava
TIA — transient ischemic attack
VC — vena cava
VCG — vectorcardiogram
VHD — valvar heart disease
VSD — ventricular septal defect
WPW — Wolff-Parkinson-White (syndrome)

ORAL READING PRACTICE

Coarctation of the Aorta

Coarctation of the aorta is one of the most interesting **congenital cardiovascular** defects amenable to surgery. It consists of a constriction of a segment of the aorta and occurs in two types. The first type is a rare condition in which the aortic obstruction is located proximal to the **ductus arteriosus.** The **lumen** of the **aorta** is atretic or completely blocked so that the impairment of the systemic circulation presents a grave problem. This defect is incompatible with life and the child dies in infancy if corrective surgery cannot be performed.

The other type of coarctation is a common form which yields to surgical intervention. There may be either a narrowing or a complete **stenosis** of the **aortic lumen distal** to the left **subclavian** artery and to the insertion of the ductus. The latter is generally **ligamentous** and **obliterated.**

The aorta near the constriction appears to be normal in size, but its major proximate branches are generally enlarged. The **intercostal** arteries distal to the obstruction, likewise, show an increase in size. The constriction of the aorta is usually limited to a short segment and permits a fair life expectancy, if not associated with other cardiovascular defects.

The outstanding diagnostic characteristic of aortic coarctation is a high blood pressure in the arms and a low blood pressure with a barely perceptible pulse in the legs. The differential diagnosis hinges on this disparity of the blood pressure in the extremities and the diminished or absent **femoral** pulse. Since the oxygenated blood reaches the systemic circulation, the patient's color remains normal. Hypertension may lead to **cerebrovascular** accident. In addition infection presents a constant threat to the **debilitated** patient since nutritional deficiency may accompany the impoverished systemic circulation.

When a short aortic segment is constricted, the clinical symptoms are absent or so minimal that they may escape notice, especially in childhood. In adolescence, symptoms of **fatigability,** decreased exercise tolerance, **epistaxis, syncope** and coldness of the feet tend to develop and cause varying degrees of disability. In untreated cases the life span rarely exceeds the fourth decade. Death may ensue from **rupture** of the aorta, **bacterial endocarditis** or **congestive** heart failure.

Efforts to relieve coarctation involve one of the most daring operations on the great vessels of the cardiovascular system. The optimum age for surgical correction is within the second decade of life according to Gross and between the ages of six and twelve years according to Hufnagel. During this period the aorta has a high degree of elasticity, works with facility, shows little or no evidence of **degenerative** changes and is in good condition for making a sizable anastomosis.

The surgical procedure consists of the removal of the constricted region and an end-to-end anastomosis of the aortic segments. Where no surgical communication of the aortic segments can be created, the left subclavian artery may be joined to the descending aorta.

Postoperatively, progress is spectacular. The blood pressure in upper and lower extremities equalizes, the femoral artery pulsation is present almost immediately and the circulation is markedly improved. The most dreaded complications are infection of the suture line resulting in leakage or dissolution of the anastomosis.[144]

Table 6

SOME CARDIOVASCULAR CONDITIONS AMENABLE TO SURGERY

Organs Involved	Diagnoses	Operations	Procedures
Heart Pulmonary artery Aorta	Patent ductus arteriosus	Complete division of ductus arteriosus	Obliteration of ductus by dividing ductus and suturing the cut ends
Heart Pulmonary artery Aorta	Complete transposition of the pulmonary artery and of the aorta	Blalock-Hanlon operation Closed heart surgery	Right thoracotomy and exposure of interatrial groove. Occlusion of vessels, application of Satinsky-type clamp, section of both atria Removal of segment and portion of septum
Heart Atria Septum	Interatrial septal defect	Repair of interatrial septal defect Open method under direct vision	Interatrial septal defect closed by direct suture or patch Extracorporeal circulation
Heart Ventricles Septum	Congenital heart disease Interventricular septal defect with pulmonary hypertension	Banding of pulmonary artery	Pulmonary artery constricted with umbilical tape in instances where direct closure is contra-indicated

Organs Involved	Diagnoses	Operations	Procedures
Heart Ventricles Septum	Interventricular septal defect	Open cardiotomy and repair of interventricular defect under direct vision	Incision into right ventricle and exposure of defect Repair with suture or ventricular patch Extracorporeal circulation with or without hypothermia

Heart
Ventricles
Pulmonary artery
	Tetralogy of Fallot
	  1. ventricular defect
	  2. pulmonic stenosis
	  3. dextroposition of arota
	  4. hypertrophy of right ventricle
		Shunting operations
		  Blalock's method
		  Potts-Smith's method
		Brock's operation
		Total correction of Tetralogy of Fallot
		Open heart surgery
			Joining right or left subclavian to pulmonary artery
			Anastomosis between pulmonary artery and aorta
			Removal of pulmonic obstruction
			Defects totally repaired using suture closure or patch for closure
			Infundibulum resected to correct pulmonary stenosis
			Cardiopulmonary bypass with or without hypothermia

Heart Atria Ventricles	Atherosclerotic, heart disease Adams-Stokes syndrome atrioventricular block	Insertion of transvenous endocardial pacemaker	Catheter electrode passed through incision in jugular vein and lodged in apex of right ventricle Subcutaneous tunnel and pocket constructed Catheter electrode fastened to pacemaker Pacemaker inserted into pocket
Heart Left ventricle	Ventricular aneurysm Left heart failure	Ventricular aneurysmectomy Open heart surgery	Transverse sternotomy with bilateral thoracotomy; heart opened Removal of aneurysm, its sac and related thrombus Reconstruction of left ventricle and closure of heart Extracorporeal circulation with or without hypothermia
Heart Right atrium	Myxoma of right atrium with progressive right heart failure	Atriotomy with excision of primary cardiac tumor Open heart surgery	Right atrium opened and myxoma removed Use of cardiopulmonary bypass with or without hypothermia
Heart Pericardium	Constrictive pericarditis Adherent pericardium	Pericardiectomy Pericardiolysis	Partial removal of pericardium Breaking up of adhesions
Heart Myocardium Coronary arteries	Obstructive coronary artery disease with myocardial ischemia and angina pectoris	**Direct Revascularization** Aortocoronary artery bypass (right) with autogenous grafts of saphenous vein Open heart surgery	Surgical creation of new ostium in ascending aorta and new openings into vessels of the aortic arch for implanting the proximal ends of the vein grafts Anastomoses of distal ends of grafts with coronary arteries to bypass occlusive lesion Extracorporeal circulation with or without hypothermia

Organs Involved	Diagnoses	Operations	Procedures
Heart Myocardium Coronary arteries	Atherosclerotic heart disease with occlusions in major coronary arteries and severe perfusion deficit	**Indirect Revascularization** Median sternotomy Vineberg-Sewell bilateral implants Open heart surgery	Sternal split incision Implantation of both internal thoracic arteries into the anterior and posterior wall of the left ventricle Extracorporeal circulation with or without hypothermia
Heart	Far advanced occlusive coronary artery disease, diffuse myocardial damage, irreversible left ventricular failure	Median sternotomy Cardiac homotransplantation	Sternal split incision Simultaneous division of aorta, pulmonary artery and atria followed by excision of donor and recipient hearts Implantation of donor heart by atrial and vascular anastomoses to recipient heart Extracorporeal circulation with or without hypothermia
Heart Pulmonary valve	Pulmonic valvar stenosis	Pulmonary valvotomy Closed method or Open heart surgery	Division and dilation of valve Extracorporeal circulation if open method used
Heart Mitral valve	Mitral stenosis due to rheumatic carditis Combined mitral stenosis and mitral insufficiency	Mitral commissurotomy Mitral valvoplasty	Separation of commissure of stenotic valve Suture or plastic repair of valve; use of prosthesis
Heart Aortic valve Mitral valve	Aortic stenosis and insufficiency Mitral stenosis and insufficiency due to rheumatic heart disease	Excision and replacement of aortic valve and mitral valve with Starr-Edwards aortic and mitral prostheses	Removal of calcified cusps of aortic valve and seating of aortic prosthesis Total removal of calcified mitral valve and insertion of mitral valve prosthesis Extracorporeal circulation, coronary artery perfusion and hypothermia
Aorta	Dissecting aneurysm of thoracic aorta	Resection of aneurysm Replacement with a plastic prosthesis	Aneurysm removed and defect bridged with prosthesis
Aorta	Atherosclerotic aortoiliac occlusion	Aortoiliac endarterectomy	Incision into left external iliac artery and removal of plaque Dissection of segmentally obstructed portion of intima of 1. common iliac arteries near bifurcation of aorta and 2. terminal aorta
Aorta	Aortic coarctation	Excision of coarctation Aortic anastomosis	Removal of constricted area and joining cut ends together with suture
Artery	Subclavian steal syndrome	Subclavian-subclavian crossover bypass graft	Extrathoracic approach Subclavian artery crossclamped Dacron graft anastomosed to vessel and tunneled subcutaneously in tissues of anterior neck Second anastomosis performed

Organs Involved	Diagnoses	Operations	Procedures
(Cont'd)	Left-sided proximal subclavian obstruction	Carotid-subclavian bypass graft	Supraclavicular approach Restoration of blood supply to the brachiocephalic region by using an autogenous saphenous vein graft
Artery	Occlusive femoropopliteal disease due to atherosclerotic lesions Pregangrenous state	Femoropopliteal arterial reconstruction by the use of reversed autogenous vein graft	Removal of the saphenous vein from knee to saphenofemoral junction Vein reversed and attached to patent vessel by end-to-end anastomosis bypassing the obstruction
Artery	Embolus in femoral artery	Embolectomy	Incision into femoral artery and removal of clot
Veins	Esophageal varices due to portal hypertension	Portacaval anastomosis	Joining the portal vein and the inferior vena cava to create a large shunt
Veins	Varicosity	Vein stripping	Ligation of saphenous vein; incision made and stripper introduced into vein; vein extirpated

REFERENCES AND BIBLIOGRAPHY

1. Anderson, R. P. *et al.* Direct revascularization of the heart: Early clinical experience with 200 patients. *Journal of Thoracic and Cardiovascular Surgery*, 63: 353-359, March, 1972.
2. Altschuler, A. Complete transposition of the great arteries. *American Journal of Nursing*, 71: 96-98, January, 1971.
3. Bain, B. Pacemakers and the patients who need them. *American Journal of Nursing*, 71: 1582-1585, August, 1971.
4. Barner, H. B., Kaiser, G. C. and Willman, V. L. Hemodynamics of carotid-subclavian bypass. *Archives of Surgery*, 103: 248-251, August, 1971.
5. Beach, P. M. *et al.* Aortic valve replacement with frozen irradiated homograft. *Circulation*, 45 (Suppl. 1): 29-35, May, 1972.
6. Benchimol, A. and Desser, K. B. Clinical application of the Doppler ultrasonic flowmeter. *American Journal of Cardiology*, 29: 540-545, April, 1972.
7. Bizer, L. S. Peripheral vascular trauma. *Postgraduate Medicine*, 49; 127-130, February, 1971.
8. Blomquist, C. G. Use of exercise testing for diagnostic and functional evaluation of patients with arteriosclerotic heart disease. *Circulation*, 44: 1120-1136, December, 1971.
9. Boukhris, R. and Becker, K. L. Calcification of the aorta and osteoporosis — A roentgenographic study. *Journal of American Medical Association*, 219: 1307-1311, March 6, 1972.
10. Bourassa, M. G. *et al.* Factors influencing patency of aortocoronary vein grafts. *Circulation*, 45 (Suppl. 1): 79-85, May, 1972.
11. Braunwald, E. *et al.* Cardiac arrhythmias. In Wintrobe, Maxwell M. (ed.). *Harrison's Principles of Internal Medicine*, 6th ed. New York: McGraw Hill Book Co., 1970, pp. 1142-1154.
12. —————. Chronic valvular heart disease. In Beeson, Paul B. and McDermott, Walsh. *Cecil-Loeb Textbook of Medicine*, 13th ed. Philadelphia: W. B. Saunders Co., 1971, pp. 996-1015.
13. Brener, E. R. Surgery for coronary artery disease. *American Journal of Nursing*, 72: 469-473, March, 1972.
14. Breslin, D. J. *et al.* Therapy of complicated arterial hypertension. *Medical Clinics of North America*, 56: 633-644, May, 1972.
15. Bucek, R. J. Intercalative angiography. *Radiology*, 76: 565-571, April, 1961.
16. Bucklin, R. Heart disease and the law. *Southern Medical Journal*, 65: 496-498, April, 1972.
17. Burch, G. E. and Giles, T. D. Ischemic cardiomyopathy. *Southern Medical Journal*, 65: 11-16, January, 1972.
18. Carnes, G. D. Understanding the cardiac patient's behavior. *American Journal of Nursing*, 71: 1187-1188, June, 1971.
19. Chatton, M. J. General symptoms. In Krupp, Marcus A. and Chatton, Milton J. *Current Diagnosis & Treatment*. LosAltos: Lange Medical Publications, 1972, pp. 1-12.
20. Chung, E. K. Guide to the interpretation of cardiac arrhythmias. *Postgraduate Medicine*, 50: 124-128, July, 1971.
21. Claudon, D. G. *et al.* Primary dissecting aneurysm of coronary artery. A cause of acute

myocardial ischemia, *Circulation*, 45: 259-266, February, 1972.

22. Cohn, P. F. Accuracy of two-step postexercise ECG. *Journal of American Medical Association*, 220: 501-506, April 24, 1972.

23. Cole, R. B. *et al.* Longterm results of aortopulmonary anastomosis for tetralogy of Fallot: Morbidity and mortality, 1946-1969. *Circulation*, 43: 263-271, February, 1971.

24. Conklin, E. F. *et al.* Use of the permanent transvenous pacemaker in 168 consecutive patients. *American Heart Journal*, 82: 4-15, July, 1971.

25. Cooley, D. A. *et al.* Ischemic contracture of the heart: "Stone heart." *American Journal of Cardiology*, 29: 575-577, April, 1972.

26. _____. Transplantation of the human heart. *Journal of American Medical Association*, 205: 480-486, August 12, 1968.

27. Cordell, A. R. *et al.* Current status of surgery for subclavian steal syndrome. *Surgical Clinics of North America*, 51: 1415-1422, December, 1971.

28. Culbert, P. and Kos, B. Teaching patients about pacemakers. *American Journal of Nursing*, 71: 504-506, March, 1971.

29. Dack, S. Acute myocardial infarction. In Conn, Howard F. (ed.). *Current Therapy 1972*. Philadelphia: W. B. Saunders Co., 1972, pp. 192-205.

30. Dale, A. W. Varicose veins. In Conn, Howard F. (ed.). *Current Therapy 1972*. Philadelphia: W. B. Saunders Co., 1972, pp. 225-229.

31. Davis, M. Z. Socioemotional component of coronary care. *American Journal of Nursing*, 72: 705-709, April, 1972.

32. Davis, R. W. and Ebert, P. A. Ventricular aneurysm. A clinical pathologic correlation. *American Journal of Cardiology*, 29: 1-6, January, 1972.

33. DeSanctis, R. W. Diagnostic and therapeutic uses of atrial pacing. *Circulation*, 43: 748-761, May, 1971.

34. DeWeese, M. S. Massive deep thrombophlebitis of the lower extremities. In Conn, Howard F. (ed.). *Current Therapy 1972*. Philadelphia: W. B. Saunders Co., 1972, pp. 219-224.

35. Dorney, E. F. The heart and collagen disease. In Hurst, J. Willis and Logue R. Bruce. *The Heart Arteries and Veins*, 2nd ed. New York: McGraw Hill Book Co., 1970, pp. 1387-1392.

36. Ebert, R. V. Use of anticoagulants in acute myocardial infarction. *Circulation*, 45: 903-910, April, 1972.

37. Eddleman, E. E. *et al.* A critical appraisal of ballistocardiography. *American Journal of Cardiology*, 29: 120-122, January, 1972.

38. Effler, D. B. Myocardial revascularization — direct or indirect? *Journal of Thoracic and Cardiovascular Surgery*, 61: 498-500, March, 1971.

39. _____. Current era of revascularization surgery. *Surgical Clinics of North America*, 51: 1009-1014, October, 1971.

40. _____. Vineberg's operation for myocardial ischemia. *Postgraduate Medicine*, 37: 304-305, March, 1965.

41. England, R. A. Treatment of ventricular arrhythmias in ambulatory patients. *Medical Clinics of North America*, 56: 615-624, May, 1972.

42. Everett, E. D. Pericarditis due to Entamoeba histolytica. *Southern Medical Journal*, 65: 501-502, April, 1972.

43. Favaloro, R. G. Direct myocardial revascularization. *Surgical Clinics of North America*, 51: 1035-1042, October, 1971.

44. Fehmers, M.C.O. *et al.* Intramuscularly and orally administered lidocaine in treatment of ventricular arrhythmias in acute myocardial infarction. *American Journal of Cardiology*, 29: 514-519, April, 1972.

45. Finkelstein, N. M. *et al.* Subclavian-subclavian bypass for the subclavian steal syndrome. *Surgery*, 71: 142-145, January, 1972.

46. Finnerty, F. A. Hypertension. In Conn, Howard F. (ed.). *Current Therapy 1972*. Philadelphia: W. B. Saunders Co., 1972, pp. 187-192.

47. Fisher, D. A. *et al.* Atherothrombotic emboli in the lower extremities. *Archives of Dermatology*, 104: 533-537, November, 1971.

48. Fleming, R. J. *et al.* Radiologic findings resulting from thoracic aortic surgery — congenital and acquired diseases. *Radiologic Clinics of North America*, 9: 253-264, August, 1971.

49. Floyd, W. L. Pericarditis. On Conn, Howard F. (ed.). *Current Therapy 1972*. Philadelphia: W. B. Saunders Co., 1972, pp. 206-209.

50. Fogarty, T. J. *et al.* Experience with balloon catheter technic for arterial embolectomy. *American Journal of Surgery*, 122: 231-237, August, 1971.

51. Frenay, Sr. Agnes C. and Pierce, G. L. The climate of care for a geriatric patient. *American Journal of Nursing*, 71: 1747-1750, September, 1971.

52. Friedberg, C. K. *Diseases of the Heart*, 3d ed. Philadelphia: W. B. Saunders Co., 1966, pp. 12-13.

53. _____. Objective manifestations of acute myocardial infarction. *Ibid.*, pp. 806-849.

54. _____. Cardiac catheterization. *Ibid.*, pp. 107-133.

55. _____. Phonocardiography and other graphic methods. *Ibid.*, pp. 74-106.

56. Gardner, Ernest, Gray, Donald and O'Rahilly, Ronan. *Anatomy — A Regional Study of Human Structure*, 3d ed. Philadelphia: W. B. Saunders Co., 1969, pp. 329-355.

57. Gaul, A. L. *et al.* Hyperbaric oxygen therapy. *American Journal of Nursing*, 72: 892-896, May, 1972.

58. Gazes, P. C. Treatment of heart failure, Part 1. *Postgraduate Medicine*, 51: 199-204, January, 1972.

59. _____. Part 2. *Ibid.*, 51: 209-212, February, 1972.

60. _____. Adams-Stokes syndrome: Indications for permanent pacemakers. *Postgraduate Medicine*, 50: 199-203, October, 1971.

61. Gilmore, H. R. The treatment of chronic hypertension. *Medical Clinics of North America*, 55: 317-324, March, 1971.

62. Goldberg, B. B. Teletransmission of ultrasonograms. *Radiology*, 103: 457-459, May, 1972.

63. Gramiak, R. *et al.* Cardiac ultrasonography. *Radiologic Clinics of North America*, 9: 469-490, December, 1971.

65. Griepp, R. B. *et al.* Determinants of operative risk in human heart transplantation. *American Journal of Surgery*, 122: 192-196, August, 1971.

66. —————. Use of antithymocyte globulin in human heart transplantation. *Circulation*, 45 (Suppl. 1): 147-153, May, 1972.

67. Hackel, D. B. *et al.* Anatomic studies of the cardiac conducting system in acute myocardial infarction. *American Heart Journal*, 83: 77-81, January, 1972.

68. Hancock, E. W. *et al.* Valve replacement in active bacterial endocarditis. *Journal of Infectious Diseases*, 123: 106, January, 1971.

69. Hansing, C. E. Tricuspid insufficiency — a study of hemodynamics and pathogenesis. *Circulation*, 45: 793-799, April, 1972.

70. Hockberg, H. M. Effects of electrical current on heart rhythm. *American Journal of Nursing*, 71: 1390-1394, July, 1971.

71. Hokanson, D. E. *et al.* Ultrasonic arteriography. A noninvasive method of arterial visualization. *Radiology*, 102: 435-436, February, 1972.

72. Howell, T. R. *et al.* Radiologic and other diagnostic clues in congenital and acquired heart disease. *Radiologic Clinics of North America*, 9: 397-443, December, 1970.

73. Huang, T. Y. Cardiac pathology of transverse pacemakers. *American Heart Journal*, 83: 469-472, April, 1972.

74. Hunt, C. E. *et al.* Banding in pulmonary artery. *Circulation*, 43: 395-406, March, 1971.

75. Hurst, J. W. and Schlant, R. C. Examination of the veins. In Hurst, J. Willis and Logue, R. Bruce. *The Heart Arteries and Veins*, 2d ed. New York: McGraw-Hill Book Co., 1970, pp. 182-192.

76. Hurst, J. Willis. Diseases of the aorta. In Beeson, Paul B. and McDermott, Walsh, (eds.). *Cecil-Loeb Textbook of Medicine*, 13th ed. Philadelphia: W. B. Saunders Co., 1971, pp. 1107-1119.

77. Jackson, B. S. Chronic peripheral arterial disease. *American Journal of Nursing*, 72: 928-934, May, 1972.

78. Jackson, D. R. Living homologous saphenous vein in geriatric femoropopliteal bypass grafting. *Vascular Surgery*, 5: 6-11, January-February, 1971.

79. Jackson, F. C. Directional flow patterns in portal hypertension. *Archives of Surgery*, 87: 307-319, August, 1963.

80. Judkins, M. P. Selective coronary arteriography. *Radiology*, 89: 815-824, November, 1967.

81. Judy, K. L. *et al.* Vascular complications of thoracic outlet syndrome. *American Journal of Surgery*, 123: 521-531, May, 1972.

82. Kaminski, D. L., Barnes, H. B. Dorighi, J. A., Kaiser, G. C. and Willman, V. L. Femoraltibial bypass grafting. *Archives of Surgery*, 104: 527-531, April, 1972.

83. Kantor, G. L. *et al.* Cytomegalvirus-induced postperfusion syndrome. *Seminars in Hematology*, 8: 261-265, July, 1971.

84. —————. Cytomegalovirus infection associated with cardiopulmonary bypass. *Archives of Internal Medicine*, 125: 488-492, March, 1970.

85. Karliner, J. S. *et al.* Present status of digitalis treatment of acute myocardial infarction. *Circulation*, 45: 891-902, April, 1972.

86. Karpman, L. The murmur of aortocoronary bypass. *American Heart Journal*, 83: 179-181, February, 1972.

87. Kartchner, M. M. Retrograde arterial embolectomy for limb salvage. *Archives of Surgery*, 104: 532-535, April, 1972.

88. Kay, C. F. Cardiac arrhythmias. In Beeson, P. B. and McDermott, Walsh, (eds.). *Cecil-Loeb Textbook of Medicine*, 13th ed. Philadelphia: W. B. Saunders Co., 1971, pp. 1066-1082.

89. Keller, J. W. *et al.* Rhythm anomalies in contemporary demand pacing. *American Journal of Cardiology*, 29: 572-574, April, 1972.

90. Killen, D. A. *et al.* Subclavian steal syndrome due to anomalous isolation of the left subclavian artery. *Archives of Surgery*, 104: 342-344, March, 1972.

91. King, D. L. Cardiac ultrasonography. A stop-action technique for imaging intracardiac anatomy. *Radiology*, 103: 387-392, May, 1972.

92. Kirklin, J. W. Pulmonary atrial banding in babies with large ventricular defects. *Circulation*, 43: 321-322, March, 1971.

93. Konno, S. *et al.* Catheter biopsy of the heart. *Radiologic Clinics of North America*, 9: 491-510, December, 1971.

94. Krakauer, J. S. *et al.* Clinical management ancillary to phase-shift balloon pumping in cardiogenic shock. *American Journal of Cardiology*, 27: 123-128, February, 1971.

95. Kraus, K. R. *et al.* Acute coronary insufficiency — course and followup, *Circulation*, 45 (Suppl. 1): 66-71, May, 1972.

96. Kukral, J. C. and Paulissian, E. B. Acute limb ischemia. *Surgical Clinics of North America*, 52: 125-143, February, 1972.

97. Lang, E. K. Arteriography and venography in the assessment of thoracic outlet syndromes. *Southern Medical Journal*, 65: 129-136, February, 1972.

98. Lasseter, K. C. Treatment of arrhythmias: Basic considerations. *Medical Clinics of North America*, 55: 435-444, March, 1971.

99. Lawrence, M. S. Endocarditis due to group C streptococci. *Southern Medical Journal*, 65: 487-489, April, 1972.

100. Lehman, J. S. Selective coronary arteriography. *Radiology*, 83: 836-853, November, 1964.

101. Levine, H. D. *et al.* Electrocardiogram and vectorcardiogram in myocardial infarction. *Circulation*, 45: 457-470, February, 1972.

102. Libretti A. *et al.* A cardiac murmur depending on Wolff-Parkinson-White syndrome. *American Heart Journal*, 83: 532-534, April, 1972.

103. Loop, F. D. Myocardial revascularization by internal mammary artery grafts: A technique without optical assistance. *Journal of Thoracic*

and Cardiovascular Surgery, 63: 674-680, April, 1972.

104. _____. Ventricular aneurysmectomy. *Surgical Clinics of North America,* 51: 1071-1079, October, 1971.

105. Luisida, A. Cardiac catheterization. *Hospital Medicine,* 2: 21-26, November, 1965.

106. Malach, M. Peritoneal dialysis for intractable heart failure in acute myocardial infarction. *American Journal of Cardiology,* 29: 61-63, January, 1972.

107. Mark, H. *et al.* Treatment of Wolff-Parkinson-White syndrome. *American Heart Journal,* 83: 565-569, April, 1972.

108. Master, A. M. Silent coronary artery disease: Two-step exercise test for diagnosis. *Postgraduate Medicine,* 50: 104-108, December, 1971.

109. Mayer, J. Nutrition and heart disease: National Commission Report. *Postgraduate Medicine,* 49: 257-259, February, 1971.

110. McDonough, J. J. and Altemeier, W. A. Subclavian venous thrombosis secondary to indwelling catheters. *Surgery Gynecology & Obstetrics.* 133: 397-400, September, 1971.

111. McHenry, P. L. *et al.* Cardiac arrhythmias observed during maximal treadmill exercise testing in clinically normal men. *American Journal of Cardiology,* 29: 331-336, March, 1972.

112. Meltzer, Lawrence E., Pinneo, R. and Kitchell, J. R. The electrocardiographic basis of arrhythmias — Arrhythmias. In *Intensive Coronary Care,* 2d ed. New York: The Charles Press Publishers Inc., 1970, pp. 109-180.

113. _____. The electrical treatment of arrhythmias — cardiac pacing — precordial shock. *Ibid.,* pp. 181-204.

114. Mendlowitz, M. A practical approach to the diagnosis and treatment of hypertension. *Geriatrics,* 27: 105-110, January, 1972.

115. Midell, A. I. and DeBoer, A. Multiple valve replacement. *Archives of Surgery,* 104: 471-476, April, 1972.

116. Mitchell, S. C. Congenital heart disease in 56,109 births. *Circulation,* 43: 323-332, March, 1971.

117. Morgan, C. V. *et al.* Permanent cardiac pacing for sinoatrial bradycardia. *Journal of Thoracic and Cardiovascular Surgery,* 63: 453-457, March, 1972.

118. Motamed, H. A. Fundamental aspects of post-multiple injury fat embolism. *Clinical Orthopaedics and Related Research,* 82: 169-181, January-February, 1972.

119. Mudd, Gerard, M. D. Personal communications.

120. Mullins, C. B. Heartblock. In Conn, Howard F. (ed.). *Current Therapy 1972.* Philadelphia: W. B. Saunders Co., 1972, pp. 159-164.

121. Murray, J. A. *et al.* Left ventricular function following internal mammary implantation. *American Heart Journal,* 83: 41-49, January, 1972.

122. Ochsner, J. L. Surgery for myocardial revascularization. *Postgraduate Medicine,* 49: 127-129, April, 1971.

123. Oldham, H. N. Cardiac arrest. In Conn, Howard F. (ed.). *Current Therapy 1972.* pp. 151-154.

124. Pfaffenberger, R. S. Prevention of heart disease. *Postgraduate Medicine,* 51: 74-78, January, 1972.

125. Portsmann, W. *et al.* Catheter closure of patent ductus arteriosus: 62 cases treated without thoracotomy. *Radiologic Clinics of North America,* 9: 203-218, August, 1971.

126. Rabinow, K. *et al.* Roentgen diagnosis of venous thrombosis in the leg. *Archives of Surgery,* 104: 134-144, February, 1972.

127. Rashkind, W. J. Atrioseptostomy by balloon catheter in congenital heart disease. *Radiologic Clinics of North America,* 9: 193-202, August, 1971.

128. Razavi, M. Indirect myocardial revascularization. *Surgical Clinics of North America,* 51, 1059-1069, October, 1971.

129. Read, M. and Mallison, M. External arteriovenous shunts. *American Journal of Nursing,* 72: 81-85, January, 1972.

130. Reul, G. J. Experience with coronary artery bypass grafts in the treatment of coronary artery disease. *Surgery,* 71: 586-593, April, 1972.

131. Robbins, S. L. *Textbook of Pathology,* 3d ed. Philadelphia: W. B. Saunders Co., 1967, p. 573.

132. Rogel, S. and Mahler, Y. The universal pacer: A synchronized-demand pacemaker. *Journal of Thoracic and Cardiovascular Surgery,* 61: 466-471, March, 1971.

133. Ross, R. S. Ischemic heart disease. In Wintrobe, M. M. (ed.) *Harrison's Principles of Internal Medicine,* 6th ed. New York: McGraw-Hill Book Co., 1970, pp. 1210-1211.

134. Russek, H. J. Etiologic factors in ischemic heart disease: The elusive role of emotional stress. *Geriatrics,* 27: 81-86, January, 1972.

135. Russell, T. *et al.* Late hemodynamic function of cloth covered Starr-Edwards valve prostheses. *Circulation,* 45 (Suppl. 1): 8-13, May, 1972.

136. Rutledge, D. I. The management of paroxysmal atrial fibrillation. *Medical Clinics of North America,* 56: 611-614, May, 1972.

137. Sarachek, N. S. and Leonard, J. J. Familial heart attack and sinus bradycardia. *American Journal of Cardiology,* 29: 451-458, April, 1972.

138. Segal, B. L. *et al.* Echocardiography. *Journal of American Medical Association,* 195: 161-166, January, 1966.

139. Selzer, A. Atrial fibrillation. In Conn, Howard F. (ed.). *Current Therapy 1972.* Philadelphia: W. B. Saunders Co., 1972, pp. 154-157.

140. Selzer, A. *et al.* Natural history of mitral stenosis — a review. *Circulation,* 45: 878-890, April, 1972.

141. Shaffer, J. G. Serodiagnostic tests other than syphilis. In Davidson, Israel and Henry, John B. (ed.). *Todd-Sanford Clinical Diagnosis by Laboratory Methods,* 14th ed. Philadelphia: W. B. Saunders Co., 1969, pp. 1131-1150.

142. Sheldon, W. C. *et al.* Direct myocardial revascularization: Venous autograft technique. *Surgical Clinics of North America,* 51: 1043-1049, October, 1971.

143. Sheps, S. G. Hypertensive crisis. *Postgraduate Medicine,* 49: 95-99, May, 1971.

144. Shumway, N. E. and Griepp, R. B. Cardiac homotransplants. In Sabiston, David C. (ed.).

Davis-Christopher Textbook of Surgery, 10th ed. Philadelphia: W. B. Saunders Co., 1972, pp. 511-522.

145. Sigel, B. *et al.* Diagnosis of lower limb venous thrombosis by Doppler ultrasound technique. *Archives of Surgery*, 104: 174-179, February, 1972.

146. Sobel, B. E. Serum enzymes determinations in the diagnosis and assessment of myocardial infarction. *Circulation*, 45: 471-482, February, 1972.

147. Sokolow, M. and Jawetz, E. Congenital heart diseases. In Krupp, Marcus A., Chatton, Milton J. and Associate Authors. *Current Diagnosis & Treatment*, 11th ed. Los Altos: California: Lange Medical Publications, 1972, pp. 149-155.

148. _____. Disturbances of rate and rhythm. *Ibid.*, pp. 192-199.

149. _____. Disturbances of conduction. *Ibid.*, pp. 199-201.

150. _____. Acquired heart diseases. *Ibid.*, pp. 155-178.

151. Soloff, L. A. On the electrocardiogram and clinical improvement after myocardial aneurysmectomy. *American Heart Journal*, 83: 237-243, February, 1972.

152. Stein, P. D. Velocity and flow measurements by electromagnetic techniques. *American Journal of Cardiology*, 29: 401-407, March, 1972.

153. Sway, P. S. *et al.* Dietary salt and essential hypertension. *American Journal of Cardiology*, 29: 33-38, January, 1972.

154. Thomas, K. T. *et al.* Single homograft aortic cusp replacement. *Circulation*, 45 (Suppl. 1): 25-28, May, 1972.

155. Thomas, M. L. Phlebography. *Archives of Surgery*, 104: 145-151, February, 1972.

156. Thomas, T. V. Surgical implications of saphenous venography. *American Journal of Surgery*, 123: 515-520, May, 1972.

157. Timmis, G. C. and Ramos, R. G. Transvenous pacing. Part a: Clinical experience with permanent units in elderly patients. *Griatrics*, 26: 89-94, December, 1971.

158. Toole, J. F. *Diagnosis and Management of Stroke*. New York: American Heart Association, 1968.

159. Tynan, M. Tricuspid incompetence after the Mustard operation for transposition of the great arteries. *Circulation*, 45 (Suppl. 1): 111-115, May, 1972.

160. Tyson, R. R. *et al.* Femorotibial bypass for salvage of the ischemic lower extremity. *Surgery Gynecology & Obstetrics*, 134: 771-776, May, 1972.

161. Veeani, M. S. Myocardial infarction associated with Wolff-Parkinson-White syndrome. *American Heart Journal*, 83: 684-687, May, 1972.

162. Viamonte, M. Innovations in angiography. *Radiologic Clinics of North America*, 9: 361-368, December, 1971.

163. Vincent, G. M. *et al.* QRS wave detector evaluation. *American Heart Journal*, 83: 475-480, April, 1972.

164. Walker, J. A. *et al.* Determinants of angiographic patency of aortocoronary vein bypass grafts. *Circulation*, 45 (Suppl. 1): 86-90, May, 1972.

165. Waxler, E. B. Right atrial myxoma: Echocardiographic, phonocardiographic and hemodynamic signs. *American Heart Journal*, 83: 251-257, February, 1972.

166. Willman, V. L. and Barner, H. B. Carotid occlusive disease. In Sabiston, David C. (ed.). *Davis-Christopher Textbook of Surgery*, 10th ed. Philadelphia: W. B. Saunders Co., 1972, pp. 1683-1692.

167. Willman, Vallee L., M.D. Personal communications.

168. Witham, A. C. and Hurst, J. W. Myocardial disease — Cardiomyopathy (Myocardosis). In Hurst, J. Willis and Logue, R. Bruce. *The Heart Arteries and Veins*, 2d ed. New York: McGraw-Hill Book Co., 1970, pp. 1189-1212.

169. Winsberg, F. *et al.* Continuous ultrasound visualization of the pulsating abdominal aorta. *Radiology*, 103: 455-456, May, 1972.

170. Winter, T. Q. *et al.* Current status of the Starr-Edwards cloth-covered prosthetic cardiac valves. *Circulation*, 45 (Suppl. 1): 14-24, May, 1972.

171. Wolk, M. J. *et al.* Heart failure complicating acute myocardial infarction. *Circulation*, 45: 1125-1138, May, 1972.

172. Yacoub, M. *et al.* Results of mitral valve replacement using unstented fresh semilunar valve homografts. *Circulation*, 45 (Suppl. 1): 44-51, May, 1972.

173. Yao, S. T. *et al.* Detection of proximal vein thrombosis by Doppler ultrasound flow detection method. *The Lancet*, 1: 1-4, January, 1972.

174. Yonkman, F. F. (ed.). Heart transplantation. In *Heart — The Ciba Collection on Medical Illustrations*, Vol. 5. Summit, New Jersey: Ciba, 1969, pp. 263-266.

175. Young, M. D. Congenital malformations of the heart. In Conn, Howard F. (ed.). *Current Therapy 1972*. Philadelphia: W. B. Saunders Co., 1972, pp. 168-174.

176. Zukowski, C. F. What's new in surgery. Transplantation. *Surgery Gynecology & Obstetrics*, 134: 280-283, February, 1972.

Chapter VI

Disorders of the Blood and Blood-Forming Organs

BLOOD

A. Origin of Terms:

1. blast (G) — germ
2. cyto (G) — cell
3. emia (G) — blood
4. erythro (G) — red
5. hemo (G) — blood
6. leuko (G) — white

7. osis (G) — increase, condition
8. penia (G) — decrease, poverty
9. phage (G) — to eat
10. polymorph (G) — many forms
11. reticulum (L) — network

B. Hematologic Terms:[11]

1. erythroblasts — immature red blood cells, possess a nucleus and are present in fetal blood.
2. erythrocytes — red blood cells; mature cells have no nucleus.
3. erythropoiesis — the production of red blood cells.
4. hematopoiesis, hemopoiesis — the development of the various cellular elements of the blood — erythrocytes, leukocytes, platelets, others.
5. hemoglobin — a chemical component of erythrocytes containing two substances: globin and hematin, an iron pigment which is responsible for the transport of oxygen to the cells.
6. leukocytes — white blood cells divided according to structure into granulocytes, lymphocytes and monocytes.
7. leukocytes of granulocytic series — the cytoplasm contains granules. This series includes
   a. polymorphonuclear neutrophils — cytoplasmic granules stainable with a neutral dye.
      Schilling's **hemogram** or **differential leukocyte count** distinguishes 4 age groups:
      (1) neutrophilic myelocytes — youngest neutrophils, nucleus round or ovoid-shaped.
      (2) neutrophilic metamyelocytes, junge kernige — immature cells in which the nucleus has become indented.
      (3) neutrophilic band or staff cells — immature non-filamented cells in which the nucleus is T, V or U-shaped without division into segments.
      (4) neutrophilic lobocytes or polymorphonuclear neutrophils — filamented mature cells with distinct segmentation.
   b. polymorphonuclear eosinophils — cytoplasmic granules of cells take an acid stain.
   c. polymorphonuclear basophils — cytoplasmic granules of cells take an alkaline stain.

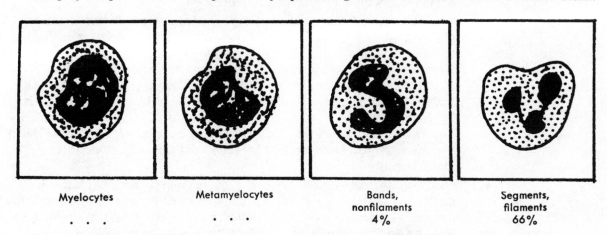

Myelocytes   Metamyelocytes   Bands,   Segments,
                                            nonfilaments   filaments
                                               4%   66%

Fig. 40 — Developmental phases of neutrophils from immature to mature cells. Eosinophils, basophils, monocytes and lymphocytes make up the remaining 30% of leukocytes.

8. lymphocytes — leukocytes derived from lymphoid tissue. The cytoplasm contains no granules or only a few.

9. monocytes — mononuclear leukocytes. The cytoplasm contains no granules or only a few.

10. myelopoiesis — the formation of blood cells and tissue elements from bone marrow.

11. myeloproliferative — referring to an increased production of myelopoietic cells and tissue.

12. phagocytes — two classes of white cells.
    a. the macrophages which absorb dead cells and tissues.
    b. the microphages which ingest bacteria.

13. plasma — liquid portion of blood without cellular elements.

14. plasma cells, plasmacytes — leukocytes, normally absent in blood film, occasionally seen in infection but rarely present in circulating blood. Their function is to synthesize immunoglobulins.[1]

15. platelets, thrombocytes — round or oval disks which control clot formation and clot retraction.

16. polymorphonuclear — having nuclei of variable shape.

17. reticulocytes — immature red cells in intermediary stage of development between nucleate and anucleate forms. They contain a fine intracellular network and are normally present in the blood in small numbers.[42]

18. serum — liquid portion of the blood after fibrinogen has been consumed in the process of clotting.[42]

C. Diagnostic Terms:

1. Conditions primarily affecting the red cells:

   a. anemia — blood disorder characterized by a reduction in erythrocyte count, hemoglobin and hematocrit, although not all 3 findings may be present.
   It is usually a manifestation or a complication of a disease, not a diagnosis.[42]
   A condensed version of Wintrobe's etiologic classification of anemia is presented:[46]

      (1) anemia of blood loss — disorder develops subsequent to an acute or chronic hemorrhage.

      (2) deficiency factors in red cell production (erythropoiesis)

         (a) iron deficiency anemia — depletion of body's iron storage, which may be followed by an inadequate production of hemoglobin and a reduction of the oxygen carrying capacity of the blood.[6]

         (b) megaloblastic anemias — the common denominator is a disordered synthesis of DNA (deoxyribonucleic acid) due to deficiency of vitamin B_{12} or folic acid.
         Normally dietary vitamin B_{12} interacts with a mucoid secretion of the gastric fundus, the intrinsic factor of Castle. In the absence of this factor, B_{12} cannot be absorbed by the ileum and nutritionally utilized by the body.[20]
         Folic acid (B_{12}) deficiency may be caused by malnutrition, malabsorption, increased requirement or loss of folic acid and defective folate metabolism.[40]

         (c) pernicious anemia — prototype of a megaloblastic anemia, usually associated with marked vitamin B_{12} deficiency caused by failure of gastric mucosa to secrete an intrinsic factor. Laboratory findings reveal a very low red count, often below 2,000,000, a hemoglobin relatively less reduced and achylia gastrica (absent or diminished gastric juice).
         Anorexia, sore tongue, weakness, fatigue, a waxy pallor and neurologic damage are common clinical manifestations.[47]

Table 7

MODIFIED SCHILLING'S HEMOGRAM — DIFFERENTIAL LEUKOCYTE COUNT

Type of Count	Percentage									
	Neutrophils						Eosinophils	Basophils	Lymphocytes	Monocytes
	Myeloblasts	Myelocytes	Metamyelocytes	Bands, nonfilaments	Segments, filaments	Total Neutrophils				
Normal Range	....	....	....	2 - 6	50 - 70	52 - 76	1 - 4	0 - 1	20 - 40	2 - 8
Shift to left; for example, infections	....	....	4	12	69	85	....	....	12	3
Shift to left; for example, chronic myelocytic leukemia	1	4	10	20	40	75	11	9	3	2
Shift to right; for example, pernicious anemia	....	....	....	2	78	80	....	....	16	4

In most infections the differential leukocyte count reveals a shift to the left. Characteristically, a few metamyelocytes (juveniles or junge kernige) and an abnormally high number of bands are found in the blood smear. The more immature the cells are, the more serious is the condition, as may be gleaned from the shift to the left in myelocytic leukemia. In pernicious anemia there is a shift to the right and the mature neutrophils are polysegmented filaments.

    (3) failure of bone marrow
        (a) aplastic anemia — markedly reduced production of red cells due to almost complete depression of bone marrow function. It may be idiopathic or caused by toxic drugs or ionizing irradiation.[48]
        (b) Fanconi syndrome, congenital pancytopenia — idiopathic anemia that develops in early infancy, appears to be hereditary and is associated with congenital abnormalities of the bones, heart, kidneys, eyes, microcephaly and an olive brown skin. The dominant hematologic finding is pancytopenia in which there is a profound depression of the cellular elements of the blood.[48]

    (4) excessive destruction of erythrocytes
        (a) hemolytic anemias — congenital or acquired blood disorders characterized by a shortened life span and an excessive destruction of mature red corpuscles.[17]
        (b) hemolytic disease of the newborn, erythroblastosis fetalis — reduction of the life span of red cells, usually resulting from a hemolytic reaction of the Rh positive infant to the sensitized Rh negative mother. Uncontrolled high bilirubin levels may result in brain damage evidenced by lethargy, characteristic spasms and sharp cries.[29]
        (c) hereditary spherocytosis, spherocytic anemia — familial type of hemolytic anemia characterized by the presence of sphere-shaped red cells, reticulocytosis, increased osmotic fragility, splenomegaly and jaundice. Sudden crises may result from an acceleration of the hemolytic process or transient failure in blood production with rapidly developing anemia.[42]

    (5) both, increased destruction and decreased production of erythrocytes
        (a) sickle cell anemia — genetic abnormality of red blood cells due to the presence of the gene Hb S* (homozygous genotype). Hemoglobin S produces progressive hemolysis and sickling of cells as the oxygen tension is lowered and deoxygenation increases. The resultant circulatory impairment may lead to vascular occlusions by plugs of sickled red cells causing thrombosis, infarction and leg ulcers. The disease is found among American negroes.[18]
        (b) thalassemias — a group of hereditary, familial anemias of the hypochromic microcytic type due to a genetic defect which results in a reduced synthesis of adult hemoglobin (Hb A). They comprise:
            (1) thalassemia major, Cooley's anemia — the homozygous genotype (both parents transmit defect) usually causes severe anemia, enlargement of the spleen and liver, jaundice and mongoloid facies.
            (2) thalassemia minor — heterogenous genotype (one parent transmits thalassemia trait to offspring) results in mild anemia.
            (3) other syndromes of thalassemia.[42, 43, 18]
b. polycythemia — disorder in which the outstanding characteristics are highly increased red cell mass and hemoglobin concentration.[34]

    (1) primary polycythemia, polycythemia rubra vera, erythremia — chronic blood condition of unknown cause characterized by hyperplasia of bone marrow, abnormally high red cell count, hemoglobin and hematocrit which may be associated with a high platelet count, leukocytosis and leukemia.

    (2) secondary polycythemias — various blood disorders in which tissue hypoxia is a significant feature. The abnormally reduced oxygen supply to the tissues stimulates an excessive production of erythropoietin which in turn increases bone marrow activity and thus red cell formation.[34]

---

    * Many other abnormal hemoglobins produce sickling without clinical symptoms. Hb S inherited from *one* parent may be asymptomatic.

2. Conditions primarily resulting from a defective mechanism of coagulation. The various substances involved in the clotting of the blood are called coagulation factors, designated by Roman numerals I to XIII. According to Wintrobe factor III, tissue thromboplastin, and factor IV, calcium, are rarely used and factor VI does not exist. Effective hemostasis is dependent upon the integrity of the factors below, cellular components of the blood and the walls of the blood vessels. A final step in the complex coagulation process involves the conversion of fibrinogen to fibrin. The coagulation factors are according to **International Nomenclature:***

factor I — fibrinogen

factor II — prothrombin

factor V — proaccelerin, labile factor, accelerator globulin, thrombogen
(AcG)

factor VII — proconvertin, stable factor, serum prothrombin conversion accelerator
(SPCA)

factor VIII — antihemophilic factor or antihemophilic globulin
(AHF) or (AHG)

factor IX — plasma thromboplastin component or Christmas factor
(PTC) or (CF)

factor X — Stuart factor or Prower factor

factor XI — plasma thromboplastin antecedent, antihemophilic factor C
(PTA)

factor XII — Hagemann factor
(HF)

factor XIII — fibrin stabilizing factor, Laki-Lorand factor, fibrinase.[3]
(LLF)

Bleeding disorders are present in

a. Christmas disease — familial disorder of blood coagulation attributed to a deficiency of the plasma thromboplastin component (factor IX). The clinical picture of the disease resembles that of hemophilia.[33]

b. hereditary hemorrhagic telangiectasia, Rendu-Osler-Weber syndrome — a congenital defect in the vascular hemostatic mechanism usually complicated by iron deficiency anemia. Localized dilatations of venules and capillaries are visible on the skin and mucous membranes. Epistaxis is common and bleeding may occur from digestive, urinary and respiratory tracts. The elderly tend to develop spiderlike skin lesions.[16]

c. hemophilia — well-known hereditary disease in which a sex-linked trait is transmitted by females, while the hemorrhagic disorder develops exclusively in males. In its classic form there is marked deficiency of the antihemophilic factor VIII leading to spontaneous bleeding episodes or prolonged bleeding after minor injury.[39]

d. purpura — disorder characterized by pinpoint extravasations or petechiae and larger skin lesions, the ecchymoses. Bleeding may occur spontaneously particularly from mucous membranes and internal organs.[4]

e. thrombocytopenia purpura, idiopathic (cause unknown) — disorder resulting from a marked degree of platelet reduction. Symptoms vary from insignificant purpuric spots to serious bleeding from any body orifice or into any tissue.[38]

f. von Willebrand's disease, pseudohemophilia, vascular hemophilia — life-long inherited bleeding disorder affecting both sexes, characterized by factor VIII deficiency and prolonged bleeding time. Abnormal bruising and bleeding into the skin and mucosa are usually of the purpuric type.[22]

---

* Maxwell M. Wintrobe (ed.). *Harrison's Principles of Internal Medicine*, 6th ed. New York: McGraw-Hill Book Co., 1970, p. 318.

3. Conditions primarily affecting the white blood cells.

    a. leukemia — a neoplastic disease which primarily involves the bone marrow, lymphatic and reticuloendothelial systems. It is usually characterized by an overproduction of leukocytes. The more common forms are presented.

        (1) acute leukemia — abrupt onset or a more gradual ushering in of fever, pallor, prostration, bleeding, joint and bone pains. Immature leukocytes usually abound in the peripheral blood and bone marrow. Anemia and thrombocytopenia may coexist.[28]

        (2) chronic lymphocytic leukemia — a great excess of lymphocytes, about 90 per cent of 50,000 - 250,000 white cells, enlargement of lymphnodes and spleen, anemia and bleeding episodes.[50]

        (3) chronic myelocytic leukemia — predominence of myelocytes in blood picture, white count ranging between 100,000 - 500,000 cells per cu mm of blood, anemia, pallor, weakness, dyspnea, cachexia, pain and hemorrhagic tendencies.[28, 8]

        (4) leukemoid reaction — blood disorder simulating leukemia because of its highly increased white count.

    b. leukopenia, granulocytopenia, agranulocytosis — a low white count of less than 5000 leukocytes per cu mm, caused by certain infections, nutritional deficiencies, hematopoietic disorders, chemical agents and ionizing radiation.[8]

4. Conditions primarily affecting cells produced by myelopoietic tissue of the bone marrow:

    a. chronic granulomatous disease (CGD) — a defect in neutrophil bacteriocidal function, characterized by recurrent infections, enlarged liver, spleen and lymph nodes, eczema and formation of granulomas. Death usually ensues in the first decade of life.[10]

    b. myeloproliferative disorders — conditions which have their origin in bone marrow and in varying degrees show an overgrowth of bone marrow cells. Examples are chronic polycythemia vera and granulocytic leukemia.[8]

    c. myelosclerosis — the classical form of this myeloprolific disorder reveals a triad of findings: (1) increasing marrow fibrosis, (2) a huge spleen and enlarged liver and (3) progressive anemia. The patient may experience a dragging sensation and intense pain in the splenic area.[8]

5. Conditions primarily concerned with an unbalanced proliferation of cells, usually plasma cells, and associated with an abnormality of immunoglobulins (gamma globulins).[30]

    a. amyloidosis — the presence of amyloid infiltrates in body tissues. Amyloid is a complex substance, principally containing protein and carbohydrates. It is imperfectly understood and undergoing further investigation.

        (1) primary systemic (or local) amyloidosis — a plasma cell dyscrasia and genetic metabolic disorder characterized by cardiac and gastrointestinal involvements, arthropathy, peripheral neuropathy and paresthesias.

        (2) secondary parenchymatous amyloidosis — condition usually associated with infection and chronic tissue breakdown of underlying disease particularly as that seen in multiple myeloma. Amyloid deposits are found in the spleen, kidney, adrenals, liver, lymphnodes and pancreas.[36]

    b. multiple myeloma, plasma cell myeloma — malignant neoplastic disease characterized by widespread bone destruction, intense bone pain, an excess of atypical plasma cells in the bone marrow, abnormal immunoglobulins, anemia and recurrent pneumonia or other bacterial infections related to defective antibody synthesis. Renal damage may be associated with elevated calcium levels in blood and urine.[25]

    c. Waldenstrom's macroglobulinemia — a plasma cell dyscrasia in which the production of gamma M globulin is greatly accelerated. Bone marrow findings resemble those of chronic lymphocytic leukemia and multiple myeloma. Anemia and low hemoglobin levels are present in symptomatic disease. There may be involvement of the heart, nerves, muscles and joints.[26]

D. Terms Related to Transfusions:[44, 45]

1. blood preparations — human tranfusion media standardized by the **National Institute of Health** (NIH) or **United States Pharmacopeia** (USP) or both.
   a. whole blood
      (1) banked whole blood, citrated whole blood, USP — normal blood collected in acid citrate dextrose solution (ACD), USP to prevent coagulation; primarily used for restoring or maintaining blood volume.
      (2) heparinized whole blood — normal blood in heparin solution to prevent coagulation; chiefly used for priming heart-lung machine to maintain extracorporeal circulation in open heart surgery.
   b. blood cells
      (1) packed red cells — concentrated suspension of red blood cells (70%) in ACD solution with plasma removed; indicated in the treatment of anemia.
      (2) platelet concentrates — platelet-rich whole blood, freshly drawn from polycythemic donor for platelet transfusion; useful as replacement therapy in platelet deficiency.
   c. blood plasma
      (1) dried plasma — vacuum drying of plasma to prevent bacterial growth, stable for seven years, stored at room temperature, reconstituted with sterile water for injection, USP prior to use, especially valuable in restoring blood volume in shock.
      (2) fresh, frozen plasma — liquid plasma, undelayed freezing and storage at a continuous temperature of — 18°C, stable for seven years; of therapeutic value in hemophilia.
      (3) normal human plasma, USP — cell-free plasma obtained by sedimentation or centrifugation of about equal portions of pooled citrated blood from eight or more donors. Banked plasma is used in coagulation disorders.
   d. blood proteins — plasma fractions
      (1) antihemophilic human plasma, USP — normal human plasma, promptly processed for preserving antihemophilic globulin, factor VIII, a component of fresh plasma. It is indicated in the treatment of hemophilia.[7, 27]
      (2) normal human serum albumin, USP — preparation of 25 Gm of human albumin in 100 ml of sterile water or normal saline. It aids in combating protein deficiencies.
2. transfusion — the transfer of blood or blood components into the bloodstream of a recipient.
3. transfusion reaction — untoward response to intravenous infusion of a blood preparation. It may be caused by air embolism, allergy, bacterial contaminants, circulatory overload and hemolysis due to incompatibility of red cells. Reactions vary in degree from mild to life-threatening; chills, fever, malaise and headache are common warning signals.[27, 42]

E. Symptomatic Terms:

1. anisocytosis — variation in size of red cells, seen in pernicious anemia.
2. blood dyscrasia — morbid blood condition.
3. erythrocytosis — abnormal increase in red blood cells.
4. erythropenia — abnormal decrease in red blood cells.
5. fibrinolysis — dissolution of fibrin; blood clot becomes liquid.
6. hemochromatosis — intracellular iron overload associated with organic damage.[15]
7. hemolysis — destruction of red cells and subsequent escape of hemoglobin into blood plasma.
8. leukocytosis — abnormally high white count.
9. leukopenia — abnormally low white count.
10. macrocytosis — abnormally large erythrocytes in the blood.
11. megaloblastosis — large, usually oval shaped, embryonic red corpuscles found in bone marrow and blood.

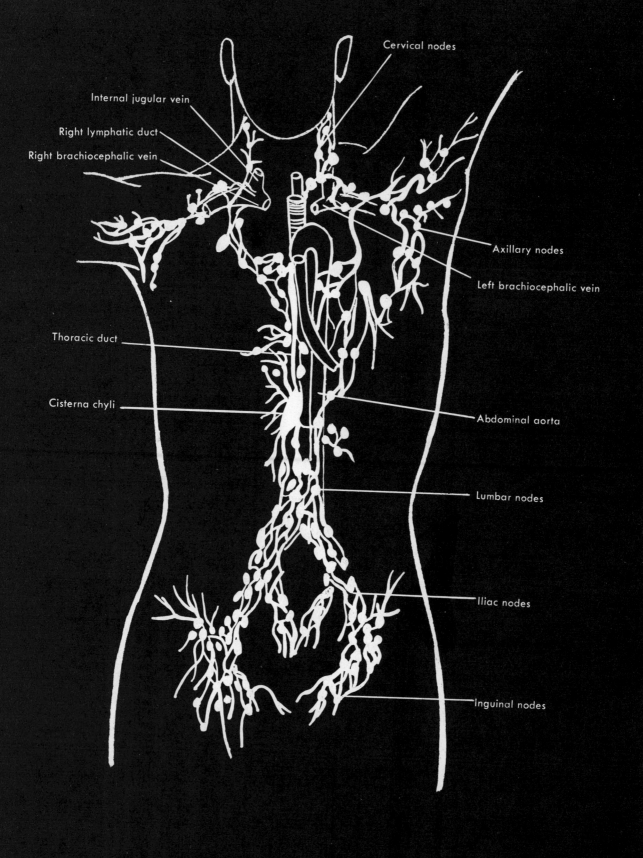

Cervical nodes

Internal jugular vein

Right lymphatic duct

Right brachiocephalic vein

Axillary nodes

Left brachiocephalic vein

Thoracic duct

Cisterna chyli

Abdominal aorta

Lumbar nodes

Iliac nodes

Inguinal nodes

Fig. 41 — Main lymphatics and lymph nodes.

12. microcytosis — abnormally small erythrocytes present in the blood.
13. neutropenia — excessively low neutrophil count.
14. neutrophilia — increase in neutrophils including immature forms, seen in pyogenic infections.
15. pancytopenia — an abnormal reduction of all blood cells: erythrocytes, leukocytes and platelets.
16. poikilocytosis — irregularly shaped red cells in the blood seen in pernicious anemia.
17. proliferation — increase in reproduction of similar forms or cells.
18. pseudoagglutination — clumping of red blood cells, not due to antibodies.
19. reticulocytosis — increase in reticulocytes in the peripheral blood.
20. rouleaux formation, pseudoagglutination — false agglutination in which the erythrocytes look like stacks of coins. It is seen in plasma cell dyscrasias such as multiple myeloma.[37]

LYMPHATIC CHANNELS AND LYMPH NODES

A. Origin of Terms:

1. lymphaden (G) — lymph gland
2. lymphangi (G) — lymph vessel

B. Anatomical Terms:

1. lymph — a clear or sometimes milky liquid found in lymphatics.
2. lymph nodes — encapsulated lymphoid tissue scattered along the lymphatics in chains or clusters. They act as filters against harmful and nonharmful substances.
3. lymphatics — thin-walled vessels widely distributed throughout the body and containing many valves.
4. lymphatic duct, right — duct which drains into the right brachiocephalic vein or one of its tributaries.
5. thoracic duct — duct which drains into the left brachiocephalic vein or one of its tributaries.

C. Diagnostic Terms:

1. bubo, inguinal — a suppurating lymph gland in the groin.
2. Burkitt's lymphoma — a malignant neoplasm of lymphoid tissue which usually involves the facial bones and abdomen of young children. The etiologic factor is thought to be the Epstein Barr virus.[13]
3. Hodgkin's disease — a fatal, probably neoplastic disease, producing lymph node involvement in the neck and axilla, enlargement of the spleen and liver and involvement of the lungs and bones.[24] According to recent investigations it is thought to be a unique example of an excessive immune response. The patient experiences exacerbations and remissions.
4. lymphadenitis — inflammation of the lymph glands.
5. lymphangitis — inflammation of the lymphatics.
6. lymphangioma — tumor composed of lymphatics.
7. lymphoma — tumor composed of lymph tissue.
8. lymphosarcoma — malignant lymph tissue, seen in the terminal phase of Hodgkin's disease.[23]

D. Operative Terms:

1. biopsy of lymph node — removal of small piece of lymphoid tissue for microscopic study.
2. lymphadenectomy — excision of lymph nodes.
3. lymphadenotomy — incision and drainage of lymph gland.

E. Symptomatic Terms:

1. lymphocytosis — abnormal increase of lymphocytes in the blood.
2. lymphocytopenia — deficient number of lymphocytes in the blood.
3. Pel-Ebstein type of fever — seen in Hodgkin's disease. Fever rises to about 102° for five or six days, then remains normal for five or six days and continues the same cycle.

SPLEEN

A. Origin of Terms:

1. splen (G) — spleen

2. lien (L) — spleen

B. Anatomical Term:

spleen — a lymphoid organ located in the left hypochondriac region. It is active in the destruction of red blood cells and the manufacture of lymphocytes and phagocytes.

C. Diagnostic Terms:

1. accessory spleens — additional spleens, performing the same function as the spleen. The condition is very common.
2. asplenia — absence of spleen.
3. chronic congestive splenomegaly, hepatolienal fibrosis, Banti's syndrome — condition characterized by longstanding congestion and enlargement of the spleen usually due to liver disease associated with portal or splenic artery hypertension. Leukopenia, anemia and gastrointestinal bleeding are common manifestations.[35]
4. Gaucher's disease — a hereditary metabolic defect resulting in faulty lipid storage. Abnormal reticuloendothelial (Gaucher) cells proliferate and cause progressive splenomegaly, pigmentation of the skin, anemia, and frequently lung and bone involvement.[21]
5. hypersplenism, hypersplenic syndrome — excessive splenic activity associated with highly increased blood cell destruction leading to anemia, leukopenia and thrombocytopenia.
6. splenic infarcts — relatively common lesions usually caused by embolism, thrombosis or infection.
7. splenitis, lienitis — inflammation of the spleen.
8. splenoptosis — downward displacement of the spleen.
9. splenorrhexis — rupture of spleen due to injury or advanced disease.

D. Operative Terms:

1. splenectomy — removal of the spleen.
2. splenopexy — fixation of a movable spleen.
3. splenorrhaphy — suture of a ruptured spleen.
4. splenotomy — incision into the spleen.

E. Symptomatic Terms:

1. autosplenectomy — small fibrotic spleen in adult with sickle cell anemia. Multiple splenic infarctions result in shrinkage of the organ.[42]
2. splenomegaly, splenomegalia — enlargement of the spleen.

RADIOLOGY

A. Terms Related to Therapeutic Radiology in General:

1. irradiation — subjection of a patient or a substance to the action of light, x-ray or other radiant energy.
2. radiation — emission of any form of radiant energy in various directions.
3. radiation therapy, radiotherapy, curietherapy — use of all forms of radiant energy in the treatment of disease. Radiotherapy is frequently the treatment of choice in leukemia, polycythemia vera and Hodgkin's disease.
4. radiocurable — capable of being restored to health by the therapeutic use of radiant energy.
5. sterilization with radiotherapy — destruction of a tumor or lesion by the use of radiant energy so that its recurrence is greatly diminished or eliminated.

B. Terms Related to Forms of Therapy:

1. external irradiation.
   a. total body — including entire torso and extremities.
   b. segmental — confined to local areas.
2. internal radiation.
   a. interstitial — insertion of radon containing capillary tubes or needles into a tissue; for example, to shrink a tumor or destroy a cancerous growth.

CLINICAL LABORATORY

A. Terms Related to Hematology:

1. aspirin tolerance test — determination of bleeding time before and two hours after an adult has taken 0.65 gram and a child 0.33 gram of aspirin. The test aids in the detection of von Willebrand's disease.[49]
2. bleeding time — duration of bleeding from a standardized wound. It measures the platelet function and the integrity of the vessel wall.
3. capillary fragility tourniquet test — procedure measuring the resistance of the capillaries to pressure and stress. A blood pressure cuff is applied to the upper arm and kept inflated at 80 mm pressure for 5 minutes. If a number of purpuric spots appear below the cuff area a few minutes after the cuff is released, the test is positive.[49]
4. coagulant — substance contributing to clot formation.
5. coagulation time, clotting time — time taken for venous blood to clot.
6. coagulum, blood clot — a lumpy mass formed in static blood in the laboratory and composed of platelets, red and white cells, irregularly scattered in fibrin network.[12]
7. clotlysis — dissolution of a clot.
8. clot retraction — formation of a clot and the exuding of serum: a qualitative platelet function test. Normally the retraction of blood begins within 30 to 60 minutes from the time it was drawn.
9. hematocrit — measurement of the volume of packed red cells in venous blood.
10. hemoglobin determination — measurement of the amount of hemoglobin, the oxygen carrier of the blood.
11. mean corpuscular hemoglobin (MCH) — weight of hemoglobin in average red blood cells, expressed in micromicrograms.[19]
12. mean corpuscular hemoglobin concentration (MCHC) — per cent of hemoglobin concentration in the average red blood cell.[19]
13. mean corpuscular volume (MCV) — mean volume of the average red blood cell, expressed in cubic microns.[19]

14. osmotic fragility — measurement of the power of red cells to resist hemolysis in a hypotonic salt solution.
15. prothrombin — coagulation factor II present in blood plasma.
16. prothrombin consumption test — determination of a patient's capacity to produce thromboplastin. When a blood sample from a normal individual clots, prothrombin is converted to thrombin and little or no prothrombin remains in the serum. However, if there is a deficiency in the factors which form thromboplastin, only a portion of the prothrombin will be converted. This will result in a high residual prothrombin in the serum.[32]
    Normal findings:
    more than 20 seconds . . . . signifying that the major portion of prothrombin has been converted by the patient's plasma thromboplastin to thrombin. Therefore the prothrombin time in this test is prolonged.
    Abnormal findings:
    less than 20 seconds . . . . indicating the presence of residual prothrombin which causes the prothrombin time to be shortened. This shows a deficiency of thromboplastic activity in the patient's plasma.[32]
17. prothrombin time — time in seconds required for thromboplastin to coagulate plasma.
    Normal findings:
    Quick's method . . . . 11-16 seconds
    Prolonged prothrombin time in vitamin K deficiency, hypoprothrombinemia and obstructive jaundice.
18. thromboplastin — coagulation factor III, thought to initiate clotting by converting prothrombin to thrombin in the presence of calcium ions. Tissue thromboplastin is chiefly found in the brain, thymus, placenta, testes and lungs.[49]
    a. complete thromboplastins — substances causing clot formation as quickly with hemophilic as with normal blood.
    b. partial thromboplastins — substances causing clot formation less quickly with hemophilic than with normal blood.[9]
    c. partial thromboplastin time (PTT) — valuable screening test for abnormalities of blood coagulation measuring coagulation factors involved in the intrinsic pathways.
        Normal findings:
        comparable to normal control.
        Increase in vitamin K deficiency, hepatic disease, von Willibrand's disease, presence of circulating anticoagulants and others.[49]
19. thrombus — structure formed in circulating blood, chiefly composed of a head of agglutinated platelets and white cells and a tail of fibrin and entrapped red cells.[12]

Table 8
CELLULAR CONSTITUENTS OF BLOOD

Constituents	Normal Range Per Cubic Millimeter of Blood[a]	Pathological Increase	Pathological Decrease
Erythrocytes — Male Erythrocytes — Female	4,500,000 to 6,000,000 4,000,000 to 5,500,000	Polycythemia vera	Anemias
Reticulated erythrocytes	Usually 1 per cent or less of total erythrocytes	Hemolytic jaundice	Purpura hemorrhagic
Leukocytes	4,000 to 10,000	Infections, leukemias	Agranulocytosis influenza typhoid fever
Platelets or thrombocytes	200,000 to 400,000	. . . .	Thrombocytopenic purpura acute leukemia

[a] Opal Hepler, *Manual of Clinical Laboratory Methods*, 4th ed. Springfield, Illinois: Charles E. Thomas Publisher, 1955, p. 33.

Table 9

SOME HEMATOLOGICAL FINDINGS IN DISEASE

Test	Normal Values	Diagnostic Aid in Disease[a]	Pathologic Response

Bleeding time
  Duke
  Ivy
	1-6 minutes
	2-3 minutes
		Thrombocytopenia
		von Willebrand's disease
		Coagulation defects
			Increase

Clotting time
  Lee White
  Silicone
	7-12 minutes
	2 hours
		Hemophilia purpura
		Hemorrhage of newborn
			Increase

Clot retraction time	1-24 hours	Thrombocytopenic purpura	No restriction
Osmotic fragility	0.4-0.2% of Na Cl	Congenital hemolytic jaundice Aplastic anemia	Increase

Capillary
  fragility
  (tourniquet
  test)
	0-10 petechiae
	per unit of
	area*
		Thrombocytopenic purpura,
		Purpura associated with
		Severe infections,
		Systemic vascular diseases
			Increase

Hemoglobin
  Sahli
  Males
  Females
	14-18 gm/100 ml
	12-16 gm/100 ml[a]
		Polycythemia vera, dehydration
		Anemias.........................
			Increase
			Decrease

Mean
  corpuscular
  hemoglobin
  MCH
	27-32 micro-
	micrograms
	29.5 average[a]
		Hyperchromic anemias.............
		Hypochromic anemias................
			Increase
			Decrease

Mean
  corpuscular
  volume
  MCV
	82-92 cubic
	microns[a]
		Macrocytic anemias.............
		Normacytic hypochromic anemia
		Microcytic hypochromic anemia
			Increase
			Decrease
			Decrease

Mean
  corpuscular
  hemoglobin
  concentration
  MCHC
	32-36%
	34% average[a]
		Macrocytic hypochromic anemia
		Microcytic hypochromic anemia
			Decrease
			Decrease

Hematocrit
  Males
  Females
  Pregnant
  women
	40-54%
	37-47%
	
	23-34%[a]
		Polycythemia vera................
		Prolonged severe hemorrhage
			Increase
			Decrease

[a] *Ibid.,* pp. 40-45 and 84-91.

B. Terms Related to Blood Grouping:[41]

1. ABO system — the international system of Landsteiner in which the 4 main blood groups are designated by the letters A, B, AB and O. This system is universally used.
2. agglutination — clumping of erythrocytes when mixed with incompatible blood or antisera.
3. agglutinin — a specific antibody in blood serum which causes agglutination.
   a. autoagglutinin — resembles cold agglutinin, reacts at temperature below 37°C with person's own cells and those of other groups.
   b. cold agglutinin — antibody causes clumping of human group O red cells at zero 5°C or below 37°C temperature.[42]
4. agglutinogen — a substance which stimulates the production of agglutinins when introduced into the body.

5. antigen — a substance which causes the formation of antibodies.

6. blood factor or hemagglutinogen — serological factor which occurs on the surface of red blood corpuscles.

7. blood group or blood type — inherited characteristic of human blood which remains unchanged throughout life.

8. blood grouping systems — the classification of bloods based on hemagglutinogens in red blood corpuscles. There are different types of blood factors (hemagglutinogens) requiring special methods of typing. The blood group systems refer to these serological factors: for example:

   ABO system to A, B, AB and O factors
   MN system to M, N, MN factors
   Rh-Hr system to Rh and Hr factors . *

   The recent discovery of subgroups (e.g.: A_1, A_2, A_3, A_4 and others for the ABO system) explains why incompatibility of types of blood may occur within the same blood group.
   a. incompatible blood — blood not capable of being mixed without causing hemolysis or clumping of red blood cells.
   b. type-O — universal donor — blood has no agglutinogens, hence no clumping.[41]

9. cross-matching — procedure done to determine the compatibility between the recipient's blood and donor's blood in order to prevent blood transfusion reaction.[41]

10. MN system — classification based on the presence of MN factors in erythrocytes. This system is used in genetic blood group analysis and in medicolegal paternity studies when parental claims are disputed.

11. Rh-Hr system — a system of complex antigenic structure. The Rh factor is an agglutinogen which occurs in the red blood corpuscles of 87% of white people. Originally only Rh positive and Rh negative agglutinogens were known; at present subgroups of Rh factors are recognized. The Rh determinations are of clinical importance in blood transfusion and obstetrics. There is a reciprocal relationship between Hr and Rh factors.

Table 10
COMPATIBILITY OF BLOOD FOR TRANSFUSION[a]

Recipient's Blood	Donor's Blood
A	A or O
B	B or O
AB	AB, A, B, or O
O	O only

[a] Rh studies are done routinely on all blood transfusions. In addition, subgroups may be checked to prevent reactions. Universal donor blood is only used for recipients of group A or B or AB in emergency when their respective type is not available.

C. Terms Related to Miscellaneous Blood Tests:

1. blood gas determinations[14] — sensitive indicators of physiological changes of lung function and tissue perfusion in acute illness. Measurements are obtained from hydrogen, carbon dioxide and oxygen tensions (pressures) of arterial or venous blood. The "p" refers to partial pressure.
   a. Pco_2 — pressure or tension of carbon dioxide measured in millimeters of mercury.
      Normal values
      arterial Pco_2 . . . . 34-45 mm Hg
      venous Pco_2 . . . . 31-42 mm Hg

---

* For information on other blood group systems (Lewis, Kell, P, Duffy, MNS, Kidd, Lutheran, Ii and Vel) consult Israel Davidsohn and John Bernard Henry (eds.). *Clinical Diagnosis by Laboratory Methods*, 14th ed. Philadelphia: W. B. Saunders Co., 1969, pp. 333-347.

Increase in hypercarbia.

CO_2 retention in respiratory acidosis and metabolic alkalosis.

Decrease in hypocarbia.

Excessive loss of carbon dioxide in hyperventilation due to respiratory alkalosis or metabolic acidosis.

b. pH — hydrogen ion concentration or acidity value of blood (or urine).

Normal values

arterial pH 7.37-7.44

venous pH 7.35-7.45

Increase in acidosis.

Decrease in alkalosis.

c. Po_2 — pressure or tension of oxygen expressed in millimeters of mercury.

Normal values

arterial Po_2 .... 80-90 mm Hg

venous Po_2 .... 25-40 mm Hg

Patients with chronic lung disease may normally have an arterial Po_2 of 70 mm Hg or less.

Decreased values

arterial Po_2 in advanced lung or heart disease.

venous Po_2 due to inadequate blood volume, exchange of gases, cardiac output and tissue perfusion.

2. fibrindex — a rapid semiquantitative test for fibrinogen using thrombin.

Normal fibrinogen index — Method of Bonsnes and Sweeney[5]

after 5-10 seconds .... beginning clot formation

after 30, 45, 60 seconds .... solid, firm clot formation

Subnormal fibrinogen index

after 60 seconds .... absence of firm clot or minimal gel formation

3. fibrinogen determination — test measures the concentration of fibrinogen in the blood plasma.

Normal values

circulating fibrinogen in plasma ...... 0.2 - 0.4 gm per 100 ml

Decrease in some blood diseases, nutritional deficiency and liver damage.

4. serum iron determination — test measures the serum concentration of iron

Normal value — Method of Barkan and Walker

serum iron level .... 50-150 micrograms per 100 ml

Decrease in iron-deficiency anemia.[31]

ABBREVIATIONS

A. Related to Hematology

ACD — acid-citrate-dextrose

AHF — antihemophilic factor VIII

AHG — antihemophilic globulin, factor VIII

bas — basophils

CBC — complete blood count

CF — Christmas factor, factor IX

eos — eosinophils

ESR — erythrocytic sedimentation rate

Hb, Hgb — hemoglobin

Hb A — adult hemoglobin

Hb F — fetal hemoglobin

Hb S — sickle cell hemoglobin

Ht — hematocrit

ITP — ideopathic thrombocytopenic purpura

lymph — lymphocytes

MCH — mean corpuscular hemoglobin

MCT — mean circulation time

mon — monocytes
PA — pernicious anemia
PCT — plasmacrit test
PCV — packed cell volume
PMN — polymorphonuclear neutrophils
PTA — plasma thromboplastin
    antecedent, factor XI

PTC — plasma thromboplastin
    component, factor IX
RBC — red blood count
RCS — reticulum cell sarcoma
RES — reticuloendothelial system
SI — saturation index
VI — volume index
WBC — white blood count

B. Related to Organizations:

AABB — American Associations of
    Blood Banks

ASCP — American Society of Clinical
    Pathologists

C. Related to Measurements:

cc — 1 cubic centimeter (1/1000 liter)
cm — 1 centimeter
gtt — guttae, drops
kg — 1 kilogram
L — 1 liter
m — 1 meter
mEq/L — 1 milliequivalent per liter
mg, mgm — 1 milligram (1/1000 gram)

cu mm — 1 cubic millimeter
gm, Gm — 1 gram (1/1000 kilogram)
min — minim
ml — 1 milliliter
mm — 1 millimeter
mm^3 — 1 cubic millimeter (same as cu mm)
μ — 1 micron (1/1,000,000 meter)
μg, μgm — 1 microgram (1/1,000,000 gram)

ORAL READING PRACTICE

Hodgkin's Disease

This peculiar and interesting disease is characterized by a painless enlargement of the lymph nodes which is initially confined to one group, frequently those located in the cervical region. From there the lymph node involvement spreads to the axillary and **inguinal** regions and progressively assumes systemic proportions. If **mediastinal** spread and **infiltration** of the lung **parenchyma** and pleura occur, the patient may experience **substernal** pain, cough, **dyspnea** and **stridor**.

Retroperitoneal lymph node involvement may lead to the formation of a mass which presses on the stomach and produces a sense of fullness. This type of involvement tends to exert a deleterious effect resulting in a dislodgment of the kidneys, compression of the **ureters** and **inferior vena cava** and **infiltrations** into the neighboring structures, the spinal nerves and **vertebrae**. **Splenomegaly** and **hepatomegaly** are common signs and may be associated with progressive **anemia, obstructive jaundice** and **ascites**.

Lesions of Hodgkin's disease are sometimes found in the reproductive system. Osteolytic and osteoplastic changes may occur in the ribs, vertebrae, femur and pelvis and cause bone tenderness or intense pain. As the disease progresses to the terminal phase, the patient manifests high fever and a marked degree of **lassitude, debility, pallor** and **cyanosis**.

The diagnostic feature of Hodgkin's disease is the **Reed-Sternberg** cell, a tumor cell containing irregular shaped **cytoplasm**, a large **nucleus**, heavy clumps of **chromatin** and **distinctive nucleoli**, surrounded by a clear halo.[2, 35, 24, 23]

The prognosis is invariably fatal, although **irradiation** and chemotherapy may induce remissions and a prolongation of life. Dramatic results have been obtained from the judicious use of **radiotherapy,** and **cobalt-60,** particularly in reducing or controlling cervical and **axillary lymph adenopathy.** **Cancerocidal** agents such as **nitrogen mustard** and **chlorambucil** as well as **adrenal corticoids** have been employed with some success, but require great caution because of their potential **toxicity**.

REFERENCES AND BIBLIOGRAPHY

1. Abramson, N. *et al.* The phagocytic plasma cells. *New England Journal of Medicine,* 283: 248-250, July 30, 1970.

2. Ackerman, Laureen V. and del Regato, Juan A. *Cancer — Diagnosis, Treatment and Prognosis,* 4th ed. St. Louis: The C. V. Mosby Co., 1970, pp. 978-984.

3. Bithell, T. C. and Wintrobe, M. M. Hematologic alterations. In Wintrobe Maxwell M (ed.). *Harrison's Principles of Internal Medicine,* 6th ed. New York: McGraw-Hill Book Co., 1970, pp. 318-319.

4. _____. The purpuras. In Wintrobe, Maxwell M. (ed.). *Harrison's Principles of Internal Medicine,* 6th ed. New York: McGraw-Hill Book Co., 1970, pp. 1646-1652.

5. Bonsnes, R. W. *et al.* A rapid semiquantitative test for fibrinogen employing thrombin. *American Journal of Obstetrics and Gynecology,* 70: 334-340, August, 1955.

6. Charlton, R. and Bothwell, T. H. Iron deficiency anemia. *Seminars in Hematology,* 7: 78-79, January, 1970.

7. Dallman, P. R. and Pool, J. G. Treatment of hemophilia with factor VIII concentrates. *New England Journal of Medicine,* 278: 199-202, January 25, 1968.

8. Dameshek, William and Gunz, Frederick. *Leukemia,* 2nd ed. New York: Grune and Stratton, 1964, pp. 356-357 and 360-361.

9. Davidsohn, Israel and Henry, John B. (eds). *Todd-Sanford Clinical Diagnosis by Laboratory Methods,* 14th ed. Philadelphia: W. B. Saunders Co., 1969, p. 401.

10. Davis, W. C., Douglas, S. D. and Fudenberg, H. H. A selective neutrophil dysfunction syndrome: Impaired killing of staphylococci. *Annals of Internal Medicine,* 69: 1237-1243, December, 1968.

11. DiFlore, Mariano, S. H. *Atlas of Human Histology,* 3rd ed. Philadelphia: Lea & Febiger, 1967, pp. 52-57.

12. Douglas, A. S. Management of thrombotic diseases. *Seminars in Hematology,* 8: 95, April, 1971.

13. Epstein, M. A., Achong, B. G. and Barr, Y. M. Virus particles in cultured lymphoblasts from Burkitt's lymphoma. *Lancet,* 1: 702-703, March 28, 1964.

14. Gambino, S. R. *Workshop Manual on Blood pH, Pco$_2$, Oxygen Saturation and Po$_2$,* 3rd ed. American Society of Clinical Pathologists, 1967, pp. 41-59. (Some texts use pO$_2$ and pCO$_2$ instead of Po$_2$ and Pco$_2$.)

15. Greenberg, M. S. and Grace, N. D. Folic acid deficiency and iron overload. *Archives of Internal Medicine,* 125: 140. January, 1970.

16. Harrington, W. J. Hemorrhagic disorders. In Beeson, Paul B. and McDermott, Walsh, (eds.). *Cecil-Loeb Textbook of Medicine,* 13th ed. Philadelphia: W. B. Saunders Co., 1971, p. 1597.

17. Haut, A. and Wintrobe, M.M. Hemolytic anemias. In Wintrobe, Maxwell M. (ed.). *Harrison's Principles of Internal Medicine,* 6th ed. New York: McGraw-Hill Book Co., 1970, pp. 1602 and 1615-1616.

18. _____. Sickle cell anemia and other homozygous abnormal hemoglobin states. In Wintrobe, Maxwell M. (ed.). *Harrison's Principles of Internal Medicine,* 6th ed. New York: McGraw-Hill Book Co., 1970, pp. 1627-1629.

19. Hepler, Opal. *Manual of Clinical Laboratory Methods,* 4th ed. Springfield, Illinois: Charles E. Thomas Publisher, 1955, pp. 40-45.

20. Jandl, J. H. Megaloblastic anemias. In Beeson, Paul B. and McDermott, Walsh (eds.). *Cecil-Loeb Textbook of Medicine,* 13th ed. Philadelphia: W. B. Saunders Co., 1971, pp. 1464-1465.

21. Krupp, Marcus A. and Chatton, Milton J. *Current Diagnosis and Treatment.* Los Altos, California: Lange Medical Publications, 1972, p. 713.

22. Leslie, J. and Ingram, G. I. The diagnosis of longstanding bleeding disorders. *Seminars in Hematology,* 8: 151, April, 1971.

23. Lipton, A. *et al.* Prognosis of stage X lymphosarcoma and reticulum-cell sarcoma. *New England Journal of Medicine,* 284: 230-233, February 4, 1971.

24. MacMahon, B. *et al.* Hodgkin's disease one entity or two? *Lancet,* 1: 240-241, January 30, 1971.

25. McArthur, J. R. *et al.* Melphalan and myeloma. *Annals of Internal Medicine,* 72: 665-670, May, 1970.

26. McAllister, B. D. *et al.* Primary macroglobulinemia. *American Journal of Medicine,* 43: 394-434, September, 1967.

27. Mollison, Patrick. *Blood Transfusion in Clinical Medicine,* 4th ed. Philadelphia: F. A. Davis Co., 1967, pp. 553-611.

28. Moore, C. V. The leukemias. In Beeson, Paul B. and McDermott, Walsh (eds.). *Cecil-Loeb Textbook of Medicine,* 13th ed. Philadelphia: W. B. Saunders Co., 1971, p. 1542.

29. Nelson, Waldo E., Vaughn, Victor C. and McKay, R. James. *Textbook of Pediatrics,* 9th ed. Philadelphia: W. B. Saunders Co., 1969, p. 1060.

30. Osserman, E. T. Plasma cell dyscrasias. In Beeson, Paul B. and McDermott, Walsh (eds.). *Cecil-Loeb Textbook of Medicine,* 13th ed. Philadelphia: W. B. Saunders Co., 1971, pp. 1574-1587.

31. Page, Lot B. and Culver, Perry J. *A Syllabus of Laboratory Examinations in Clinical Diagnosis,* 2nd ed. Cambridge, Massachusetts: Harvard University Press, 1960, p. 6.

32. Pohala, M. J. and Singher, H. O. Procedure for prothrombin consumption test as used in the coagulation laboratory of the Ortho Research Foundation, Rariton, New Jersey.

33. Ratnoff, O. D. Coagulation defects. In Beeson, Paul B. and McDermott, Walsh (eds.). *Cecil-Loeb Textbook of Medicine,* 13th ed. Philadelphia: W. B. Saunders Co., 1971, p. 1542.

34. Reinhard, E. H. Polycythemia. In Beeson, Paul B. and McDermott, Walsh (eds.). *Cecil-Loeb Textbook of Medicne,* 13th ed. Philadelphia: W. B. Saunders Co., 1971, pp. 1521-1525.

35. Robbins, Stanley L. *Pathology,* 3rd ed. Philadelphia: W. B. Saunders Co., 1967, p. 688 and p. 675.

124

36. Samter, Max (ed.). *Immunological Diseases*, 2nd ed. Boston: Little, Brown and Co., 1971, pp. 1073-1075.

37. *Stedman's Medical Dictionary*, 22nd ed. Baltimore: The Williams and Wilkins Co., 1972, p. 1033.

38. Steinberg, A. D. *et al.* Thrombotic thrombocytopenia purpura complicating Sjögren's syndrome. *Journal of American Medical Association*, 215: 257-261, February 1, 1971.

39. Stormorken, H. and Owren, P. A. Physiopathology of hemostasis. *Seminars in Hematology*, 8: 3-29, January, 1971.

40. Streiff, R. R. Folic acid deficiency anemia. *Seminars in Hematology*, 7: 23-29, January, 1970.

41. *Technical Methods and Procedures of the American Association of Blood Banks*, 5th ed. Chicago: American Association of Blood Banks, 1970, pp. 49-81.

42. Tucker, Eugene, F., M.D. Personal communications.

43. Wai Kan, Y. *et al.* Globin chain synthesis in the alpha thalassemia syndromes. *Journal of Clinical Investigation*, 47: 2515, 1968.

44. Widman, F. K. Give the patient what he needs. 1. Blood component therapy: red cell concentrates. *Postgraduate Medicine*, 49: 47-50, January, 1971.

45. _____. Give the patient what he needs. 2. Blood component therapy: platelets, plasma proteins, and white cells. *Postgraduate Medicine*, 49: 55-59, February, 1971.

46. Wintrobe, M. M. Hematologic alterations — pallor and anemia. In Wintrobe, Maxwell M. (ed.). *Harrison's Principles of Internal Medicine*, 6th ed. New York: McGraw-Hill Book Co., 1970, pp. 309-310.

47. Wintrobe, M. M. and Lee, G. R. Pernicious anemia and other megaloblastic anemias. In Wintrobe, Maxwell M. (ed.). *Harrison's Principles of Internal Medicine*, 6th ed. New York: McGraw-Hill Book Co., 1970, p. 1595.

48. Wintrobe, M. M. and Bithell, T. C. Bone marrow failure. In Wintrobe, Maxwell M. (ed.). *Harrison's Principles of Internal Medicine*, 6th ed. New York: McGraw-Hill Book Co., 1970, pp. 1634-1635.

49. Wintrobe, Maxwell M. (ed.). *Clinical Hematology*, 6th ed. Philadelphia: Lea & Febiger, 1967, pp. 322-325.

50. Zacharski, L. R. *et al.* Chronic lymphocytic leukemia versus chronic lymphosarcoma cell leukemia. *American Journal of Medicine*, 47: 75, July, 1969.

Chapter VII

Respiratory Disorders

NOSE

A. Origin of Terms:

1. choane (G) — a funnel
2. concha (L) — a shell
3. meatus (L) — a passage
4. osme (G) — sense of smell
5. rhin- (G) — nose
6. septum (L) — partition

B. Anatomical Terms:

1. choana (pl. choanae), posterior aperture — opening of the nasal cavity into the naso-pharynx.
2. concha (pl. conchae), turbinate — one of the scroll-like bony projections on the lateral wall of the nasal cavity.
3. naris (pl. nares) — nostril.
4. nasal meatus (pl. meatuses) — space beneath each concha of the nose.
5. nasal septum — partition between the two halves of the nasal cavity.
6. nasopharynx — an open chamber located behind the nasal fossa and below the base of the skull.[1]

C. Diagnostic Terms:

1. atresia of choanae — pathological closure of posterior nares or congenital absence of the same.
2. coryza — cold in head.
3. deflection of septum — deviation of septum (deviation: departure from normal).
4. nasopharyngeal cancer — usually an epidermoid carcinoma or lymphosarcoma of the nasopharynx which may spread by direct extension to the meninges, compress cranial nerves and cause cranial nerve paralyses, ptosis of the eyelid and eventually loss of sight. Invasion of lymph nodes occurs frequently. The incidence of nasopharyngeal cancer is high among the Chinese and Maylays and low in Caucasians.[1, 64, 44, 29]
5. nasopharyngitis — inflamed condition of the nasopharynx.
6. rhinitis — inflammation of the nasal mucosa.[21]
7. rhinolith — nasal concretion.

D. Operative Terms:

1. rhinoplasty — plastic reconstruction of the nose.
2. septectomy, submucous resection — excision of the nasal septum or part of it.
3. turbinectomy — excision of a turbinate bone.
4. turbinotomy — surgical incision of a turbinate bone.

E. Symptomatic Terms:

1. anosmia — absence of sense of smell.
2. epistaxis — nosebleed.
3. rhinorrhea — thin, watery discharge from nose.[24]

PARANASAL SINUSES

A. Origin of Terms:

1. antrum (L) — cavity
2. ethmo (G) — sieve
3. front (L) — brow
4. maxilla (L) — jawbone
5. sinus (L) — hollow
6. sphen (G) — wedge

B. Anatomical Terms:

1. ethmoidal sinus — a collection of small cavities or air cells in the ethmoidal labyrinth between the eye socket (orbit) and nasal cavity.
2. frontal sinus — air space in the frontal bone above each orbit.

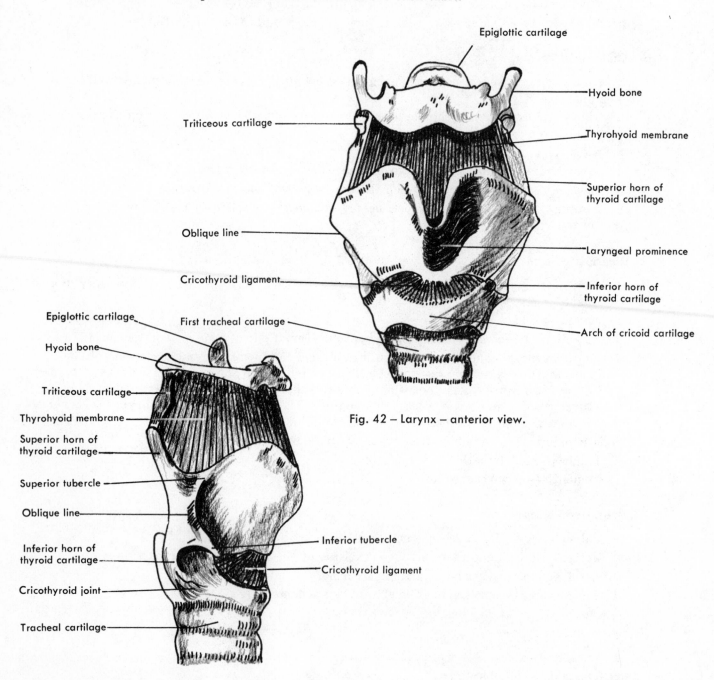

Fig. 42 – Larynx – anterior view.

Fig. 43 – Larynx – right lateral view.

3. maxillary sinus, antrum of Highmore — large air sinus of the maxillary bone.
4. sphenoidal sinus — air space, variable in size, in the sphenoid bone. It is divided into right and left halves by a septum.

C. Diagnostic Terms:

1. actinomycosis of sinus — fungus infection in sinus.
2. pansinusitis — inflammation of all the sinuses.
3. sinusitis — inflammation of a sinus or sinuses.[45]

D. Operative Terms:

1. antrotomy — opening of antral wall.
2. Caldwell-Luc operation — radical maxillary antrotomy.
3. ethmoidectomy — excision of ethmoid cells.
4. lavage of sinus — washing out a sinus for removal of purulent material.

LARYNX

A. Origin of Terms:

1. chondros (G) — cartilage, gristle
2. cricoid (G) — ringlike
3. glottis (G) — aperture of larynx
4. larynx (G) — voice box
5. phono- (G) — voice
6. vox (L) — voice

B. Anatomical Terms:

1. cricoid cartilage — ring-shaped cartilage of lowest part of larynx.
2. endolarynx — interior of larynx divided into a supraglottic portion, the glottis and a subglottic portion.[2]
3. epiglottis — thin, leaf-shaped cartilage partially covered with mucous membrane. It closes the entrance to the larynx during swallowing.
4. glottis — two vocal folds with the rima glottidis between them.[2, 8]
5. larynx — tone-producing organ, the voice box, composed of muscle and cartilage. Its interior surface is lined with mucous membrane.
6. rima glottidis — narrowest portion of laryngeal cavity between the vocal folds.[8]
7. vocal folds, vocal cords — mucosal folds each containing a vocal ligament and muscle fibers.

C. Diagnostic Terms:

1. endolaryngeal carcinomas — malignant epithelial tumors of various laryngeal structures such as the glottis, subglottis or supraglottis. Hoarseness is the presenting symptom in cancer of the vocal cord.[2, 68, 55]
2. epiglottitis — inflammation of the epiglottis.[61]
3. hypoplasia of epiglottis — defective development of epiglottis.
4. laryngitis — inflammation of larynx.[21]
5. laryngospasm, laryngismus, laryngeal stridor — adduction of laryngeal muscles and vocal cords resulting in obstruction of airway, marked by sudden onset of inspiratory dyspnea. It is common in children.
6. laryngotracheobronchitis — inflammation of the mucous membrane of larynx, trachea and bronchi.
7. perichondritis — inflammation of the perichondrium, a membrane of fibrous connective tissue which surrounds the cartilage.
8. stenosis of larynx — a narrowing or stricture of the larynx.[70]

D. Operative Terms:

1. dilatation of the larynx — instrumental stretching of the larynx.
2. laryngectomy — removal of the larynx for carinoma.
3. laryngoplasty — plastic repair of the larynx.[9, 73]
4. laryngoscopy — examination of interior larynx with a laryngoscope.
5. laryngostomy — establishing a permanent opening through the neck into the larynx.

E. Symptomatic Terms:

1. aphonia — loss of voice due to local disease, hysteria or injury to recurrent laryngeal nerve.
2. dysphonia — difficulty in speaking, hoarseness.

TRACHEA

A. Origin of Terms:

1. furca (L) — fork
2. steno- (G) — narrow
3. trachea (G) — windpipe, rough

B. Anatomical Terms:

1. bifurcation — division into two branches.
2. carina — ridge between the trachea at the bifurcation.
3. trachea — windpipe composed of about 18 C-shaped cartilages, held together by elastic tissue and smooth muscle and extending from the larynx to the bronchi.

C. Diagnostic Terms:

1. calcification of tracheal rings — deposit of calcium in trachea.
2. stenosis of trachea — contraction or narrowing of lumen of trachea.
3. tracheoesophageal fistula — communication of esophagus with trachea, a congenital or acquired anomaly.
4. tracheopleural fistula — communication of trachea with the pleura which may be due to postoperative injury or to pressure necrosis of inflated cuff of a tracheostomy tube.[51, 40]

D. Operative Terms:

1. tracheoplasty — plastic operation on trachea.
2. tracheoscopy — inspection of interior of trachea by means of a reflected light.
3. tracheostomy — formation of a more or less permanent opening into the trachea, usually for insertion of a tube. Tracheostomy (or laryngostomy) is absolutely imperative prior to total laryngectomy, to establish an open airway. It may be necessary after thyroidectomy, brain or lung surgery, to overcome a tracheal obstruction.
4. tracheotomy — incision into the trachea.[21, 51, 40]

BRONCHI

A. Origin of Terms:

1. bronchus (L) — bronchus, windpipe
2. bronchiolus (L) — air passage
3. plasia (G) — to form
4. scope (G) — to examine

B. Anatomical Terms:

1. bronchi, main — the two primary divisions of the trachea resembling it structurally.
   a. right main bronchus is shorter and more vertical than the left and is, therefore, more prone to lodge foreign bodies when aspirated. Its upper and lower parts provide the air passages for the three lobes of the right lung.

    b. left main bronchus gives rise to two lobar bronchi which supply the lobes of the left lung.

  2. bronchioles, bronchioli (sing, bronchiole, bronchiolus) — the smaller subdivisions of the bronchial tubes which do not have cartilage in their walls.

C. Diagnostic Terms:

1. aplasia of bronchus — undeveloped bronchus.
2. bronchiectasis — dilation of a bronchus or bronchi, secreting large amounts of offensive pus.[65]
3. bronchiectasic — pertaining to bronchiectasis.
4. bronchiogenic carcinoma — lung cancer arising in the mainstem bronchus in 75% of patients with this malignant tumor. Metastasis occurs readily because the great vascularity, rich network of pulmonary lymph nodes and constant lung movements facilitate spread to neighboring and remote structures such as the brain, liver and other organs.[3, 47]
5. bronchitis — inflammation of the bronchial mucous membrane; endobronchial tuberculosis or tuberculous bronchitis due to tubercle bacillus.[7]
6. bronchopleural fistula — open communication between a bronchus, a cavity and the pleura. This may be a complication of pulmonary resection.
7. chronic airway obstruction — disorder of respiratory tract resulting from generalized bronchial narrowing and destruction of functional lung tissue. It is usually characterized by severely impaired expiratory outflow which responds poorly to therapy. Asthma, chronic bronchitis and emphysema are primary respiratory disorders in which chronic airway obstruction is a dominant feature.[37, 15, 58, 81, 34]

D. Operative Terms:

1. bronchoplasty — plastic operation for closing fistula.
2. bronchoscopy — examination of the bronchi through a bronchoscope.
3. bronchotomy — incision into a bronchus.
4. closure of bronchopleural fistula — bronchoplasty with postoperative drainage of pleural cavity.

LUNGS

A. Origin of Terms:

1. alveolus (L) — little tub
2. apex (L) — tip
3. phthisis (G) — a wasting
4. pneumo- (G) — air
5. pulmo-, pulmon (L) — lung
6. segment (L) — a portion

B. Anatomical Terms:

1. alveoli (sing. alveolus) — air cells of the lungs in which the exchange of gases takes place.
2. apex of lung — most superior part of the lung above the clavicle.
3. base of lung — inferior part of the lung above the diaphragm.
4. bronchopulmonary segment — one of the subdivisions of a pulmonary lobe, supplied with a bronchial tube and blood and lymph vessels. The right lung has ten and the left lung nine segments.
5. bronchopulmonary tree — the lung compared to a hollow tree upside down in the thorax. The tree trunk is the trachea kept open and stiffened by C-shaped bars of cartilage. The main bronchi are two large branches which ramify into smaller and smaller ones until they become leaf stems or bronchioles. These, in turn, form tiny airways, the alveolar ducts, which lead to countless clusters of air cells surrounded by capillaries. There the exchange of gases takes place.

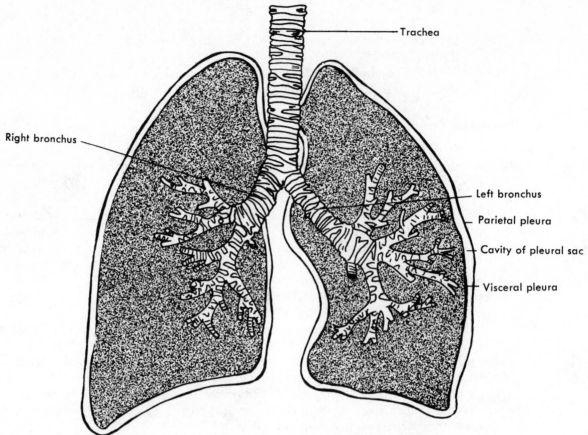

Fig. 44 – Trachea, bronchi, lungs and pleural sacs.

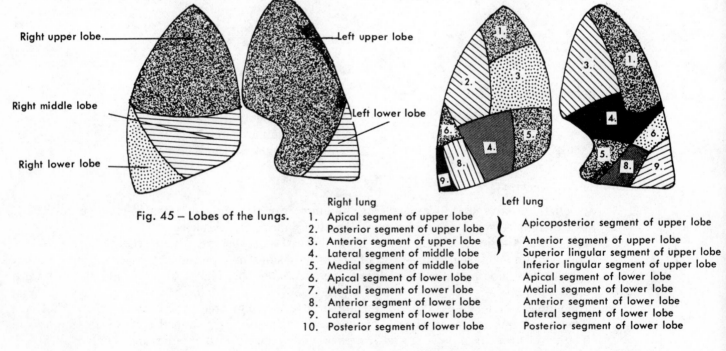

Fig. 45 – Lobes of the lungs.

Right lung

1. Apical segment of upper lobe
2. Posterior segment of upper lobe
3. Anterior segment of upper lobe
4. Lateral segment of middle lobe
5. Medial segment of middle lobe
6. Apical segment of lower lobe
7. Medial segment of lower lobe
8. Anterior segment of lower lobe
9. Lateral segment of lower lobe
10. Posterior segment of lower lobe

Left lung

Apicoposterior segment of upper lobe

Anterior segment of upper lobe
Superior lingular segment of upper lobe
Inferior lingular segment of upper lobe
Apical segment of lower lobe
Medial segment of lower lobe
Anterior segment of lower lobe
Lateral segment of lower lobe
Posterior segment of lower lobe

Fig. 46 – Bronchopulmonary segments of lungs.

6. hilus — triangular depression on the medial surface of the lung which contains the hilar lymph nodes and the entrance or exit of blood and lymph vessels, nerves and bronchi. They form the root of the lung.

7. lobe — a major division of the lung composed of bronchopulmonary segments.

8. parenchyma — the functional tissue of any organ, for example: the respiratory bronchioles, alveolar ducts, sacs and alveoli which participate in respiration.

C. Diagnostic Terms:

1. abscess of lung — a localized area of suppuration in the lung with or without cavitation. It is accompanied by necrosis of tissue.[77]

2. acute respiratory failure — a life-threatening condition characterized by excessively high carbon dioxide tension or abnormally low oxygen tension of the arterial blood.
   It may be caused by blockage of air passages by tenacious secretions from lung infection, by exposure to atmospheric smog or other irritant inhalants or by brain damage to the respiratory center.[37, 56, 42, 13]

3. anthracosis — a disease of the lungs caused by the prolonged inhalation of fine particles of coal dust.

4. aplasia of lung — incomplete development of the lung.

5. asbestosis — occupational disease due to protracted inhalation of asbestos particles.

6. atelectasis — a functionless, airless lung or portion of a lung.[67, 19]

7. blast injury — internal trauma of lungs, ears, and intestines due to high pressure waves following explosion. It may result in extreme bradycardia, severe cyanosis, dyspnea, hemorrhage and deafness.

8. carcinoma of the lung, primary, secondary or metastatic — malignant new growth and the most important of the neoplastic diseases of the lung.[43, 57, 16, 33, 27]

9. cystic disease of the lungs — condition characterized by the presence of air or fluid containing spaces within the lung. Most cystic lesions are secondary to obstructive emphysema, partial bronchial obstruction and tuberculous infection.
   Air cysts may enlarge tremendously and form tension cysts due to the development of a check-valve mechanism in the draining bronchus. Solitary cysts occasionally balloon to such a large size that they dislocate the mediastinal structures and produce dyspnea and cyanosis. Rupture of the cyst leading to pneumothorax is not infrequent.

10. histoplasmosis — fungus disease caused by Histoplasma capsulatum; sometimes associated with calcified pulmonary lesions.[31, 80, 78]

11. pneumoconiosis — a disease of the lungs due to injury by dust from any source.

12. pneumonia — inflammation of the lungs with exudation into lung tissue and consolidation. Predominent etiological agents are pneumococci and mycoplasmas or pleuropneumonia-like organisms (PPLO). Many other bacteria may cause pneumonia.[48, 22]
    a. bronchopneumonia — inflammation of bronchioli and air vesicles with scattered areas of consolidation.
    b. lobar pneumonia — acute inflammation of one or more lobes of the lung or lungs.
    c. primary atypical pneumonia — infection due to Mycoplasma pneumoniae varying from mild to fatal disease.[32]
    Etiology of pneumonia: the pneumococcus is generally the source of the infection, but sometimes respiratory viruses and tubercle bacilli cause the disease and, rarely, streptococci and staphylococci are the etiological bacteria.

13. pneumonitis — inflammation of the lung; a virus form of pneumonia.

14. pneumonocele, pneumocele — a pulmonary hernia.

15. pulmonary edema — excess of intra-alveolar and intrabronchial fluid in the lungs inducing cough and dyspnea; common in left heart failure.[25]

16. pulmonary embolism — lodgment of a clot or foreign substance in a pulmonary arterial vessel cutting off the circulation.[39, 82]

17. pulmonary or vesicular emphysema — overdistention of alveoli and smaller bronchial tubes with air.[72, 49, 26, 30]

18. pulmonary hypertension — condition due to increased pressure in the pulmonary artery resulting from obstruction by pulmonary embolism or thrombosis, tuberculosis, emphysema or pulmonary fibrosis.[36]

19. pulmonary infarction — necrosis of functional lung tissue (parenchyma) due to loss of blood supply usually caused by embolism.

20. pulmonary thrombosis — clot formation in any pulmonary blood vessel resulting in circulatory obstruction.

21. pulmonary tuberculosis, phthisis — a specific inflammatory disease of the lungs caused by tubercle bacillus and characterized anatomically by a cellular infiltration which subsequently caseates, softens, and leads to ulceration of lung tissue; manifested clinically by wasting, exhaustion, fever and cough.[50, 59, 63, 52, 60, 20]
    a. classification according to extent of lesions:[23]
       (1) minimal — the lesions are of moderate density without cavitation and either limited to one lung or affecting both lungs. The total extent of these tuberculous infiltrations, regardless of their distribution, does not exceed the equivalent of lung tissue which lies above the level of the second rib.
       (2) moderately advanced — either unilateral or bilateral lung involvement is present. The extent of the lesions is limited to
          (a) the dissemination of infiltrates throughout one lung, or its equivalent in both lungs.
          (b) confluent, dense infiltrations which do not exceed one-third of the volume of one lung.
          (c) cavitation less than 4 cm in diameter.
       (3) far advanced — lesions are more extensive, dense and confluent and cavitation exceeds 4 cm in diameter.
    b. some forms of tuberculosis:
       (1) endobronchial tuberculosis — implantation of tubercle bacilli in the bronchial mucosa followed by the development of irregular necrotic ulcers or by extensive fibrosis with a gradual occlusion of the bronchial lumen.
       (2) fibrocaseous, fibroulcerative tuberculosis — form characterized by reparative fibrous and destructive caseous elements representing the two extremes in the way of healing and progression — the most frequent form of tuberculosis in the ages of 20 to 40.
       (3) miliary tuberculosis — symmetrical distribution of minute tubercles in both lungs — generally hematogenous in origin. Seeding elsewhere may occur resulting in dissemination of tubercles in various organs.[54, 23]

22. silicosis — occupational disease due to inhalation of silica dust usually over a period of ten years or more.[10, 79]

D. Operative Terms:

1. biopsies:
   a. lung biopsy — small specimen of lung tissue used for pathologic, bacteriologic and spectrographic studies to aid diagnosis.[23]
   b. lymph node biopsy — removal of tissue from scalene or supraclavicular lymph nodes for gross or microscopic examination to aid in the detection of cancer, tuberculosis or other disease.[3, 69, 11]
   c. percutaneous needle biopsy — procedure used when tissue diagnosis is needed to plan radiation therapy and chemotherapy. The area to be biopsied is detected by television fluoroscopy. A biopsy needle is inserted through a small skin incision and cells aspirated are used for cytologic and bacteriologic diagnosis.[41]

2. bronchofiberscopy — endoscopic examination of the tracheobronchial tree using a flexible bronchofiberscope to view the carina and right and left mainstem of bronchus. A 35 mm camera, attached to the bronchofiberscope provides photographic documentation.[6]
3. collapse surgery — surgical procedure which aims to put the diseased lung at rest by causing it to relax. The tuberculous lesion remains within the lung, but becomes non-active and rarely develops into a focus of reinfection. Most collapse procedures have been abandoned since the advent of antituberculous chemotherapy. The only operations occasionally performed are
    a. extrapleural thoracoplasty — multiple rib resection without entering the pleural space.
        (1) primary — to effect permanent collapse of the diseased lung and cavity closure.
        (2) postlobectomy or postpneumonectomy — to obliterate dead space subject to infection or to reduce empyema space.
    b. plombage — packing the space between chest wall and lung with foreign material to collapse the lesion.[47]
4. excisional surgery (extirpative, definitive) — partial or complete removal of the diseased lung.
    a. lobectomy — removal of a pulmonary lobe.
    b. lung resection, pulmonary resection — partial excision of the lung, such as
        (1) segmental resection — removal of a bronchopulmonary segment.
        (2) subsegmental resection — removal of a portion of a segment.
    c. pneumonectomy — removal of an entire lung.
    d. wedge resection — removal of a triangular portion of the lung, usually a small peripheral lesion, such as a tuberculoma.[12, 75]

E. Symptomatic Terms:

1. anoxemia — deficient oxygen tension in arterial blood.
2. anoxia — oxygen want in tissues and organs.
3. apnea, apnoea — temporary absence of respiration — also seen in Cheyne-Stokes respiration.
4. bronchial or tubular breathing — harsh breathing with a prolonged high pitched expiration which may have a tubular quality.
5. Cheyne-Stokes respiration — irregular breathing beginning with shallow breaths which increase in depth and rapidity to a certain degree; then they gradually decrease and cease altogether. After 10-20 seconds of apnea, the same cycle is repeated.
6. cyanosis — bluish color of skin due to deficient oxygenation.
7. dyspnea, dyspnoea — difficult breathing.
8. expectoration — act of coughing up and spitting out material from the lungs, trachea and mouth.
9. hemoptysis — expectoration of blood.
10. hiccough, hiccup, singultus — spasmodic lowering of the diaphragm followed by spasmodic, periodic closure of the glottis.
11. hypercapnia, hypercarbia — an excess of carbon dioxide in the circulating blood, abnormally high carbon dioxide tension (Pco_2) causing overstimulation of respiratory center.[17]
12. hyperpnea — respirations increased in rate and depth.
13. hyperventilation, hyperaeration — excessive movement of air in and out of the lungs.
14. hyperventilation syndrome — prolonged heavy breathing and long sighing respirations causing marked apprehension, palpitation, dizziness, muscular weakness, paresthesia and tetany. The attack may result from biochemical changes in neuromuscular and neurovascular function or from acute anxiety.[35]
15. hypoxia — oxygen want due to decreased amount of oxygen in organs and tissues.
16. orthopnea, orthopnoea — breathing only possible when person sits or stands.
17. rales — bubbling sounds heard in bronchi at inspiration or expiration.

PLEURA AND MEDIASTINUM

A. Origin of Terms:

1. paries (L) — wall
2. phren (G) — diaphragm, mind
3. pleura (G) — pleura
4. pyon (G) — pus
5. thorax (G) — breast plate, chest
6. viscus, viscer (L) — flesh, vital organ

B. Anatomical Terms:

1. mediastinum — the interpleural space containing the pericardium, heart, major vessels, esophagus and thoracic duct.[8]
2. pleura (pl. pleurae) — a thin sac of serous membrane which is invaginated by the lung and lines the mediastinum and thoracic wall. Each lung has its own pleural sac.
   a. parietal pleura — the costal, mediastinal and diaphragmatic parts of the pleura and the cupola which covers the apex of the lung.[8]
   b. visceral pleura, pulmonary pleura — pleura which invests the lungs and lines the interlobar fissures.
3. pleural cavity — potential space between the parietal and visceral pleurae, lubricated by a thin film of serum.

C. Diagnostic Terms:

1. empyema of pleura, pyothorax — pus in pleural cavity.[71]
2. hemothorax — blood in pleural cavity due to trauma or ruptured blood vessel.
3. hydropneumothorax — watery effusion and air in pleural cavity.
4. pleural effusion — excessive formation of serous fluid within the pleural cavity.[46]
5. pleurisy, pleuritis — inflammation of the pleura.[76]
6. pyopneumothorax — pus and air in the pleural cavity.
7. spontaneous pneumothorax — entrance of air into the pleural cavity resulting in a collapse of a lung.
8. tension or valvular pneumothorax — entrance of air into pleural cavity on inspiration; air exit blocked by valve-like tissue on expiration; enlargement of pleural cavity and collapse of lung as positive pressure increases resulting in mediastinal shift and depression of diaphragm.

D. Operative Terms:

1. artificial or therapeutic pneumothorax — the introduction of a measured amount of air into the pleural cavity through a needle in order to give the diseased lung temporary rest.
2. biopsies.
   a. mediastinal node biopsy — resection of small piece of tissue from regional lymph node for microscopy and culture.[23]
   b. pleural biopsy — aspiration of cells from parietal pleura with biopsy needle for bacteriologic and histologic studies.
3. cervical mediastinotomy — small incision into the mediastinum in the neck region to obtain biopsy specimen from lymph node for diagnostic evaluation.[23]
4. mediastinoscopy — examination of the mediastinal organs by a mediastinoscope under direct vision to aid in the diagnosis of disease and in assessing the resectability of bronchogenic carcinoma.[5]
5. pleurectomy:
   a. partial — removal of a portion of the pleura.
   b. complete — removal of the entire pleura. This is generally associated with pneumonectomy.

6. pulmonary decortication — removal of fibrinous exudate or pleural peel from the visceral surface of the imprisoned lung to restore its functional adequacy.

7. thoracentesis — tapping of the pleural cavity to remove pleural effusion for diagnostic or therapeutic purposes.

E. Symptomatic Terms:

1. pleural adhesions — fibrous bands which bind the visceral pleura to the parietal pleura. They may be loose, elastic, avascular or firm, inelastic and vascular.

2. pleural effusion — abnormal accumulation of fluid within the pleural space.

3. pleural exudate — pus or serum accumulating in the pleural cavity. Fibrinous exudate may lead to the formation of adhesions.

4. pleural peel — abnormal layer of fibrous tissue adherent to the visceral pleura and underlying diseased lung. The ever thickening peel may inhibit respiratory function.

5. pleuritic pain, pleurodynia — sharp, intense pain felt in intercostal muscles.

RADIOLOGY

A. General Terms Used in X-Ray Reports:

1. aerated — filled with air.

2. calcification — deposit of lime salts in the tissues.

3. consolidation — solidification of the lung as in pneumonia.

4. density — the compactness of structure of a substance.

5. discrete — well-defined and clear-cut in appearance.

6. fibrosis — replacement of normal tissue with fibrous tissue.

7. infiltration — the permeation of a tissue with substances that are normally absent.

8. infraclavicular — below the clavicle or collar bone.

9. infrascapular — below the scapula or shoulder plate.

10. inspissated — thickened by absorption of fluid content.

11. peribronchial — pertaining to area around the bronchial tubes.

12. rarefaction — process of decreasing density.

13. rarefied area — area of lessened density.

14. subdiaphragmatic — below the diaphragm.

15. substernal — below the sternum or breast bone.

B. Terms Related to X-Ray Examination of Chest:

1. bronchial brushing — safe and reliable method of establishing a definite diagnosis in patients with inoperable pulmonary lesion before radiotherapy is instituted. Under fluoroscopic guidance and topical anesthesia a radiopaque catheter is passed into the bronchial segment where the lesion is located and its proper position is confirmed by spot films. Minute flexible nylon brushes are then inserted through the catheter to an optimal position. The lesion is brushed by vigorous, short strokes. Brush scrapings are used for cytologic and bacteriologic examinations. A biopsy forceps, passed through the catheter, provides tissue specimens for histologic study of the lesion which is helpful in the identification of benign tumors. After slightly withdrawing the catheter, selective bronchography is performed.[66, 41]

2. bronchography — radiographic examination of the bronchial tree following the intratracheal injection of an opaque solution.

3. laminograms of lung — body section radiograms which delineate sharply a thin layer of lung tissue; thus, the structures lying anteriorly and posteriorly are more or less blurred out. Laminograms demonstrate the presence of a cavity and many other lung lesions.[74]

4. planigrams, tomograms of lung — same as laminograms.
5. selective segmental bronchography — bronchographic examination of selected parts of the lungs; for example, the apices. Under local anesthesia a Metras catheter is inserted for the injection of a radiopaque substance. Aided by fluoroscopic guidance, the contrast medium is allowed to fill the bronchial branches of the pulmonary segments. Abnormalities are recorded instantly by spot-films.[74]
6. teleradiography — x-ray pictures obtained with the tube at a distance of 2 meters from the body.

CLINICAL LABORATORY

A. Terms Related to Some Essential Bacteriological Studies:

1. examination of sputum and gastric washings — tests for demonstrating pathogenic organisms. Three methods are used:
   a. animal inoculation — injection of prepared material from specimen into a laboratory animal; for example, either a guinea pig or a white mouse. Smears are made from sacrificed animal after a definite time has elapsed.
   b. culture — material inoculated into an appropriate medium for the purpose of growth and possible identification of the organism.
   c. smear — material spread on a slide for microscopic study of organisms.[23, 50, 4, 53]
2. sensitivity studies — tests for determining the susceptibility of the patient's bacteria to various antimicrobial agents in an effort to evaluate the effectiveness of the therapeutic regime. Results indicate:
   a. drug sensitivity or
   b. drug resistance.[23]
3. skin tests — tests for detecting previous exposure and sensitization to tubercle bacilli.
   a. Heaf — intradermal tuberculin test by multiple puncture technique.
   b. Mantoux — intradermal tuberculin test.
   c. Tine — intradermal tuberculin test by puncture with four tines dip-dried with old tuberculin.[14]
4. vaccine for tuberculosis, BCG — attenuated vaccine composed of avirulent tubercle bacilli. BCG vaccination produces immunity against tuberculosis, variable in effect and duration.

B. Terms Related to the Evaluation of Lung Function:

1. bronchospirometry — graphic recording of the relative participation of the two lungs in ventilation and oxygen uptake.[18, 28]
2. pulmonary function studies — specific tests for determining the ability of the lungs to perform respiration as compared to the normal for a given age, height and weight. They are primarily concerned with the evaluation of lung volumes, ventilation, the distribution of ventilation and diffusion or oxygen consumption.[83]

ABBREVIATIONS

A. General:

ACD — anterior chest diameter
AFB — acid fast bacillus
A&P — auscultation and percussion
AP — anterior-posterior
    (projection of x-rays)
ARD — acute respiratory disease
BCG — bacillus Calmette Guerin,
    vaccine for tuberculosis

BS — breath sounds
COPD — chronic obstructive
    pulmonary disease
FRC — functional residual
    capacity
IPPB — intermittent positive
    pressure breathing
IS, ICS — intercostal space

LSB — left sternal border
MCL — midcostal line
MSL — midsternal line
OT — old tuberculin
PA — posterior-anterior
PAP — primary atypical pneumonia
PPD — purified protein derivative
PPLO — pleuropneumonia-like

organisms
RD — respiratory disease
RM — respiratory movement
TB — tuberculosis
TF — tactile fremitus
URI — upper respiratory
 infection
VF — vocal fremitus

B. Organizations:

ALA — American Lung Association
ALS — American Lung Society

HEW — US Health, Education and
 Welfare Department

ORAL READING PRACTICE

Bronchial Asthma

Bronchial asthma is a condition characterized by **paroxysmal** attacks of dyspnea in which the breathing is wheezy, the expiration is prolonged and the normal **vesicular** murmur is obscured by loud, musical rales.

In some instances nasal **polypi, hypertrophy** of the **conchae;** or **ethmoiditis** provoke the disease. An essential factor in many cases is a peculiar susceptibility or **hypersensitivity** to some special protein which is inhaled or ingested. In some cases of asthma **focal** infection is the essential **etiologic** factor. Physical overexertion, emotional excitement, seasonal changes and **intercurrent** infections favor the occurrence of attacks.

The paroxysms are excessive at night. The patient is seized with intense **dyspnea** and a feeling of impending **suffocation** which compel him to sit upright. The face is anxious, sometimes livid and the skin is covered with cool perspiration. The respirations are labored and noisy. Cough is usually present and is associated with the **expectoration** of viscid **mucus.**

During the attack the chest is fixed in full inspiratory expansion. **Percussion** gives **hyperresonance** in chronic **emphysematous** cases. On **auscultation** there are numerous **rales** especially during **expectoration.**[37, 62]

Table 11

SOME RESPIRATORY CONDITIONS AMENABLE TO SURGERY

Organs Involved	Diagnoses	Operations	Operative Procedures
Nasal septum	Deflection of nasal septum, congenital or post-traumatic	Septectomy or submucous resection	Removal of nasal septum, partial or complete
Nasal mucosa	Mucous polyp	Excision of lesion	Removal of polyp
Maxillary sinus (antrum of Highmore)	Maxillary sinusitis due to streptococcus	Maxillary sinusotomy, antrum window operation	Opening of the antrum
Larynx	Papilloma or cyst of larynx	Laryngoscopy with excision of lesion	Endoscopic examination with removal of neoplasm
Larynx Epiglottis Vocal cords	Squamous carcinoma of larynx	Total laryngectomy	Removal of entire larynx

Organs Involved	Diagnoses	Operations	Operative Procedures
Trachea	Carcinoma of larynx	Tracheostomy (preliminary step to laryngectomy)	Fistulization of trachea
Bronchi	Endobronchial tuberculosis	Bronchoscopy with aspiration of bronchial secretions	Endoscopic examination of bronchi
Bronchopulmonary segment	Cystic disease of lung, tension air cyst	Segmental resection, lateral segment, middle lobe	Removal of segment including tension air cyst of lung
Bronchopulmonary segment	Moderately advanced tuberculosis with cavitation	Segmental resection, upper lobe	Removal of two segments of upper lobe
Bronchus, Bronchioli Lung	Bronchiectasis, post-infectional	Lobectomy, middle lobe	Removal of middle lobe of lung
Lobe	Tuberculoma	Wedge resection, upper lobe	Excision of triangular shaped tuberculoma
Lung Visceral pleura	Far advanced fibrocaseous tuberculosis Fibrinous pleurisy, lower lobe	Lobectomy, upper lobe Decortication, lower lobe	Removal of upper lobe Excision of thickened fibrotic lesion of visceral pleura
Lung Visceral pleura	Carcinoma of lung or unilateral far advanced tuberculosis	Pneumonectomy, Pleurectomy	Removal of lung including visceral pleura
Lung Thorax	Excessive pleural effusion, empyema	Postpneumonectomy thoracoplasty	Multiple rib resection in two stages

REFERENCES AND BIBLOGRAPHY

1. Ackerman, Lauren V. and del Regato, Juan A. Nasopharynx. In *Cancer*, 4th ed. St. Louis: The C. V. Mosby Co., 1970, pp. 254-275.
2. ——————. Endolarynx. *Ibid.*, pp. 308-329.
3. ——————. Lung. *Ibid.*, pp. 329-376.
4. Ackerman, L. V. and Rosai, J. The pathology of tumors. Part three: frozen section, gross and microscopic examination, ancillary studies. *Ca — A Cancer Journal for Clinicians*, 21: 270-281, September-October, 1971.
5. American Thoracic Society. Diagnostic mediastinoscopy. *American Review of Respiratory Disease*, 105: 487-489, March, 1972.
6. Amikam, B. *et al.* Bronchofiberscopic observations of the tracheobronchial tree during intubation. *American Review of Respiratory Disease*, 105: 747-755, May, 1972.
7. Anderson, W. H. Chronic bronchitis. In Conn, Howard F. (ed.). *Current Therapy 1972*. Philadelphia: W. B. Saunders Co., 1972, pp. 100-102.
8. Anson, Barry J. (ed.). *Morris' Human Anatomy*, 12th ed. New York: McGraw-Hill Book Co., 1966, pp. 1424-1440.
9. Asai, R. Laryngoplasty after total laryngectomy. *Archives of Otolaryngology*, 95: 114-119, February, 1972.
10. Becklake, M. R. Chemical and physical irritants. In Beeson, Paul B. and McDermott, Walsh (eds.). *Cecil-Loeb Textbook of Medicine*, 13th ed. Philadelphia: W. B. Saunders Co., 1971, pp. 881-899.
11. Berger, R. L. *et al.* Dissemination of cancer cells by needle biopsy of the lung. *Journal of Thoracic and Cardiovascular Surgery*, 63: 430-432, March, 1972.
12. Bonfils-Roberts, E. A. *et al.* Contemporary indications for pulmonary resections. *Journal of Thoracic and Cardiovascular Surgery*, 63: 433-438, March, 1972.
13. Boyd, D. R. Monitoring patients with posttraumatic pulmonary insufficiency. *Surgical Clinics of North America*, 52: 31-46, February, 1972.
14. Browder, A. A. *et al.* Tuberculin Tine tests on medical wards. *American Review of Respiratory Disease.* 105: 299-301, February, 1972.
15. Burrows, B. Chronic airway obstruction. In Conn, Howard F. (ed.). *Current Therapy 1972.* Philadelphia: W. B. Saunders Co., 1972, pp. 90-95.
16. Caceres, J. *et al.* Double primary carcinomas of the lung. *Radiology*, 102: 45-50, January, 1972.
17. Cherniack, R. M. Acute respiratory failure. In Conn, Howard F. (ed.). *Current Therapy 1972.* Philadelphia: W. B. Saunders Co., 1972, pp. 84190.

18. Cohen, C. A. *et al.* Respiratory symptoms, spirometry and oxidant air pollution in non-smoking adults. *American Review of Respiratory Disease,* 105: 251-261, February, 1972.

19. Collart, M. and Brenneman, J. K. Preventing postoperative atelectasis. *American Journal of Nursing,* 71: 1982-1987, October, 1971.

20. Council on Drugs, American Medical Association. Evaluation of a new antituberculous agent. *Journal of American Medical Association,* 220: 414-415, April 17, 1972.

21. Deatch, W. W. Ear nose & throat. In Krupp, Marcus A., Chatton, Milton J. and Margen, Sheldon. *Current Diagnosis & Treatment,* 10th ed. LosAltos, California: Lange Medical Publications, 1971, pp. 93-109.

22. Denny, F. W. *et al.* Mycoplasma pneumoniae disease: Clinical spectrum, pathophysiology, epidemiology and control. *Journal of Infectious Diseases,* 123: 747-92, January, 1971.

23. *Diagnostic Standards and Classification of Tuberculosis,* 12th ed. New York: National Tuberculosis Association, 1969, pp. 30-76.

24. Douglas, R. G. Viral respiratory infections. In Conn, Howard F. (ed.). *Current Therapy 1972.* Philadelphia: W. B. Saunders Co., 1972, pp. 140-142.

25. Ebert, R. V. Diffuse lung disease. In Beeson, Paul B. and McDermott, Walsh (eds.). *Cecil-Loeb Textbook of Medicine,* 13th ed. Philadelphia: W. B. Saunders Co., 1971, pp. 903-910.

26. —————. Abnormal air spaces. *Ibid.,* pp. 899-903.

27. Feinstein, A. R. Neoplasms of the lung. In Beeson, Paul B. and McDermott, Walsh (eds.). *Cecil-Loeb Textbook of Medicine,* 13th ed. Philadelphia: W. B. Saunders Co., 1971, pp. 923-929.

28. Gimeno, F. Spirometry-induced bronchial obstruction. *American Review of Respiratory Disease,* 105: 68-74, January, 1972.

29. Goldman, M. L. and Miller, D. Antibody to Epstein-Barr virus in American patients with carcinoma of the nasopharynx. *Journal of American Medical Association,* 216: 1618-1622, June 7, 1971.

30. Goldsmith, J. R. Prevention of chronic lung disease. *Postgraduate Medicine,* 51: 93-99, January, 1972.

31. Goodwin, R. A. Histoplasmosis. In Conn, Howard, F. (ed.). *Current Therapy 1972.* Philadelphia: W. B. Saunders Co., 1972, pp. 111-113.

32. Griffin, J. P. *et al.* Viral and mycoplasmal pneumonias. In Conn, Howard F. (ed.). *Current Therapy 1972.* Philadelphia: W. B. Saunders Co., 1972, pp. 120-123.

33. Grimes. O. F. Neuromuscular syndrome in patients with lung cancer. *American Journal of Nursing,* 71: 752-755, April, 1971.

34. Henderson, R. L. Respiratory manifestations of hashish smoking. *Archives of Otolaryngology,* 95: 248-251, March, 1972.

35. Heyman, A. Syncope and hyperventilation. In Beeson, Paul B. and McDermott, Walsh. *Cecil-Loeb Textbook of Medicine,* 13th ed. Philadelphia: W. B. Saunders Co., 1971, pp. 167-171.

36. Hickam, J. B. Pulmonary hypertension. In Beeson, Paul B. and McDermott, Walsh (ed.). *Cecil-Loeb Textbook of Medicine,* 13th ed. Philadelphia: W. B. Saunders Co., 1971, pp. 937-946.

37. Howell, J. B. L. Airway obstruction. In Beeson, Paul B. and McDermott, Walsh (eds.). *Cecil-Loeb Textbook of Medicine,* 13th ed. Philadelphia: W. B. Saunders Co., 1971, pp. 881-899.

38. Hyde, L. Clinical significance of the tuberculin test. *American Review of Respiratory Disease,* 105: 453-454, March, 1972.

39. Israel, H. L. Acute pulmonary embolism. In Conn, Howard F. (ed.). *Current Therapy 1972,* Philadelphia: W. B. Saunders Co., 1972, pp. 123-124.

40. Jacquette, G. To reduce hazards of tracheal suctioning. *American Journal of Nursing,* 71: 2363-2364, December, 1971.

41. Janower, M. L. and Land, R. E. Lung biopsy — bronchial brushing and percutaneous puncture. *Radiologic Clinics of North America,* 9: 73-83, April, 1971.

42. Kamada, R. O. *et al.* The phenomenon of respiratory failure in shock: The genesis of shock lung. *American Heart Journal,* 83: 1-3, January, 1972.

43. Langston, H. T. Lung cancer — a projection. *Journal of Thoracic and Cardiovascular Surgery,* 63: 412-415, March, 1972.

44. Lin, T. M. *et al.* Antibodies to herpes-type virus in nasopharyngeal carcinoma and control groups. *Cancer,* 29: 603-609, March, 1972.

45. Lockwood, W. R. *et al.* Sinusitis. In Conn, Howard F. (ed.). *Current Therapy 1972.* Philadelphia: W. B. Saunders Co., 1972, pp. 127-129.

46. Maher, G. G. *et al.* Massive pleural effusion: Malignant and nonmalignant causes in 46 patients. *American Review of Respiratory Disease,* 105: 458-460, March, 1972.

47. Manson, R. M. *et al.* Respiratory tract & mediastinum. In Krupp, Marcus A., Chatton, Milton J. and Margen, Sheldon. *Current Diagnosis & Treatment,* 10th ed. Los Altos, California: Lange Medical Publications, 1971, pp. 110-152.

48. McCall, C. E. Bacterial pneumonia. In Conn, Howard F. (ed.). *Current Therapy 1972.* Philadelphia: W. B. Saunders Co., 1972, pp. 116-120.

49. Mittman, C. Summary of symposium on pulmonary emphysema and proteolysis. *American Review of Respiratory Disease,* 105: 430-448, March, 1972.

50. Moulding, T. Tuberculosis and atypical mycobacteria. In Conn, Howard F. (ed.). *Current Therapy 1972.* Philadelphia: W. B. Saunders Co., 1972, pp. 131-140.

51. Mulder, D. S. Tracheopleural fistula — A complication of the cuffed tracheostomy tube. *Journal of Thoracic and Cardiovascular Surgery,* 63: 416-418, March, 1972.

52. Mushlin, I. M. Big city approach to tuberculosis control. *American Journal of Nursing,* 71: 2342-2345, December, 1971.

53. Myers, J. A. Elderly people and their tubercle bacilli. *Geriatrics,* 26: 77-83, December, 1971.

54. Neff, T. A. *et al.* Miliary tuberculosis and carcinoma of the lung. Successful treatment with chemotherapy and resection. *American Review of Respiratory Disease,* 105: 111-113, January, 1972.

55. Olofsson, J. *et al.* Radiotherapy vs conservative surgery in the treatment of selected supraglottic

carcinomas. *Archives of Otolaryngology*, 95: 240-242, March, 1972.

56. Pontoppidan, H. *el al.* Acute respiratory failure. In Welch, Claude E. *et al. Advances in Surgery*, Vol. 4. Chicago: Year Book Medical Publishers, Inc., 1970, pp. 163-248.

57. Pool, J. L. *Primary lung cancer.* In Conn, Howard F. (ed.). *Current Therapy 1972.* Philadelphia: W. B. Saunders Co., 1972, pp. 105-109.

58. Quaife, M. A. *et al.* Correlation of the ventilation and perfusion aspects of chronic obstructive pulmonary disease. *Chest*, 61: 459-464, May, 1972.

59. Raffel, S. Tuberculosis. In Samter, M. (ed) *Immunological Diseases*, 2d ed. Boston: Little, Brown and Co., 1971, pp. 601-629.

60. Raleigh, J. W. Rifampin in treatment of advanced pulmonary tuberculosis. *American Review of Respiratory Disease*, 105: 397-409, March, 1972.

61. Reeves, K. R. Acute epiglottitis — pediatric emergency. *American Journal of Nursing*, 71: 1539-1541, August, 1971.

62. Reisman, R. E. Bronchial asthma. In Conn, Howard F. (ed.). *Current Therapy 1972.* Philadelphia: W. B. Saunders Co., 1972, pp. 536-542.

63. Ribi, E. Currents in tuberculosis research. *Journal of Infectious Diseases*, 123: 562-565, May, 1971.

64. Rubin, P. Cancer of the head and neck — nasopharyngeal cancer. *Journal of American Medical Association*, 220: 390-408, April 17, 1972.

65. Ruth, W. E. Bronchiectasis. In Conn, Howard F. (ed.). *Current Therapy 1972.* Philadelphia: W. B. Saunders Co., 1972, pp. 97-100.

66. Sagel, S. S. Current practices in chest roentgenography. In Welsh, Calude E. *et al.* (eds.). *Advances in Surgery*, Vol. 5. Chicago: Year Book Medical Publishers, Inc., 1971, pp. 51-87.

67. Satterfield, J. V. Atelectasis. In Conn, Howard F. (ed.). *Current Therapy 1972.* Philadelphia: W. B. Saunders Co., 1972, pp. 95-96.

68. Schindel, J. *et al.* Late-appearing (radiation induced) carcinoma. *Archives of Otolaryngology*, 95: 205-210, March, 1972.

69. Schmidt, F. E. *et al.* Biopsy of apical pulmonary tumors: An open technique with needle biopsy. *Surgery*, 70: 614-615, October, 1971.

70. Schofield, J. Conservative treatment of subglottic stenosis of the larynx. *Archives of Otolaryngology*, 95. 457-459, May, 1972.

71. Sealy, W. C. Empyema thoracis. In Conn, Howard F. (ed.). *Current Therapy 1972.* Philadelphia: W. B. Saunders Co., 1972.

72. Senior, R. M. Pulmonary emphysema. In Conn, Howard F. (ed.). *Current Therapy 1972.* Philadelphia: W. B. Saunders Co., 1972, pp. 102-105.

73. Shaia, F. T. Laryngeal trauma. *Archives of Otolaryngology*, 95. 104-108, February, 1972.

74. Simon, G. *Principles of Chest X-Ray Diagnosis*, 3d ed. New York: Appleton-Century-Grofts, 1971, pp. 243-244.

75. Stafford, E. G. *et al.* Postpneumonectomy empyema: Neomycin instillation and definitive closure. *Journal of Thoracic and Cardiovascular Surgery*, 63: 771-775, May, 1972.

76. Stead, W. W. Diseases of the pleura. In Beeson, Paul B. and McDermott, Walsh (eds.). *Cecil-Loeb Textbook of Medicine*, 13th ed. Philadelphia: W. B. Saunders Co., 1971, pp. 929-936.

77. Stein, K. M. *et al.* Occult lung abscess complicating high-dosage corticosteroid therapy. *Postgraduate Medicine*, 51: 97-101, April, 1972.

78. Sutliff, W. D. Histoplasmosis-cooperative study. *American Review of Respiratory Disease*, 105: 60-67, January, 1972.

79. Theodos, P. A. Silicosis. In Conn, Howard F. (ed.). *Current Therapy 1972.* Philadelphia: W. B. Saunders Co., 1972, pp. 124-127.

80. Vanek, J. *et al.* The gamut of histoplasmosis. *American Journal of Medicine*, 50: 89-104, January, 1971.

81. Vassallo, C. L. Exercise-induced hypocapnia and acidosis. *American Review of Respiratory Disease*, 105: 42-49, January, 1972.

82. Wenger, N. K. Massive acute pulmonary embolism. *Journal of American Medical Association*, 220: 842-844, May 8, 1972.

83. Williams, M. H. Ventilatory function. In Beeson, Paul B. and McDermott, Walsh (eds.). *Cecil-Loeb Textbook of Medicine*, 13th ed. Philadelphia: W. B. Saunders Co., 1971, pp. 866-869.

Chapter VIII
Digestive Disorders

MOUTH

A. Origin of Terms:

1. bucca (L) — cheek
2. cheilos (G) — lip
3. dent- (L) — tooth
4. gingiva (L) — gum
5. glossa (G) — tongue
6. labium (L) — lip
7. lingua (L) — tongue
8. odont- (G) — tooth
9. os, pl. ora (L) — mouth
10. staphyle (G) — bunch of grapes
11. stoma (G) — mouth
12. uvula (L) — little grape

B. Anatomical Terms:

1. alveolus — bony tooth socket.
2. hard palate, bony palate — anterior part of roof of mouth.
3. oral cavity — the mouth.
4. soft palate — posterior part of palate partially separating the oral from the nasal part of the pharynx.
5. uvula — small, cone-shaped downward projection from the free lower edge of the soft palate in midline.

C. Diagnostic Terms:

1. aphthous stomatitis — small ulceration of the mucous membrane of the mouth.
2. ankyloglossia — tongue-tie.
3. candidiasis, moniliasis, thrush — curd-like creamy patches in the mouth due to overgrowth of Candida albicans. Pain, fever, and lymphadenopathy may be present. The fungal growth is prone to occur when antibiotic therapy or acute illness upsets the balance of the normal flora.[27]
4. cancer of the mouth — malignant lesions of the lips, gums and tongue.[6, 74, 92, 114]
5. cavity of tooth — loss of tooth structure due to decay process, attrition, abrasion, erosion or developmental defect.
6. chilitis, cheilitis — inflammation of the lips.
7. chilosis — morbid condition of the lips due to vitamin deficiency.
8. cleft lip, harelip — congenital anomaly of upper lip consisting of a vertical fissure often associated with cleft palate.
9. cleft palate — a congenital fissure of the roof of the mouth due to nonunion of bones.
10. dental caries — localized progressive decay of tooth structure.
11. epulis, giant cell epulis — a reparative lesion of gingiva which develops in response to trauma or hemorrhage.[116]
12. gingivitis — inflammation of the gums.
13. glossitis — inflammation of the tongue.
14. leukoplakia of the mouth — white patches on the mucous membrane of the tongue and buccal mucosa.[27, 50]
15. periapical abscess — abscessed tooth, due to dental decay leading to infection of the pulp.
16. periodontal disease — dental disorders characterized by inflammation of the gums, destruction of alveolar bone, degeneration of periodontal ligament and periodontal pocket formation.[102, 12]
17. stomatitis — inflammation of the mucosa of the mouth and an oral manifestation of systemic disease, allergy or toxic drug effect. Multiple ulcerations and fissures of the corners of the mouth may be present.[27]
18. Vincent's infection, trench mouth — a painful, inflammatory condition of the gums usually associated with fever, ulcerations, bleeding and lymphadenopathy.[27]

D. Operative Terms:

1. cheiloplasty — plastic repair of a lip.
2. cheilostomatoplasty — plastic repair of lip and mouth for cleft lip.
3. clipping of frenum linguae — clipping of membranous fold below tongue to relieve tongue-tie.
4. electrocoagulation for oral cancer — application of electrode to lesion to destroy it.[42, 25]
5. glossectomy, complete — removal of entire tongue generally done for carcinoma.
6. glossectomy, partial, hemiglossectomy — resection of the tongue.
7. glossorrhaphy — suture of an injured tongue.
8. palatoplasty — repair of cleft palate.[153]
9. staphylorrhaphy — suture of cleft palate.
10. stomatoplasty — plastic repair of mouth.

SALIVARY GLANDS

A. Origin of Terms:

1. mandible (L) — lower jaw
2. parotid (G) — beside the ear
3. ptyalin (G) — saliva, spittle
4. sialon (G) — saliva, spittle
5. sialaden (G) — salivary gland
6. sialangi (G) — salivary duct

B. Anatomical Terms:

1. chief salivary glands — 3 pairs of glands with ducts opening into the oral cavity. They secrete saliva which moistens, dissolves and transports food and produces a starch-splitting enzyme, amylase.
   a. parotid gland and duct (Stensen's duct) located below the ear.
   b. sublingual gland and 10 to 30 ducts situated on the floor of the mouth beneath the tongue; some of the ducts open into the submandibular duct.
   c. submandibular gland and duct (Wharton's duct), situated mainly below the mandible.
2. small salivary glands — numerous glands in tongue, cheeks, lips.

C. Diagnostic Terms:

1. carcinoma of a salivary gland — malignant neoplasm arising from the glandular epithelium of a salivary gland.[48, 90]
2. parotitis — inflammation of parotid gland.
3. ptyalith, sialolith — stone in salivary gland.
4. ptyalocele — cystic tumor of a salivary gland.
5. sialadenitis — inflammation of salivary gland.

D. Operative Terms:

1. sialadenectomy — removal of a salivary gland.
2. sialolithotomy — removal of a stone from a salivary gland.

E. Symptomatic Terms:

1. halitosis — offensive odor of breath.
2. ptyalism, salivation — excessive secretion of saliva.

PHARYNX

A. Origin of Terms:

1. fauces (L) — throat
2. palatum (L) — palate
3. pharynx (G) — throat
4. tonsilla (L) — almond, tonsil

B. Anatomical Terms:

1. crypts — follicles or pits in tonsils.
2. palatine tonsil, faucial tonsil — a collection of lymphoid tissue lodged in the tonsillar fossa on either side of the oral part of the pharynx.
3. pharyngeal tonsil — a collection of lymphoid tissue located in the posterior wall of the nasal part of the pharynx.
4. pharynx — fibromuscular tube lined with mucous membrane and divided into oral, nasal and laryngeal parts. It extends from the nose and mouth to the esophagus and serves as a common pathway for food and air.

C. Diagnostic Terms:

1. adenoids — enlarged pharyngeal tonsils.
2. hypertrophy of tonsils — enlarged palatine tonsils.
3. peritonsillar abscess, quinsy — localized collection of pus around the tonsil.
4. pharyngitis — inflammation of pharynx.
5. tonsillitis — inflammation of the tonsils.

D. Operative Terms:

1. tonsillectomy — removal of tonsils.
2. adenoidectomy — removal of adenoids.

E. Symptomatic Terms:

1. aphagia — inability to swallow.
2. deglutition — swallowing.
3. dysphagia — difficulty in swallowing.

ESOPHAGUS

A. Origin of Terms:

1. esophagus (G) — food-carrier, gullet

B. Anatomical Terms:

1. cervical esophagus — portion of esophagus in the neck.
2. thoracic esophagus — portion of esophagus which passes through the thorax.

C. Diagnostic Terms:

1. atresia of esophagus — congenital absence or pathological closure of the esophagus.
2. carcinoma of esophagus — malignant neoplasm, commonly an epidermoid carcinoma, arising from the epidermis or squamous epithelium; metastatic spread to other organs is a frequent occurrence.[143]
3. dilatation of esophagus, achalasia — a common disorder due to failure of cardiac sphincter to relax. It is characterized by a dilated and hypertrophied esophagus except for the distal segment which is atrophied.[27, 20]

4. diverticula of esophagus (sing. diverticulum) — outpouching of esophageal wall. Two kinds:

    a. pulsion or true diverticula — consist of a bulging of mucosa through weakened parts of the esophageal wall.

    b. traction or false diverticula are due to pull exerted by diseased neighboring structures.

5. esophageal reflux ulceration — ulceration of the esophagus resulting from reflux of acid-peptic secretions into the esophagus due to incompetence of the gastroesophageal sphincter.[111]

6. esophageal trauma — injury to esophagus.[16]

    a. esophageal perforation — a hole in esophageal wall usually due to mechanical injury by ingestion of foreign body, gunshot wound or other causes.[42, 16, 80]

    b. esophageal stricture — narrowing of the esophageal lumen, usually due to chemical injury such as lye ingestion or other caustic agents.[16]

7. esophagitis — inflammation of the esophagus.

8. varices (sing. varix) of esophagus — swollen, tortuous esophageal veins which may burst and result in massive hemorrhage. Condition is usually secondary to portal hypertension.[42]

D. Operative Terms:

1. bougienage for esophageal stricture — dilation of esophagus with bougies, flexible instruments resembling sounds, used to diagnose and treat strictures of tubular passages.[144]

2. esophageal diverticulectomy — excision of diverticulum and closure of the resulting defect.

3. esophagojejunostomy — formation of a communication between the esophagus and jejunum.

4. esophagoplasty — reconstruction or plastic repair of esophageal defect.

5. esophagoplasty with reversed gastric tube — a physiological method of esophageal replacement using the patient's own stomach to avoid immune reactions caused by rejection of transplants.[65]

6. esophagorrhaphy — suture of injured or ruptured esophagus.

7. fundic patch operation — surgical procedure for repair of ruptured esophagus or acid-peptic stricture and in the treatment of advanced achalasia.[64]

8. fundoplication — operative procedure to relieve gastroesophageal reflux of large amounts of acid-peptic juice and to restore gastroesophageal competence.[47, 145]

9. Heller's operation — surgical procedure for achalasia of the cardia.[10]

10. radical resection for esophageal cancer — excision of tumor bearing portion of esophagus and regional lymph nodes, followed by restoration of continuity by anastomosis or interposition of loop of colon or jejunum.[42]

11. resection for esophageal stricture — removal of extensive narrow segment followed by colonic bypass. The right colon with terminal ileum and ileocecal valve is tunneled into the neck and anastomosed with the proximal esophagus. The operation is indicated when chronic stricture is unresponsive to bougienage.[144]

E. Symptomatic Terms:

1. dysphagia — difficulty in swallowing.

2. regurgitation — backflow of gastric contents into the mouth.[42]

STOMACH

A. Origin of Terms:

1. fundus (L) — base
2. gaster (G) — stomach, belly
3. omentum (L) — membrane enclosing bowel
4. pyloros (G) — gatekeeper
5. ruga (L) — fold, crease
6. sphincter (G) — binder

B. Anatomical Terms:

1. cardiac orifice — opening at the junction of the esophagus with the stomach.
2. curvatures of stomach:
   a. lesser — right and superior margin of the stomach.
   b. greater — left and inferior margin of the stomach.
3. fundus of stomach — enlarged portion to the left located above the level of the cardiac orifice.
4. omenta (sing. omentum) — peritoneal sheets connecting the stomach with other viscera as the liver, spleen and transverse colon.
5. pyloric sphincter — circular muscle around pylorus.
6. pylorus — opening between stomach and duodenum.
7. rugae (sing. ruga) — irregular folds of the mucous membrane of the stomach in which gastric glands are embedded.

C. Diagnostic Terms:

1. gastric neoplasms, benign — new growths of the stomach that rarely interfere with gastric peristalsis.
   a. adenoma — tumor derived from glandular epithelium.
   b. papilloma — circumscribed hypertrophy of gastric mucosa.
   c. polyp, polypus — pedunculated outgrowth of mucous membrane.[27]
2. gastric neoplasms, malignant:
   a. carcinoma — usually adenocarcinoma; a malignant new growth of glandular epithelium.
   b. sarcoma — frequently lymphosarcoma, arising from lymphoid tissue.
3. gastric ulcers — localized erosions of gastric mucosa which may result from the digestive action of acid gastric secretion. Secondary involvement of muscle tissue may occur.[26]
4. gastritis — inflammation of the gastric mucosa.
5. gastrocele — hernia of stomach; example, diaphragmatic gastric hernia.
6. gastrocolitis — inflammation of stomach and colon.
7. gastroduodenitis — inflammation of stomach and duodenum.
8. gastroenteritis — inflammation of stomach and intestine.
9. gastroptosis, Glenard's disease — downward displacement of stomach.
10. hiatal hernia, hiatus hernia — protrusion of part of the stomach through the esophageal opening of the diaphragm.[152]
11. hypertrophic, pyloric stenosis, congenital — condition seen in the newborn characterized by an overgrowth of muscle fibers which markedly diminishes the lumen of the pyloric canal and gives rise to obstruction.
12. Zollinger-Ellison syndrome — excessive gastric secretion, rapidly worsening refractory peptic ulceration and hyperplasia of pancreatic islet cells.[76]

Table 12

GASTRIC TYPES IN RELATION TO ARCHITECTURAL STRUCTURES OF INDIVIDUALS[a]

Type of Stomach	Description of Type of Stomach	Tonicity of Stomach	Graphic Description
Hypersthenic individual stocky short	Stomach high, wide above, narrow below, transverse position, pylorus to the right	Hypertonic Increased tone	
Sthenic individual well-built	Stomach tubular in shape, as wide above as it is below, pylorus to the right, well above the umbilicus	Orthotonic Normal tone	
Hyposthenic individual more slender	Stomach longer, narrower at the top; a tendency to sag below the greater curvature near the umbilicus; pylorus swinging to the left	Hypotonic Decreased tone	
Asthenic individual still more slender	Stomach sags far down below the umbilicus, being almost collapsed above, expanding into large sac below	Atonic Weak tone	

[a] L. R. Sante. *Principles of Roentgenological Interpretation*, 10th ed. Ann Arbor, Michigan: Edwards Brothers, Inc., 1956, p. 368.

D. Operative Terms:

1. anastomosis — surgical formation of a passage or opening between two hollow viscera or vessels; for example, gastrojejunostomy.[139]

2. gastrectomy — partial or complete removal of stomach.

3. gastric freezing — cryotherapy for peptic ulcers, usually consisting of a 50 minute gastric freeze to produce a semipermanent alteration of the gastric glands' ability to secrete hydrochloric acid. Currently procedure is rarely used.

4. gastric resection — usually the removal of 50-75% of the stomach combined with one of the following procedures:
   a. gastroduodenal anastomosis, Billroth I — joining the resected stomach to the duodenum.
   b. gastrojejunal anastomosis, Billroth II — joining the remaining stomach to the jejunum by either the
      (1) Polya technique — anterior anastomosis, large stoma or
      (2) Hofmeister technique — posterior anastomosis, small stoma.[42, 34, 81]

5. gastrojejunostomy — creation of a communication between the stomach and jejunum.

6. gastrostomy — external fistulization of the stomach. This may be done for the purpose of maintaining nutrition.

7. mucosal antrectomy — complete removal of gastrin secreting antral mucosa to provide protection against recurrent peptic ulceration.[84]

8. pyloromyotomy, Fredet-Ramstedt operation — incision of the hypertrophic pyloric muscle down to the mucosa.[33]

9. pyloroplasty — revision of pyloric stoma.[42]

10. repair of hiatus hernia — several different methods are used either by the transthoracic or transabdominal approach, for example: freeing the esophagus at the cardia and attaching the region of the esophagogastric junction to the defect in the diaphragm.[42, 17, 112 ,152]

11. vagotomy — section of the vagus nerve fibers before they enter the stomach to eliminate the nerve impulses stimulating gastric acid secretion.[31, 11, 75]

E. Symptomatic Terms:

1. achlorhydria — absence of hydrochloric acid in the gastric juice.
2. achylia gastrica — absent or reduced gastric secretion due to atrophy of the mucosa of the stomach.
3. anorexia — loss of appetite.
4. bulemia — excessive appetite.
5. cyclic vomiting — periodic vomiting.
6. dumping syndrome — symptoms occurring after meals following gastrectomy. The patient experiences sweating, flushing, warmth, faintness and sometimes diarrhea.[4]
7. dyspepsia — imperfect digestion.
8. epigastric pain — pain over the pit of the stomach.
9. eructation — belching.
10. hematemesis — vomiting blood.
11. hyperchlorhydria — excessive amount of hydrochloric acid in the gastric juice.
12. hypochlorhydria — deficient amount of hydrochloric acid in the stomach.
13. intrinsic factor, Castle's intrinsic factor — factor normally present in gastric mucosa and gastric juice and required for absorption of vitamin B_{12}. It is absent in pernicious anemia.[150]
14. polyphagia — excessive food intake.

SMALL AND LARGE INTESTINES

A. Origin of Terms:

1. appendix (L) — appendage
2. cecum (L) — blind gut
3. colon (G) — large intestine
4. duodenum (L) — twelve, duodenum
5. enteron (G) — intestine
6. ileum (G) — to twist
7. jejunum (L) — empty
8. procto- (G) — anus
9. rectum (L) — straight
10. vermiform (L) — shape of worm

B. Anatomical Terms:

1. small intestine — proximal portion of intestine from pylorus to ileocecal junction.
   a. duodenum — first part of small intestine; extends from pylorus to jejunum.
   b. jejunum — second part of small intestine; extends from duodenum to ileum.
   c. ileum — third part of small intestine; extends from jejunum to cecum.
   d. mesentery — peritoneal fold which carries the blood supply and attaches the jejunum and ileum to the posterior abdominal wall.[39, 42]
2. large intestine — distal portion of intestine including cecum, appendix, colon, rectum and anal canal.
   a. anus — outlet or orifice of anal canal.
   b. appendix vermiformis — an intestinal diverticulum projecting from cecum 3 - 13 cm and ending blindly.[39]
   c. cecum — blind pouch of large intestine at and below level of ileocecal junction.
   d. colon — large intestine from cecum to rectum including the ascending colon, transverse colon, descending colon and sigmoid or pelvic colon.
   e. flexures of colon[39]
      (1) right colic flexure, formerly hepatic flexure — bend of colon near liver.
      (2) left colic flexure, formerly splenic flexure — bend of colon near spleen.
   f. mesocolon — mesentery attaching the colon to the posterior abdominal wall.

C. Diagnostic Terms:

1. appendicitis — inflammation of the appendix.
2. colitis:
   a. ischemic colitis — a spontaneous reduction of the arterial blood flow of large intestine associated with abrupt onset of abdominal pain, frequent bloody stools and radiographic changes of colon.[117]
   b. mucous colitis — inflammatory condition marked by large amount of mucus in stool.
   c. ulcerative colitis — inflammation and multiple erosions of the intestinal mucosa leading to hemorrhage and perforations, clinically noted for frequent evacuations of watery, purulent and bloody stools.
3. congenital megacolon, Hirschsprung's disease — excessive enlargement of the colon associated with an absence of ganglion cells in the narrowed bowel wall distally. The aganglionic segment of the colon is the pathological lesion.[42, 136, 126]
4. diverticulitis — inflammation of a diverticulum or diverticula.[154, 22, 28]
5. diverticulosis — presence of diverticula in the intestinal tract.
6. duodenal ulcer — circumscribed erosion of duodenal wall which may involve full thickness and is usually located near the pylorus.[83, 78, 108, 99]
7. dysentery — inflammation of the intestinal mucosa characterized by frequent small stools, chiefly of blood and mucus. It is due to specific bacillus or ameba.
8. fecal fistula — abnormal communication of the intestine to the surface or another hollow viscus.[42]
9. fistula in ano, anal fistula — abnormal communication from anal canal to skin near anus.
10. enteritis — inflammation of the intestine.
11. hemorrhoids, piles — dilated varicose veins of the anal canal and at anal orifice.[42, 89, 148]
12. ileitis — inflammation of the ileum.
    a. tuberculous ileitis — caused by tubercle bacilli.
    b. regional ileitis, Crohn's disease — inflammatory process of ileum associated with cicatrization (scar formation), perforation, fistulae and abscesses.[93, 45]
13. intestinal obstruction, ileus — obstruction of small intestine associated with variable symptoms: abdominal distention, colicky pain, nausea, vomiting, obstipation or diarrhea. Interference with the blood flow to the obstructed intestine demands emergency surgery.
    a. adynamic (paralytic) ileus — paralysis of intestinal muscles, absence of bowel sounds. It may be due to electrolyte imbalance or operative handling of intestine.
    b. dynamic (mechanical) ileus — intestinal occlusion from adhesions, strangulated hernia, volvulus, intussusception, emboli or thrombi.[105, 7]
14. intussusception — telescoping of intestine; usually ileum slips into cecum which leads to intestinal obstruction.
15. Meckel's diverticulum — a congenital pouch or sac which usually arises from the ileum and may cause strangulation, intussusception or volvulus.
16. multiple polyposis — polyps or tumors derived from mucous membrane; scattered throughout intestine and rectum; may undergo malignant degeneration.
17. perforated viscus — a ruptured internal organ due to advanced disease, malignancy, trauma, drugs, gunshot or stab wound. It may be complicated by hemorrhage, shock and peritonitis.[122, 134]
18. pilonidal cyst — congenital anomaly, a cyst of the sacral area. It usually is a teratomatous (hair containing) cyst.[21]
19. proctitis — inflammation of rectum.
20. prolapse of rectum — downward displacement of rectum, seen in infants and old people.[40]
21. pruritus ani — itching sensation around the anus.
23. rectal cancer — malignant tumor of the rectum or rectosigmoid.[32, 120, 62, 113]
24. rectocele — herniation of rectum into vagina.
25. volvulus — twisting of the bowel upon itself leading to obstruction.[103]
26. Whipple's disease — rare disorder characterized by malabsorption of lipids (fat) with resultant steatorrhea, diarrhea, abdominal distress, fever, anemia, lymph node involvement and bouts of arthralgia.[130]

D. Operative Terms:

1. abdominal perineal resection — combined laparotomy and perineal operation for partial or complete removal of colon and rectum.[129]
2. appendectomy — removal of appendix.
3. cecectomy — excision of cecum.
4. cecostomy — external fistulization of the cecum for intestinal obstruction.
5. colon resection and end-to-end anastomosis — excision of involved colon with or without adjacent lymph glands; joining segments of colon.
6. colostomy — formation of an abdominal anus by bringing a loop of the colon to the surface of abdomen.
7. excision of pilonidal cyst — removal of cyst.
8. exteriorization of pilonidal cyst, marsupialization — laying open the cyst cavity and all its channels.
9. diverticulectomy — removal of diverticulum including resection of involved bowel.
10. hemorrhoidectomy — removal of hemorrhoids.
11. ileostomy — external fistulization of ileum often with total colectomy for ulcerative colitis.
12. jejunoileal bypass — creation of a bypass of a considerable portion of the small intestine by joining the proximal jejunum to the terminal ileum and the distal end of the bypassed segment to the cecum. The procedure reduces the absorptive capacity of small intestine and induces weight loss. Various techniques are used to control morbid obesity and hyperlipidemia.[23, 123, 124, 19, 18, 101]
13. operations for aganglionic megacolon (Hirschsprung's disease)
    a. modified Duhamel procedure — side-to-side anastomosis of colon and rectum.
    b. modified Soave procedure — endorectal pull-through of ganglionated bowel to anus.[136, 121]
14. proctoplasty — plastic repair or reconstruction of rectum or anus.
15. reduction of intussusception — normal intestinal continuity restored either by barium enema or if unsuccessful by laparotomy.[42]
16. reduction of volvulus — untwisting of lesion by manipulation.
17. tube cecostomy — surgical decompression of the colon by tube drainage of the cecum.[35]

E. Symptomatic Terms:

1. borborygmus — rumbling or splashing sound of bowels.
2. colic — spasm of any tubular hollow organ associated with pain.
3. diarrhea — frequency of bowel action, soft or liquid stools.
4. fecalith — a fecal concretion.
5. melena — black stool, also black vomit due to blood.
6. obstipation — extreme constipation, often due to obstruction.
7. steatorrhea — increased fat content in feces as in malabsorption syndrome or in pancreatitis.

LIVER, BILIARY SYSTEM, PANCREAS, PERITONEUM

A. Origin of Terms:

1. bile (L) — bile, gall
2. celi- (G) — abdomen
3. cholangi (G) — bile duct
4. chole (G) — bile, gall
5. cholecyst (G) — gallbladder
6. choledoch (G) — bile duct
7. cirrho- (G) — yellow, tawny
8. hepato- (G) — liver
9. laparo- (G) — abdominal wall
10. peritoneum (G) — stretching over

B. Anatomical Terms:

1. bile duct — duct formed by union of common hepatic duct and cystic duct, carries bile into duodenum.
2. common hepatic duct — duct formed by union of right and left hepatic ducts which receive bile from liver.

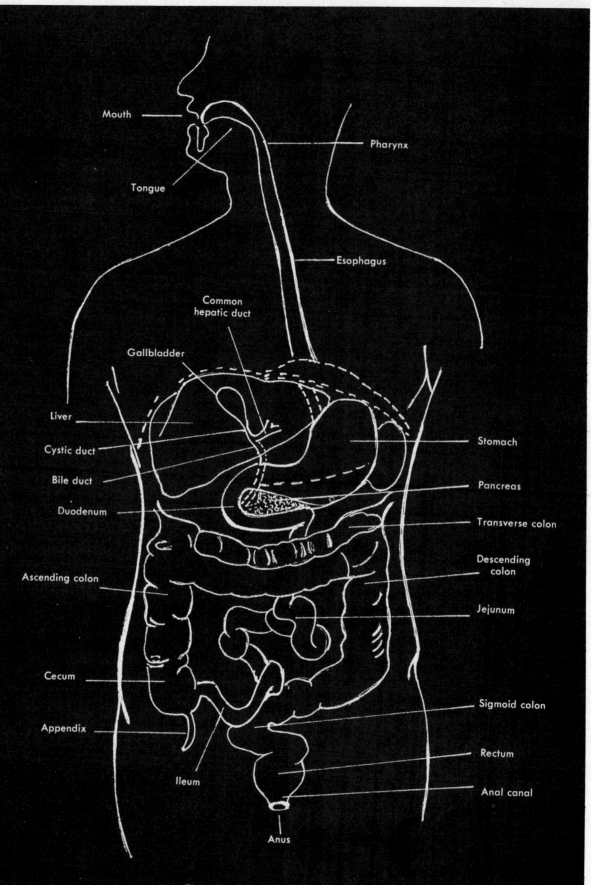

Mouth

Pharynx

Tongue

Esophagus

Common
hepatic duct

Gallbladder

Liver

Stomach

Cystic duct

Bile duct

Pancreas

Duodenum

Transverse colon

Descending
colon

Ascending colon

Jejunum

Cecum

Sigmoid colon

Appendix

Rectum

Anal canal

Ileum

Anus

Fig. 47 – Scheme of digestive tract.

3. cystic duct — passageway for bile from gallbladder to bile duct.
4. gallbladder — pear-shaped, sac-like organ which serves as reservoir for bile.
5. pancreas — large endocrine and exocrine gland, its right extremity or head lying within the duodenal curve, its left extremity or tail ending near the spleen.
6. pancreatic duct — main passageway for pancreatic juice containing enzymes; runs from left to right and empties into duodenum.
7. pancreatic islets, islets of Langerhans — clusters of cells producing the hormone insulin.
8. peritoneum — a sac of serous membrane composed of a parietal peritoneum which lines the abdominal wall and a visceral peritoneum which invests most viscera and holds them in position.
9. portal circulation — venous blood collected by the portal vein from gastrointestinal canal, spleen, gallbladder and pancreas enters the liver, passes through sinusoids and leaves the liver by the hepatic veins to pour into the inferior vena cava.
10. sphincter of bile duct (of Oddi) — circular muscle fibers around the end of the bile duct.
11. sphincter of hepatopancreatic ampulla — circular muscle fibers around end of ampulla (the union of the bile duct and main pancreatic duct).

C. Diagnostic Terms:

1. liver:
   a. abscess of liver — circumscribed area of suppuration. Infection brought to liver via portal vein, hepatic artery or bile ducts.[91]
   b. acute infective hepatitis, viral hepatitis.
      (1) infectious hepatitis caused by virus A (IH virus) demonstrable in stools, duodenal contents and in blood prior to the icteric period; incubation period from twenty to forty days.[53, 118]
      (2) serum hepatitis caused by virus B (SH virus) demonstrable in blood only; virus transmitted by blood transfusions, contaminated syringes and needles; incubation period from 60 to 160 days.[37, 141, 56, 69, 54, 30]
   c. acute yellow atrophy of liver — any severe form of hepatitis marked by shrinkage and necrosis of liver.
   d. Budd-Chiara syndrome — a rare disease characterized by occlusion of hepatic veins usually accompanied by ascites, hepatomegaly and pain in abdomen.[71, 36, 135, 44]
   e. cirrhosis of the liver — organ diffusely nodular and firm.
      (1) portal cirrhosis — Laennec's cirrhosis the most common form, frequently associated with alcoholism and nutritional deficiency.
      (2) biliary cirrhosis — obstructive form is characterized by chronic jaundice and liver failure due to obstruction and inflammation of bile ducts.[51]
   f. hemachromatosis — excess of iron absorption and presence of iron containing deposits (hemosiderin) in liver, pancreas, kidneys, adrenals and heart. It may be associated with hepatic enlargement and insufficiency and esophageal bleeding from varices.[27]
   g. hepatic calculi — stones originating in extrahepatic biliary tract or solely in the liver. They are also found in liver cysts.[9, 32, 95]
   h. hepatic coma, cholemia — peculiar syndrome characterized by slow or rapid onset of bizarre behavior, disorientation, flapping tremors of extended arms, hyperactive reflexes, later lethargy and coma. It seems to be caused by intoxication with ammonia, a product of protein digestion which the diseased liver fails to convert into urea.[1, 2]
   i. hepatic trauma — liver injury resulting from blunt trauma or penetrating wounds.[94]
   j. hepatorenal syndrome — combined liver and kidney failure usually due to serious injury to the liver associated with hemorrhage, shock and acute renal insufficiency.[15]
   k. portal hypertension — a portal venous pressure above 20 mm Hg associated with splenomegaly, increased collateral circulation, varicosity, bleeding and ascites. Portal hypertension may result from
      (1) intrahepatic block — block within the liver or
      (2) extrahepatic block — block within the portal vein.[73]

2. biliary system:[131]
   a. carcinoma of gallbladder — scirrhous (hard) type most common; early invasion of adjacent structures.
   b. cholangitis — inflammatory disease of bile ducts.[147]
   c. cholecystitis — inflammatory disease of the gallbladder, frequently associated with the presence of gallstones.[38, 128]
   d. cholelithiasis, biliary calculi — the presence of gallstones in the gallbladder.[14, 132]
   e. empyema of gallbladder — pus in the gallbladder.
   f. hydrops of gallbladder — distention of gallbladder with clear fluid.

3. pancreas:
   a. carcinoma of pancreas — neoplasm usually derived from glandular epithelium and involving the head of the pancreas (65%).[24]
   b. cystic fibrosis of pancreas, pancreatic fibrosis, mucoviscidosis — a hereditary, familial disease seen in children and adolescents and characterized by a more or less extensive involvement of the exocrine glands, especially those secreting mucus and sweat.
      It includes a variety of clinical conditions:
      (1) meconium ileus causing intestinal obstruction.
      (2) chronic pulmonary disease often leading to fatal complications.
      (3) pancreatic insufficiency resulting in malnutrition.
      (4) cirrhosis of liver with or without portal hypertension, the latter terminating in uncontrolled hemorrhages.
      (5) abnormally raised levels of sweat electrolytes causing salt depletion and cardiac collapse in hot weather.[87]
   c. islet cell tumors — neoplasms originating from the islets of Langerhans: may be benign, malignant and metastasizing.[49, 88]
   d. pancreatitis — inflammation of pancreas.
      (1) acute form — serious inflammatory reaction marked by excruciating pain.[55, 115]
      (2) chronic form — progressive destruction of pancreas associated with recurrent attacks of severe pain in abdomen.

4. peritoneum:
   a. ascites — collection of fluid within the peritoneal cavity.
   b. hemoperitoneum — blood within the peritoneal cavity.
   c. hernia — rupture or protrusion of a part from its normal location; for example, an intestinal loop through a weakened area in the abdominal wall.[42]
      (1) location:
         (a) femoral — organ passes through femoral ring.
         (b) inguinal — organ protrudes through inguinal canal.
         (c) umbilical — hernia occurs at the navel.
      (2) types:
         (a) incarcerated — hernia causes complete bowel obstruction.
         (b) postoperative — hernia complicates surgical intervention.
         (c) strangulated — hernia cuts off circulation so that gangrene develops if emergency operation is not performed.[42]
   d. peritonitis — inflammation of peritoneum.

D. Operative Terms:

1. liver:
   a. biopsy of liver — removal of small piece of tissue for microscopic study.
   b. hepatic lobectomy — removal of lobe of liver.
   c. hepatotomy — incision into liver substance.
   d. shunts for portal hypertension — surgical method of diverting a considerable amount of blood of the hypertensive portal system into the normal systemic venous system in order to prevent hemorrhages from varices.[72, 57, 133]

      (1) direct portal vein to vena cava anastomosis for intrahepatic block due to cirrhosis of the liver.

      (2) splenectomy followed by splenorenal shunt (end-to-end) for extrahepatic block due to thrombosis of the portal vein.

2. biliary system:

    a. cholecystectomy — removal of the gallbladder.

    b. cholecystostomy — surgical creation of a more or less permanent opening into the gallbladder. This operation is indicated where removal of the gallbladder would be unduly hazardous.

    c. choledochoduodenostomy — surgical joining of the common bile duct to the duodenum.[140]

    d. choledocholithotomy — incision into bile duct for removal of gallstones.

    e. choledochoplasty — plastic repair or reconstruction of bile duct.

3. pancreas:

    a. pancreatectomy — partial or total removal of pancreas; for example, for islet cell tumor.

    b. pancreatojejunostomy — anastomosis of pancreas to jejunum. May be done for carcinoma of the ampulla of Vater.

4. peritoneum:

    a. exploratory laparotomy — surgical opening of abdomen for diagnostic purposes.

    b. hernioplasty, herniorrhaphy — repair of hernia.[96]

    c. incision and drainage of peritoneal abscess or retroperitoneal abscess or subphrenic abscess.

E. Terms Related to Special Procedures:

1. endoscopy with flexible fiberscope — visualization of a hollow organ using an endoscope with a tip for remote control and a biopsy channel for tissue sampling and histologic study of lesion.[13]

    a. colonoscopy, colonofiberoscopy — a method of examining the colon by using a colonic fiberscope with a 4 way controlled tip to facilitate traversing the flexures of the sigmoid and transverse colon under fluoroscopic guidance. It may permit the removal of polyps up to the ascending colon.[13, 151]

    b. duodenoscopy — the introduction of a flexible duodenoscope into the first part of the duodenum, visualization and cannulation of papilla of Vater. Contrast material is injected into the orifice of the ampulla through a minute cannula to obtain a retrograde cholangiogram or pancreatogram.[13]

    c. esophagogastroscopy — visualization of the esophagus, stomach and duodenal bulb using a flexible fiberscope with provision for target biopsy and color photography through the scope. Benign or malignant lesions, bleeding points and hemorrhagic gastritis may be detected by direct vision.[13]

    d. fiber optic gastroscopy — use of an end-viewing fiberscope as the usual method of choice for visualizing the esophagus, stomach, antrum, pylorus, duodenal bulb and an anastomosis after surgery. In addition to the fiber optic light source the scope contains a channel for biopsies, for suction and air or water instillation and for endoscopic photography.[59,67]

    e. peritoneoscopy — procedure for visualization of the peritoneal cavity using a peritoneoscope with a fiber optic light source. It is possible to perform a percutaneous liver biopsy under direct vision, to photograph the lesions, to irrigate the peritoneal cavity, to aspirate ascitic fluid for cytoanalysis and finally to arrive at a diagnosis of obscure abdominal disease by peritoneoscopy.[104]

2. exchange transfusion for hepatic coma — exchange of equal volume of blood using a closed transfusion circuit for the purpose of clearing bilirubin, improving the clotting mechanism and reversing coma. Fresh blood is used and electrolytes are added as needed.[2]

3. hepatic arterial ligation — tying a hepatic artery to control a massive hemorrhage from liver injury.[43]

4. hyperalimentation — long-term intravenous nutrition with an amino acid-glucose infusate using disposable tubing and infusion pump to maintain a constant infusion rate. A large intravenous catheter is inserted through a central vein and its proper position is radiographically confirmed. Hyperalimentation should be reserved for patients with severe digestive abnormalities.[125, 70]

5. liver perfusion — method of providing extracorporeal support to liver in hepatic coma using regional heparinization and a disposable perfusion circuit primed with 250 to 300 ml of blood. Under aseptic precautions fresh blood is obtained from healthy baboons or from human cadaver, chilled with electrolyte solution and used for liver perfusion until consciousness is restored.[1]

6. selective intra-arterial infusion of vasopressor — method of controlling variceal hemorrhage by injecting a vasopressor such as vasopressin (Bitressin) into the superior mesenteric artery.[43]

E. Symptomatic Terms:[73]

1. alopecia, pectoral and axillary — absence of hair on chest and axillae (arm pits) in liver damage.

2. arterial spiders, spider nevi — cutaneous vascular lesions occurring on face, neck and shoulders in advanced hepatic disease, also in malnutrition and pregnancy. Each lesion consists of a central arteriole from which many small vessels radiate.

3. caput medusae — dilatation of the abdominal veins around the umbilicus seen in severe portal hypertension with liver damage.

4. fetor hepaticus — a musty, sweet odor to the breath, characteristic of hepatic coma.

5. flapping tremor, liver flap — involuntary movements, elicited in the extended hand by supporting the patient's forearm. It consists of bursts of quick, irregular movements at the wrist similar to waving goodbye. The protruded tongue and dorsiflexed feet may likewise be affected. Flapping tremors occur in severe liver disease and signal impending hepatic coma.

6. icterus, jaundice — yellow discoloration of skin, sclera (white of eyes), membranes and secretions due to excess bilirubin in the blood.

7. palmar erythema, liver palms — a bright or mottled redness of the palms and finger tips seen in liver disease. Palmar erythema also occurs in malnutrition and rheumatoid arthritis.

RADIOLOGY

A. Terms Related to Examinations of Digestive Tract:[98]

1. air contrast enema, double contrast enema — examination of the colon using a small amount of barium to coat the walls of the mucosa and air to distend the colon. This procedure may demonstrate intestinal polyps.

2. barium enema examination — fluoroscopic and radiographic examination of the colon after administering a barium sulfate mixture. The colon may be spot-filmed while the enema is effective. Barium enemas are also used in the treatment of intussusception, which is often reduced by the rectal instillation of barium under fluoroscopic guidance.

3. contour — surface configuration or outline of an organ or part; for example, that of the stomach.

4. duodenal cap — freely movable triangular part of the duodenum distal to the pyloroduodenal junction.

5. Hampton maneuver — examination of the upper gastrointestinal tract with fluoroscopy and radiography using a barium mixture, but without applying pressure to abdomen. This technique is usually employed in patient with upper gastrointestinal hemorrhage.

6. portography, portovenography — radiography of the portal vein after injection of radiopaque material.
7. scout film — a preliminary radiogram of the abdomen before the administration of a radiopaque substance.
8. sialogram — radiographic visualization of the main salivary glands and ducts following the injection of radiopaque material.[97]
9. small intestine series — serial radiograms during the passage of barium through the small intestines.
10. splenoportogram — injection of radiopaque material into the spleen for radiographic study of the splenic and portal veins.
11. spot film — radiogram of small isolated areas taken during fluoroscopy. Example: sigmoid colon.

B. Terms Related to Gallbladder Examinations:[98]

1. cholangiography — the introduction of radiopaque material into the bile ducts for x-ray examination of the biliary system.
2. cholecystography — x-ray examination of the gallbladder after rendering the bile radiopaque.
   a. intravenous administration of radiopaque material or
   b. oral administration of Telepaque or any other suitable contrast medium.
      Both methods permit adequate gallbladder visualization.
3. operative cholangiography — visualization of the ductal system by filling it with a contrast medium and taking radiograms at the time of the operation. This examination seeks to detect the presence of congenital anomalies, neoplasms and elusive gallstones.[3, 61]
4. cinecholedochography — the routine films combined with cineradiography for visualization of the entire biliary ductal system.
5. cineradiography, cineroentgenography — the making of motion pictures by radiography.

CLINICAL LABORATORY

A. Terms Related to Tests of the Digestive System:

1. amylase (amyl: starch - ase: enzyme) — digestive enzyme acting on starches. It is found in salivary glands, pancreatic juice, liver and adipose tissue.
2. amylolytic — starch-splitting.
3. biliary drainage, medical — a diagnostic and therapeutic measure. Magnesium sulfate, injected through duodenal tube, relaxes the sphincter of Oddi and stimulates bile drainage. Normally, the following distinctions are noted:
   a. the first specimen designated as "A" bile is golden yellow and is collected from the common bile duct.
   b. the second specimen known as "B" bile is green to yellow brown and directly aspirated from the gallbladder.
   c. the third specimen, "C" bile is light yellow and freshly secreted by the liver.
   Bacteriological studies are done on the second specimen.[66]
4. diastase (syn. amylase) — enzyme digesting starches.
5. duodenal drainage — diagnostic aid in detecting biliary infection. The procedure is the same as that of biliary drainage except that no magnesium sulfate is injected.
6. gastric analysis (tube) — aspiration of gastric contents for the purpose of determining the secretory ability and motility of the stomach.[119, 63]

   Normal values

fasting free HCL	0 - 30 degrees per 100 ml.
total HCl	10 - 50 degrees per 100 ml.
free acid, one hour after histamine	30 - 85 degrees per 100 ml.
time for emptying	3 - 6 hours.

Increase of acidity in gastric and duodenal ulcers.

Decrease or absence of HCl in gastric carcinoma, pernicious anemia and simple achlorhydria.

7. gastric analysis (tubeless) — use of diagnex blue to determine whether the stomach contains free hydrochloric acid.

Normal values of HCl .... greater than 0.6 mg in 2 hours.
Doubtful .... 0.3 - 0.6 mg in 2 hours.
Anacidity .... 0 - 0.3 mg in 2 hours.

8. guaiac test — test for occult blood in feces (also in urine).

Negative reaction — no blood .... no greenish to blue color.
Positive reaction — blood present ..... greenish to blue color.
Ulcerated carcinomas of colon or stomach always yield a positive reaction.
Nonmalignant gastric ulcers intermittently yield a positive reaction.

9. intragastric photography — diagnostic procedure accomplished by a minuscule gastrocamera swallowed by the patient to provide color photographs of the interior of the stomach. The procedure is valuable in the detection of ulcers, tumors, polyps and gastritis.

10. intestinal absorption tests — these studies require further development. They are:
    a. D-xylose absorption test (oral)
    b. serum carotene level
    c. vitamin A tolerence test.[109]

11. proteolytic — protein-splitting.

12. serum diastase (amylase) determination — test of diagnostic value in pancreatic conditions. Any interference with the outflow of diastase (amylase) causes a rise of the enzyme level.

Normal values — Method of Somogyi.
serum diastase .... 80-150 units per 100 ml.
Increase in acute pancreatitis, chronic recurrent pancreatitis and carcinoma of the head of the pancreas and parotitis.
Decrease in carcinoma of liver and pancreatic insufficiency.

13. serum leucine aminopeptidase determination (LAP) — measurement of leucine aminopeptidase, a protein splitting enzyme. Persistent high enzyme levels suggest carcinoma of the pancreas.[109]

14. serum lipase determination — test of usefulness in the early detection of pancreatic cancer.

15. stool examination — macroscopic and microscopic studies, chemical analysis and examinations for parasites and protozoa as diagnostic aids, especially for detecting diseases of the digestive tract.

16. sweat test — diagnostic test in cystic fibrosis of pancreas or mucoviscidosis. Excessively high sweat chloride levels confirm the diagnosis.

Normal values of sweat chloride range between 4 - 60 mEq/L.
The finger prints or hand print technique of the sweat test is a simplified method for screening children and their relatives. Silver chromate paper moistened with distilled water is used for the test.
Normal values — imprints of fingers or hand are light and indistinct. In mucoviscidosis imprints of fingers or hand are heavy and distinct. The red silver chromate changes to white silver chloride.

17. transaminase (SGPT) — a valuable diagnostic aid and sensitive index in acute hepatic disease.

Normal values (spectrophotometrically)
transaminase (SGPT) .... 8 - 25 units.
(serum glutamic pyruvic transaminase)
Increase in acute liver disease .... 600 - 700 units.
This rise usually occurs within 25 days after onset of disease. A return to normal is very gradual within 40-80 days.[109]

B. Terms Related to Liver Function:

Liver function tests are of great importance, not only in discovering the severity of hepatic disease, but also in determining the amount of liver damage caused by pathological conditions of the gallbladder and pancreas. The liver is the largest gland in the body. Essential tests for detecting hepatic impairment are presented.

Table 13

LIVER FUNCTION TESTS

Hepatic Function	Tests	Normal Values
1. Excretory function chiefly related to bile pigments	a. Bromsulphalein (BSP) Retention of dye indicative of liver damage, metastatic carcinoma of liver and others	Method of Goebler Dye excreted within 45 minutes with 5 mg/kg dose
	b. Serum Alkaline Phosphatase Elevated in obstructive jaundice, liver abscess and cancer of liver	Method of Bodansky 1.5- 4 units (adults) 5.0-12 units (children) Hepler, op. cit., 312.
	c. Serum Bilirubin 1-minute reaction time of serum bilirubin . . . . total serum bilirubin . . . . Increased in hepatogenous jaundice, obstructive jaundice, portal cirrhosis, hepatic carcinoma	Method of Malloy and Evelyn 0-0.26 mg/100 ml of serum 0-1.00 mg/100 ml of serum Reference Page, op. cit, 5.
	d. Bilirubin in Urine Present in hepatitis, hepatogenous and obstructive jaundice	Methods Foam . . . . .negative Harrison spot . . . . .0.1+ Meth. blue . . . . .0.4 drops
	e. Urobilinogen in Urine Present in hepatogenous jaundice and obstructive jaundice	Method of Watson 0-1.0 Ehrlich unit of 2 hour sample
	f. Urobilinogen in Feces Increase in hemolytic jaundice Decrease in obstructive jaundice	130-250 Ehrlich units/100 gm. Reference Hepler, op. cit., 118
2. Regulation of composition of blood	a. Prothrombin Determination Increased in seconds . . . . Decreased in per cent . . . . in obstructive jaundice, liver cell damage, vitamin K deficiency	Method of Quick 11-15 seconds 70-100% Reference Ibid., 87.
3. Protein metabolism	a. Total Serum Proteins . . . . Serum Albumin . . . . Serum Globulin . . . . A/G ratio . . . . Increase of globulin in infectious hepatitis Decrease of total proteins and albumin in liver disease	Method of Kjeldahl 6.0-8.0 gm/100 ml 3.2-5.6 gm/100 ml 1.3-3.2 gm/100 ml of serum 1.5:1 to 2.5:1 Reference Ibid., 277.

Hepatic Function	Tests	Normal Values
4. Inhibitory action of albumin on gamma globulin and others	a. Cephalin Cholesterol Flocculation Test Grade of flocculation reflecting liver damage	Method of Hanger no flocculation
	b. Thymol Turbidity and Flocculation Test Increased in cirrhosis and infectious hepatitis	Method of Neefe 0-5 units of turbidity 0-1 + flocculation in 18 hours Reference Ibid., 121-122.
	c. Zinc Sulfate Turbidity Altered in prolonged degeneration of liver cells	2.0-12 units of turbidity Reference Page, op. cit., 421.
5. Carbohydrate metabolism	a. Oral Galactose Test Excretion in a 5 hour period Increased in toxic hepatitis and galactosemia	0-3 gm
	b. Oral Glucose Tolerance Test Excretion of glucose within 30-60 minutes Increased in obstructive jaundice	Method of Janney-Isaacson 120-160 mg/100 ml Return to normal within 2 hours Reference Hepler, op cit., 119, 269.
6. Fat metabolism	a. Determination of Cholesterol........................	Method of Bloor 150-280 mg/100 ml
	b. Determination of Cholesterol Esters.................... Both increased in obstructive jaundice Both decreased in liver failure and hepatic necrosis	50-65% of total cholesterol Reference Page, op. cit., 409.
7. Enzyme activity	a. Serum Cholinesterase Decreased in liver disease, slightly low in obstructive jaundice, very low in poisoning from some insecticides	Method of Michel 0.5 pH units or over per hour for serum Reference Ibid., 5.
	b. Serum Glutamic Oxalacetic Transaminase (SGOT)............... Increased in infectious hepatitis and serum hepatitis	Method of Karmen 10-40 units
	c. Serum Glutamic Pyruvic Transaminase (SGPT)............... Highly elevated in acute hepatitis, toxic hepatitis and hepatocellular damage	8-25 units. Reference Bulletin Lab. Med. 6, No. 7, 1957.

ABBREVIATIONS

AC, ac — before meals (ante cibos)
Ba — barium
BID, bid — twice a day
BSP — bromsulphalein
CCF — cephalin cholesterol flocculation
COH — carbohydrate
FBS — fasting blood sugar
5-HIAA — 5-hydroxyindole acetic acid
HAA — hepatitis Australia antigen, hepatitis associated antigen
GI — gastrointestinal

HCl — hydrochloric acid
HS, hs — at bedtime
IH — infectious hepatitis
LAP — leucine amino peptidase
OD, od — once a day
PC, pc — after meals (post cibos)
PP — postprandial
prn — as often as necessary
QID, qid — four times a day
SH — serum hepatitis
sos — if necessary
TID, tid — three times a day

ORAL READING PRACTICE

Malignant Neoplasms of the Oral Cavity

Carcinomas of the mouth include malignant tumors of the lips, tongue and floor of the oral cavity. **Neoplastic** growth may be preceded by gradual development of irregular, white, raised patches known as **leukoplakia.** This condition starts as a chronic, painless inflammation of the **oral mucosa.** It is usually considered a premalignant lesion. Although its **etiology** is unknown, the relationship of tobacco and leukoplakia is a well established fact, since leukoplakia seen in heavy smokers tends to disappear after smoking has been discontinued. The white patches are due to a **keratinization** of the **epithelium.** Fissuring or **ulceration** in a leukoplakic area may be a diagnostic sign that malignant changes are in progress.[6]

Tumors of the upper lip are generally **basal cell carcinomas** which tend to invade adjacent structures, but rarely metastasize. Prompt treatment is imperative.

Carcinoma of the lower lip may show a widespread involvement of the **epidermoid (squamous cell)** type. In its early phase there is a fissure, flat ulcer or chronic leukoplakia which readily forms a **fungating** mass, malignant in character.[6, 74]

Carcinoma of the tongue begins as a fissured ulcer with raised borders. Pain is not present until the cancer may have progressed and metastasized. The areas of **induration** are prone to extend with time. Spontaneous bleeding occurs from ulcerating crevices and is distressing to the patient. With increasing **infiltration** the movement of the tongue becomes restricted. Metastatic **adenopathy** may develop early or late and generally involves the **cervical** and **submaxillary** lymph nodes.[114]

Any ulcer or newgrowth of the lips, tongue or floor of the mouth that does not heal with treatment in a three weeks' period should be **biopsied.** Suspicious lesions must receive prompt attention since progression to inoperability occurs before the patient feels pain.

The treatment of choice in carcinoma of the mouth is surgical removal of the lesion with or without irradiation or, if inoperable, **palliative** radiotherapy alone. For cancer of the lip a V-excision of the malignant lesion may be done to provide relief from discomfort and overcome disfigurement. Roentgen therapy and interstitial radiotherapy using needles of low radium content have been employed in the postoperative regime with considerable success.[92, 50]

Table 14

SOME DIGESTIVE CONDITIONS AMENABLE TO SURGERY

Organ Involved	Diagnoses	Operations	Operative Procedures
Lip	Cleft lip	Cheiloplasty	Plastic repair of lip
Lip (lower)	Squamous cell carcinoma of lower lip	Eslander operation for carcinoma of the lower lip	V-excision of lesion-defect filled by a flap from the upper lip
Lip (upper)	Squamous cell or basal cell carcinoma of upper lip	Eslander operation for carcinoma of the upper lip	V-excision and replacement of operative defect by a triangular flap from the lower lip
Tongue	Epidermoid carcinoma and/or metastatic cervical adenopathy	Partial glossectomy Radical neck dissection or Cautery excision with radon seed implantation in selected cases	Wide excision of malignant lesion including the removal of the jugular vein, muscles of the neck, submaxillary and cervical lymph nodes

Organ Involved	Diagnoses	Operations	Operative Procedures
Parotid gland	Parotid tumor	Resection of parotid gland and tumor under direct vision	Y-shaped incision and dissection for skin flaps Partial removal of parotid gland with tumor keeping facial nerve intact
Parotid gland Facial nerve	Parotid tumor widely infiltrating, facial nerve embedded in tumor	Total parotidectomy Elective excision of facial nerve	Removal of entire gland and tumor including main trunk of facial nerve with plexus
Palate	Cleft palate	Staphylorrhaphy Palatoplasty	Suture of a cleft palate Reconstruction of a cleft palate
Floor of the mouth	Squamous cell carcinoma	Excision of lesion and/or Radiation therapy	Removal of neoplasm and/or irradiation
Tonsils, palatine	Hypertrophy of tonsils Chronic tonsillitis	Tonsillectomy	Removal of tonsils
Tonsils, pharyngeal	Adenoids	Adenoidectomy	Removal of adenoids
Esophagus	Esophageal lesion	Esophagoscopy with biopsy	Direct visualization of the esophagus with removal of bits of tissue
Esophagus	Diverticulum of esophagus	Diverticulectomy	Extirpation of the diverticulum
Esophagus Stomach	Carcinoma of esophagus of the midthoracic portion	Radical resection of the carcinomatous segment of the esophagus Esophagogastric anastomosis or interposition of segment of bowel	Excision of malignant lesion and regional lymph nodes Anastomosis of remaining esophagus and stomach or using a bowel segment as a substitute
Esophagus Stomach	Recurrent hiatus hernia	Repair of hiatus hernia, abdominal or thoracic approach	Direct vision reduction; sac sutured to under surface of diaphragm; inclusion of gastric wall in fixation
Stomach Pyloric muscle	Congenital hypertrophic stenosis of pyloric sphincter	Pyloromyotomy Fredet-Ramstedt operation	Section of hypertrophic pyloric muscle down to mucosa
Stomach	Gastric carcinoma, resectability unknown	Exploratory laparotomy	Opening the abdomen to determine operability of lesion
Stomach Duodenum Jejunum	Early carcinoma of stomach Malignant gastric lesion in upper stomach	Subtotal gastrectomy Gastroduodenostomy or Gastrojejunostomy or Esophagojejunostomy	Partial removal of stomach including lymph glands Joining remaining portion of stomach and duodenum Joining remaining portion of stomach and jejunum Transthoracic approach and esophagojejunal anastomosis
Stomach Duodenum Jejunum	Chronic or recurrent gastric ulcer with obstruction or hemorrhage	Gastric resection Billroth I or Billroth II Polya modification or Hofmeister modification	Partial removal of stomach and gastroduodenal anastomosis or gastrojejunal anastomosis using anterior approach or posterior approach

Organ Involved	Diagnoses	Operations	Operative Procedures
Stomach Duodenum	Duodenal ulcer	Selective vagotomy	Complete vagal denervation of the stomach
		Mucosal antrectomy[a]	Excision of entire gastrin-secreting antral mucosa
Duodenum	Progressive duodenal ulcer with obstruction or hemorrhage	Complete bilateral vagotomy	Section of vagus nerve fibers before they enter the stomach
		Pyloroplasty	Surgical repair of pyloric muscle
Duodenum Jejunum	Large duodenal perforation	Surgical reconstruction of perforated duodenum	Excision of duodenal ulcer
			Full thickness jejunal pedicle graft for closure of large duodenal defect
Jejunum Ileum	Morbid obesity Hyperlipidemia	Jejunoileal bypass[b]	Division of jejunum a few inches distal to ligament of Treitz, and ileum a few inches proximal to ileocecal valve
			End-to-end anastomosis to restore continuity Closure of distal jejunum
			Implantation of proximal ileum into transverse colon or into left colon
Ileum Colon	Regional enteritis	Resection of involved ileum and colon Enteroanastomosis	Radical extirpation of bowel involved in regional enteritis Surgical joining of remaining parts
Colon Ileum	Chronic ulcerative colitis with hemorrhage	Permanent ileostomy with total colectomy	Surgical creation of an ileal stoma for fecal drainage and removal of colon
Colon Cecum	Intestinal obstruction Cancer of left colon	Cecostomy Gibson's technique	Creating a communication between cecum and body surface for fecal drainage
		Transverse colostomy	Diverting fecal content to the body surface
Appendix	Appendicitis	Appendectomy	Removal of appendix
Colon Rectum	Aganglionic megacolon (Hirschsprung's disease)	Modified Duhamel procedure or Modified Soave procedure[c]	Side-to-side colorectal anastomosis
			Endorectal pull-through of ganglionated bowel to anus
Rectosigmoid	Rectal hemorrhage, cause unknown	Rectosigmoidoscopy	Endoscopic examination of the rectosigmoid
Rectosigmoid	Carcinoma of rectum and low sigmoid	Abdomino-perineal resection Miles' operation	Sectioning of bowel above the tumor — creation of permanent colostomy — removal of bowel above and below tumor — excision of anus
Rectum	Hemorrhoids, internal anal or external	Hemorrhoidectomy	Removal of hemorrhoids

Organ Involved	Diagnoses	Operations	Operative Procedures
Peritoneum	Hernia, inguinal femoral umbilical ventral	Hernioplasty	Surgical repair of hernia
Liver	Hepatic necrosis Hepatic failure Hepatic coma	Exchange transfusion[d] (fresh blood)	Construction of arteriovenous shunt Priming the exchange transfusion circuit Exchange of equal volume of blood
Gallbladder	Cholecystitis Cholelithiasis	Cholecystectomy	Removal of gallbladder
Bile duct	Benign stricture of bile duct	Repair of biliary stricture by end-to-end anastomosis of bile duct	Excision of constricted part and surgical communication of the two ends of the bile duct

[a] R. M. Kirk et al. Vagotomy and mucosal antrectomy in the elective treatment of duodenal ulcers. *American Journal of Surgery*, 123: 323-328, March, 1972.

[b] A. B. Brill *et al.* Changes in body composition after jejunoileal bypass in morbidly obese patients. *American Journal of Surgery*, 123: 49-56, January, 1972.

[c] R. T. Soper *et al.* Hirschsprung's disease. *Archives of Surgery*, 104: 249-437, April, 1972.

[d] G. M. Abouna. Improved technique of exchange transfusion for hepatic coma. *Surgery Gynecology & Obstetrics*, 134: 658-662, April, 1972.

REFERENCES AND BIBLIOGRAPHY

1. Abouna, G. M. Treatment of acute hepatic coma by ex vivo baboon and human liver perfusions. *Surgery*, 71: 537-546, April, 1972.

2. _____. Improved technique of exchange transfusion for hepatic coma. *Surgery Gynecology & Obstetrics*, 134: 658-662, April, 1972.

3. Adams, J. D. Operative cholangiography. Its value in the unsuspected choledochal stone. *Surgical Clinics of North America*, 52: 333-340, April, 1972.

4. Adson, M. A. *et al.* Management of gastrointestinal dysfunction after gastric surgery. *Surgical Clinics of North America*, 51: 915-926, August, 1971.

5. Alshuler, A. Esophageal varices in children. *American Journal of Nursing*, 72: 687-693, April, 1972.

6. Baker, H. W. Diagnosis of oral cancer. Part one. *Ca — A Cancer Journal for Clinicians*, 22: 31-39, January-February, 1972.

7. Baker, J. W. Intestinal obstruction. In Conn, Howard F., (ed.). *Current Therapy 1972*. Philadelphia: W. B. Saunders Co., 1972, pp. 343-345.

8. Baker, R. J. Acute surgical diseases of the pancreas. *Surgical Clinics of North America*, 52: 239-256, February, 1972.

9. Balasegaram, M. Hepatic calculi. *Annals of Surgery*, 175: 149-154, February, 1972.

10. Barker, J. R. and Franklin, R. H. Heller's operation for achalasia of the cardia. *British Journal of Surgery*, 58: 466-468, June, 1971.

11. Beahrs, O. H. Surgical management of peptic ulceration recurring postoperatively. *Surgical Clinics of North America*, 51: 863-870, August, 1971.

12. Bender, J. B. *et al.* The effect of periodontal disease on the pulp. *Oral Surgery Oral Medicine & Oral Pathology*, 33: 458-475, March, 1972.

13. Berci, G. Endoscopy today. Flexible fiber endoscopes. *Postgraduate Medicine*, 51: 111-113, March, 1972.

14. Berk, J. E. Cholecystitis and cholelithiasis. In Conn, Howard F. (ed.). *Current Therapy 1972*. Philadelphia: W. B. Saunders Co., 1972, pp. 309-311.

15. Better, O. S. *et al.* Traumatic hepatorenal failure: Supportive treatment with simultaneous hemodialysis and exchange transfusion. *Archives of Surgery*, 104: 347-348, March, 1972.

16. Bombeck, C. T. Esophageal trauma. *Surgical Clinics of North America*, 52: 219-230, February, 1972.

17. Boyd, D. P. Transabdominal repair of hiatal hernia. *Surgical Clinics of North America*, 51: 597-606, June, 1971.

18. Brasch, J. W. The surgical treatment of obesity. A study of applied physiology. *Surgical Clinics*

of North America, 51: 667-673, June, 1971.

19. Brill, B. *et al.* Changes in body composition after jejunoileal bypass in morbidly obese patients. *American Journal of Surgery*, 123: 49-56, January, 1972.

20. Brindley, G. V. Neuromuscular disorders of the esophagus. *Surgical Clinics of North America*, 52: 319-331, April, 1972.

21. Broadrick, G. L. *et al.* Simplified treatment of pilonidal disease on an outpatient basis. *Surgery*, 70: 635-637, October, 1971.

22. Broders, C. W. Bleeding from diverticula of the colon. *Surgical Clinics of North America*, 52: 315-318, April, 1972.

23. Buchwald, H. and Varco, R. L. A bypass operation for obese hyperlipidemic patients. *Surgery*, 70: 62-70, July, 1971.

24. Buck, B. A. Carcinoma associated with pancreatic cyst. *Surgery Gynecology & Obstetrics*, 134: 44-46, January, 1972.

25. Cady, B. Carcinoma of the oral cavity. *Surgical Clinics of North America*, 51: 537-552, June, 1971.

26. Cameron, A. J. Medical treatment of gastric ulcer. *Surgical Clinics of North America*, 51: 893-900, August, 1971.

27. Carbone, J. V. *et al.* Gastrointestinal tract & liver. In Krupp, Marcus A., Chatton, Milton J. and Associate Authors. *Current Diagnosis and Treatment*, 11th ed. Los Altos, California: Lange Medical Publications, 1972, pp. 300-364.

28. Carpenter, W. S. *et al.* Fistulas complicating diverticulitis of the colon. *Surgery Gynecology & Obstetrics*, 134: 625-628, April, 1972.

29. Chaitin, H. Cholecystostomy in geriatric surgery. *Geriatrics*, 26: 57-60, August, 1971.

30. Cherubin, C. E. *et al.* Chronic liver disease in asymptomatic narcotic addicts. *Annals of Internal Medicine*, 76: 391-396, March, 1972.

31. Chong, G. C. and Kelly, K. A. Surgical management of acute gastric and doudenal stress ulcers. *Surgical Clinics of North America*, 51: 863-870, August, 1971.

32. Chung-chieh, W. Intrahepatic stones: A clinical study. *Annals of Surgery*, 175: 166-177, February, 1972.

33. Chung, E. P. *et al.* Pyloromyotomy technique in conjunction with esophagectomy or repair of hiatus hernia with vagotomy. *Journal of Thoracic and Cardiovascular Surgery*, 61: 282-286, February, 1971.

34. Clagett, O. T. The surgical management of gastric ulcer. *Surgical Clinics of North America*, 51: 901-906, August, 1971.

35. Clark, D. D. *et al.* Tube cecostomy: An evaluation of 161 cases. *Annals of Surgery*, 175: 55-61, January, 1972.

36. Club, A. W. Budd-Chiari syndrome after oral contraceptives. *British Medical Journal*, 1: 252, January 27, 1968.

37. Cossart, Y. E. What determines the incidence of serum hepatitis after blood transfusion? *American Journal of Diseases of Children*, 123: 354-356, April, 1972.

38. Crichlow, R. W. *et al.* Cholecystitis in adolescents. *Digestive Diseases*, 17: 68-72, January, 1972.

39. Crouch, James E. *Functional Anatomy*, 2d ed. Philadelphia: Lea & Febiger, 1972, pp. 369-373.

40. Davidson, V. A. Transsacral repair of rectal prolapse. *American Journal of Surgery*, 123: 231-235, February, 1972.

41. Dingmann, R. O. and Grabb, W. C. A rational program for surgical management of bilateral cleft lip and cleft palate. *Plastic and Reconstructive Surgery*, 47: 239-242, March, 1971.

42. Doyle, Charles, M. D. Personal communications.

43. Drapanas, T. What's new in surgery. Gastrointestinal and biliary tracts. *Surgery Gynecology & Obstetrics*, 134: 263-266, February, 1972.

44. Drill, V. A. *et al.* Oral contraceptives and thromboembolic disease. *Journal of American Medical Association*, 206: 77-84, September 30, 1968.

45. Eade, M. N. Clinical and hematologic features of Crohn's disease. *Surgery Gynecology & Obstetrics*, 134: 643-646, April, 1972.

46. Ebbels, B. J. Peptic ulcer. In Conn, Howard F. (ed.). *Current Therapy 1972*. Philadelphia: W. B. Saunders Co., 1972, pp. 348-351.

47. Ellis, F. H. Gastroesophageal reflux. Indication for fundoplication. *Surgical Clinics of North America*, 51: 575-588, June, 1971.

48. Evans, R. W. *et al.* *Epithelial Tumors of the Salivary Glands*. Philadelphia: W. B. Saunders Co., 1970.

49. Ferris, D. O. *et al.* Recent advances in management of functioning islet cell tumor. *Archives of Surgery*, 104: 443-446, April, 1972.

50. Fuchihata, H. Radiotherapy of carcinoma developed from leukoplakia. *Oral Surgery Medicine & Oral Pathology*, 33: 137-143, January, 1972.

51. Galambos, J. T. Cirrhosis. In Conn, Howard F. (ed.). *Current Therapy 1972*. Philadelphia: W. B. Saunders Co., 1972, pp. 312-318.

52. Georgiade, N. G. Improved technique for one stage repair of bilateral cleft lip. *Plastic and Reconstruction Surgery*, 48: 318-324, October, 1971.

53. Giles, J. P. *et al.* Viral hepatitis. *American Journal of Diseases of Children*, 123: 281-282, April, 1972.

54. Ginsberg, A. L. *et al.* Prevention of endemic HAA-positive hepatitis with gamma globulin. *New England Journal of Medicine*, 286: 562-566, March 16, 1972.

55. Given, B. and Simmons, S. Acute pancreatitis. *American Journal of Nursing*, 71: 934-939, May, 1971.

56. Grady, G. F. *et al.* Risk of posttransfusion hepatitis in the United States. *Journal of American Medical Association*, 220: 692-701, May 1, 1972.

57. Graham, K. J. The results of shunt operation for bleeding varices due to intrahepatic obstruction. *Surgery Gynecology & Obstetrics*, 134: 47-50, January, 1972.

58. Greenstein, A. J. *et al.* Interrelationship of intussusception and the integumentary system. *Surgery Gynecology & Obstetrics*, 133: 999-1002, December, 1971.

59. Gregg, J. A. *et al.* Fiber optic examination of the digestive tract. *Surgical Clinics of North America*, 51: 633-640, June, 1971.

60. Griffin, J. M. and Starkloff, G. B. Surgery of

chronic pancreatitis. *American Journal of Surgery*, 122: 18-21, July, 1971.

61. Guiberteau, M. J., Hersh, T. and Goyal, R. K. Transhepatic cholangiography in the differential diagnosis of jaundice. *Postgraduate Medicine*, 51: 201-206, March, 1972.

62. Hardin, W. J. Unusual manifestation of malignant disease of the large intestine. *Surgical Clinics of North America*, 52: 287-298, April, 1972.

63. Harrison, A. M. Gastric analysis in the absence of demonstrable gastric pathology. *American Journal of Surgery*, 123: 132-136, February, 1972.

64. Hatafuka, T. *et al.* Fundic patch operation in the treatment of advanced achalasia of the esophagus. *Surgery Gynecology & Obstetrics*, 134: 617-624, April, 1972.

65. Heimlich, H. J. Esophagoplasty with reversed gastric tube. Review of fifty-three cases. *American Journal of Surgery*, 123: 80-92, January, 1972.

66. Hepler, Opal E. *Manual of Clinical Method*, 4th ed. Springfield, Illinois: Charles C. Thomas, Publisher, 1955, pp. 98-99.

67. Higgins, J. A. Gastroscopy of peptic ulceration. *Surgical Clinics of North America*, 51: 961-968, August, 1971.

68. Hitchens, E. M. Benign gastric ulcer as a cause of gastrocolic fistula: Report of a case and review of the literature. *Archives of Surgery*, 104: 108-110, January, 1972.

69. Holder, J. B. Serum hepatitis. *Lawyer's Medical Journal*, 6: 79-89, May, 1970.

70. Host, W. R. *et al.* Hyperalimentation in cirrhotic patients. *American Journal of Surgery*, 123: 57-62, January, 1972.

71. Hoyumpa, A. M. *et al.* Budd-Chiara syndrome in women taking oral contraceptives. *American Journal of Medicine*, 50: 137-138, January, 1971.

72. Hsu, K. Y. Portal systemic shunt for portal hypertension. Importance of bromsulphalein retention for prediction of survival. *Annals of Surgery*, 175: 569-576, April, 1972.

73. Jeffries, G. H. Diseases of the liver. In Beeson, Paul B. and McDermott, W. *Textbook of Medicine*, 13th ed. Philadelphia: W. B. Saunders Co., 1971, pp. 1377-1404.

74. Jesse, R. H. *et al.* Cancer of the oral cavity. *American Journal of Surgery*, 120: 505-508, October, 1970.

75. Johnson, C. L. and Judd, E. S. The usefulness of vagotomy in treatment for gastric ulcer. *Surgical Clinics of North America*, 51: 907-914, August, 1971.

76. Johnston, D. P. *et al.* Diagnosis of stomal ulceration. *Surgical Clinics of North America*, 51: 871-877, August, 1971.

77. Jones, S. A. and Smith, L. S. A reappraisal of sphincteroplasty. *Surgery*, 71: 565, 575, April, 1972.

78. Judd, E. S. Selection of treatment for patients with duodenal ulcer disease. *Surgical Clinics of North America*, 51: 843-851, August, 1971.

79. Kelley, M. L. Diverticula of the alimentary tract. In Conn, Howard F. (ed.). *Current Therapy 1972*. Philadelphia: W. B. Saunders Co., 1972, pp. 325-329.

80. Kelly, D. L. *et al.* Spontaneous intramural esophageal perforation. *Journal of Thoracic and Cardiovascular Surgery*, 63: 504-508, March, 1972.

81. Kelly, K. A. Gastric motility and ulcer surgery. *Surgical Clinics of North America*, 51: 927-934, August, 1971.

82. Kelsey, J. R. *et al.* Cancer of the colon and rectum. In Conn, Howard F. (ed.). *Current Therapy 1972*. Philadelphia: W. B. Saunders Co., 1972, pp. 351-353.

83. Kettering, R. F. Current concepts in the medical treatment of duodenal ulcer. *Surgical Clinics of North America*, 51: 835-842, August, 1971.

84. Kirk, R. M. *et al.* Vagotomy and mucosal antrectomy in the elective treatment of duodenal ulcers. *American Journal of Surgery*, 123: 323-328, March, 1972.

85. Kirsner, J. B. Acid-peptic disease. In Beeson, Paul B. and McDermott, Walsh. *Textbook of Medicine*, 13th ed., Philadelphia: W. B. Saunders Co., 1971, pp. 1259-1284.

86. —————. Ulcerative colitis. In Conn, Howard T. (ed.). *Current Therapy 1972*. Philadelphia: W. B. Saunders Co., 1972, pp. 356-367.

87. Knowlessar, O. D. Diseases of the pancreas. In Beeson, Paul B. and McDermott, Walsh. *Cecil-Loeb Textbook of Medicine*, 13th ed., Philadelphia: W. B. Saunders Co., 1971, pp. 1312-1327.

88. Koutras, P. and White, R. R. Insulin-secreting tumors of the pancreas — A diagnostic and therapeutic challenge. *Surgical Clinics of North America*, 52: 299-314, April, 1972.

89. Kratzer, G. L. Anal fissure, anal fistula and hemorrhoids. In Conn, Howard F. (ed.). *Current Therapy 1972*. Philadelphia: W. B. Saunders Co., 1972, pp. 331-334.

90. Leafstedt, S. W. *et al.* Adenoid cystic carcinoma of major and minor salivary glands. *American Journal of Surgery*, 122: 756-762, December, 1971.

91. Lee, J. F. and Black, G. E. The changing clinical pattern of hepatic abscesses. *Archives of Surgery*, 104: 465-470, April, 1972.

92. Leffall, L. D. Head and neck cancer. *Ca — A Cancer Journal of Clinicians*, 21: 288-291, September-October, 1971.

93. Levin, E. Crohn's disease. In Conn, Howard F. (ed.). *Current Therapy 1972*, Philadelphia: W. B. Saunders Co., 1972, pp. 329-330.

94. Linn, R. C. *et al.* Liver trauma — Current method of management. *Archives of Surgery*, 104: 544-550, April, 1972.

95. Maki, T. *et al.* A reappraisal of surgical treatment for intrahepatic gallstones. *Annals of Surgery*, 175: 155-165, February, 1972.

96. Maloney, G. E. Darning inguinal hernias. *Archives of Surgery*, 104: 129-130, February, 1972.

97. Mandel, L. and Baurmash, H. The role of sialography in utraparotid disease. *Journal of Oral Surgery*, 31: 164, 1971.

98. Margulis, A. R. Interventional diagnostic roentgenology. In Welsh, Claude E. *et al.* (eds.). *Advances in Surgery*, Vol. 5. Chicago: Year Book Medical Publishers, Inc., 1971, pp. 88-102.

99. McDonough, J. M. *et al.* Factors influencing

prognosis of perforated peptic ulcer. *American Journal of Surgery*, 123: 411-416, April, 1972.

100. McElroy, R. *et al.* Hereditary pancreatitis in a kinship associated with portal vein thrombosis. *American Journal of Medicine*, 52: 228-241, February, 1972.

101. McGill, D. B. *et al.* Cirrhosis and death after jejunoileal shunt. *Gastroenterology*, 63: 872-877, November, 1972.

102. **Mergenhangen, S. E. Periodontal disease: A model for the study of inflammation.** *Journal of Infectious Diseases*, 123: 676-677, June, 1971.

103. Myers, J. R. *et al.* Cecal volvulus: A lesion requiring resection. *Archives of Surgery*, 104: 594-599, April, 1972.

104. Mosenthal, W. T. Peritoneoscopy. A neglected aid in the diagnosis of general medical and surgical disease. *American Journal of Surgery*, 123: 421-428, April, 1972.

105. Moyer, Carl A. *et al.* *Surgery Principles and Practices*, 3d ed. Philadelphia: J. B. Lippincott Co., 1965, pp. 1116-1117.

106. Nelson, R. S. Tumors of the stomach. In Conn, Howard F. (ed). *Current Therapy 1972*. Philadelphia: W. B. Saunders Co., 1972, pp. 354-356.

107. Neuer, Otto. A simple procedure for the closure of a large palatal perforation. *Plastic and Reconstructive Surgery*, 47: 296-298, March, 1971.

108. Onstad, G. R. *et al.* Jaundice as a complication of duodenal ulcer. *Surgical Clinics of North America*, 51: 885-892, August, 1971.

109. Page, Lot B. and Culver, Perry J. *Syllabus of Laboratory Examinations*. Cambridge, Massachusetts: Harvard University Press, 1960, pp. 258-423.

110. Palmer, E. D. Fistula secondary to unoperated benign gastroduodenal ulcer. *Postgraduate Medicine*, 51: 107-110, April, 1972.

111. Payne, W. S. Esophageal reflux ulceration: Causes and surgical management. *Surgical Clinics of North America*, 51: 935-944, August, 1971.

112. Pearson, F. G. *et al.* Gastroplasty and Belsey hiatus hernia repair: Operation for management of peptic stricture with acquired short esophagus. *Journal of Thoracic and Cardiovascular Surgery*, 61: 50-62, January, 1971.

113. Peterson, M. L. Neoplastic diseases of the alimentary tract. In Beeson, Paul B. and McDermott, W. (eds.). *Textbook of Medicine*, 13th ed. Philadelphia: W. B. Saunders Co., 1971, pp. 1358-1376.

114. Pichler, A. G. *et al.* Carcinoma of the tongue in childhood and adolescence. *Archives of Otolaryngology*, 95: 178-179, February, 1972.

115. Renning, J. A. Pancreatitis after renal transplantation. *American Journal of Surgery*, 123: 293-296, March, 1972.

116. Robbins, Stanley L. *Pathology* 3d ed. Philadelphia: W. B. Saunders Co., 1967, p. 806.

117. Ross, S. T. Ischemic colitis. *Postgraduate Medicine*, 51: 71-74, April, 1972.

118. Rossi, E. A. Clinical aspects of acute forms of viral hepatitis. *American Journal of Diseases of Children*, 123: 277-281, April, 1972.

119. Rovelstad, R. A. *et al.* Gastric analysis. *Surgical Clinics of North America*, 51: 969-978, August, 1971.

120. Sanfelippo, P. M. Factors in the prognosis of adenocarcinoma of the colon and rectum. *Archives of Surgery*, 104: 401-406, April, 1972.

121. Satomura, K. A simplified endorectal pull-through operation for the treatment of Hirschsprung's disease. *Surgery*, 71: 345-351, March, 1972.

122. Schumer, W. *et al.* The perforated viscus: Diagnosis and treatment. *Surgical Clinics of North America*, 52: 231-238, February, 1972.

123. Scott, H. W. *et al.* Experience with a new technic of intestinal bypass in the treatment of morbid obesity. *Annals of Surgery*, 174: 560-572, October, 1971.

124. Scott, H. W. Metabolic surgery for hyperlipidemia and atherosclerosis. *American Journal of Surgery*, 123: 3-12, January, 1972.

125. Segwick, C. E. and Viglotti, J. Hyperalimentation. *Surgical Clinics of North America*, 51: 681-686, June, 1971.

126. Shandling, B. Aganglionic megacolon. In Conn, Howard F. (ed.). *Current Therapy 1972*. Philadelphia: W. B. Saunders Co., 1972, pp. 345-347.

127. Shepherd, J. A. Familial polyposis of the colon with special reference to regression of rectal polyposis after subtotal colectomy. *British Journal of Surgery*, 58: 85-91, February, 1971.

128. Sigwart, U. *et al.* Cholecystitis associated with Haemophilus influenza. *Southern Medical Journal*, 65: 503-504, April, 1972.

129. Slanetz, C. A. *et al.* Anterior resection versus abdominoperineal resection for cancer of the rectum and rectosigmoid. *American Journal of Surgery*, 123: 110-117, January, 1972.

130. Sleisenger, M. H. Diseases of malabsorption. In Beeson, Paul B. and McDermott, W. (eds.). *Textbook of Medicine*, 13th ed. Philadelphia: W. B. Saunders Co., 1971, pp. 1285-1312.

131. _____. Diseases of the gallbladder. In Beeson, Paul B. and McDermott, W. (eds.). *Textbook of Medicine*, 13th ed. Philadelphia: W. B. Saunders Co., 1971, pp. 1405-1419.

132. Small, D. M. Gallstones: diagnosis and treatment. *Postgraduate Medicine*, 51: 187-193, January, 1972.

133. Smith, G. W. Splenectomy and coronary vein ligation for the control of bleeding esophageal varices. *American Journal of Surgery*, 119: 122-131, February, 1970.

134. Snyder, C. J. Bowel injuries from automobile seat belts. *American Journal of Surgery*, 123: 312-316, March, 1972.

135. Somayaji, B. N. *et al.* Budd-Chiara syndrome after oral contraceptives. *British Medical Journal*, 1: 53-54, January, 1968.

136. Soper, R. T. *et al.* Hirschsprung's disease. *Archives of Surgery*, 104: 429-437, April, 1972.

137. Spiro, R. H. and Strong, E. W. Epidermoid carcinoma of the mobile tongue. Treatment by partial glossectomy alone. *American Journal of Surgery*, 122: 707-710, December, 1971.

138. Stanley, H. R. Aphthous lesions. *Oral Surgery Oral Medicine & Oral Pathology*, 33: 407-416, March, 1972.

139. Stempien, S.J. *et al.* The role of distal gastrec-

tomy with or without vagotomy in the control of cephalic secretion and peptic ulcer disease. *Surgery*, 71: 110-117, January, 1972.

140. Stuart, M. S. and Hoerr, S. O. Late results of side-to-side choledochoduodenostomy and transduodenal sphincterotomy for benign disorders. *American Journal of Surgery*, 123: 67-72, January, 1972.

141. Sudnick, A. I. Australia antigen, posttransfusion hepatitis and the chronic carrier state. *American Journal of Diseases of Children*, 123: 392-400, April, 1972.

142. Sugawa, C. and Lucas, C. E. Therapeutic implications of disturbed gastric physiology in patients with stress ulcerations. *American Journal of Surgery*, 123: 25-34, January, 1972.

143. Suzuki, H. *et al.* Diagnosis of early esophageal cancer. *Surgery*, 71: 99-103, January, 1972.

144. Talbert, J. L. Corrosive strictures of the esophagus. In Sabiston, David C. (ed.). *Davis-Christopher Textbook of Surgery*, 10th ed. Philadelphia: W. B. Saunders Co., 1972, pp. 755-760.

145. Thomas, T. S. Restoration of cardioesophageal competence. *Postgraduate Medicine*, 51: 171-175, March, 1972.

146. _____. Subcostosternal diaphragmatic hernia. *Journal of Thoracic and Cardiovascular Surgery*, 63: 279-283, February, 1972.

147. Thompson, B. W. *et al.* Sclerosing cholangitis. *Archives of Surgery*, 104: 460-464, April, 1972.

148. Turell, R. A modern look at the problem of hemorrhoids. *American Journal of Surgery*, 123: 245-246, March, 1972.

149. Uchida, J. I. A new approach to the correction of cleft lip and nasal deformities. *Plastic and Reconstructive Surgery*, 47: 454-458, May, 1971.

150. Wallerstein, R. O. Anemias. In Krupp, Marcus A. and Chatton, Milton J. *Current Diagnosis and Treatment*, 11th ed. Los Altos, California: Lange Medical Publications, 1972, pp. 256-261.

151. Wolff, W. I. *et al.* Colonfiberoscopy. A new and valuable diagnostic modality. *American Journal of Surgery*, 123: 180-184, February, 1972.

152. Woodward, E. F. Hiatus hernia. In Sabiston, David C. (ed.). *Davis-Christopher Textbook of Surgery*, 10th ed. Philadelphia: W. B. Saunders Co., 1972, pp. 743-755.

153. Yules, Richard B. *Atlas for Surgical Repair of Cleft Lip, Cleft Palate and Noncleft Velopharyngeal Incompetence.* Springfield, Illinois: Charles C. Thomas, Publisher, 1971.

154. Zetzel, L. Inflammatory diseases of intestines. In Beeson, Paul B. and McDermott, W. (eds). *Cecil-Loeb Textbook of Medicine*, 13th ed. Philadelphia: W. B. Saunders Co., 1971, pp. 1327-1353.

Chapter IX
Urogenital Disorders

KIDNEYS

A. Origin of Terms:

1. calyx (G) — cup
2. cortex (L) — rind, outer portion
3. glomerulus (L) — little skein
4. medulla (L) — marrow, inner portion
5. nephron (G) — kidney
6. ren (L) — kidney

B. Anatomical Terms:

1. kidneys — paired, bean-shaped organs situated behind the peritoneum on either side of the lumbar spine. Their function is to preserve the ionic balance of the blood and extract its waste products.
2. nephron, renal tubule — the functional unit of the kidney which is composed of a
   a. glomerular capsule, Bowman's capsule — a double-layered envelope of epithelium which encloses a capillary tuft. It filters water and solutes out of the blood into the tubule.
   b. glomerulus (pl. glomeruli) — capillary cluster or tuft which is concerned with the initial phase of urine formation.
   c. renal corpuscle — both glomerular capsule and glomerulus.
   d. secretory tubule — tubule which completes urine formation and is functionally divided into a proximal tubule, a thin segment and a distal tubule or thick segment.[34]
   e. collecting tubule — tubule which conveys urine to the renal pelvis.[22]
3. renal cortex — outer portion of the kidney.
4. renal medulla — inner portion of the kidney containing the renal pyramids which include collecting tubules and parts of the secretory tubules.[34]
5. renal papillae — apices of the pyramids which indent the calices.
6. renal pelvis — funnel-shaped enlargement of the ureter as it leaves the kidney. It contains
   a. calices, formerly calyces (sing. calyx)[43] — cuplike indentations in the kidney pelvis. The collecting tubules open into the calices.
   b. hilus — a notch on the medial surface of the kidney through which the ureter and blood vessels enter or leave the kidney.

C. Diagnostic Terms:

1. acute renal failure — clinical state marked by a sudden decrease in glomerular filtration rate and cessation of renal function subsequent to severe kidney damage due to toxins, disease or trauma. Renal tubular necrosis is a dominant characteristic. The lumen of the renal tubules is occluded by debris usually containing protein, epithelial cells and hemoglobin. If the initial oliguric phase is followed by a diuretic phase the patient recovers. Residual damage is common.[53, 80, 67, 44, 79, 125]
2. arteriolar nephrosclerosis — renal disorder characterized by an intimal thickening of the afferent glomerular arterioles resulting in a narrowing of the arteriolar lumen and reduced blood supply to nephrons.[53]
3. congenital anomalies of kidneys:[104]
   a. agenesis — absence of one kidney.
   b. dysplasia — multicystic kidney forming an irregular mass.
   c. ectopy — low position, kidney failed to ascend.

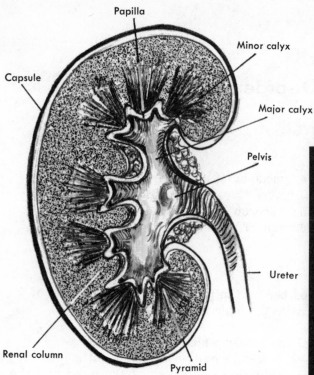

Fig. 48 – Longitudinal section of kidney.

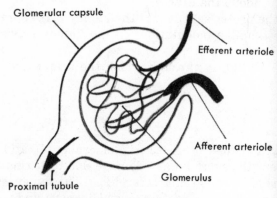

Fig. 49 – Structure of renal corpuscle.

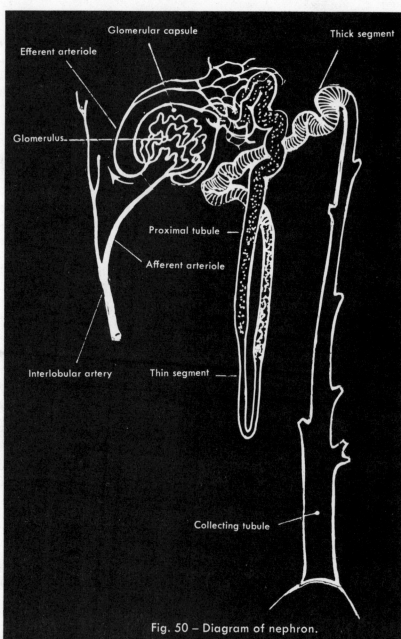

Fig. 50 – Diagram of nephron.

    d. medullary sponge kidney — cystic dilatation of the distal collecting tubules, generally affecting both kidneys.

    e. polycystic kidneys — nearly always an enlargement of both kidneys caused by multiple cysts that replace normal tissue.[100]

    f. simple cyst — usually a solitary cyst of one kidney which may compress functional tissue.

    g. vascular abnormalities — aberrant arteries or veins sometimes compressing the ureter thus causing hydronephrosis.[104]

4. glomerulonephritis — form of nephritis involving the renal glomeruli of both kidneys. There is evidence that the glomeruli may be injured by antigen-antibody complexes which develop from the immune responses to streptococcal infection. Headache, malaise, puffiness around the eyes, oliguria, blood, protein and casts in the urine are common clinical findings.[53, 132, 92, 12]

5. hydronephrosis — accumulation of fluid chiefly in pelvis and calices, resulting in enlargement of kidney and pressure atrophy. If fluid becomes infected, pyonephrosis develops.

6. hypertrophy of kidney — increase of size and functional capacity of organ.

7. infections of the kidney:

    a. abscess of kidney — usually a focal suppuration of the cortex.

    b. perinephric abscess, perinephritis — infection around the kidney.

    c. pyelonephritis — bacterial kidney infection.

        (1) acute form, commonly caused by gram-negative enteric bacilli

        (2) chronic form, generally no symptoms of urinary infection present.[4, 55]

8. injuries to the kidney — uncommon pathologic lesions usually due to athletic, occupational and traffic accidents. They comprise:

    a. contusions — simple bruising of functional tissue of kidney.

    b. ecchymoses — black and blue spots of kidney substance due to escape of blood.

    c. fissures — slits in renal capsule or pelvis, may cause hematuria.

    d. hematoma — a local mass of clotted blood which may develop especially after injury to renal pelvis.

    e. lacerations — tears may involve renal pelvis and renal capsule and result in severe hematuria.

    f. rupture — an extensive tear of the kidney may be the cause of massive bleeding and death.[103]

9. neoplasms of kidney:

    a. benign tumors: adenoma, fibroma, lipoma.

    b. malignant tumors:

        (1) adenocarcinoma and lymphosarcoma of kidney; renal tumors in the adult.

        (2) nephroblastoma, Wilm's tumor in children, infrequent in adults. It arises in the cortex and exerts pressure on the functional renal tissue of the medulla.

10. nephritis, Bright's disease — acute or chronic renal disease of unknown etiology. It is characterized by the presence of protein, casts and sometimes blood in the urine, resulting from a renal dysfunction. Edema, hypertension and nitrogen retention are prominent symptoms.

11. nephrolithiasis, renal calculi — stones in the kidney, generally in the pelvis and calices. They may be caused by renal tubular syndromes, enzyme disorders, hypercalcemia, increased uric acid and other factors.[121, 119, 102, 133]

12. nephroptosis — a movable, floating kidney which is displaced downward.

13. nephrotic syndrome — clinical state characterized by massive edema, excessive loss of protein in urine and low albumin blood levels. It may develop during the course of glomerulonephritis, a collagen disease, toxic drug reaction or specific allergy.[117, 132]

14. obstructive uropathy — obstruction occurring anywhere along the urinary tract from the renal pelvis to the external urethral meatus, causing changes in renal function, volume of

urine and amount of protein and sediment in urine.   Obstructive lesions include renal, ureteral, vesical and urethral calculi, strictures, prostatic lesions all of which may lead to hydronephrosis and renal failure.[91]

15. renal artery occlusion — acute blockage of renal artery due to embolus, thrombus or other cause.   The kidney is deprived of its blood supply when the occlusion is complete. Renal infarction and renal failure are rare complications.[124]

16. renal calcinosis, nephrocalcinosis — scattered foci of calcification within functional renal tissue.[121]

17. renal hypertension, renovascular hypertension — high blood pressure of kidney resulting from marked thickening of arteriolar walls or stenosis of renal artery by atheromatous plaques and thrombi.   It is not known why the ischemic kidney elevates the blood pressure.[41, 85, 105, 35, 8]

18. renal medullary necrosis, renal papillary necrosis — tissue death of renal papillae and medulla, usually a complication of pyelonephritis.[4]

19. renal tuberculosis — degeneration of kidney substance due to infection with tubercle bacilli.

20. renal vein thrombosis — occlusion of the renal vein by a thrombus which may result in an elevation of the renal pressure, excessive proteinuria and other manifestations of the nephrotic syndrome.   A complete occlusion of the renal vein may be complicated by a hemorrhagic infarction of the kidney.[132]

21. uremia — syndrome resulting from greatly reduced excretory function in progressive bilateral kidney disease.   Clinical symptoms vary widely from lassitude and depression in the early phase to anuria, uremic frost and peripheral neuropathy in the terminal phase.

D. Operative Terms:

1. nephrectomy — excision of kidney primarily for advanced calculous pyonephrosis, hydronephrosis or malignant tumor.

2. nephrolithotomy — incision into kidney for removal of stones.

3. nephrolysis — surgical destruction of renal adhesions.

4. nephropexy — surgical fixation of a displaced kidney.

5. nephrorrhaphy — suture of an injured kidney.

6. nephrostomy — surgical creation of a renal fistula for drainage.

7. nephrotomy — incision into kidney.

8. nephroureterectomy — removal of ureter and kidney for tumor of the renal pelvis or for malignant tumor of the ureter.[115, 48]

9. pyelolithotomy — incision into renal pelvis for removal of calculi.

10. pyeloplasty — plastic repair of renal pelvis.

11. pyelotomy — incision into renal pelvis.

12. renal biopsy, kidney biopsy, percutaneous renal biopsy — removal of renal tissue by a pronged biopsy needle.   The procedure, usually performed under fluoroscopic control, aids in the diagnosis and prognosis of renal disease and serves as guide in its therapeutic management.[7]

13. renal transplantation, kidney transplantation — a form of replacement surgery in which a healthy donor kidney is implanted in a patient after his irreversibly diseased kidneys have been removed.   The renal homograft may be obtained from a living donor or from a cadaver of a person who met with a fatal accident.   Bilateral nephrectomies are imperative since invariably the donor transplant will develop the disease of the collateral recipient's kidney if only one kidney has been removed.   After the donated homograft is placed extraperitoneally, vascular anastomoses to the iliac vessels and hypogastric artery are performed and an opening is surgically created between a ureter and the

bladder (ureteroneocystostomy). A splenectomy may be included in this complex surgical procedure.[122, 120, 51, 49, 3, 127, 25, 81, 23, 11, 45, 69, 88, 135]

surgery for renovascular hypertension — operative procedures for the restoration of normal blood flow to the kidney:

a. bypass grafting for unilateral or bilateral renal artery stenosis
b. excision of occluded lesion of renal artery followed by end-to-end anastomosis.
c. renal endarterectomy or surgical removal of intimal plaques from renal artery with or without patch grafting.[82, 105]

E. Symptomatic Terms

1. anuria — total suppression of urine due to renal failure or blockage of urinary tract.
2. azotemia — nitrogenous substances present in the blood.
3. Dietl's crisis — recurrent attacks of lumbar and abdominal pain, nausea and vomiting, caused by ureteral kinking or by vascular tension in cases of hypermobile kidney.
4. renal insufficiency, renal shut-down, lower nephron nephrosis — severe disturbance of excretory kidney function in renal disease or following surgery or trauma. Anuria may develop from blood transfusions, overhydration and electrolyte imbalance.
5. renal pain — various degrees from dull, aching to severe, stabbing or throbbing pain in lumbar region.
6. uremic frost — powdery deposit of urea on the skin due to the excretion of urea through perspiration.

URETERS

A. Origin of Terms:

1. junction (L) — joining
2. pyelo- (G) — pelvis, tub
3. pyo- (G) — pus
4. ureterovesical junction — meeting point

B. Anatomical Terms:

1. ureter — muscular, distensible tube lined with mucous membrane. It carries urine from each kidney to the bladder.
2. ureteric orifice — opening of the ureter at the outer, upper angle of the trigone (base) of the urinary bladder.
3. ureteropelvic junction — meeting point between ureter and renal pelvis.
4. ureterovesical junction — meeting point between ureter and urinary bladder.

C. Diagnostic Terms:

1. calculus in ureter — ureteral stone causing obstruction.
2. congenital malformations of the ureter:[106]
   a. duplication of ureters — the most common ureteral abnormality.
      There are 2 kinds:
      (1) complete duplication — usually complicated by vesicoureteral reflux, ureteral dilatation and hydronephrosis.[73]
      (2) incomplete duplication — common Y type; no interference with normal function.
   b. ectopic ureteral orifice — displaced opening, a developmental defect seen more frequently in women than men. It may result in incontinence.[14]

    c. incomplete ureter — embryonic development ceased before ureter reached kidney. Kidney may be absent or multicystic.

    d. stricture of ureter — abnormal narrowing of the duct, usually at the
        (1) uteropelvic junction or
        (2) ureterovesical orifice.
        It may be complicated by ureteral dilatation and hydronephrosis. The condition may be acquired.[2, 14]

    e. ureterocele — cystic protrusion or ballooning of lower end of ureter into bladder. It may be asymptomatic or obstructive, complicated by ureteral dilatation and hydronephrosis.[106]

3. hydroureter — ureter overdistended with urine due to obstruction.

4. injuries to ureter — uncommon pathological states which may be due to external trauma, be associated with pelvic fractures or occur inadvertently during surgery. A penetrating wound from a bullet may perforate a ureter and result in leakage of urine into the peritoneal cavity.[103, 24, 33, 47]

5. obstruction of ureter — blocking of ureter, usually resulting from pressure. It interferes with passage of urine.

6. occlusion of ureter — complete or partial closure of ureter.

7. pyoureter — infection in the ureter, generally secondary to infection of the bladder or kidney.

8. ureteritis — inflammation of the ureter.

D. Operative Terms:

1. ureteral resection — local incision of benign tumor of ureter.[115, 89]

2. ureterectomy — partial or complete removal of ureter.

3. ureterocystostomy, ureteroneocystostomy — reimplantation of ureter into bladder.

4. ureterolithotomy — incision into ureter for removal of calculi.

5. ureterolysis — freeing the ureter from adhesions to relieve secondary obstruction.

6. ureteropelviplasty — plastic operation at the ureteropelvic junction.

7. ureteropyelostomy — anastomosis of ureter and renal pelvis.

8. ureterostomy, cutaneous — transplantation of ureter to skin.

9. ureterovesicoplasty — corrective surgery for persistent reflux by repair of the ureterovesical junction.[109, 116]

E. Symptomatic Terms:

1. ureteral colic — excruciating, stabbing pain usually caused by the passage of a stone or large clot into the ureter. It may be accompanied by prostration, diaphoresis, shock and collapse.

2. ureteral spasm — contraction of ureter, frequently resulting from painful overdistention of ureter by stone.

BLADDER AND URETHRA

A. Origin of Terms:

1. cysto- (G) — bladder
2. trigone (G) — triangle
3. urethra (G) — urethra
4. vesica (L) — bladder

B. Anatomical Terms:

1. bladder, urinary — a hollow, muscular, distensible organ. It serves as a temporary reservoir for urine.

2. detrusor urinae muscle — a muscular network with bundles of muscle fibers running in various directions, intermingling and decussating. Their contraction effects the expulsion of urine from the bladder.[34]

3. neck of bladder — lowest angle of bladder.

4. vesical sphincter — thickened detrusor muscle fibers which surround the bladder neck.

5. trigone — triangular internal surface of the posterior wall of the bladder.

6. urethra — fibromuscular channel of communication between the urinary bladder and external urethral orifice.
   a. female urethra — passageway for urine.
   b. male urethra — passageway for urine and seminal fluid. It is composed of a
      (1) prostatic portion — passes through prostate.
      (2) membranous portion — passes through the pelvic and urogenital diaphragms.[34]
      (3) spongy portion — passes through the penis.

C. Diagnostic Terms:

1. atony of bladder — enormous distention of bladder associated with reduced expulsive force. It occurs in some diseases of the central nervous system.

2. bladder neck obstruction — blockage of the lumen of the bladder outlet resulting in over-distention of the urinary bladder, frequency, dysuria, persistent pyuria, retention with overflow and urinary back flow, dilatation of the ureters, hydronephrosis, renal pain, stone formation and chronic pyonephrosis. The obstruction may be due to
   a. contracture of vesical outlet, congenital or acquired — a form of urethral stricture. The bladder neck may be narrowed by hypertrophic muscle, fibrous tissue or chronic inflammatory disease or
   b. obstructive lesions of vesical outlet — blood clots, calculi, diverticula, tumors, prostatic enlargement.[15]

3. calculus (pl. calculi) of bladder — bladder stone.[121, 102]

4. cord bladder — bladder dysfunction due to injury or lesion of spinal cord. Residual urine, incontinence and vesicoureteral reflux are usually present.

5. cystitis, acute or chronic — inflammation of bladder due to infection.[20]

6. exstrophy of bladder — a congenital absence of the lower abdominal and anterior vesical walls with eversion of the bladder; absence of closure or formation of the anterior one half of the bladder.[15]

7. injuries to
   a. urinary bladder — direct trauma to the distended bladder may cause vesical compression or rupture; a bony spicule of a fractured bone may pierce the bladder; blood and urine may spill into the peritoneal cavity; a hematoma may form. Accidental perforation of the bladder may occur during surgery.
   b. urethra — injury to the posterior urethra may be more serious than to the bladder including contusions, lacerations and rupture associated with extravasation of urine and blood and formation of hematoma. Shearing injuries are likely to be complicated by urethral stricture.[103, 19]

8. interstitial cystitis, submucous fibrosis of bladder, Hunner's ulcer — a bladder disorder predominantly seen in middle-aged women. Fibrosis of the vesical wall reduces the bladder capacity which is clinically manifested by frequency, nocturia, distention of the bladder and suprapubic tenderness or pain.[107, 110]

9. megalocystis, megabladder — enormous dilatation of urinary bladder.

10. neoplasms:
    a. benign: papilloma, polyp, others.
    b. malignant: transitional cell carcinoma, epidermoid carcinoma, others.[42, 9, 26]

11. neurogenic bladder — there are 2 main types:
    a. flaccid atonic type — condition caused by lower motor neuron lesion due to trauma, ruptured intervertebral disk, meningomyelocele or other disorders and resulting in vesical dysfunction. The bladder has a large capacity, low intravesical pressure and a mild degree of trabeculation (hypertrophy) of the bladder wall.
    b. spastic automatic type — condition caused by upper motor neuron lesion due to injury, multiple sclerosis or other factors. The bladder capacity is reduced, the intravesical pressure is high, there is marked hypertrophy of the bladder wall and spasticity of the urinary sphincter.[107]
12. prolapse of bladder — a downward displacement of the bladder.
13. stress incontinence — incontinence resulting from a mechanical failure in the voluntary inhibition of the impulse to void.[64, 13]
14. stricture of urethra — narrowing of lumen of urethra, due to infection or trauma.[131]
15. stricture of vesicourethral orifice — narrowing of the opening between the bladder and urethra.
16. syphilis of bladder and urethra — venereal infection due to Treponema pallidum.
17. Trichomonas infection — a parasitic infection which may occur in bladder and male urethra.
18. trigonitis — inflammation of the trigone, the triangular base of the bladder.
19. urethritis, acute or chronic — inflammation of urethra which may be due to gonococcic infection.[16]
20. vesical fistulas — pathological openings of bladder leading to adjacent organs:
    a. vesicoenteric fistula — sinus tract between bladder and intestine.
    b. vesicorectal fistula — fistulous connection between bladder and rectum.
    c. vesicovaginal — pathological opening between bladder and vagina.[16]

D. Operative Terms:

1. cold punch transurethral resection of the vesical neck — endoscopic procedure for relief of bladder neck obstruction using a cold punch resectoscope for transurethral resection of tumor tissue, calcareous deposit or cicatrix. The new Kaplan resectoscope permits:
    a. fiber optic illumination
    b. magnification and sharp visualization of surgical area
    c. the free flow of irrigation fluid and
    d. controlled movement of the knife.[46]
2. cystectomy — excision of bladder.
    a. partial — resection of bladder.
    b. complete — removal of entire viscus.
3. cystolithotomy — incision into bladder for removal of stones.
4. cystoplasty — surgical repair of the bladder.
5. cystorrhaphy — suture of a ruptured or lacerated bladder.
6. cystoscopy — endoscopic examination of the bladder.
7. cystostomy — surgical creation of a cutaneous bladder fistula for urinary drainage.
8. meatotomy — incision of urinary meatus to increase its caliber.
9. multiple detrusor myotomy — a series of detrusor incisions around the bladder in an effort to reduce detrusor hypertrophy and hypercontractability and thereby to control severe juvenile urinary incontinence.[62, 63]
10. suprapubic vesicourethral suspension, Marshall-Marchetti repair — elevation and immobilization of the bladder neck and urethra by suturing them to the pubis and rectus muscles for the establishment of urinary control.[65, 86]
11. transurethral resection of the bladder neck — endoscopic resection of the bladder neck for removal of inelastic tissue using the transurethral approach.

12. ultraviolet cystoscopy — endoscopic examination with ultraviolet light source for the detection of bladder cancer following a two-day oral administration of tetracycline. Ultraviolet fluorescence reveals certain deeply invasive malignant lesions in bladder mucosa that appear normal or inflamed by visible light cystoscopy.[129]
13. urinary diversion operations for incapacitated bladder
    a. ileal conduit, ureteroileostomy — transplantation of both ureters to an isolated segment of the ileum. The urine drains through an external ileal stoma into a bag glued to the skin. Candidates for an elective ileal conduit may be children with bladder exstrophy and incontinence or adults with neurogenic bladders due to injury or neurological disease or victims of a vesical carcinoma. In malignancy and persistent bladder infection a cystectomy is done with ileal conduit.[21, 32]
    b. sigmoid bladder, neobladder, colocystoplasty — replacement of bladder by creating a substitute bladder. A sigmoid segment is isolated and the ureters and urethra are implanted in the segment.

E. Symptomatic Terms:[108]

1. albuminuria, proteinuria — albumin or protein in urine.
2. automatic bladder — vesical control reestablished following cord injury by having patient empty bladder at regular intervals.
3. autonomous bladder — condition due to spinal cord injury. It is characterized by a lack of bladder control manifested by urinary leakage and residual urine.
4. dysuria — difficult or painful urination.
5. enuresis — incontinence or involuntary discharge of urine.
6. frequency of urination — voiding at close intervals, more often than every two hours. This is normal in infancy.
7. glycosuria — sugar in urine.
8. hematuria — blood in urine.
9. hesitancy — dysuria due to nervous inhibition or to obstruction of vesical outlet.
10. hyperuropiresia — "an abnormal urodynamic state characterized by pathological elevations in hydraulic pressure within the urinary system." (David T. Mahoney)[63]
11. micturition — urination.
12. nocturia — frequent voiding during the night, may be due to renal inability to concentrate urine.
13. obstruction in bladder or urethra — blockage causing backflow of urine and renal damage.
14. oliguria — scanty urinary output.
15. overflow incontinence — involuntary urination caused by overdistention of bladder.
16. polyuria — excessive urinary output.
17. pyuria — pus in the urine.
18. residual urine — inability to empty bladder at micturition resulting in urinary retention and vesical overdistention.
19. spinal shock — sequela of complete transverse injury to cord. It causes autonomous bladder paralysis and later automatic voiding.[110]
20. suprapubic discomfort — uncomfortable sensation which may be due to interstitial cystitis, ulceration of the vesical mucosa or other disorders. It is usually present when the bladder fills and disappears when the bladder empties.[108]
21. tenesmus of vesical sphincter — painful spasm at the end of micturition.
22. urethral discharge — clear, thin, mucoid or purulent, scanty or profuse excretion from the urethra.
23. urgency — intense need to urinate at once.
24. urinary retention — inability to expel urine. This may be acute or chronic, complete or incomplete. It is frequently caused by obstruction of urinary outflow due to stone, stricture, tumor and the like.
25. vesicoureteral reflux — black flow of urine into kidney, usually due to bladder neck obstruction. It may cause severe renal damage.[28, 97, 7, 109, 116]

F. Terms Related to Special Procedures:

1. air cystometry — determination of vesical innervation and the elasticity of the bladder wall by infusing nonfiltered room air into the bladder. Intravesical pressure changes are recorded by a calibrated transducer. Detrusor reflex contraction and reflex inhibition are noted.[70, 71]

2. cystometry — measurement of intravesical pressure during filling of the urinary bladder with fluid.

3. cystometrogram — a graphic record of pressure reactions while the patient's bladder is being filled with water. Bladder capacity, residual urine and sensory responses are checked. In cord bladders sensations are absent.[110]

4. dialysis — the passage of solutes back and forth across a semipermeable membrane placed between two solutions. Each solute moves toward the fluid in which its concentration is lower. Dialysis is used in acute renal failure to remove urea from the body and terminate electrolyte imbalance. Hemodialysis and peritoneal irrigation are the methods of choice.[52]

5. extracorporeal hemodialysis — circulation established outside the body with the artificial kidney. The blood of the patient who is connected to the renal machine passes from a cannulated vein into a coil of cellophane, immersed in a bath or rinsing fluid. The cellophane substitutes for the glomerular membrane. The concentration of solutes in the blood differs from that in the bath to promote a solute transfer through the cellophane which restores the electrolyte balance. After the solute exchange has taken place, the blood reenters the patient's vein.[54, 74]

6. peritoneal dialysis, peritoneal lavage, intermittent method — perfusion of the peritoneum using commercially prepared electrolyte solutions, special catheters and a closed system of infusion and drainage in the treatment of renal failure. The peritoneum functions basically as an inert semipermeable membrane permitting the exchange of solutes in both directions.[87]

7. prophylactic dialysis — the use of peritoneal dialysis to prevent renal failure.

MALE GENITAL ORGANS

A. Origin of Terms:

1. balano- (G) — glans
2. deferens (L) — carrying away
3. didymos (G) — testis, twin
4. orchido- (G) — testis
5. semen (L) — seed
6. vas (L) — vessel, duct

B. Anatomical Terms:

1. penis — a highly vascular organ containing three erectile tissue components. The distal end is the glans penis over which is folded the prepuce or foreskin.

2. prostate — organ composed of smooth muscle, fibrous and glandular tissue and divided into two lateral lobes and one median lobe. The prostate is structurally an extension of the urinary bladder. It is pierced by the prostatic urethra and ejaculatory ducts. Its secretion is part of the seminal fluid.[22]

3. scrotum — sac of loose redundant skin which encloses the testes and epididymides.

4. testes (sing. testis) — paired male reproductive glands lying in the scrotum and divided into lobules by septa which are inward extensions of the outer covering. The lobules contain threadlike coils, the seminiferous tubules. The testes produce spermatozoa, part of the seminal fluid and androgen, the male hormone responsible for the secondary sex characteristics. Three ducts share in the transport of spermatozoa on each side:

a. epididymis (pl. epididymides) — structure lying on top and at the side of the testis and composed of head, body and tail. It stores spermatozoa before they are emitted. The greatly coiled duct of the epididymis, about six meters in length, merges into the ductus deferens.

b. ductus deferens, vas deferens — duct conveying spermatozoa from the epididymis to the ejaculatory duct.

c. ejaculatory duct — duct formed by union of ductus deferens with duct of seminal vesicle. Its fluid is carried into the urethra.

5. tunica vaginalis testis — double-layered serous sheath partially covering the testis and epididymis. An abnormal collection of serum between the layers is known as hydrocele.[34]

C. Diagnostic Terms:

1. actinomycosis — a fungus disease which may affect the genital organs.

2. adenocarcinoma — malignant tumor of glandular epithelium. It most commonly involves the prostate, less commonly the other genital organs. Metastases to bone occur frequently.[134, 77]

3. anorchism — absence of testes.

4. balanitis — inflammation of the glans penis.

5. cryptorchism — improperly descended testis, descent arrested.[111]

6. ectopy of testicle — testicle outside the path of normal descent.[111]

7. epididymitis — inflammation of the epididymis.

8. hydrocele
   a. tunica vaginalis — a collection of fluid within the tunica of the testis.
   b. spermatic cord — a collection of fluid along the spermatic cord usually within the inguinal canal.

9. hypertrophy of prostate, benign — a diffuse enlargement of the prostate, frequently seen in elderly men. The gland interferes with micturition and eventually results in hydronephrosis and dilatation of ureters.[18]

10. orchitis — inflammation of the testes.

11. paraphimosis — foreskin retracted behind the glans with subsequent edema preventing restoration to normal position.[14]

12. phimosis — stenosis of the orifice of the prepuce or foreskin. It may be congential or due to infection. The opening may be pinpoint or absent.

13. polyorchism, polyorchidism — more than 2 testes present.[101]

14. prostatitis — inflammation of the prostate gland.

15. syphilis — venereal disease due to Treponema pallidum. Involvement of genital organs is common.

16. tuberculosis — systemic, contagious disease caused by tubercle bacilli. Involvement of genital organs is infrequent.

17. varicocele — swelling and distention of veins of spermatic cord.[111]

D. Operative Terms:

1. circumcision — removal of an adequate amount of prepuce to permit exposure of the glans.

2. epididymectomy — excision of the epididymis.[60]

3. excision of hydrocele — evacuation of serous fluid or removal of serous tumor from tunica vaginalis.[60, 128, 39]

4. excision of varicocele — removal of varicose veins of the spermatic cord.

5. orchiectomy, orchectomy, orchidectomy — removal of testis.

6. orchiopexy — suturing an undescended testis in the scrotum.[60, 84]

7. orchioplasty — plastic repair of a testis.

178

8. prostatectomies:
    a. perineal prostatectomy — removal of prostate through an incision in the perineum.[6]
    b. retropubic prostatectomy — a form of extravesical removal of prostate with partial or complete resection of gland.[94]
    c. suprapubic prostatectomy — removal of gland through an opening into the bladder from above.[78]
    d. transperineal urethral resection of the prostate — endoscopic resection of prostate combined with perineal urethrotomy to avoid the formation of a postoperative urethral stricture.[30]
    e. transurethral cryogenic prostatectomy — use of special endoscope and freezing technique for destruction of prostatic tumor.[27, 118]
    f. transurethral prostatectomy — removal of obstructing glandular tissue using a special endoscope and electrocautery.[76]
9. vasectomy — removal of a short segment of the vas deferens and ligation of the severed ends.[14, 60]
10. vasoligation — tying the vas deferens with ligature to produce sterility or to prevent epididymitis.
11. vasovasostomy, epididymovasostomy — anastomosis of the vas deferens to epididymis to produce fertility by circumventing the obstructive lesion in the vas.[60]

E. Symptomatic Terms:

1. edematous swelling — enlargement of an organ or part resulting from its infiltration with an excessive amount of tissue fluid.
2. lumbosacral pain — pain felt in the small of the back.
3. mucopurulent discharge — drainage of mucus and pus.
4. prodromal pain — initial pain signalling that a more severe attack is approaching.
5. prostatism — urinary difficulty resulting from obstruction at the bladder neck by hypertrophy of prostate gland or other causes.
6. strangury — painful urination, drop by drop, due to spasmodic muscular contraction of bladder and urethra.

RADIOLOGY

A. Terms Related to Diagnosis by Urography:

1. plain urogram, scout urogram — radiogram made **without** injection of air or radiopaque solution to serve as contrast media. This is done as a preliminary step.
2. urogram — any radiogram either of the entire urinary tract or of a particular organ. A radiopaque solution is used for the visualization of the organs.[56, 112]
    a. cystogram — urogram of bladder.[66]
    b. nephrogram — comparative study of urograms of both kidneys in order to detect urinary obstruction, if present.
    c. pyelogram — urogram of kidney pelvis.
    d. ureterogram — urogram of ureter.
    e. urethrogram — urogram of urethra and prostate.
    f. voiding cystogram, voiding cystourethrogram — urogram made while patient voids the contrast medium.[56, 112]
3. urographic medium (pl. media) — a radiopaque solution used for the visualization of the various organs of the urinary tract. The following contrast media of low toxicity are used:

Conray — Hypaque — Renografin

These media may also be employed in the x-ray examination of other organs.[56, 112]

4. urography — radiography concerned with the detection of urological conditions.   Some special procedures are:
   a. air pyelography — injection of air as contrast medium into the renal pelvis through a ureteral catheter to demonstrate relatively nonopaque stones.
   b. cineradiography of urinary tract (cinecystogram) — urographic motion pictures to demonstrate transient or persistent vesicoureteral reflux after having gradually filled the bladder with a radiopaque medium.[112]
   c. drip infusion pyelography — intravenous infusion of a large volume of dilute contrast medium in conjunction with nephrotomograms to provide detailed visualization of renal pelves and ureters.   The procedure is of special value in the detection of renal cysts.[96]
   d. excretory, intravenous pyelography — the intravenous injection of a contrast medium followed by radiography of ureters and renal pelves.[56, 112]
   e. nephrotomography — body section radiography of the kidney.[90]
   f. pneumocystography — radiographic examination of the urinary bladder after it has been filled with air.   This method aids in the detection of vesical tumors.
   g. renal artery infusion urography — infusion of radiopaque medium into renal artery to demonstrate the state of the renal cortex and parenchyma which cannot be seen in retrograde pyelography.[38, 50, 29]
   h. retrograde pyelography — x-ray examination of the urinary tract after the injection of opaque solution which is introduced through ureteral catheters during cystoscopy. The calices, pelves and ureters are usually well demonstrated.[56]
   i. retroperitoneal pneumography — delineation of retroperitoneal organs by presacral insufflation using carbon dioxide as contrast medium.[56]
   k. urea washout test — urographic study for the detection of renal ischemia.
      Normal findings — the radiopaque fluid is washed out in 15 minutes.
      Positive for renal ischemia — the affected kidney retains the radiopaque medium 6 to 9 minutes longer than its mate.[112]

B. Terms Related to Diagnosis by Ultrasound:

1. nephrosonography — the delineation of deep renal structures by measuring the transmission of ultrasonic vibrations.[123]
2. renal sonogram, nephrosonogram — a record of ultrasonic waves passing through the renal tissue for the purpose of determining the size and location of the kidney.   Sonograms may detect congenital anomalies: horseshoe kidney, agnesis, renal ectopy, aid in differentiating between hydronephrosis, unilateral multicystic kidney and polycystic kidney and demonstrate cyst-tumor deformity.[123, 58, 99]
3. ultrasonic laminograms of kidney — sonographic renal section studies which delineate thin layers of renal tissue and are a valuable adjunct to other diagnostic modalities.[123]

C. Terms Related to Therapy:

1. radiation therapy for tumors of the urinary tract:
   a. carcinoma of the urinary bladder — favorable response to external radiation reported when tumors were located near the ureteral orifice and trigone.   Implantation of gold radon seeds through cystoscope has been used for papillomatous neoplasms.
   b. adenocarcinoma of kidney — beneficial results may be obtained from courses of therapy after the surgical removal of the tumor.
   c. Wilm's tumor — temporary relief from symptoms following deep x-ray therapy may result.[1]
2. radiation therapy of prostate gland —
   a. in primary carcinoma value is doubtful.
   b. in metastatic carcinoma the relief from pain is remarkable.[1]

CLINICAL LABORATORY

A. Terms Concerned with Urine Findings:

1. urinalysis — examination of physical and chemical properties of urine. Physical properties comprise quantity, color, specific gravity, odor and others. Chemical properties are concerned with quantitive or qualitative tests dealing with protein, glucose, bile pigments, ketone bodies, blood, calculi and the like. In conditions of the urinary system albumin and casts are frequently present and the pH concentration is altered.
   a. Albumin occurs in kidney and febrile diseases and the toxemias of pregnancy. It is due to increased permeability of the glomerular filter.
   b. Casts are formed in the renal tubules and appear in the urine as hyaline, granular, epithelial, blood and pus casts.
   c. Hydrogen ion concentration (chemical symbol pH) refers to the reaction of the urine.
      (1) pH concentration ...... 7 .... normal neutrality.
      (2) pH concentration below 7 .... acid in reaction.
      (3) pH concentration above 7 .... alkaline in reaction.
      In acidosis the urine is strongly acid; in chronic cystitis and in urinary retention the urine is usually alkaline in reaction.[113, 56, 72]
   d. Porphyrins (coproporphyrin, uroporphyrin, porphobilinogen) are pigments resembling bilirubin and apparently derived from the hemoglobin of the blood. Minute amounts of porphyrins are normally present in the urine. An increase is abnormal.
      (1) coproporphyrin urinary excretion — a valuable test in the detection of lead poisoning, acute porphyria, pellagra and liver damage.
      (2) uroporphyrin urinary excretion — diagnostic aid in acute porphyria and acute intermittent porphyria.[40]
   e. Urinary calculi are stones found in the pelvis of the kidney, ureter and bladder in the form of
      (1) cystine stones — white or pale yellow granules.
      (2) oxalate stones — crystalline structure.
      (3) phosphate and carbonate stones — compact balls.
      (4) uric acid stones — smooth round pebbles.[40]

B. Terms Related to Proprietary Urine Tests:

1. acetest — test for acetone in urine; present in acidosis, starvation, diabetic coma.
2. bumintest — test for albumin in urine; present in renal conditions and others.
3. clinitest — test for sugar in urine; present in uncontrolled diabetes mellitus.
4. hematest — test for occult blood in urine (also in feces, pleural fluid and others); present in disease of the urogenital system and others.
5. ictotest — test for bile in urine; present in liver disease, biliary tract obstruction and others.
6. nitrazine test — test determining the pH of the urine.

C. Terms Related to Renal Function Studies:

1. blood urea nitrogen (BUN) — a renal function test which measures the concentration of urea in the blood. In health the blood levels are low since urea, an end-product of protein metabolism, is freely excreted in the urine. In renal impairment and failure urea nitrogen accumulates in the blood and the patient may lapse into coma.
   Normal values 8-18 mg of urea nitrogen per 100 ml of blood.
   Increase in nephritis, urinary obstruction, uremia.
   Decrease in amyloidosis, nephrosis, pregnancy.[113, 56, 72]
2. concentration and dilution test — this test measures the functional capacity of the kidney to concentrate and dilute urine.

Normal values   **Specific Gravity**

Concentration phase .... 1.022 - 1.026.

Dilution phase .... 1.003 - 1.016.

Failure to concentrate urine indicates kidney damage. It may be partially caused by a faulty mechanism of the antidiuretic hormone (ADH) released from the pituitary gland.[113, 56, 72]

3. creatinine determination — a renal function test comparable to blood urea nitrogen. Creatinine is derived from catabolism (breakdown) of creatine phosphate from muscle tissue. It is eliminated by glomerular filtration and excreted in the urine. In a healthy individual the amount of creatinine remains almost constant from day to day.[56]

Table 15

CREATININE AND CREATINE IN HEALTH AND DISEASE

Test	Normal Values	Increased Values	Decreased Values[a]
Creatinine Serum (Folin's Method) Urine	0.8-2.0 mg/100 ml 0.7-2.0 gm/24 hrs	Nephritis Urinary obstruction Intestinal obstruction Diabetes mellitus Pneumonia Tetany Typhoid fever	Amyotonia congenita (Oppenheim's disease) Advanced nephritis Muscular atrophy Anemia Leukemia
Creatine-Creatinine Urine	0.0- 50.0 mg/24 hrs-M 0.0-100.0 mg/24 hrs-F	Muscular disorders Carcinoma of liver Diabetes mellitus Hyperthyroidism	

a Values taken from Hepler, *op. cit.*, 286-288.

4. Howard test, excretion of water, salt and creatinine — renal function study to detect ischemia of the kidney due to stenosis of the renal artery or its branch or to chronic pyelonephritis with arteriolar involvement. A low urine volume, low sodium and high creatinine concentrations are positive findings and indicate that the patient may benefit by renovascular surgery.[114]

5. nonprotein nitrogen (NPN) — a kidney function test which measures the nitrogenous waste products from protein metabolism chiefly urea. An abnormally high NPN level in the blood signals kidney damage.

Normal values — NPN .... 25 - 35 mg per 100 ml.

Increase in renal insufficiency, glomerulonephritis, urinary obstruction, dehydration, uremia and others.

Decrease may occur in normal pregnancy and diabetes.[40]

6. phenolsufonphthalein (PSP) — a dye test for the detection of kidney impairment. About 90% of the PSP is eliminated through the renal tubules and only 10% through glomerular filtration.

Normal values — PSP.....first hour 40 - 60%; second hour 20 - 25%

A low urinary excretion of the dye of 40% or less in 2 hours is usually associated with nitrogen retention in the blood. Elimination of the dye is delayed in hypertrophy of prostate gland complicated by hydronephrosis, in malignant hypertension, and cystitis with urinary retention.[40]

7. Stamey test — sodium chloride-urea-ADH-PAH test designed to demonstrate abnormal reabsorption of water by the ischemic kidney by revealing its reduced urine volume and elevated PAH concentration in comparison with its urate.[114]

8. urea clearance — test measures the glomerular function of the kidneys to remove urea from the blood. It is calculated as plasma cleared of urea in one minute. Two tests are used: standard clearance and maximum clearance, the latter being the more reliable test.

    Normal value .... urea clearance ..... above 60%

    Renal impairment .... urea clearance ..... below 60%.[40]

9. uroflowmetry — the use of an electronic uroflowmeter for recording the flow of urine as:

    a. a screening test for assessing the degree of obstruction in the lower urinary tract.

    b. an aid for evaluating the results of urologic surgery.

    c. a guide for planning postoperative follow-up care.[56]

D. Terms Related to Tests for Metastases:

1. serum acid phosphatase — test measures acid phosphatase, an enzyme freely present in the normal prostate gland which produces it and releases a small amount into the blood serum.

    Normal value — Method of Gutman and King-Armstrong

    Serum acid phosphatase is .... 1.0 to 4 units per 100 ml.

    Increase is seen in metastatic carcinoma of the prostate gland. The test aids in the detection of obscure bone lesions.

2. serum alkaline phosphatase — test measures the activity of alkaline phosphatase, a prostatic enzyme which is found in small quantity in the blood serum.

    Normal value — Method of Bodansky

    Serum alakaline phosphatase is 1.5 to 4 units per 100 ml.

    Increase may occur in metastases of prostatic carcinoma to bone, in bone growth and repair, bone injury, Paget's disease, biliary tract blockage and liver disease.[40, 68, 61, 10]

3. urinary exfoliative cytology — cytologic study of urinary sediments to detect malignant cells in the urine as an aid in the diagnosis of cancer.[98]

ABBREVIATIONS

ADH — antidiuretic hormone
AG — albumin/globulin (ratio)
BNO — bladder neck obstruction
BNR — bladder neck resection
BPH — benign prostatic hypertrophy
BUN — blood urea nitrogen
CBI — continuous bladder irrigation
CC — chief complaint
CUG — cystourethrogram
Cysto — cystoscopic examination
DL — danger list
ERPF — effective renal plasma flow
GBM — glomerular basement membrane
GFR — glomerular filtration rate
GU — genitourinary
ICU — intensive care unit

IVP — intravenous pyelogram
KUB — kidney, ureter, bladder
NPN — nonprotein nitrogen
NPO — nothing by mouth
PAH — p-aminohippuric acid
pH — hydrogen ion concentration
PPC — progressive patient care
PSP — phenolsulfonphthalein
PU — prostatic urethra
RER — renal excretion rate
RPF — renal plasma flow
RTA — renal tubular acidosis
TPUR — transperineal urethral resection
TUR — transurethral resection
UP — urine/plasma (ratio)
VCUG — voiding cystourethrogram

ORAL READING PRACTICE

Hydronephrosis

This condition is a byproduct of mechanical obstruction of the urinary tract. When the interference with the outflow of urine is below the bladder, as in **urethral stricture** or **hypertrophy** of the prostate gland, **bilateral hydronephrosis** develops. When above the bladder, as in **unilateral, ureteral stricture, calculus** or **neoplasm,** the condition affects only one kidney. In addition, pressure from tumors, adhesions or the **pregnant uterus** outside the urinary tract may interfere with the flow of urine and lead to **hydronephrosis. Congenital anomalies** of the **ureter** or **urethra** may also be responsible for this condition.[17, 53]

There are various degrees of **dilatation** of the **renal pelvis** and ureter. In the initial phase of the disease the pathological changes are slight. As the condition progresses, the amount of fluid increases, the **papillae** assume a flattened appearance, the **renal cortex** becomes thinned and the pyramids of the medulla undergo atrophic changes. The kidney resembles a hollow shell filled with fluid. In extreme cases several liters of fluid may accumulate in the renal pelvis leading to a complete loss of physiological capacity. If the **hydronephrosis** is unilateral, the healthy kidney undergoes compensatory hypertrophic changes to adapt itself to the increased functional work load. In this case renal insufficiency does not develop. However, in the presence of advanced bilateral hydronephrosis, the downhill clinical course is steady and terminates in fatal uremia.[53, 57]

The fluid in the kidney differs from normal urine in its reduced content of urea. Since it is locked up in the renal shell and unable to escape to its proper destination, it becomes easily a breeding place for invading bacterial organisms.[55] Another deleterious **sequela** of fluid retention in the kidney is the formation of **renal calculi** which adds insult to injury and completes the physiological destruction of the organ.[102]

In the early phase of hydronephrosis symptoms may be absent or so mild that they escape notice. As the condition progresses, the kidney becomes palpable, tender and painful. With unrelieved obstruction continued over weeks, the only symptom may be a dull pain. If intermittent obstruction occurs, attacks of pain develop periodically and are accompanied by oliguria which is promptly reversed to **polyuria** when the obstruction is abolished. Should the damaged kidney become infected, **leukocytosis**, fever and **pyuria** signal the onset of **pyonephrosis**.[91]

The treatment of hydronephrosis consists in removing the cause of obstruction such as the ureteral stricture or compressing **prostatic** or vesical tumor. If done early, the kidney may be saved. In advanced cases the presence of irreparable damage demands the excision of the diseased organ since it serves no useful function and is a constant threat of focal infection.[17, 57, 5]

Table 18

SOME UROGENITAL CONDITIONS AMENABLE TO SURGERY

Organs Involved	Diagnoses	Operations	Operative Procedures
Kidneys	Chronic glomerulo-nephritis, preterminal Irreversible renal failure	Renal homotrans-plantation including a. bilateral nephrectomy b. splenectomy c. revascularization of homograft d. ureterocystostomy	Removal of both kidneys and spleen Extraperitoneal donor homo-grafting with vascular anastomoses to iliac and hypogastric vessels Creation of an opening between a ureter and bladder
Kidney	Nephroptosis	Nephropexy	Fixation or suspension of movable or displaced kidney
Kidney	Posttraumatic fistula of kidney	Nephrorrhaphy	Suture of kidney
Kidney	Bilateral nephrolithiasis Unilateral calculous pyonephrosis and infection of ureter	Nephrolithotomy Nephrectomy Ureterectomy	Removal of stones from better kidney first Removal of kidney and ureter
Kidney Ureter	Calculous anuria due to acute ureteral obstruction	Nephrostomy Pyelostomy	Creation of a communication between the kidney and the skin for drainage

Organs Involved	Diagnoses	Operations	Operative Procedures
Kidney Ureter	Adenocarcinoma of kidney Papillary carcinoma of kidney pelvis Carcinoma of ureter	Total nephrectomy Nephroureterectomy Partial cystectomy	Removal of kidney Removal of kidney, ureter and bladder cuff
Kidney Ureter	Hydronephrosis due to obstruction from impacted ureteral calculus Dilatation of infected ureter	Total nephrectomy Ureterectomy	Excision of severely damaged kidney and ureter
Renal pelvis	Calculus in renal pelvis, small	Pyelolithotomy	Removal of calculus from renal pelvis
Ureter	Calculus in ureter associated with renal obstruction	Ureterolithotomy	Incision into ureter with removal of calculus
Ureter	Postinfectional stricture of ureter	Ureteroplasty	Plastic repair of ureter
Bladder	Diverticulum of bladder	Diverticulectomy of urinary bladder	Local excision of diverticulum
Bladder	Cystocele	Cystoplasty	Plastic repair of cystocele
Bladder	Hemorrhage from urinary bladder	Cystoscopy with evacuation of blood clots	Endoscopic examination of the bladder
Bladder	Early carcinoma of urinary bladder, no metastasis	Partial cystectomy with wide local excision of tumor	Removal of bladder wall including the carcinoma and a surrounding cuff of normal bladder wall
Bladder	Papilloma encroaching on ureteral orifice	Suprapubic cystostomy with excision of tumor Ureterocystostomy	Surgical opening of the bladder above the symphysis pubis and removal of tumor Anastomosis of ureter to bladder and reimplantation of ureter into bladder
Bladder	Rupture of bladder due to injury	Cystorrhaphy	Suture of bladder
Bladder Ureters	Bladder neck obstruction, vesicoureteral reflux	Bladder neck reconstruction (Y-V plasty) Ureteroneocystostomy	Surgical bladder neck revision and reimplantation of ureters into bladder to correct vesicoureteral reflux
Bladder Ureters	Neurogenic bladder associated with vesical calculi and recurrent pyelonephritis Carcinoma of bladder Exstrophy of bladder	Ureteroileostomy (Ileal conduit) Cystectomy	Transplantation of both ureters to an isolated segment of the ileum for conveying urine to an external stoma Removal of bladder in vesical malignancy and uncontrolled infection

Organs Involved	Diagnoses	Operations	Operative Procedures
Bladder Ureters Urethra	Carcinoma of bladder	Cystectomy Colocystoplasty (Neobladder or Sigmoid bladder)	Excision of urinary bladder Creation of a new bladder by isolating a sigmoid segment and implanting the ureters and urethra in the segment
Prostate	Hypertrophy of prostate	Transurethral resection of prostate cryosurgery of prostate	Partial removal of prostate using a special endoscope and the electrocautery or localized freezing of prostate
Prostate Seminal vesicles Vasa deferentia	Carcinoma of prostate	Retropubic prostatectomy Radical perineal prostatectomy	Radical extravesical removal of the prostate Removal of prostate, seminal vesicles and vasa deferentia through perineal incision
Testis Spermatic cord	Torsion of spermatic cord complicated by testicular gangrene	Orchiectomy Orchiopexy	Removal of testis Scrotal fixation of the opposite testis
Testes	Advanced carcinoma of the prostate gland with bone metastases	Orchiectomy, bilateral (castration for androgen control)	Removal of both testes
Testis	Undescended testis, unilateral	Orchioplasty Orchiopexy	Surgical transfer of testis to scrotum

REFERENCES AND BIBLIOGRAPHY

1. Ackerman, Lauren V. and del Regato, Juan A. Cancer of the genitourinary tract. In *Cancer*, 4th ed. St. Louis: The C. V. Mosby Co., 1970, pp. 606-690.

2. Allen, T. D. Congenital ureteral strictures. *Journal of Urology*, 104: 196-204, July, 1970.

3. Anderson, E. E. *et al.* Urologic complications in renal transplantation. *Journal of Urology*, 107: 187-192, February, 1972.

4. Beeson, P. B. Pyelonephritis. In Beeson, Paul B. and McDermott, Walsh (eds.). *Cecil-Loeb Textbook of Medicine*, 13th ed. Philadelphia: W. B. Saunders Co., 1971, pp. 1201-1205.

5. Belgrad, R. Hydration pyelography — a neglected tool in the diagnosis of intermittent hydronephrosis. *Arizona Medicine*, 29: 208-210, March, 1972.

6. Belt, E. *et al.* Total perineal prostatectomy for carcinoma of prostate. *Journal of Urology*, 107: 91-96, January, 1972.

7. Bischoff, P. F. Problems in treatment of vesicorneal reflux. *Journal of Urology*, 107: 141-142, January, 1972.

8. Bookstein, J. J. *et al.* Arteriography in renovascular hypertension. *Journal of American Medical Association*, 221: 368-373, July 24, 1972.

9. Bowles, W. T. Carcinoma of bladder: computer analysis of 516 patients. *Journal of Urology*, 107: 245-247, February, 1972.

10. Bradley, G. M. Urinary screening tests in the infant and young child. *Medical Clinics of North America*, 55: 1457-1471, November, 1971.

11. Braun, W. E. Immunologic aspects of renal transplantation. *Surgical Clinics of North America*, 51: 1161-1173, October, 1971.

12. Bridi, G. S. *et al.* Glomerulonephritis and renal tubular acidosis in a case of chronic active hepatitis with hyperimmunoglobulinemia. *American Journal of Medicine*, 52: 267-278, February, 1972.

13. Brocklehurst, J. C. Treatment of urinary incontinence in the elderly. *Postgraduate Medicine*, 51: 184-187, April, 1972.

14. Byrne, John E., M.D. Personal communications.

15. Campbell, M. F. Anomalies of the bladder. In Campbell, Meredith F. and Harrison, J. Hartwell (eds.). *Urology*, 3d ed. Philadelphia: W. B. Saunders Co., 1970, pp. 1543-1572.

16. Campbell, M. F. Surgery of the bladder. In Campbell, Meredith, F. and Harrison J. Hartwell (eds.). *Urology*, 3d ed. Philadelphia: W. B. Saunders Co., 1970, pp. 2338-2404.

17. Campbell, M. F. Urinary obstruction — hydronephrosis. In Campbell, Meredith F. and Harrison, J. Hartwell (eds.). *Urology*, 3rd ed. Philadelphia: W. B. Saunders Co., 1970, pp. 1772-1793.

186

18. Castro. J. E. *et al.* Urinary dynamics of benign prostatic hypertrophy. *Journal of Urology*, 107: 289-292, February, 1972.

19. Clark, S. S. *et al.* Lower urinary tract injuries associated with pelvic fractures: Diagnosis and management. *Surgical Clinics of North America*, 52: 183-202, February, 1972.

20. Comarr, A. E. Intermittent catheterization for the traumatic cord bladder patient. *Journal of Urology*, 108: 79-81, July, 1972.

21. Cordonnier, J. J. and Bowles, W. T. Surgery of the ureter and urinary conduits. In Campbell, Meredith F. and Harrison, J. Hartwell (eds.). *Urology*, 3rd ed. Philadelphia: W. B. Saunders Co., 1970, pp. 2289-2337.

22. Crouch, James E. *Functional Anatomy*, 2nd ed. Philadelphia: Lea & Febiger, 1972, pp. 414-448.

23. David, D. S. *et al.* Viral syndromes and renal homograft rejection. *Annals of Surgery*, 175: 257-259, February, 1972.

24. Del Villar, R. G. Ureteral injury owing to external trauma. *Journal of Urology*, 107: 29-30, January, 1972.

25. Deodhar, S. D. *et al.* Pathology of human renal allograft rejection. *Surgical Clinics of North America*, 51: 1141-1159, October, 1971.

26. DeWeerd, J. H. Invasive vesical carcinoma treated by preoperative radiotherapy and operation. *Journal of Urology*, 107: 51-55, January, 1972.

27. Dow, J. A. The technique of cryosurgery of the prostate. *Journal of Urology*, 105: 286-290, February, 1971.

28. Elo, J. Vesicoureteral reflux in children. *Journal of Urology*, 106: 603-605, October, 1971.

29. Evans, John A. and Bosnik, M. A. *The Kidney —Atlas of Tumor Radiology*. Chicago: Year Book Medical Publishers Inc., 1971, pp. 6-134.

30. Flanagan, M. J. Transperineal urethral resection of the prostate. *Journal of Urology*, 107: 1028-1031, June, 1972.

31. Frankson, C. *et al.* Renal carcinoma (hypernephroma) occurring in 5 siblings. *Journal of Urology*, 108: 58-61, July, 1972.

32. Frenay, Sr. Agnes Clare. A dynamic approach to the ileal conduit patient. *American Journal of Nursing*, 64: 80-84, January, 1964.

33. Gangai, M. P. Ureteral injury incident to lumbar disc surgery. *Journal of Neurosurgery*, 36: 90-96, January, 1972.

34. Gardner, Ernest, Gray, Donald and O'Rahilly, Ronan. *Anatomy — A Regional Study of Human Structure*, 3rd ed. Philadelphia: W. B. Saunders Co., 1969, pp. 424-490.

35. Gill, W. B. *et al.* Renovascular hypertension developing as complication of selective renal arteriography. *Journal of Urology*, 107: 922-924, June, 1972.

36. Grabstald, H. *et al.* Renal pelvic tumors. *Journal of American Medical Association*, 218: 845-854, November 8, 1971.

37. Greenberg, M. *et al.* Neurogenic bladder in Parkinson's disease. *Southern Medical Journal*, 65: 446-448, April, 1972.

38. Hare, W. Renal artery infusion urography. *Radiology*, 90: 569, March, 1968.

39. Hendrick, J. W. and Bohne, A. W. Treatment of testicular tumors. *Southern Medical Journal*, 64: 873-881, July, 1971.

40. Hepler, Opal E. *Manual of Clinical Laboratory Methods*, 4th ed. Springfield, Illinois: Charles C. Thomas, Publisher, 1955, pp. 13-28 and pp. 312-315.

41. Honari, J. and Ing, T. S. Renovascular hypertension. *Medical Clinics of North America*, 55: 1429-1438, November, 1971.

42. Holtz, F., Fox, J. E. and Abell, M. R. Carcinoma of the urinary bladder. *Cancer*, 29: 294-304, February, 1972.

43. International Anatomical Nomenclature Committee. *Nomina Anatomica*, 2nd ed. New York: Excerpta Medica Foundation, 1961, p. 29 and p. 67.

44. Ireland, G. W. Recognition and management of acute high output renal failure. *Journal of Urology*, 108: 40-43, July, 1972.

45. Jonasson, O. Emergencies in renal transplantation. *Surgical Clinics of North America*, 52: 257-264, February, 1972.

46. Kaplan, J. H. A new cold punch resectoscope. *Journal of Urology*, 107: 1054-1055, June, 1972.

47. Kaufman, J. J. and Brosman, S. A. Blunt injuries of the genitourinary tract. *Surgical Clinics of North America*, 52: 747-760, June, 1972.

48. Kim, K. H. *et al.* Primary tumors of ureter. *Journal of Urology*, 107: 955-958, June, 1972.

49. Kiser, W. S. *et al.* Surgical complications of renal transplantation. *Surgical Clinics of North America*, 51: 1133-1140, October, 1971.

50. Koehler, P. R. Angiography of the transplanted kidney. *Radiology*, 102: 443-444, February, 1972.

51. Konnak, J. W. Bilateral nephrectomy prior to renal transplantation. *Journal of Urology*, 107: 9-12, January, 1972.

52. Krumlovsky, F. A. Dialysis in treatment of neomycin overdosage. *Annals of Internal Medicine*, 76: 443-446, March, 1972.

53. Krupp, M. A. Genitourinary tract. In Krupp, Marcus A. and Chatton, Milton J. *Current Diagnosis & Treatment*, 11th ed. Los Altos, California: Lange Medical Publications, 1972, pp. 477-504.

54. Kuruvila, K. C. *et al.* Arteriovenous shunts and fistulas for hemodialysis. *Surgical Clinics of North America*, 51: 1219-1234, October, 1971.

55. Lang, G. R. and Levin, S. Diagnosis and treatment of urinary tract infections. *Medical Clinics of North America*, 55: 1439-1456, November, 1971.

56. Leader, A. J. *et al.* Urologic diagnosis and the urologic examination. In Campbell, Meredith, F. and Harrison, J. Hartwell (eds.). *Urology*, 3rd ed. Philadelphia: W. B. Saunders Co., 1970, pp. 197-294.

57. Leary, D. J. Preoperative aortography in hydronephrosis. *Journal of Urology*, 107: 542-546, April, 1972.

58. Leopold, G. R. Renal transplant size measured by reflected ultrasound. *Radiology*, 95: 687-689, June, 1970.

59. Lome, L. G. *et al.* Urinary reconstruction following temporary cutaneous ureterostomy diversion in children. *Journal of Urology*, 108: 162-164, July, 1972.

60. MacDonald, S. A. Surgical treatment of the scrotum and its contents. In Campbell, Meredith, F. and Harrison, J. Hartwell. *Urology*, 3rd ed. Philadelphia: W. B. Saunders Co., 1970, pp. 2648-2662.

61. Mahon, F. B. *et al.* Serum enzyme determinations after transurethral resection of prostate. *Journal of Urology*, 107: 88-90, January, 1972.

62. Mohony, D. T. *et al.* Studies of enuresis. Multiple detrusor myotomy: A new operation for the rehabilitation of severe detrusor hypertrophy and hypercontractibility. *Journal of Urology*, 107: 1064-1067, June, 1972.

63. _____. Studies of enuresis. III. Vesical hyperuropiresia as a hazardous side effect of sphincter repair surgery. *Journal of Urology*, 107: 1059-1063, June, 1972.

64. Marchant, D. J. Evaluation of stress urinary incontinence. *Postgraduate Medicine*, 49: 192-196, February, 1971.

65. Marshall, V. F., Marchetti, A. A. and Krantz, K. E. Correction of stress incontinence by simple vesicourethral suspension. *Surgery Gynecology & Obstetrics*, 88: 505-518, April, 1949.

66. Matsumoto, K. Accurate roentgenographic diagnosis of vesical tumors with double contrast cystography and arteriography. *Journal of Urology*, 107: 46-48, January, 1972.

67. Matten, W. D. Oliguric acute renal failure in malignant hypertension. *American Journal of Medicine*, 52: 187-197, February, 1972.

68. Mattenheimer, H. Enzymes in the urine. *Medical Clinics of North America*, 55: 1493-1508, November, 1971.

69. Merkatz, I. R. *et al.* Resumption of female reproductive function following renal transplantation. *Journal of American Medical Association*, 216: 1749-1754, June 14, 1971.

70. Merrill, D. C. *et al.* Air cystometry. I. Technique and definition of terms. *Journal of Urology*, 106: 678-681, November, 1971.

71. _____. Air cystometry. II. A clinical evaluation of normal adults. *Journal of Urology*, 108: 85-88, July, 1972.

72. Merrill, J. P. Normal and abnormal renal function and treatment of renal failure. In Campbell, Meredith F. and Harrison, J. Hartwell (eds.). *Urology*, 3rd ed. Philadelphia: W. B. Saunders Co., pp. 39-67.

73. Miller, H. C. Ureteral reflux as genetic trait. *Journal of American Medical Association*, 220: 842-843, May 8, 1972.

74. Muehrcke, R. C. *et al.* Home hemodialysis. *Medical Clinics of North America*, 55: 1473-1491, November, 1971.

75. Murphy, G. P. Percutaneous needle biopsy of renal allotransplants. *Journal of Urology*, 107: 193-195, February, 1972.

76. Nesbit, R. M. Transurethral prostatic resection. In Campbell, Meredith F. and Harrison, J. Hartwell (eds.). *Urology*, 3rd ed. Philadelphia: W. B. Saunders Co., 1970, pp. 2479-2506.

77. Nussbaum, P. S. Carcinoma of the prostate presenting as pelvic lipomatosis. *Surgical Clinics of North America*, 52: 405-414, April, 1972.

78. O'Connor, V. J. Suprapubic prostatectomy. In Campbell, Meredith F. and Harrison, J. Hartwell (eds.). *Urology*, 3rd ed. Philadelphia: W. B. Saunders Co., 1970, pp. 2338-2404.

79. Ooi, B. S. *et al.* Multiple myeloma with massive proteinuria and terminal renal failure. *American Journal of Medicine*, 52: 538-546, April, 1972.

80. Orecklin, J. R. and Brosman, S. A. Current concepts in diagnosis of acute renal failure. *Journal of Urology*, 107: 892-896, June, 1972.

81. Popowniak, K. L. Immunosuppressive therapy in renal transplantation. *Surgical Clinics of North America*, 51: 1191-1201, October, 1971.

82. Poutasse, E. F. Renovascular surgery. In Campbell, Meredith F. and Harrison, J. Hartwell (eds.). *Urology*, 3rd ed. Philadelphia: W. B. Saunders Co., 1970, pp. 2272-2288.

83. Rabiner, S. F. Bleeding in uremia. *Medical Clinics of North America*, 56: 221-234, January, 1972.

84. Redman, J. F. A retroperitoneal approach to orchiopexy. *Journal of Urology*, 108: 107-108, July, 1972.

85. Reiss, M. D. *et al.* Complications in renovascular hypertension. *Journal of American Medical Association*, 221: 374-377, July 24, 1972.

86. Ridley, J. H. Urinary incontinence not curable by sphincter plication. In TeLinde, Richard W. and Mattingly, R. F. *Operative Gynecology*, 4th ed. Philadelphia: J. B. Lippincott Co., 1970, pp. 548-571.

87. Reichers, R. N. *et al.* Peritoneal dialysis for patients in uremia secondary to obstructive disease. *Journal of Urology*, 107: 341-344, March, 1972.

88. Penn, I. *et al.* Parenthood in renal homograft recipients. *Journal of American Medical Association*, 216: 1755-1761, June 14, 1971.

89. Petkovic, S. D. A plea for conservative operation for ureteral tumors. *Journal of Urology*, 107: 220-223, February, 1972.

90. Phister, R. C. and Shea, T. E. Nephrotomography — performance and interpretation. *Radiologic Clinics of North America*, 9: 41-62, April, 1971.

91. Pillay, V. K. G. *et al.* Clinical aspects of obstructive uropathy. *Medical Clinics of North America*, 55: 1417-1427, November, 1971.

92. Pollak, V. E. and Mendoza, N. Rapidly progressive glomerulonephritis. *Medical Clinics of North America*, 55: 1397-1415, November, 1971.

93. Salomon, M. I. Kidney biopsy. *Medical Times*, 96: 939-942, September, 1968.

94. Salvatierra, O. *et al.* Modified retropubic prostatectomy. A new technique. *Journal of Urology*, 108: 126-130, July, 1972.

95. Samuels, L. D. Scans in children with renal tumors. *Journal of Urology*, 107: 127-132, January, 1972.

96. Schencker, B. Drip infusion pyelography. *Radiography*, 83: 12-21, July 1964.

97. Schmidt, J. D. *et al.* Vesicoureteral reflux — An inherited lesion. *Journal of American Medical Association*, 220: 821-824, May 8, 1972.

188

98. Schoonees, R. *et al.* The diagnostic value of urinary cytology in patients with bladder carcinoma. *Journal of Urology*, 106: 693-696, November, 1971.

99. Schreck, W. R. *et al.* Ultrasound as a diagnostic aid for renal neoplasms and cysts. *Journal of Urology*, 103: 281-285, March, 1970.

100. Schreiner, G. E. Cysts of the kidney. In Beeson, Paul B. and McDermott, Walsh (eds.). *Cecil-Loeb Textbook of Medicine*, 13th ed. Philadelphia: W. B. Saunders Co., 1971, pp. 1223-1227.

101. Smart, R. H. Polyorchism with normal spermatogenesis. *Journal of Urology*, 107: 278-279, February, 1972.

102. Smith, Donald R. Urinary stones. In *General Urology*, 7th ed. Los Altos, California: Lange Publications, 1972, pp. 207-227.

103. _____. Injuries to the genitourinary tract. *Ibid.*, pp. 228-247.

104. _____. Disorders of the kidneys. *Ibid.*, pp. 332-352.

105. _____. Renovascular hypertension. *Ibid.*, 408-415.

106. _____. Disorders of the ureters. *Ibid.*, pp. 353-363.

107. _____. The neurogenic bladder: abnormal vesical fuction, differential diagnosis of neurogenic bladders. *Ibid.*, pp. 303-323.

108. _____. Symptoms of disorders of the genitourinary tract. *Ibid.*, pp. 29-37.

109. _____. Urinary obstruction and stasis. vesicoureteral reflux. *Ibid.*, pp. 114-140.

110. _____. The neurogenic bladder. Cystometric study. *Ibid.*, pp. 303-323.

111. _____. Disorders of the testis, scrotum and spermatic cord. *Ibid.*, pp. 392-399.

112. _____. Roentgenographic examination of the urinary tract. *Ibid.*, pp. 61-84.

113. _____. Urologic laboratory examination. *Ibid.*, pp. 46-60.

114. _____. Renovascular hypertension. *Ibid.*, pp. 408-415.

115. Smith, D. R., Schulte, J. W. and Smart, W. R. Surgery of the kidney. In Campbell, Meredith F. and Harrison, J. Hartwell (eds.). *Urology*, 3rd ed. Philadelphia: W. B. Saunders Co., 1970, pp. 2143-2239.

116. Smith, D. R. Vesicoureteral reflux and other abnormalities of the ureterovesical junction. In Campbell, Meredith F. and Harrison, J. Hartwell (eds.). *Urology*, 3rd ed. Philadelphia: W. B. Saunders Co., 1970, pp. 349-398.

117. Smith, F. G. The nephrotic syndrome: Current concepts. *Annuals of Internal Médicine*, 76: 463-477, March, 1972.

118. Smith, H. T. The advantages of cryosurgery in prostate disease. *Geriatrics*, 26: 169-173, March, 1971.

119. Smith, L. H. The diagnosis and treatment of metabolic stone disease. *Medical Clinics of North America*, 56: 977-988, July, 1972.

120. Stewart, B. H. The surgery of renal transplantation. *Surgical Clinics of North America*, 51: 1123-1131, October, 1971.

121. Straffon, R. A. *et al.* Urinary lithiasis. In Campbell, Meredith F. and Harrison, J. Hartwell (eds.). *Urology* 3rd ed. Philadelphia: W. B. Saunders Co., 1970, pp. 687-765.

122. Straffon, R. A. Current status of renal transplantation. *Surgical Clinics of North America*, 51: 1105-1110, October, 1971.

123. Stuber, J. L. *et al.* Ultrasonic evaluation of the kidneys. *Radiology*, 104: 139-144, July, 1972.

124. Tse, R. L. and Liberman, P. R. Acute renal artery occlusion: Etiology, diagnosis and treatment. Report of case with subsequent revascularization. *Journal of Urology*, 108: 32-34, July, 1972.

125. Viner, N. A. *et al.* Prolonged renal failure following allotransplantation of cadaver kidney. *Southern Medical Journal*, 65: 429-432, April, 1972.

126. Waldbaum, R. S. Management of the congenital neurogenic bladder in children. *Journal of Urology*, 108: 165-166, July, 1972.

127. Weiss, E. R. *et al.* Diagnosis of renal transplant rejection in association with acute tubular necrosis using scintillation camera. *Journal of Urology*, 107: 917-921, June, 1972.

128. Wendel, E. F. *et al.* The effect of orchiectomy and estrogens on benign prostatic hyperplasia. *Journal of Urology*, 108: 116-119, July, 1972.

129. Whitmore, W. C. Ultraviolet cystoscopy for detection of bladder cancer. *Ca — A Cancer Journal for Clinicians*, 16: 128, May, June, 1966.

130. Wilson, D. M. Metabolic abnormalities in uremia. *Medical Clinics of North America*, 55: 1381-1396, November, 1971.

131. Wise, H. A. Treatment of urethral strictures. *Journal of Urology*, 107: 269-272, February, 1972.

132. Weong, O. M. Glomerular disease. In Beeson, Paul B. and McDermott, Walsh (eds.). *Cecil-Loeb Textbook of Medicine*, 13th ed. Philadelphia: W. B. Saunders Co., pp. 1177-1199.

133. Young, J. D. and Martin, L. G. Urinary calculi associated with incomplete renal tubular acidosis. *Journal of Urology*, 107: 170-173, February, 1972.

134. Young, J. A. *et al.* Carcinoma of prostate. Treatment and survival with radical prostatectomy. *Journal of Urology*, 107: 1041-1042, June, 1972.

135. Zukowski, C. F. What's new in surgery — transplantation. *Surgery, Gynecology & Obstetrics*, 134: 280-283, February, 1972.

Chapter X
Gynecological Disorders

VULVA AND VAGINA

A. Origin of Terms:

1. colpo- (G) — vagina
2. fistula (L) — pipe, tube
3. hymen (G) — membrane
4. krauros (G) — dry
5. labia (L) — lips
6. vagina (L) — sheath
7. vestibule (L) — antechamber
8. vulva (L) — covering

B. Anatomical Terms:

1. perineum — space between vulva and anus.
2. Skene's glands — urethral glands in female.
3. vagina — musculomembranous tube which connects the uterus with the vulva. It is the lower part of the birth canal.
4. vulva, pudendum[1] — external female genital organ. Some of the vulvar structures of gynecological importance are the following:
   a. clitoris — small body of erectile tissue which enlarges with vascular congestion.
   b. hymen — membranous fold which partially covers the vaginal opening in a virgin.
   c. labia majora (sing. labium majus) — two raised folds of adipose and erectile tissue covered on their outer surface with skin.[25]
   d. labia minora (sing. labium minus) — two small folds covered with moist skin lying between labia majora.
   e. vestibular glands (greater), Bartholin's glands — two small ovoid or round glands which secrete mucus. They lie deep under the posterior ends of the labia majora.
   f. vestibule of vagina — space between the labia minora which contains the vaginal and urethral orifices and openings of greater vestibular glands.

C. Diagnostic Terms:

1. atresia of:
   a. vagina — congenital absence of vagina.
   b. vulva — congenital absence of vulva.
2. Bartholin's adenitis — inflammation of Bartholin's glands, generally due to gonococcus.
3. Bartholin's retention cysts — tumors retaining glandular secretions. They tend to undergo suppuration and form abscesses.
4. carcinoma of vagina — usually
   a. clear-cell type — cancer characterized by glands and tubules lined by clear cells (hobnail cells) clustering in solid nests and containing glycogen. It occurs in adolescents and young women.[26, 27]
   b. epidermoid type — cancer arising from epidermal cells. It occurs in women over 50 years of age. Cells are devoid of glycogen.
   Other forms of vaginal cancer are rare.
5. carcinoma of vulva — usually a squamous cell cancer which begins with a small nodule, later undergoes ulceration and may become invasive. It is the third most common of cancers of the female organs.[2, 18, 28, 37, 20]
6. condylomas — warty growths scattered over vulva.
7. fistula:
   a. rectovaginal — opening between rectum and vagina.
   b. vesicovaginal — opening between bladder and vagina.

8. kraurosis of vulva — excessive shrinkage and atrophy of vulva, commonly seen during postmenopause.

9. leukoplakia of vulva — whitish plaques on vulva which tend to form cracks and fissures. Condition results in leukoplakic vulvitis.

10. vaginitis — inflammation of vagina.[43]
    a. gonorrheal — due to gonococcal infection.[47]
    b. mycotic, monilial — due to fungus infection.
    c. senile — due to atrophic changes; occurs in elderly women.
    d. Trichomonas — due to infection with Trichomonas vaginalis.

11. vulvar Paget's disease — a form of vulvar cancer in situ, recurrent, noninvasive, spreading slowly and presenting a discrete eruption which is initially velvety, soft and red and later eczemoid and weepy with white plaques scattered about in the well localized lesion. Pruritus and burning are distressing symptoms. The presence of Paget's cells in the lesion clinches the diagnosis.[17, 5]

12. vulvovaginitis — inflammation of the vulva and vagina.

D. Operative Terms:

1. colpectomy — removal of vagina.

2. colpocleisis — closure of vagina, one indication being prolapse of vagina following total hysterectomy.[25]

3. colpoperineoplasty — repair of rectocele.

4. colpoperineorrhaphy — suture of vagina and perineum.

5. colporrhaphy — suture of vagina.
    a. anterior — repair of cystocele.
    b. posterior — repair of rectocele.

6. colposcopy — examination of the vagina and cervix uteri usually with a binocular microscope that allows the study of tissues under direct vision by magnifying the cells, makes possible colpophotography and the colposcopic selection of target biopsy sites.[12, 31, 25]

7. colpotomy — incision into the vagina to induce drainage.

8. episioplasty — plastic repair of the vulva.

9. excision of Bartholin's gland — removal of the gland.

10. marsupialization of Bartholin's gland cyst — incision and drainage of the cyst and partial excision of the cyst wall followed by suture of the cyst lining to the surrounding surface epithelium. Lubrication is preserved since the gland is not removed.[25]

11. vulvectomy:
    a. partial removal of vulva.
    b. radical removal of vulva including regional lymph nodes.

E. Symptomatic Terms:

1. leukorrhea — abnormal cervical or vaginal discharge of white or yellowish mucus.

2. pruritus vulvae — severe itching of vulva.

UTERUS AND SUPPORTING STRUCTURES

A. Origin of Terms:

1. cervix (L) — neck
2. fundus (L) — base
3. hyster (G) — womb
4. isthmus (G) — narrow passage
5. ostium (L) — small opening
6. metra (G) — womb
7. trachelo- (G) — neck
8. uterus (L) — womb

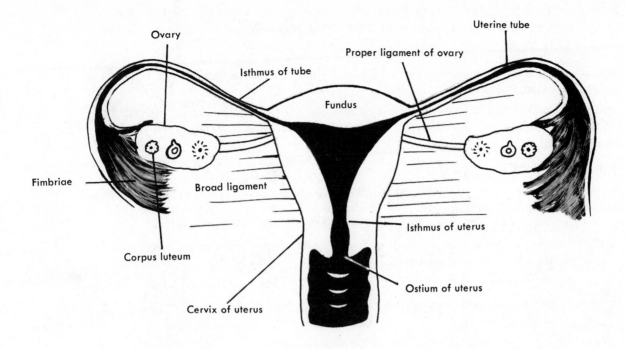

Fig. 51 — Uterus, uterine tubes and ovaries (schematic).

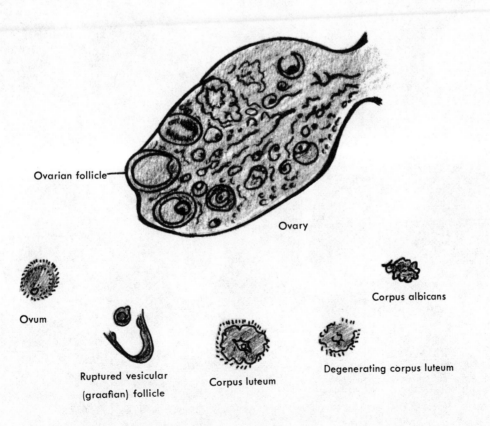

Fig. 52 — Normal ovulatory cycle.

B. Anatomical Terms:[22]

1. cul-de-sac, rectouterine pouch, Douglas' pouch — a pocket between the rectum and posterior uterus, formed by an extension of the peritoneum.

2. ligaments of uterus.

    a. broad ligaments — double-layered peritoneal sheets which extend from the side of the uterus to the lateral pelvic wall.

    b. round ligaments — two fibromuscular bands, one on each side arising anteriorly from the fundus, passing through the inguinal canal and inserting into the labia majora.[25]

3. myometrium — muscular wall of uterus.

4. uterus (nonpregnant) — a pear-shaped, thick-walled, muscular organ, situated in the pelvis between the urinary bladder and the rectum. It is about three inches (7½ cm) long and two inches (5 cm) wide in its upper segment. It is divided into a

    a. body of uterus — main part extending from fundus to isthmus of uterus.
        (1) body cavity, uterine cavity — triangular space within the body.
        (2) endometrium — mucous membrane lining the body cavity.

    b. cervix of uterus — lower part of uterus extending from isthmus to vagina.
        (1) cervical canal — passageway between uterine cavity and vagina.
        (2) ostium of uterus, external os — opening of cervix into vagina.

    c. fundus of uterus — superior dome-shaped portion of uterus above the openings of the uterine tubes into the body cavity of uterus.

    d. isthmus of uterus — constriction of uterus between body and cervix.[22]

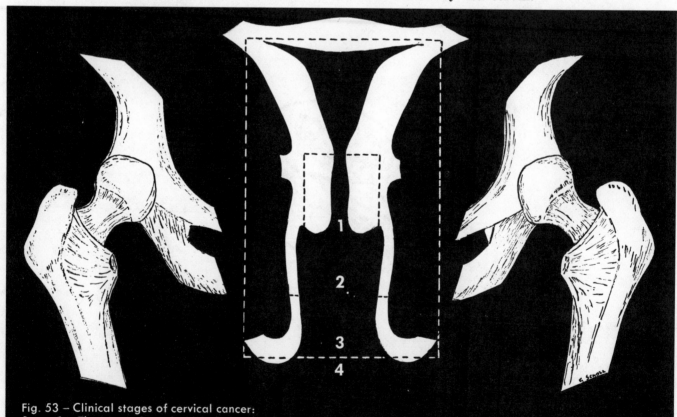

Fig. 53 – Clinical stages of cervical cancer:
Stage 1 – The cancer is exclusively limited to the uterine cervix.
Stage 2 – The cancer has spread beyond the cervix but has not reached the pelvic wall.
Stage 3 – The cancer involves the lower third of the vagina or extends to the pelvic wall.
Stage 4 – The cancer has spread to the mucous membrane of the rectum and bladder or has extended beyond the true pelvis.

(Adapted from R. W. TeLinde and R. F. Mattingly. OPERATIVE GYNECOLOGY, 4th ed. Lippincott, 1970)

C. Diagnostic Terms:

1. diseases of the cervix uteri:
    a. carcinoma of the cervix — malignant new growth.
        (1) adenocarcinoma — highly malignant cancer assuming a glandular pattern.
        (2) squamous cell or epidermoid carcinoma — most frequent form arising from squamous epithelium.[52, 10, 8]
    Terms adopted by the **International Federation of Gynecology and Obstetrics:**
        (1) invasive carcinoma — cancer of cervix including the 4 stages presented in Fig. 53.
        (2) microinvasive carcinoma — Stage IA preclinical cancer characterized by early stromal invasion. Diagnosis is based on microscopic examination from biopsy specimen.[54]
        (3) preinvasive carcinoma — Stage O intraepithelial carcinoma, carcinoma in situ.[53]
    b. cervicitis — inflammation of the cervix uteri.
        (1) acute — typically due to acute gonorrheal infection.
        (2) chronic — a common condition due to low grade infection.
    c. endocervicitis — inflammation of the mucous membrane of the cervix uteri.
    d. erosion of cervix — a red area produced by the replacement of squamous epithelium by columnar epithelium.[33]
    e. eversion of cervix, ectropion — a rolling outward of swollen mucous membrane resulting from chronic cervicitis. It may be associated with lacerations, cysts and erosions.
    f. polyps of cervix — soft, movable, pedunculated tabs that bleed readily.
2. diseases and malfunctions of the corpus uteri:
    a. dysfunctional uterine bleeding — functional bleeding not due to any local disease.[25] It may result from an irregular production of estrogen and/or progesterone by the ovary and may occur during puberty, the reproductive period of life or during menopause.[7, 1, 11, 21, 34]
    b. endometriosis — aberrant endometrial tissue found in various pelvic and abdominal organs.[30, 44, 45]
    c. endometritis — inflammation of the mucous membrane lining the corpus uteri.
    d. parametritis — cellulitis of the tissues adjacent to the uterus.
    e. perimetritis — pelvic peritonitis.
3. displacements of the uterus:
    a. anteflexion — uterus, abnormally bent forward.
    b. retroflexion — corpus uteri, abnormally bent backward.
    c. retroversion — corpus uteri, abnormally bent backward with cervix directed toward symphysis pubis.
    d. prolapse, procidentia, descensus uteri — downward displacement of the uterus which may protrude from the vagina.[56]
4. neoplasms of the uterus:
    a. benign new growths — primarily fibromas, fibromyomas and myomas.[16, 49]
    b. malignant tumors — adenocarcinomas and sarcomas. (See Part II, Chapter XVII).[36, 32, 64]

D. Operative Terms:

1. cold conization, cold knife cone biopsy of uterine cervix — cold knife removal of lining of cervical canal for locating the site of abnormal exfoliative cells in the absence of a visible lesion. The procedure is valuable in the detection of preinvasive lesions, cancer in situ and occult cancer.
2. culdocentesis — surgical puncture of the cul-de-sac used as a diagnostic procedure whenever intraperitoneal bleeding is suspected, as for example in ectopic pregnancy.
3. culdoscopy — endoscopic examination of the rectouterine pouch (cul-de-sac) and pelvic viscera to detect whether or not endometriosis, adnexal adhesions, tumors or ectopic pregnancy are present or to determine the cause of pelvic pain, sterility or other disorders.

4. dilatation and curettage — instrumental expansion of the cervix and scraping of the uterine cavity to remove
   a. endocervical tissue and endometrial tissue for diagnosis.
   b. placental tissue to control bleeding as in an incomplete abortion.
   c. small submucous fibroid, polyp or other lesion in the management of uterine bleeding.[34]

5. electrocautery of endocervix — removing the mucous lining of the cervical canal by a high frequency current to control chronic cervicitis.[25] The procedure is also used to repair an incompetent cervix so that successful pregnancy may be achieved.[63]

6. hysterectomy — removal of the uterus.
   a. partial or subtotal excision; for example, supracervical removal.
   b. total hysterectomy — excision of entire uterus and cervix.
   c. radical, Wertheim's operation — removal of entire uterus and dissection of regional lymph nodes.[57]
   d. vaginal hysterectomy — removal of the uterus by the vaginal approach.[66]

7. laparoscopy — endoscopic visualization of abdominal organs, especially the pelvic viscera: the uterus, tubes and ovaries. The procedure is of diagnostic value in primary and secondary amenorrhea, polycystic ovarian syndrome, unruptured ectopic pregnancy, pelvic inflammatory disease and other disorders.[50, 38]

8. myomectomy:
   a. abdominal approach — removal of intramural fibroid or fibroids from the uterus.
   b. vaginal approach — removal of cervical myoma from uterine cervix.[59]

9. panhysterectomy, total hysterectomy — removal of entire uterus including the cervix.

10. pelvic exenteration — radical removal of uterus, tubes, ovaries, vagina, bladder, rectum and pelvic lymphglands in recurrent cancer of the cervix when operability seems satisfactory. Urinary and fecal diversion may be achieved by ileal conduit and colostomy.[58, 13]

11. radium application — insertion of a radioactive substance into the cervix or uterus.

12. suspension of uterus — correction of retrodisplacement of the uterus:
    a. Baldy-Webster procedure — creation of a surgical opening for the passage of the round ligaments which are then sutured to the back of the uterus.[56]
    b. modified Gilliam procedure — surgical shortening of the round ligaments through the internal inguinal ring. This allows the stronger portion of the round ligament to bring the uterus forward.[56]

13. trachelectomy, cervicectomy — removal of uterine cervix.

14. tracheloplasty, Sturmdorf procedure — cone or core excision of endocervix; cervical canal covered with mucosal flap.

E. Symptomatic Terms:

1. amenorrhea — absence of menstruation.[23, 24]
2. dysmenorrhea — painful menstruation.[65]
3. menorrhagia — excessive bleeding during menstrual period.
4. metrorrhagia — bleeding from uterus not due to menses.
5. oligomenorrhea — scanty menstruation.[48]

OVARIES AND UTERINE TUBES

A. Origin of Terms:

1. albus (L) — white
2. ampulla (L) — little jar
3. dehiscere (L) — to gape
4. fimbria (L) — fringe
5. folliculus (L) — little bag
6. infundibulum (L) — funnel
7. luteum (L) — yellow
8. ovarium (L) — egg holder
9. ovum, ova (L) — egg, eggs
10. salpingo (G) — tube, trumpet

B. Anatomical Terms:

1. ova (sing. ovum) — female reproductive cells.
2. ovaries (sing. ovary) — two female reproductive glands producing ova after puberty.
   a. ovarian follicle — small excretory structure of the ovary. The primary ovarian follicle is immature consisting of a single layer of follicular cells. The vesicular ovarian or graafian follicle develops, ruptures and discharges the ovum. It also secretes the follicular hormone, estrogen.
   b. corpus luteum — small yellow body formed in ruptured ovarian follicle. It secretes the corpus luteum hormone, progesterone.
   c. corpus albicans — white body which develops from corpus luteum. It leaves a pitlike scar on ovary.
3. uterine tubes, fallopian tubes, oviducts — two muscular canals about four inches (10 cm) long which provide a passageway for the ovum to the uterus and a meeting place for the ovum and spermatozoon in fertilization. An ovum entering the tube through the abdominal opening of the fimbriated infundibulum passes through the
   a. ampulla — wider, thinner-walled longest part of the tube.
   b. isthmic portion — interstitial portion of the tube, narrower and thicker-walled than the ampulla.[25]
   c. uterine part — tube within the myometrium.
   d. uterine opening — entrance into the uterine cavity.[22]

C. Diagnostic Terms:

1. abscess, tuboovarian — localized suppuration of the uterine tube and ovary.
2. cyst of ovary — a fluid containing tumor of the ovary.
   a. graafian follicle cyst.
   b. corpus luteum cyst.
   c. corpus albicans cyst.
3. cystadenoma of ovary — cyst and glandular tumor combined.
4. dehiscence of wound, burst abdomen, evisceration, wound disruption — a bursting open of a sutured wound, followed by protrusion of intestines through the incision, a serious surgical complication; also dehiscence of a graafian follicle.
5. hydrosalpinx — uterine tube distended by clear fluid.
6. infertility, female — temporary or permanent inability to conceive or become pregnant depending on multiple etiologic factors such as
   a. anovulation
   b. defects of the luteal phase
   c. the condition of the cervix
   d. the status of the uterine tubes
   e. immunologic responses and
   f. male factors.[60, 35]
7. oophoritis, acute and chronic — inflammation of the ovary or ovaries.
8. pelvic inflammatory disease — broad terms including pelvic inflammations due to gonococcal, streptococcal postabortal infections as well as intestinal parasites in juveniles. multiple infectious organisms may coexist.[15, 62]
9. polycytic ovarian syndrome, Stein-Leventhal syndrome — a symptom complex characterized by bilateral enlarged ovaries containing multiple follicular microcysts. Amenorrhea, infertility, obesity, hypertension and hirsutism (hairiness) are common symptoms.[61, 9]
10. pyosalpinx — pus in the uterine tube.
11. ruptured tubo-ovarian abscess — a breaking open of the abscess and escape of purulent drainage into peritoneal cavity.
12. salpingitis, acute and chronic — inflammation of the uterine tube or tubes.

13. torsion of ovarian pedicle — twisting of the pedicle of an ovarian cyst resulting in circulatory disturbance and sharp persistent pain.
14. tumors of the ovary:
    The **International Federation of Gynecology and Obstetrics** classifies ovarian tumors as follows (condensed classification):
    a. benign tumors:
        (1) cystic, non-neoplastic — follicular, luteal, others.
        (2) cystic, neoplastic — epithelial, dermoid, others.
        (3) solid — fibroma, Brenner tumor, others.
    b. malignant tumors:
        (1) cystic — cystadenocarcinoma, carcinoma.
        (2) solid — carcinoma, endometrioid, mesonephroma.
        (3) other malignant tumors — teratoma, etc.
        (4) tumors with endocrine potential — feminizing or virilizing tumors.
        (5) metastatic or by direct extension.[40, 4, 19]
15. tumors of the uterine tubes:
    a. benign tumors — adenomyoma, others.
    b. malignant tumors — carcinoma, sarcoma.
    c. metastatic tumors.[41, 61]

D. Operative Terms:

1. Estes operation — implantation of ovary within the endometrial cavity for the correction of infertility.[60]
2. oophorectomy.
    a. partial removal of an ovary.
    b. complete removal of one ovary.
    c. castration, bilateral, complete removal of ovaries.
3. oophoropexy — fixation of a displaced ovary.
4. oophoroplasty — plastic repair of an ovary.
5. panhysterectomy and bilateral salpingo-oophorectomy — removal of complete uterus, both tubes and ovaries.
6. salpingectomy — partial or complete removal of the uterine tubes.
7. salpingolysis — the breaking up of peritubal adhesions which damage the fimbriated end of the tube. This procedure is considered an effective means of correcting infertility.[60]
8. salpingo-oophorectomy — removal of tubes and ovaries.
9. tubal implantation — correction of the cornual block and implantation of the unobstructed tubes into the uterine cavity, to restore tubal patency following sterilization surgery.[14]
10. tubal insufflation, uterotubal insufflation, Rubin's test — procedure used for diagnostic and therapeutic purposes:
    a. to detect whether the tubes are blocked or patent.
    b. to relieve tubal obstruction by dislodging mucous plugs and breaking up adhesions at the fimbriated ends of the tubes. Successful pregnancy may follow.
11. tubal ligation — tying the tubes to prevent pregnancy; sterilization surgery.
12. tuboplasty, salpingoplasty — reconstructive tubal surgery for the correction of infertility. The constricted or occluded end of the uterine tube is excised and the distal portion of the tube is reimplanted into the uterus. Recently the use of cone-shaped, spiral stents has been advocated as an effective method of maintaining tubal patency.[60, 46, 14]

E. Symptomatic Terms:

1. anovulation — absence of ovulation due to cessation or suspension.
2. menopause — cessation of menses and reproductive period of life.
3. ovulation — expulsion of an ovum from the ruptured graafian follicle.
4. septic shock — sudden hypotension, renal dysfunction, peripheral blood pooling and metabolic acidosis caused by gram-negative bacteremia due to septic abortion, puerperal sepsis or pelvic infection.[62]

RADIOLOGY

A. Terms Related to Radiotherapy:

1. radiotherapy — used in the management of radiosensitive tumors either alone or in conjunction with surgery. This treatment tends to reduce the operative risk by sterilizing the malignant lesion and devitalizing cancer cells. The fibrotic reaction, produced by irradiation, results in the imprisonment of cancer cells. Carcinomas of the endometrium and corpus uteri generally respond well to radiotherapy.[1]
2. irradiation — used postoperatively as a palliative or therapeutic measure in selected cases of carcinoma.

B. Terms Related to Radiation Injury:

1. overirradiation — excessive radiation therapy. It may cause a syndrome characterized by nausea, vomiting, diarrhea, anorexia and malaise within hours after overexposure followed by blood dyscrasia, within weeks or months.
2. radiation anemia — usually aplastic anemia; no red blood cells are formed due to suppression of bone marrow activity.
3. radiodermatitis — inflammation of skin resulting from exposure to radiation.
4. radioepithelitis — disintegration of epthelial tissue due to radiation, notably to that of the mucous membrane.
5. radionecrosis — disintegration or death of tissue caused by radiation.
6. radionephritis — acute condition due to overexposure of kidney to radiation. It is manifested by hypertension, edema, casts and protein in urine.
7. radioneuritis — nerve involvement resulting from overexposure to radioactivity.
8. radiation sickness — untoward effects of radiotherapy, usually manifested by nausea, vomiting and diarrhea, resulting from the breakdown of body tissue.

CLINICAL LABORATORY

A. Cytologic Studies for Gynecological Conditions:

1. Papanicolaou's smear test for cytologic diagnosis of cervical and endometrial cancer. The smear technic is based on the fact that vaginal and uterine epithelia, like all epithelial tissue, undergo continual exfoliation or shedding of cells. Similarly, tumors which reach the lining surface may exfoliate cells which fall into the vagina and become mixed with the vaginal secretion. Experts in exfoliative cytology recognize incompletely developed malignant cells which gradually and progressively change from a benign, preinvasive, preclinical stage to an early invasive and late malignant stage.
2. Cytologic studies are of particular value in the detection of tumors of the cervix and endometrium in the preinvasive state when proper treatment can be instituted. Several methods have been devised to obtain smears for cytologic diagnosis.
   a. Papanicolaou's method — a curved glass pipette with rubber bulb is used to aspirate vaginal fluid with its cellular components.
   b. Ayre's surface cell biopsy method — the smear is obtained from cervical scrapings by means of a wooden spatula.[1]
   c. Gravlee jet washer — a vacuum suction technique of intrauterine washing for collecting cytology specimens from the endometrium for an early detection of cancer.[56]

B. Cytologic Studies for Other Conditions:

Exfoliative cytology has been applied with success to various body fluids such as sputa, gastric secretions and urine, pleural, peritoneal and bronchial aspirates. Its practical significance has been confirmed in lung cancer.[1]

C. Other Tests:

1. Schiller test — test helpful in the detection of superficial cancer particularly that of the cervix. Normal epithelium is rich in glycogen and stained deeply by iodine solution. Cancerous epithelium has almost no glycogen and takes no stain. The test has its limitations.[42]
2. serum protein-bound fucose level — diagnostic aid in detecting the presence and extent of cervical and ovarian cancer in its advanced and recurrent stage.

    Normal fucose level................... less than 14.0 mg%
    F/P ratio .... less than 2.2 mg x 10⁻³

    Increase in squamous cell carcinoma of cervix
    No increase in benign gynecologic disorders.[3]

ABBREVIATIONS

A. General Terms:

CIS — carcinoma in situ
D&C — dilatation and curettage
FSH — follicle stimulating hormone
GC — gonorrhea
Gyn — gynecology
IUD — intrauterine device
HPO — hypothalamic-pituitary-
    ovarian

LH — luteinizing hormone
LTH — luteotrophic hormone
LMP — last menstrual period
MH — marital history
Path — pathology
PID — pelvic inflammatory disease
PMP — previous menstrual period
WF — white female

B. Organizations:

ACOG — American College of
    Obstetricians and
    Gynecologists
ACS — American College of
    Surgeons

FIGO — International Federation of
    Gynecology and Obstetrics

ORAL READING PRACTICE

Ovarian Neoplasms

Ovarian neoplasms may occur at any age; however, the majority develop during the reproductive period. Of these the proportion of **benign** to **malignant** neoplasms is about three to four.

The new growths tend to be larger than 6 cm in diameter. The ovaries and related **embryonic** rests are frequent sources of cyst formation. Smaller or plum-sized **cysts** occasionally are **non-neoplastic** growths. **Follicular** cysts are derived from the **graafian follicles** and vary in size from 2 to 20 mm, though sometimes are larger. They are usually **bilateral** and **multiple** and lined with flattened epithelium which is lost in some areas. Characteristically, their contents appear watery to serous, straw-colored or blood-tinged.

Simple cystadenomata of the ovary are prone to reach an enormous size, containing several gallons of fluid. They are usually globular, **lobulated** and **multilocular** with a smooth surface and a pedicle attachment through which nutrient blood vessels pass.

The lining epithelium of cystadenomas may proliferate markedly forming an irregular widespread ingrowth which contains **papillary projections** extending into the cyst cavity. The neoplasm thus formed is usually quite **vascular** and the epithelial covering of its tree-like branches is **hyperplastic** and often **anaplastic.** It may exhibit a marked tendency to **invade** adjacent structures and reach the **peritoneal** surface from which point widespread peritoneal invasion and metastasis take place. The outcome is a gelatinous **carcinomatosis** of the **peritoneum.** The same fatal complication may develop if rupture of a **papillary cystadenoma** results in freeing neoplastic cells and bits of tissue in the peritoneal cavity.

Ovarian cysts may be entirely asymptomatic. When manifestations do result, they fall into the following categories: (1) those involving functional disturbances, such as **menorrhagia** and **meteorrhagia,** (2) those resulting from mechanical factors incident to the size of the cyst, (3) those characterized by obvious enlargement of the abdomen often without associated manifestations and, finally, (4) those resulting from **torsion** of the **pedicle** of the cyst.[40, 4, 19]

Table 17

SOME GYNECOLOGICAL CONDITIONS AMENABLE TO SURGERY

Organs Involved	Diagnoses	Operations	Operative Procedures
Hymen	Atresia of hymen	Hymenotomy Hymenectomy	Incision of hymen Excision of hymen
Clitoris	Congenital hypertrophy of clitoris due to adrenal cortical hyperplasia	Reconstruction of external genitals Clitorectomy	External genitals reconstructed along normal female lines and clitoris removed
Bartholin's gland	Abscess of Bartholin's gland	Incision and drainage of Bartholin's gland	Surgical opening and evacuation of abscess
Bartholin's gland	Chronic bartholinitis and cysts of Bartholin's gland	Marsupialization of Bartholin's gland cyst	Partial excision of cyst wall Suture of cyst lining to the surrounding surface epithelium
Vulva	Leukoplakia of vulvae	Vulvectomy	Removal of vulvae
Vulva	Vulvar carcinoma, epidermoid type	Basset operation: Vulvectomy Lymphadenectomy	Excision of vulva, superficial inguinal lymph nodes and wide dissection of deep femoral and inguinal glands
Vulva Perineum	Burn of vulva and perineum	Episioperineoplasty	Plastic repair of vulva and perineum
Vagina Bladder	Vesicovaginal fistula	Closure of vesicovaginal fistula	Suture of fistula
Vagina Bladder	Urinary stress incontinence	Suprapubic vesicourethral suspension Marshall-Marchetti operation	Surgical elevation and fixation of the bladder neck and urethra by suturing them to the pubis and rectus muscles
Vagina Bladder	Urinary stress incontinence associated with cystocele	Kelly operation modified technique	Construction of a firm shelf of periurethral tissue to support bladder and urethra
Vagina Bladder	Cystocele	Colpoplasty	Plastic repair of vagina; repair of cystocele

Organs Involved	Diagnoses	Operations	Operative Procedures
Vagina Perineum	Rectocele	Colpoperineoplasty	Plastic repair of vagina and perineum; repair of rectocele
Cervix uteri	Chronic endocervicitis	Conization	Removal of mucous lining of cervical canal by high frequency current
		Sturmdorf procedure Plastic repair of cervix uteri	Conized area covered with mucosal flap
Cervix uteri	Eversion of cervix (ectropion)	Striping by cautery	Hot cautery
		Cryosurgery	Freezing technique
Cervix uteri	Squamous cell carcinoma of cervix uteri, early phase, radioresistant lesion	Radical hysterectomy Pelvic lymphadenectomy	Excision of entire uterus Removal of pelvic lymph glands
Corpus uteri	Submucous myoma	Myomectomy	Complete enucleation of myoma
Corpus uteri Tubes Ovaries	Adenocarcinoma of corpus uteri Metastasis to adnexa uteri	Panhysterectomy Salpingectomy Oophorectomy	Removal of corpus and cervix uteri, tubes and ovaries
Uterus	Prolapse of uterus	Manchester-Fothergill operation	Amputation of cervix and fixation of ligament to anterior uterus
Uterus	Severe retroversion of uterus Slight descensus uteri	Suspension of uterus Modified Gilliam procedure	Surgical shortening of the round ligaments through the internal inguinal ring
Uterine tube	Tuboövarian abscess	Incision and drainage of abscess	Surgical opening and evacuation of abscess
Ovary	Torsion of ovarian pedicle	Oophorectomy	Excision of ovary
Ovary	Cystadenocarcinoma, serous type	Panhysterectomy Bilateral salpingo-oophorectomy	Removal of entire uterus, both tubes and ovaries, including regional lymph nodes

REFERENCES AND BIBLIOGRAPHY

1. Ackerman, Lauren V. and del Regato, Juan A. *Cancer Diagnosis Treatment and Prognosis*, 4th ed. St. Louis: The C. V. Mosby Co., 1970, pp. 755-803.
2. Averette, H. E. Carcinoma of the vulva. In Conn, Howard F. (ed.). *Current Therapy 1972*. Philadelphia: W. B. Saunders Co., 1972, pp. 782-783.
3. Barlow, J. J. *et al.* Serum protein-bound fucose in patients with gynecologic cancers. *Obstetrics and Gynecology*, 39: 727-734, May, 1972.
4. Benson, R. C. Ovarian tumors in childhood and adolescence. *Postgraduate Medicine*, 50: 230-235, November, 1971.
5. Boehm, F. and Morris, J. Paget's disease and apocrine gland carcinoma of the vulva. *Obstetrics and Gynecology*, 38: 185-192, August, 1971.
6. Boutselis, J. G. Radical vulvectomy for invasive squamous cell carcinoma of the vulva. *Obstetrics and Gynecology*, 39: 827-835, June, 1972.
7. Buttram, V. C. Dysfunctional uterine bleeding. In Conn, Howard F. (ed.). *Current Therapy 1972*. Philadelphia: W. B. Saunders Co., 1972, pp. 763-766.
8. Christopherson, W. M. The changing patterns of cervix cancer. *Ca-A Cancer Journal for Clinicians*, 21: 283-287, September-October, 1971.
9. Cooke, C. *et al.* Polycystic ovarian syndrome with

unilateral cystic teratoma. *Obstetrics and Gynecology*, 39: 789-794, May, 1972.

10. Creasm, W. T. Carcinoma in situ of the cervix. An analysis of 861 patients. *Obstetrics and Gynecology*, 39: 373-380, March, 1972.

11. Cyernobilsky, B. Utero-ovarian pathology in dysfunctional uterine bleeding. *Clinical Obstetrics and Gynecology*, 13: 416-433, June, 1971.

12. Davis, H. J. Colposcopy. In TeLinde, Richard W. and Mattingly, Richard F. *Operative Gynecology*, 4th ed. Philadelphia: J. B. Lippincott Co., 1970, pp. 722-723.

13. Deckers, P. J. *et al.* Pelvic exenteration for primary carcinoma of the uterine cervix. *Obstetrics and Gynecology*, 37: 647-659, May, 1971.

14. deMaria, F. J. Recent advances in surgery of the fallopian tubes. *Postgraduate Medicine*, 50: 114-149, December, 1971.

15. Dennis, E. J. Pelvic inflammatory disease. In Conn, Howard F. (ed.). *Current Therapy 1972*. Philadelphia: W. B. Saunders Co., 1972, pp. 775-777.

16. Dunn, L. J. Uterine myomas. In Conn, Howard F. (ed.). *Current Therapy 1972*. Philadelphia: W. B. Saunders Co., 1972, pp. 777-778.

17. Fetherston, W. C. *et al.* The origin and significance of vulvar Paget's disease. *Obstetrics and Gynecology*, 39: 735-744, May, 1972.

18. Franklin, E. W. Epidemiology of epidermoid carcinoma of the vulva. *Obstetrics and Gynecology*, 39: 165-172, February, 1972.

19. Freedman, S. I. Adenofibrocarcinoma of the ovary. *Obstetrics and Gynecology*, 39: 795-801, May, 1972.

20. Friedrich, E. G. Vulvar carcinoma in situ in identical twins. An occupational hazard. *Obstetrics and Gynecology*, 39: 837-841, June, 1972.

21. Garcia, C. R. Endocrine approach in the management of dysfunctional uterine bleeding. *Clinical Obstetrics and Gynecology*, 13: 460-473, June, 1971.

22. Gardner, Ernest, Gray, Donald and O'Rahilly, Ronan. *Anatomy — A Regional Study of Human Structure*, 3rd ed. Philadelphia: W. B. Saunders Co., 1969. pp. 490-502.

23. Gold, J. J. Amenorrhea. In Conn, Howard F. (ed.). *Current Therapy 1972*. Philadelphia: W. B. Saunders Co., 1972, pp. 766-769.

24. Golditch, I. M. Postcontraceptive amenorrhea. *Obstetrics and Gynecology*, 39: 903-908, June, 1972.

25. Hamilton, Eugene G., M.D. Personal communications.

26. Herbst, A. L. and Scully, R. E. Adenocarcinoma of the vagina in adolescence. A report of 7 cases including 6 clear-cell carcinomas. *Cancer*, 25: 745-757, April, 1970.

27. Herbst, A. L. *et al.* Adenocarcinoma of the vagina. Association of maternal stilbestrol therapy with tumor appearance in young women. *New England Journal of Medicine*, 284: 878-881, April 22, 1971.

28. Hughes, R. R. Early diagnosis and management of premalignant lesions and early invasive cancer of the vulva. *Southern Medical Journal*, 64: 1490-1492, December, 1971.

29. Kanbour, A. *et al.* The Gravlee jet washer: Evaluation of the reflux into the fallopian tubes. *Acta Cytologica*, 16: 199-202, May-June, 1972.

30. Krieger, J. S. Endometriosis. In Conn, Howard F. (ed.). *Current Therapy 1972*. Philadelphia: W. B. Saunders Co., 1972, pp. 762-763.

31. Krumholz, B. A. *et al.* Colposcopic selection of biopsy sites. *Obstetrics and Gynecology*, 39: 22-26, January, 1972.

32. Lash, A. F. *et al.* Cancer of the uterus. In Conn, Howard F. (ed.). *Current Therapy 1972*. Philadelphia: W. B. Saunders Co., 1972, pp. 778-782.

33. Mier, Thomas M., M.D. Personal communications.

34. Mikuta, J. J. Surgical management of dysfunctional bleeding. *Clinical Obstetrics and Gynecology*, 13: 451-459, June, 1971.

35. Moghissi, K. S. The function of the cervix in fertility. *Fertility and Sterility*, 23: 295-306, April, 1972.

36. Moltz, A. *et al.* Adenocarcinoma of the endometrium. *Obstetrics and Gynecology*, 39: 199-201, February, 1972.

37. Morrow, C. P. *et al.* Melanoma of the vulva. *Obstetrics and Gynecology*, 39: 745-752, May, 1972.

38. Neuwirth, R. S. A method of bilateral ovarian biopsy at laparoscopy in infertility and chronic anovulation. *Fertility and Sterility*, 23: 361-366, May, 1972.

39. Novak, Edmund R. and Woodruff, J. Donald. Benign lesions of the cervix. In *Novak's Gynecologic and Obstetric Pathology with Clinical and Endocrine Relations*, 6th ed. Philadelphia: W. B. Saunders Co., 1967, pp. 62-77.

40. ——————. Classification of ovarian tumors. *Ibid.*, pp. 309-389.

41. ——————. Tumors of the tube, parovarium and uterine ligaments. *Ibid.*, pp. 272-285.

42. ——————. Carcinoma of the cervix. *Ibid.*, pp. 78-114.

43. Palladino, A. Vaginitis. In Conn, Howard F. (ed.). *Current Therapy 1972*. Philadelphia: W. B. Saunders Co., 1972, pp. 772-775.

44. Ramney, B. Endometriosis II. Emergency operations due to hemoperitoneum. *Obstetrics and Gynecology*, 36: 437-442, September, 1970.

45. ——————. Endometriosis IV. Hereditary tendency. *Obstetrics and Gynecology*, 37: 734-737, May, 1971.

46. Roland, M. *et al.* Tuboplasty in 130 patients. Improved results due to stents and preoperative endoscopy. *Obstetrics and Gynecology*, 39: 57-64, January, 1972.

47. Schroeter, A. L. and Lucas, J. B. Gonorrhea — diagnosis and treatment. *Obstetrics and Gynecology*, 39: 274-285, February, 1972.

48. Smith, R. A. Investigation and classification of oligomenorrhea and amenorrhea. *Medical Clinics of North America*, 56: 931-940, July, 1972.

49. Stearns, C. H. Uterine myomas: Clinical and pathologic aspects. *Postgraduate Medicine*, 51: 165-168, April, 1972.

50. Stenger, V. G. What's new in surgery: gynecology and obstetrics. *Surgery Gynecology & Obstetrics*, 134: 267-268, February, 1972.

51. TeLinde, Richard W. and Mattingly, Richard F. Complete perineal lacerations and rectovaginal fistulas. In *Operative Gynecology*, 4th ed. Philadelphia: J. B. Lippincott Co., 1970, pp. 641-661.

52. —————. Carcinoma in situ of the cervix. *Ibid.*, pp. 708-731.

53. —————. Invasive carcinoma of the cervix. *Ibid.*, pp. 733-770.

54. —————. Microinvasive carcinoma. *Ibid.*, pp. 724-731.

55. —————. Nonmalignant cervical lesions and their treatment. *Ibid.*, pp. 387-424.

56. —————. Malpositions of the uterus, cervical stump and vagina. *Ibid.*, pp. 469-533.

57. —————. Radical Wertheim hysterectomy. *Ibid.*, pp. 750-752.

58. —————. Pelvic exenteration. *Ibid.*, pp. 771-788.

59. —————. Myomata uteri. *Ibid.*, pp. 143-191.

60. —————. Infertility. *Ibid.*, pp. 293-310.

61. —————. Adnexal tumors. Bilateral polycystic ovaries: Stein-Leventhal syndrome. *Ibid.*, pp. 817-856.

62. —————. Pelvic inflammatory disease and its complications. *Ibid.*, pp. 230-269.

63. Vogel, E. H. Electrocautery in the treatment of incompetent cervix. *Obstetrics and Gynecology*, 39: 27-36, January, 1972.

64. Wakonig-Vaartaja, T. Cytogenetics of gynecologic neoplasms. *Clinical Obstetrics and Gynecology*, 13: 813-830, December, 1970.

65. Weingold, A. B. Dysmenorrhea. In Conn, Howard F. (ed.). *Current Therapy 1972*. Philadelphia: W. B. Saunders Co., 1972, pp. 769-770.

66. White, S. C. *et al.* Comparison of abdominal and vaginal hysterectomies. A review of 600 operations. *Obstetrics and Gynecology*, 37: 530-536, April, 1971.

Chapter XI
Maternal, Antenatal and Neonatal Conditions
PREGNANCY, DELIVERY, PUERPERIUM

A. Origin of Terms:

1. gravida (L) — pregnancy
2. multi (L) — many
3. nulli (L) — none
4. pario (L) — to bear
5. pelvis (L) — basin
6. placenta (L) — cake
7. primi (L) — first
8. puer (L) — boy, child

B. General Terms:

1. basal body temperature — body temperature taken under basal conditions before arising in the morning. Relatively lower levels are present in the preovulatory phase than in the postovulatory phase.
2. biphasic curve — curve referring to the two basic general temperature levels in the menstrual cycle:
   a. the lower temperature level, known as the estrogenic phase, extends from the onset of menstruation to a short period after ovulation. The woman's basal temperature is usually **below 97.9°F (36.6°C)** orally. The early part of this estrogenic phase is non-fertile. The time and extent of this period of infertility can be approximated (see rhythm).
   b. the higher temperature level follows ovulation. The woman's basal temperature is usually **above 97.9°F (36.6°C)**. Since the life of an ovum is limited, the period which follows the first 3 days of the rise is nonfertile.[31, 111]
3. gravida — a pregnant woman.
4. high risk gravida — there are multiple reasons for considering a pregnant woman a high risk patient. She may be too young or too old, underweight or overweight, have diabetes, hypertension, urinary infection, rubella, hepatitis, Rh incompatibility, alcoholic or narcotic addiction and many other health hazards. By identifying the problem during early gestation appropriate treatment may be instituted to protect the mother and growing fetus.
5. multipara — a woman who has given birth to two or more children.
6. natural childbirth — childbirth in a normal physiological manner without anesthetic or instruments. The woman participates actively and consciously in her delivery.
   a. Read's method, childbirth **without fear** — antenatal program for the mother-to-be including education, psychological conditioning, exercises and **relaxation** techniques preparatory to the 3 stages of labor. The relaxation is active and may induce sleep and amnesia. A minimum of pain is experienced during delivery.
   b. psychoprophylactic method as practiced by Lamaze, childbirth **without pain** — verbal analgesia based on antenatal training of the expectant mother. Words are used as therapeutic agents to create in the woman's mind a chain of conditioned reflexes applicable to childbirth (Pavlov's second system). The mother-to-be learns to give birth: to breathe, push and relax effectively and to bring forth the child in a mentally alert state. The couple's united efforts make childbirth without pain a victory for both, since the husband plays an active part in the entire program.[110]
7. parturient — woman in labor.
8. primipara — a woman who has given birth to her first child.
9. puerpera — a woman who has just delivered a child.
10. rhythm — in obstetrics the alternating periods of sterility and fertility in the menstrual cycle. Since fertilization depends on the availability of the ovum, pregnancy can be avoided by practicing continence a few days before and after ovulation. Rhythm is a means of determining the approximate time of ovulation. It is based on the length of a series of a woman's menstrual cycles.[80, 51, 111, 31, 32]

C. Anatomical Terms:

1. pelvis (pl. pelves) — bony ring adapted to childbearing in female. It is composed of sacrum, coccyx and hip bones.
    a. false pelvis — bounded posteriorly by lumbar vertebrae; serves to support pregnant uterus.
    b. true pelvis — bounded posteriorly by sacrum, of practical significance in child bearing.
    c. pelvic brim, pelvic inlet — upper opening into true pelvic cavity.
    d. pelvic outlet — the lower opening of the pelvis.
    e. promontory of the sacrum — the upper projecting part of the sacrum.
2. placenta — vascular structure which provides nutrition for the fetus.
3. secundines, afterbirth — fetal membranes and placenta; their expulsion occurs in third stage of labor.

D. Diagnostic Terms:

1. abortion — expulsion of the product of conception before the fetus has attained viability.[33, 104]
    a. habitual abortion — 3 or more consecutive, spontaneous abortions.[33]
    b. imminent, threatened abortion — vaginal bleeding with or without pain, and cervical dilatation, usually terminating in expulsion of fetus.
    c. incomplete abortion — fetal expulsion with retention of total or partial placenta and subsequent bleeding.
    d. induced abortion — voluntary expulsion of fetus, brought about by mechanical means or drugs.
    e. inevitable abortion — rupture of membranes associated with cervical dilatation and followed by fetal expulsion.
    f. missed abortion — fetus dead, but retained in utero for days or weeks.[33, 104]
    g. septic abortion — abortion with fever without any other known cause for temperature elevation, usually referred to as septic. Patients who have had interference, even if afebrile, may have a septic abortion. A foul smelling vaginal discharge is a dominant feature.[104, 29]
2. choriocarcinoma — highly malignant, invasive tumor derived from trophoblasts. Neoplastic cells infiltrate the myometrium and readily metastasize to the liver, lungs, brain and pelvic organs. Choriocarcinoma may be a complication of a hydatidiform mole.[35]
3. ectopic pregnancy — fertilized ovum implanted outside of uterine cavity: in tube, ovary or free in abdomen attached to a viscus.[34, 81, 113]
4. hydatidiform mole — developmental abnormality of the placenta characterized by the conversion of chorionic villi into a mass of vesicles that resemble hanging grapes. Abortion or surgical removal of the mole is imperative.[35]
5. hyperemesis gravidarum — severe nausea and vomiting during the first months of pregnancy which may cause dehydration and serious metabolic disturbances in mother and fetus.
6. hypertensive disorders of pregnancy — high blood pressure of 140/90 and above preceding pregnancy or developing during gestation or in early puerperium. Proteinuria, edema, convulsions and coma may be present.[73, 36, 54]
    a. eclampsia — major disorder of pregnancy and puerperium manifested by high blood pressure, convulsions, renal dysfunction, headache, edema and severe cases of coma.
    b. preeclampsia — usually a disorder of a first pregnancy but may also occur in multiparas who are severely hypertensive or diabetic. Characteristically there is an upward trend in high blood pressure, sudden and excessive weight gain related to fluid retention and kidney dysfunction, proteinuria or albuminuria.[35, 36, 73]
7. involution of uterus — postpartum return of uterus to its former shape and size.
8. oligohydramnios — deficient amount of amniotic fluid.

9. phlegmasia alba dolens — phlebitis of femoral vein; may occur postpartum.
10. placenta ablatio, placenta abruptio — premature detachment of the placenta generally causing severe hemorrhage.
11. placenta previa — a displaced placenta, implanted in lower segment of uterine wall.
   a. marginal insertion — placenta comes up to the ostium uteri, but does not cover it.
   b. partial placenta previa — placenta covers the ostium uteri incompletely.
   c. complete or central placenta — placenta entirely obstructs the ostium uteri.

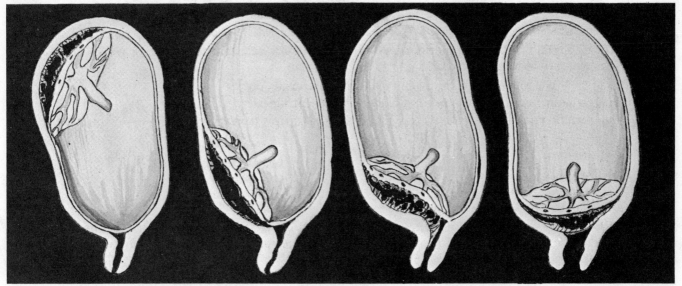

Fig. 54 – Normal placenta. Fig. 55 – Marginal placenta previa. Fig. 56 – Partial placenta previa. Fig. 57 – Complete placenta previa.

(Adapted from J. W. Huffman, Gynecology and Obstetrics, Saunders, 1962 with permission of publisher).

12. polyhydramnios, hydramnios — excessive amount of amniotic fluid.
13. puerperal hematoma — escape of blood into the mucosa or subcutaneous tissues of the external genitalia forming painful vaginal or vulvar hematomas (blood tumors).[39] They may also form in broad ligaments.[29]
14. puerperal infection, puerperal fever, childbed fever, puerperal septicemia, puerperal sepsis — infection of the genital tract occurring within the postpartum period. Fever is the dominant characteristic of puerperal infection; however, the puerpera may have fever from other causes, e.g. kidney or lung infections.[39]
15. rupture of uterus, hysterorrhexis, metrorrhexis — laceration of uterus, a torn uterus. Hellman gives the following classification:
   a. rupture of previous uterine scar
   b. spontaneous rupture of intact uterus
   c. traumatic rupture of the intact uterus.[40]
16. subinvolution — failure of the uterus to reduce to its normal size after delivery.
17. uteroplacental apoplexy, Couvelaire uterus — sudden, severe retroplacental bleeding into the myometrium.
18. various conditions associated with pregnancy or puerperium — disorders or states affecting the nonpregnant women may also affect the gravida and puerpera.[37, 109, 57, 39, 8, 97, 94, 64, 77, 98, 30]

E. Operative Terms:

1. Cesarean section — removal of the fetus through an incision into the uterus.[7, 87]
   a. classical — incision into corpus uteri.[112]
   b. lower uterine segment — incision into the lower segment of the uterus.[16]
   c. Cesarean hysterectomy — delivery of the child by section, followed by supravaginal or supracervical hysterectomy.
   d. vaginal hysterectomy, colpohysterectomy — removal of the uterus through the vagina.

2. breech extraction — method of delivery when the presenting parts are the buttocks or feet. The fetus is pulled out.
3. episiotomy — incision of perineum to facilitate delivery and prevent perineal laceration.
    a. median episiotomy — midline incision of perineum.
    b. mediolateral episiotomy — the incision is directed toward one side of the midline.[41, 29]
4. forceps operations — instrumental delivery of child.
    a. low forceps — application of forceps when head is on perineum.
    b. high forceps — application of forceps before head has passed through the pelvic inlet.
    c. mid-forceps — application of forceps when head is at level of ischial spines.[29]
5. saline abortion — intra-amniotic injection of hypertonic salt solution after 14 weeks of gestation to induce abortion.[12, 75, 100, 83, 26, 5, 101]
6. version — the process of turning the fetus in the uterus.
    a. cephalic version — the head is made the presenting part.
    b. podalic version — the breech is made the presenting part.

F. Symptomatic Terms:

1. attitude, obstetric — the intrauterine position of the fetus.
2. ballottement — method of detecting pregnancy or testing for engagement of fetal head. The examiner sharply taps against the lower uterine segment with his forefinger in the vagina and tosses the embryo upward.[19]
3. Bandl's ring — a groove seen on the abdomen between pubis and umbilicus after hard labor.
4. Braxton Hick's sign — painless contractions of the uterus throughout gestation. They occur periodically and last to term.[29]
5. bruit of placenta — blowing sound heard on auscultation. It is due to maternal circulation.[29]
6. Chadwick's sign — violet discoloration of the vaginal mucosa, presumptive evidence of pregnancy.[19]
7. colostrum — yellowish fluid secreted by the mammary gland during pregnancy and for the first 2 or 3 days postdelivery.
8. dilatation of cervix — gradual opening of the cervix to permit passage of fetus.
9. dystocia — difficult birth.[42, 43, 44]
10. effacement — obliteration of cervix; the process of thinning and shortening of the uterine cervix.
11. engagement — descent of the fetal head through the pelvic inlet.
12. engorgement — excessive venous and lymph stasis of lactating breasts, usually referred to as caked breasts.[19]
13. gestation — pregnancy.
14. Goodell's sign — softening of the uterine cervix, indicative of pregnancy.
15. Hegar's sign — softening of lower uterus; occurs in pregnancy.[19]
16. hemorrhage — excessive blood loss.
    a. antepartum — before birth.
    b. intrapartum — during delivery.
    c. postpartum — after delivery.
17. labor — normal uterine contractions which result in the delivery of the fetus.
    a. missed labor — a few contractions at full-term, then cessation of labor and fetal retention, usually due to death of fetus in utero or extrauterine pregnancy.
    b. precipitate labor — hasty labor.
    c. premature labor — before full-term.
    d. protracted labor — unduly prolonged.[45, 24, 65]

18. labor — 3 stages:
   a. cervical dilatation — first stage begins with uterine contractions terminates with complete cervical dilatation.
   b. expulsion — second stage, from complete dilatation of the cervix to the birth of the baby.[65]
   c. placental separation and expulsion — third stage, from delivery of neonate to expulsion of the placenta.
19. lochia — discharge from the birth canal following delivery.
20. pica — peculiar cravings of the pregnant woman for strange foods or nonedibles.
21. presentation or lie — the relation which the long axis of the fetus bears to that of the mother. Accordingly, distinction is made between longitudinal and transverse presentations. Longitudinal presentation occurs in 99.5% of cases and includes the following varieties:
   a. breech presentation — presentation of the fetal buttock.
      (1) complete breech — thighs flexed on abdomen and legs flexed upon thighs.
      (2) footling — the foot presents.
      (3) frank breech — legs extended over ventral body surface.
      (4) knee — the knee presents.
   b. face presentation — presentation of the fetal head.
      (1) brow — the forehead presents.
      (2) sinciput — the large fontanel presents.
      (3) vertex — the upper and back part of the head presents. This is the most common variety.[74, 46]
   Transverse presentation occurs in 0.5% of cases.
22. quickening — the pregnant woman's first perception of fetal life.
23. sterility — infertility, reproductive failure.[71, 66]

THE ANTENATAL PERIOD

A. Origin of Terms:

1. amnion (G) — membrane around fetus
2. antigen (G/L) — against begetting
3. chorion (G) — membrane around fetus
4. fetus (L) — offspring

B. Anatomical Terms:

1. amnion — the innermost fetal membrane which forms the bag of waters and encloses the fetus.
2. amniotic fluid — fluid contained in the amniotic sac.
3. chorion — outer envelope of the fetus.
4. embryo — the product of conception, especially during the first three months of life.
5. fetus — the unborn child after the first three months of development.

C. Diagnostic Terms:

1. fetal anoxia, intrauterine asphyxia — oxygen want of the fetus which may result from prolapse of the cord, placenta abruptio, compression of the umbilical vein or other causes. Death is inevitable if fetus is not delivered promptly.
2. fetal distress — a life threatening condition due to fetal anoxia, hemolytic disease or other causes.
3. fetal hemolytic disease — blood disorder caused by antibody antigen reaction in ABO, Rh or other blood group incompatibility. Maternal antibodies cross the placenta, agglutinate fetal blood cells and destroy them. Fetal anemia develops.[29]
4. prolapse of cord — premature descent of the umbilical cord, a cause of fetal death.

D. Terms Related to Special Procedures:

1. amniocentesis — puncture of the amniotic cavity:[90, 22, 96]
   a. to aspirate fluid for amniotic fluid analysis.[1, 52, 11]
   b. to inject radiopaque substance for amniography.[6, 10]
   c. to administer intrauterine transfusions to the fetus with severe hemolytic disease.[91, 22]
   d. to determine pressure changes of amniotic fluid which permit the continuous monitoring of uterine contractibility.[90]
   e. to monitor the fetal heart rate.[90]
   f. to detect possible genetic disorder antenatally.[79, 89]
   g. to induce abortion.[12, 75, 100]

2. amniography — radiography of amniotic cavity after injecting a radiopaque substance into the sac. The procedure permits an accurate evaluation of the fetus, the presence or absence of scalp edema, a protuberant abdomen, flaccid extremities and other signs.[7, 10, 91]

3. anti-D antibody injection — preparation for passive immunization of Rh negative mothers of D-positive babies administered intramuscularly or intravenously within 72 hours after delivery. Its purpose is to prevent Rh isoimmunization and fetal hemolytic disease in future pregnancies. The individual sterile vaccine vials are prepared from plasma obtained from severely sensitized Rh-negative women who had still-born hydropic fetuses or from gamma globulin from naturally or artificially sensitized donors.[27, 28, 29]

4. fetal electrocardiography — a method of detecting and recording electrical impulses of the fetal heart. In contradistinction to the larger, slower deflections of the maternal heart, the normal fetal heart beat yields smaller and, more rapid deflections. Fetal distress may be evidenced by a delay in the conduction time.[60, 29]

5. fetal monitoring — continuous recording of fetal heart rate (FHR) patterns from a direct fetal electrocardiogram (FECG) electrode and uterine contractions using a transcervical catheter. Indications are clinical signs of fetal distress, FHR changes, suspected cephalopelvic disproportions and high risk pregnancies.[84, 85, 68]

6. fetal phonocardiography — the detection of fetal heart sounds by means of a phonocardiograph.

7. fetal telemetry — a wireless radio transmission which provides remote recordings of the fetal electrocardiography or other data.

8. intrauterine transfusion — the injection of red cell concentrate prepared from Rh-negative whole blood (packed erythrocytes) into the peritoneal cavity of the fetus to combat fetal hemolytic anemia and prevent fetal death.

9. ultrasound monitoring of mother and fetus — continuous recording by a Doppler ultrasound instrument with one transducer placed over the fundus to monitor uterine contractions and the other transducer placed in a location to monitor the fetal heart tones.[9, 29]

THE NEONATAL PERIOD

A. Origin of Terms:

1. natus (L) — birth
2. neo (G) — new, recent
3. neonate (L) — newborn
4. umbilicus (L) — naval

B. Anatomical Terms:

1. fontanel, fontanelle — the junction point of cranial sutures which remains widely open in the newborn.
2. umbilical cord — cord connecting placenta with fetal umbilicus. At birth chiefly composed of one umbilical vein and two umbilical arteries surrounded by gelatinous substance.

C. Diagnostic Terms:

1. asphyxia neonatorum — lack of oxygen in the blood of the newborn.
2. atelectasis neonatorum — failure of the lungs to expand at birth.
3. caput succedaneum — tumor-like edema of presenting part of child's head.
4. cerebral hemorrhage — brain hemorrhage due to birth injury or coagulation defects resulting in anoxia, cyanosis and convulsions.
5. congenital stridors — breathing disorders associated with a crowing or stridulous noise from birth or first week of life due to malformation, abnormal position or functioning of glottis, trachea or vocal cords.[95]
6. cord hemorrhage — bleeding from umbilical cord.
7. Down's syndrome, mongolism, trisomy G_{21} — a chromosome aberration characterized by mental retardation and many physical features such as slanting eyes, flat facial profile, thick, fissured tongue protruding from open mouth, pudgy, broad neck, hypotonia and absence of the Moro reflex in the newborn.[20, 48, 103]
8. drug addiction in neonate — withdrawal symptoms in the newborn appearing soon after birth. The infant is restless, has a shrill cry, tremors, twitchings and convulsions. Its manifestations may closely parallel those of adult withdrawal, such as yawning, sneezing, anorexia and diarrhea.
9. erythroblastosis fetalis — hemolytic disease of the newborn.
    a. anemic type — damage to bone marrow liver and spleen, excessive hemolysis.
    b. hydropic type — extremely edematous, stillborn or neonatal death.
    c. icteric type — marked jaundice, may be followed by kernicterus.[47]
10. hydrocephalus — abnormal fluid collection in the ventricles of the brain resulting in an enlargement of the head.[48]
11. hyperbilirubinemia, neonatal — abnormally high bilirubin content of the circulating blood predisposing the newborn to kernicterus due to unconjugated bilirubin concentration within brain tissue.[47, 88]
12. idiopathic respiratory distress syndrome, hyaline membrane disease — serious breathing difficulty due to hyaline material, a sticky exudate, filling the alveolar ducts and alveoli, thus obstructing the airway and preventing oxygenation. The condition, which occurs primarily in premature infants, may be fatal.[20]
13. imperforate anus, atresia of anus — rectum ending in a blind pouch.
14. infections of the newborn:
    a. epidemic diarrhea — loose, yellow green stools, dehydration and acidosis.
    b. impetigo contagiosa — skin disease, appearance of vesicles which changes to pustules and later to crusts. It is caused by staphylococci.
    c. ophthalmia neonatorum — purulent conjunctivitis.
    d. thrush — fungus infection of oral mucous membrane forming white patches or aphthae.[20]
15. kernicterus, nuclear jaundice, biliary encephalopathy — irreparable brain damage complicating severe erythroblastosis. Excess serum bilirubin, liberated by destroyed erythrocytes and not converted into an excretable form, stains the brain nuclei and results in mental retardation, cerebral palsy or deafness. The most severe cases die within a few days. Kernicterus can be prevented by exchange transfusions.[20, 47]
16. meningocele — meninges protruding through a defect in the spine or skull.
17. phocomelia — congenital deformities such as absence or stunting of extremities. Infants, born of mothers, who took thalidomide during the first trimester of pregnancy, developed these malformations.[20, 47]
18. prematurity — infant born before his development is complete. A birth weight below 2500 Gm marks prematurity according to the World Health Organization.
19. retrolental fibroplasia — disorder seen in premature infants who receive continuous oxygen therapy. The retina becomes edematous and detached. Partial or total blindness develops.
20. tongue-tie, ankyloglossia — short frenulum linguae preventing neonate from taking feeding.
21. umbilical hernia, omphalocele — rupture of the umbilicus associated with protrusion of intestine. It occurs in the first weeks of life.[92]

D. Operative Terms:

1. exchange transfusion — replacing the blood of a neonate who has a severe antibody-antigen reaction due to hemolytic disease with blood devoid of the offending antigen.[29]
2. clipping of frenulum linguae — minor operation to relieve tongue-tie.
3. repair of imperforate anus — surgical creation of an opening.

E. Symptomatic Terms:

1. Apgar score — assessing a neonate's physical condition by evaluating his heart rate, respiratory effort, reflex irritability and skin color according to a scoring system.[49, 62]
2. Chvostek's sign — facial irritability in tetany evoked by a slight tap over the facial nerve. The spasm is unilateral.
3. congenital — born with a certain condition.
4. eructation — belching.
5. meconium — black stools of the newborn.
6. Moro reflex, startle reflex — reflex indicating an awareness of balance in the neonate. The reflex is stimulated by a sudden jarring of the crib or jerking of a blanket. The infant draws up his legs and throws his arms symmetrically forward.[20]
7. premature — before the proper time, in obstetrics before full term.
8. pylorospasm — spasm of circular muscle of lower end of stomach.[29]
9. vernix caseosa — fatty substance which covers the newborn.

RADIOLOGY

A. Terms Related to Reproductive Organs and Pelvis:

1. hysterosalpingography, uterotubal radiography, uterosalpingography — introduction of a contrast medium under pressure into the uterus and uterine tubes. This procedure is done under radiographic control to determine the patency of the tubes in reproductive failure.[55, 105]
2. pelvimetry — radiographic measurement of various obstetrical diameters of the bony pelvis.
3. pelvimetry and cephalometry — radiographic measurement of the relationship of the size of the fetal head to the size of the pelvic diameters.
4. sonograms — ultrasonics by the pulse-echo Sonar method to delineate soft tissue planes for diagnosis. Sonograms reveal size and shape of tissue boundaries, sonic transparency of organs, growths and cysts, distortion of organs such as the uterus and bladder.[99, 23, 69]

B. Terms Related to the Placenta:

1. cystographic placentography — radiography for diagnosis of placenta previa in pregnancy. The urinary bladder is filled with an opaque medium and a radiogram is made. The diagnosis is based on the distance of the bladder from the fetal head.
2. intravenous placentography — radiographic visualization of placenta after intravenous injection of contrast medium to determine whether placenta previa is the cause of bleeding in the third trimester of pregnancy.
3. placentography — radiography of the placenta after the injection of a contrast medium or without opaque substance using a compensating filter to even up the x-ray exposure of the pregnant uterus.[93, 15]

CLINICAL LABORATORY

A. Terms Related to Pregnancy Tests:

1. biologic pregnancy tests — bioassays for pregnancy using various test animals. They require technical skill and results are delayed for days. Examples are:
   a. frog test (Wiltberger-Miller) — injection of the patient's serum or urine into a female frog.
   Positive reaction: Eggs are excreted by the frog.
   b. mouse test (Aschheim-Zondek) — injection of the patient's urine into immature female mice.
   Positive reactions:
   (1) Hyperemia and swelling of the graafian follicles are noted (Reaction 1).
   (2) The ripened follicles show hemorrhages (Reaction 2).
   c. rabbit test (Friedman) — injection of the patient's serum or urine into a virgin female rabbit.
   Positive reaction: Follicles ripen and bleed.
   d. rat test, ovarian hyperemia test (Beck *et al.*) — injection of the patient's urine or serum into an immature rat.
   Positive reaction: Ovary of immature rat shows gross hyperemia.
   e. toad test (Galli Mainini) — injection of the patient's urine or serum into male toad.
   Positive reaction: Sperms are excreted by toad.
2. immunologic pregnancy tests — immunoassays for pregnancy, sensitive tests for human chorionic gonadotrophin (HCG) in serum and urine. Excess chorionic gonadotrophin is present in pregnancy. Techniques are simple and results are read in 2 hours or less (actually in 5 minutes). The tests are designed for office use.
   However, immunologic tests as well as the biologic tests yield positive results in choriocarcinoma and hydatidiform mole. In menopause elevated pituitary gonadotrophin may produce a falsely positive test.[50, 61, 13] The following commercial immunologic pregnancy tests are in current use:
   a. hemagglutination-inhibition tube tests:
   (1) Pregnosticon tube test.
   (2) Pregnosticon Accuspheres (a free-dried reagent).
   (3) UCG test (urinary chorionic gonadotrophin).
   b. latex inhibition slide tests:
   (1) HCG test (human chorionic gonadotrophin).
   (2) Pregnosticon slide test.
   (3) Pregnosticon Dri-Dot (a dried reagent).[50, 61, 67, 13]
3. Other hormone tests:
   a. human placental lactogen (HPL) determination — serum assay shows that HPL levels rise progressively during pregnancy, are very high in diabetes and low in placental insufficiency.[96]
   b. urinary estriol determination, Tekid method — a pregnancy urinary estrogen assay for monitoring high risk pregnancies. Estriol excretion during pregnancy reflects the condition of the fetus.[63, 96]

B. Terms Related to Fertility Studies:

1. biopsy:
   a. endometrial biopsy and histologic study — method of determining evidence of ovulation. If absent, the ovarian factor is thought to be the cause of sterility.[55] However the biopsy does not indicate whether the ovary is primarliy or secondarily involved.[29]
   b. ovarian biopsies, bilateral — removal of ovarian tissue under laparoscopic control for infertility, evaluation and resumption of ovarian function. Large ovarian biopsies with use of Palmer biopsy forceps may be done under laparoscopic control.[78]

2. laparoscopy — endoscopic examination of pelvic and reproductive organs for diagnostic appraisal and/or therapeutic control.

3. quantitative hydrotubation — evaluation of tubal patency by the intrauterine infusion of indigocarmine solution with a clamp on the cervix. It is observed whether the dye merely trickles through a pinpoint fimbrial opening or flows freely from both fimbriae. In addition tubal dilatation is seen as the dye passes through the lumen of the tube. The pressure, used to force the solution through the cornual ends, can also be measured. The method offers a reliable index of the functional patency of the uterine tubes.[53]

4. tubal insufflation (Rubin test) — tubal patency test in reproductive failure. Blocked tubes are a cause of sterility.[55]

B. Terms Related to Parental, Antenatal and Neonatal Tests and Procedures:

1. ABO incompatibility — incompatibility in the A,B,AB, and O blood types. Usually the mother is type O and the baby type A or B. This incompatibility occurs in a considerable number of pregnancies, but erythroblastosis develops in a relatively small percentage of them.

2. amniotic fluid analyses — spectrophotometric tracings or other determinations on amniotic fluid in the antepartum management of Rh incompatibility, diabetes, etc. Fetal involvement exists if there is an abnormal increase in the pigments that absorb light at wave lengths between 450 and 460 mμ. Repeated amniotic fluid analyses are valuable guides for timing intrauterine transfusion or induction of labor.[22, 96]

3. antiglobulin reaction, Coombs test — a test for antibodies.
   a. direct Coombs test — a test for antibody coating of erythrocytes.
      Negative reaction — direct Coombs, no antibody coating on newborn's red cells.
      Positive reaction — direct Coombs, antibody coating on newborn's red cells indicative of hemolytic disease.[106]
   b. indirect Coombs test — test determines presence of antibodies in serum.[29]

4. bilirubin — a pigment in bile derived from degenerated hemoglobin of destroyed blood cells. In newborns and particularly in premature and erythroblastotic babies the liver is unable to cope with the large amount of bilirubin liberated by destroyed erythrocytes. This results in an excess of bilirubin in the blood.

5. bilirubin determinations using cord blood of neonate.
   Normal values of serum bilirubin
   full-term newborn .... 0.2 - 1.4 mg/100 ml.
   Increase in serum bilirubin
   physiological jaundice .... 5.0 - 13.0 mg/100 ml.
   hyperbilirubinemia .... 20.0 mg/100 ml. and over.
   kernicterus .... 25.0 mg/100 ml. and over or below.[88, 96]

6. blood group analysis of prospective parents — a study of the parental blood groups in order to detect maternal and paternal grouping differences, predictive of mother-child incompatibilities. Routine procedures include ABO grouping, Rh typing and screening for irregular antibodies.

7. blood group analyses for **exclusion studies** — tests used in medicolegal practice on the basis that parental blood groups are inherited by the child.
   The American Medical Association accepts only the findings of the ABO, MN and Rh-Hr analyses for legal purposes except when experts use other systems.[102]
   Determinations are made to exclude allegation or denial of paternity. To clarify the issue an example of the MN system of blood typing should be of interest.

Disputed Father   Mother
Type M   Type N

Child
Type N — Genotype NN

Since the child does not have the gene M, the person in question is not his father.

8. glucuronyl transferase — enzyme absent from the liver of premature infants at birth and incompletely developed in full-term newborns. This enzyme lack seems to account for the liver's inability to handle the load imposed by the increased destruction of red cells in the first days of life.

9. phenylalanine — essential amino acid present in protein foods. A blocking of its conversion into tyrosine causes phenylalanine blood levels to rise and phenylketone bodies to be excreted in the urine. As a result brain development ceases. Mental retardation is preventable by early treatment with a low phenylalanine diet.

10. phenylketonuria detection — diagnostic tests for detecting PKU, an inborn error of protein metabolism.
   a. ferric chloride tests (5 or 10%) on urine:
      (1) diaper test
      (2) tube test
      (3) Phenistix reagent strip test.
      Negative reaction — no color change.
      Positive reaction — blue green or gray color of urine.
      Phenylpyruvic acid is one of the metabolites excreted in phenylketonuria.
   b. Guthrie test — a simple screening test requiring several drops of blood from the heel of the newborn before the baby is taken home from the hospital.
      Negative test — phenylketonuria unlikely to develop
      Positive test — diagnosis to be confirmed by other tests.
      In states where mandatory testing of the neonate for phenylketonuria is done, the Guthrie test is considered legally acceptable. Thus the detection of this hereditary disorder is becoming a legal as well as a professional obligation in medicine.
   c. serum phenylalanine test — procedure measures phenylalanine levels in blood serum.
      Normal level — serum phenylalanine .... 1-3mg/100 ml.
      Increase in phenylketonuria .... 60mg/100 ml and above.[20]

11. phototherapy for neonate — effective method of lowering unconjugated bilirubin levels by exposing the newborn to fluorescent or other light according to need:
   a. infants with physiologic jaundice due to mildly elevated serum bilirubin benefit by the fluorescent lighting system of the nursery.
   b. infants with hyperbilirubinemia threatening encephalopathy are exposed to intense fluorescent light therapy in special incubators to reduce their excessive serum bilirubin.[114, 4, 70, 82, 107]

12. Rh isoimmunization — sensitization that occurs when red cells containing Rh antigens, not present in the cells of the recipient, enter the circulation. This develops most commonly in Rh negative women carrying Rh positive babies or receiving transfusion with Rh positive blood. It usually occurs during the second Rh positive pregnancy or subsequent pregnancies.[29, 22, 96]

13. rubella, German measles, in early pregnancy — a relatively mild disease with fever, rash and lymph node involvement which causes serious deformities in the growing fetus when it occurs during the first trimester. Preventive measures are presented:
   a. gammaglobulin in rubella infection — prophylactic agent thought to prevent maternal and congenital rubella and rubella-induced congenital malformations.[72]
   b. hemagglutination (HI) test for rubella — routine test to be performed within 10 days of exposure to rubella. An antibody titer of 1:10 or above is usually indicative of patient being immune and will not develop rubella. An antibody titer below 1:10 suggests that the patient may develop rubella.[4]
   c. postpartum rubella immunization — procedure performed on nonimmune women during the puerperium to prevent rubella infection in future pregnancies.[59, 56, 17]

14. sickle cell disease screening tests — screening procedures for sickle cell hemoglobin (HbS) during the first months of life, preferably at the infant's first checkup. Tests primarily indicated include the tube solubility or a microscopic test for HbS and a blood smear to detect sickled cells.[14]

214

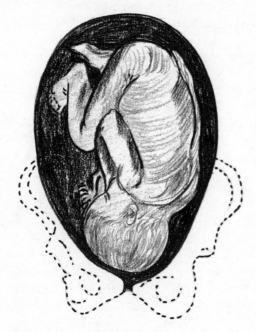

Fig. 58 – Right occiput anterior (ROA) position.

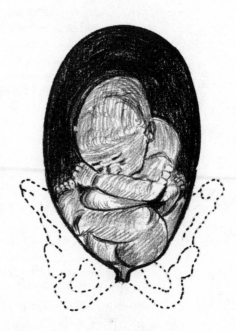

Fig. 59 – Left sacro-posterior (LSP) position.

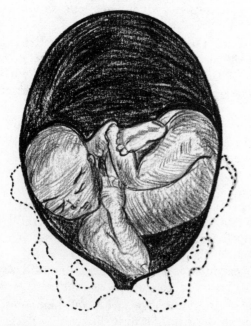

Fig. 60 – Right scapulo-posterior (RScP) position.

15. spectrophotometry — instrumental measurement of the intensity of various wave lengths of light transmitted under standardized conditions by a substance under study.[22]

ABBREVIATIONS

A. General

AZ — Ascheim-Zondek test
BBT — basal body temperature
CDC — calculated day of confinement
CS — Cesarean section
CWP — childbirth without pain
EDC — estimated day of confinement
FECG — fetal electrocardiogram
FHR — fetal heart rate
FHT — fetal heart tone
FTND — full term normal delivery
HCG — human chorionic gonadotrophin
HDN — hemolytic disease of newborn
HPL — human placental lactogen

HSG — hysterosalpingography
IU — international unit
LMP — last menstrual period
mμ — micron, micrometer, $\frac{1}{1000}$ millimeter
NB — newborn
OB — obstetrics
PPA pos. — phenylpyruvic acid positive (phenylketonuria present)
PU — pregnancy urine
RML — right mediolateral (episiotomy)
Rh neg. — rhesus factor negative
Rh pos. — rhesus factor positive
UC — uterine contractions

B. Vertex Presentations:[108]

LOA — left occipitoanterior
LOP — left occipitoposterior
LOT — left occipitotransverse

ROA — right occipitoanterior
ROP — right occipitoposterior
ROT — right occipitotransverse

C. Face Presentations:

LMA — left mentoanterior
LMP — left mentoposterior
LMT — left mentotransverse

RMA — right mentoanterior
RMP — right mentoposterior
RMT — right mentotransverse

D. Breech Presentations:

LSA — left sacroanterior
LSP — left sacroposterior

RSA — right sacroanterior
RSP — right sacroposterior

E. Transverse Presentations:

LScA — left scapuloanterior
LScP — left scapuloposterior

RScA — right scapuloanterior
RScP — right scapuloposterior

F. Organizations:

AAMIH — American Association for Maternal and Infant Health
ACNMW — American College of Nurse Midwifery
ACOG — American College of Obstetricians and Gynecologists

FSAA — Family Service Association of America
ICM — International Confederation of Midwives
MCA — Maternity Center Association
USCB — United States Children's Bureau

ORAL READING PRACTICE

Clinical Signs of Fetal Hydrops

There are three clinical types of **fetal erythroblastosis, hydrops fetalis, neonatal icterus gravis and hemolytic anemia** of the newborn. Of these types hydrops fetalis is the most serious condition since its mortality rate is one hundred per cent.

The clinical signs of fetal hydrops are manifold and are sequels of the massive destruction of blood. They include

1. anemia due to hemolysis
2. **hyperplasia** of the marrow which is thought to be a compensatory reaction of the marrow to the hemolytic process
3. foci of **extramedullary** production of red cells (**erythropoiesis**) in the spleen, liver, kidneys and other tissues, resulting in **splenomegaly, hepatomegaly** and other tissue reactions
4. a marked increase of immature erythrocytes (**erythroblasts**) in the circulation
5. anemic anoxia associated with tissue damage, particularly of the **endothelial** cells, cerebral nuclei and liver
6. hemolytic **jaundice** due to the excessive increase in blood destruction
7. **obstructive jaundice** caused by the occlusion of biliary capillaries
8. **hepatocellular jaundice** resulting from oxygen want of liver cells
9. **edema** due to **hepatic hypoproteinemia** and damage to endothelial tissues.[25, 58]

Table 18

SOME OBSTETRIC AND NEONATAL CONDITIONS AMENABLE TO SURGERY

Organs Involved	Diagnoses	Operations	Operative Procedures
Cervix uteri Endometrium	Early incomplete abortion	Dilatation and curettage	Instrumental expansion of cervix and scraping of endometrium to remove blood clots and tissue
Cervix uteri	Dystocia Cervical stenosis Carcinoma of cervix in pregnancy, viable fetus	Cesarean section	Removal of fetus through incision into uterus
Uterine tube	Ruptured ectopic pregnancy with massive hemorrhage	Salpingectomy, unilateral	Removal of one fallopian tube
Perineum	Second stage of labor, tense perineum	Episiotomy, mediolateral or midline	Incision into perineum
Perineum	Obstetrical laceration of the perineum	Perineorrhaphy	Suture of the torn perineum
Pelvis	Inlet contraction of pelvis	Cesarean section	Abdominal delivery of fetus
Pelvis	Prolonged labor, dystocia	Elective forceps delivery	Fetus delivered by horizontal traction
Uterus	Total placenta previa. antepartum or intrapartum hemorrhage	Cesarean section	Incision into corpus uteri and delivery of fetus through abdomen
Uterus	Rupture of uterus, fatal hemorrhage, maternal death	Postmortem Cesarean section	Delivery of fetus by incision through abdominal wall and uterus after death of mother

Organs Involved	Diagnoses	Operations	Operative Procedures
Cervix uteri	Obstetrical laceration of cervix	Trachelorrhaphy	Suture of torn cervix uteri
Blood of fetus	Fetal hemolytic disease, severe	Amniocentesis Intrauterine transfusion	Surgical puncture of amniotic cavity Injection of Rh negative packed red cells into the fetal peritoneal cavity
Blood of newborn	Erythroblastosis fetalis, Rh positive Hyperbilirubinemia	Exchange transfusions within 24 hours after birth	Replacing the infant's red cells by transfusing him with Rh negative erythrocytes which will remain unharmed by maternal antibodies
Intestine of newborn	Meconium ileus with intestinal obstruction due to mucoviscidosis	Intestinal resection	Surgical intervention to relieve intestinal obstruction

REFERENCES AND BIBLIOGRAPHY

1. Amstey, M. S., et al. Comparative analysis of amniotic fluid bilirubin. *Obstetrics and Gynecology*, 39: 407-410, March, 1972.

2. Anderson, D. G. Hemorrhage in late pregnancy. In Conn, Howard F. (ed.). *Current Therapy 1972.* Philadelphia: W. B. Saunders Co., 1972, pp. 736-738.

3. Bard, H. Birth asphyxia and resuscitation. In Conn, Howard F. (ed.). *Current Therapy 1972.* Philadelphia: W. B. Saunders Co., 1972, pp. 732-734.

4. Behrman, R. E. and Hsia, D. Y. Summary of a symposium on phototherapy for hyperbilirubinemia. *Journal of Pediatrics*, 75: 724-727, October, 1969.

5. Berkowitz, R. L. Electrolyte changes and serious complications after hypertonic saline instillation. *Clinical Obstetrics and Gynecology*, 14: 166-178, March, 1971.

6. Bottorf, M. K. and Fish, S. A. Amniography. *Southern Medical Journal*, 64: 1203-1206, October, 1971.

7. Brame, R. G. and Bahti, S. A. Cesarean section for fetal distress. *Southern Medical Journal*, 64: 1398-1402, November, 1971.

8. Calliet, R. Trauma to the pelvis. *Lawyer's Medical Journal*, 3: 401-426, February, 1968.

9. Case, L. L. Ultrasound monitoring of mother and fetus. *American Journal of Nursing*, 72: 725-727, April, 1972.

10. Caterini, H. R. *et al.* Amniography during subsequent pregnancy for evaluating the post-cesarean section uterine scar. *Obstetrics and Gynecology*, 39: 717-720, May, 1972.

11. Clements, J. A. *et al.* Respiratory distress syndrome. Rapid test for surfactant in amniotic fluid. *New England Journal of Medicine*, 286: 1077-1081, May 18, 1972.

12. Cronenwet, L. R. and Choyce, J. M. Saline abortion. *American Journal of Nursing*, 71: 1754-1757, September, 1971.

13. Crooke, A. C. Human gonadotrophins. In Philipp, Elliot E., Barnes, Josephine and Newton, Michael. *Scientific Foundations of Obstetrics and Gynecology.* Philadelphia: F. A. Davis Co., 1970, pp. 495-508.

14. Diggs, L. W. Screening tests for sickle cell disease, Part 2. *Postgraduate Medicine*, 51: 277-280, March, 1972.

15. Drukker, B. H. *et al.* Placental localization. A comparative evaluation of isotopic placentography and amniography. *American Journal of Obstetrics and Gynecology*, 110: 9-13, May, 1971.

16. Durfee, R. B. Low classic cesarean section: A new look at an old operation. *Postgraduate Medicine*, 51: 219-222, February, 1972.

17. Emanuel, I. Some preventive aspects of abnormal intrauterine development. *Postgraduate Medicine*, 51. 144-148, January, 1972.

18. Firor, H. V. Surgical emergencies in newborns and infants. *Surgical Clinics of North America*, 52: 77-98, February, 1972.

19. Fitzpatrick, Elise, Reeder, Sharon R. and Mastroianni, Luigi. *Maternity Nursing*, 12th ed. Philadelphia: J. B. Lippincott Co., 1971, pp. 615-623.

20. _____. Abnormalities of the fetus and newborn. Disorders of the newborn. *Ibid.*, pp. 523-554.

21. _____. Care of the newborn infant. *Ibid.*, pp. 345-401.

22. Freda, V. J. and Bowe, E. T. Hemolytic disease due to Rh sensitization. Amniocentesis and spectrophotometric scanning. In Conn, Howard F. (ed.). *Current Therapy 1972.* Philadelphia: W. B. Saunders Co., 1972, pp. 252-255.

23. Garrett, W. T. *et al.* Assessment of fetal size and growth rate by ultrasonic echoscopy. *Obstetrics and Gynecology*, 38: 525-534, October, 1971.

24. Goodlin, R. C. Importance of the lateral position during labor. *Obstetrics and Gynecology*, 37: 698-701, May, 1971.

25. Greenhill, J. P. *Obstetrics*, 13th ed. Philadelphia: W. B. Saunders Co., 1965, pp. 779-780.

26. Halbert, D. R. *et al.* Consumptive coagulopathy with generalized hemorrhage after hypertonic saline-induced abortion. *Obstetrics and Gynecology*, 39: 41-44, January, 1972.

27. Hamilton, E. G. Ten year experience with high-titer anti-D plasma for the prevention of Rh immunization. *Obstetrics and Gynecology*, 40: 692-696, November, 1972.

28. —————. High-titer anti-D plasma for the prevention of Rh isoimmunization. *Obstetrics and Gynecology*, 36: 331-340, September, 1970.

29. Hamilton, Eugene G., M.D. Personal communications.

30. Heaney, R. P. and Skillman, T. G. Calcium metabolism in normal human pregnancy. *Journal of Clinical Endocrinology and Metabolism*, 33: 661-670, October, 1971.

31. Hellman, Louis M. and Pritchard, Jack A. The ovarian cycle and its hormones. In *Williams Obstetrics*, 14th ed. New York: Appleton-Century-Crofts, 1971, pp. 58-89.

32. —————. The safe period or rhythm. *Ibid.*, pp. 1102-1103.

33. —————. Abortion and premature labor. *Ibid.*, pp. 493-534.

34. —————. Ectopic pregnancy. *Ibid.*, pp. 535-564.

35. —————. Diseases and abnormalities of the placenta and fetal membranes. *Ibid.*, pp. 564-608.

36. —————. Hypertensive disorders in pregnancy. *Ibid.*, pp. 685-747.

37. —————. Medical and surgical illnesses during pregnancy and the puerperium. *Ibid.*, pp. 748-834.

38. —————. Placenta previa and abruptic placenta. *Ibid.*, pp. 609-638.

39. —————. Abnormalities of the puerperium. *Ibid.*, pp. 971-1006.

40. —————. Injuries to the birth canal. *Ibid.*, pp. 932-955.

41. —————. Episiotomy and repair. *Ibid.*, pp. 423-429.

42. —————. Dystocia caused by anomalies of the expulsive forces. *Ibid.*, pp. 835-852.

43. —————. Dystocia caused by abnormalities in position, presentation or development of the fetus. *Ibid.*, pp. 853-893.

44. —————. Dystocia caused by pelvic contraction. *Ibid.*, pp. 894-920.

45. —————. The forces concerned in labor. *Ibid.*, pp. 349-373.

46. —————. Presentation, position, attitude and lie of the fetus. *Ibid.*, pp. 320-331.

47. —————. Diseases of the newborn. *Ibid.*, pp. 1026-1062.

48. —————. Malformation of the fetus. *Ibid.*, pp. 1063-1084.

49. —————. The newborn — evaluation of the infant. *Ibid.*, pp. 477-491.

50. —————. Diagnosis of pregnancy. *Ibid.*, pp. 277-289.

51. Holt, J. G. *Marriage and Periodic Abstinence*, 2d ed. New York: Longmans Green Co., 1960 (a scholarly exposition).

52. Horger, E. O. Amniotic fluid maturity index. *Southern Medical Journal*, 65: 299-301, March, 1972.

53. Horne, H. W. *et al.* Quantitative method of evaluating functional patency of human uterine tubes. *Obstetrics and Gynecology*, 39: 368-372, March, 1972.

54. Hotchkiss, R. L. *et al.* Renovascular hypertension in pregnancy. *Southern Medical Journal*, 64: 1256-1258, October, 1971.

55. Huffman, J. William. Reproductive failure. In *Gynecology and Obstetrics*. Philadelphia: W. B. Saunders Co., 1962. pp. 278-303.

56. Isacson, P. *et al.* Comparative study of live, attenuated rubella virus vaccines during the immediate puerperium. *Obstetrics and Gynecology*, 37: 332-337, March, 1971.

57. Jonas, S. *et al.* Chorea gravidarum and streptococcal infection. *Obstetrics and Gynecology*, 39: 77-79, January, 1972.

58. Jones, D. E. *et al.* Hydrops fetalis associated with idiopathic arterial calcification. *Obstetrics and Gynecology*, 39: 435-440, March, 1972.

59. Kelly, C. S. *et al.* Postpartum rubella immunization. Results with the HPV-77 strain. *Obstetrics and Gynecology*, 37: 338-342, March, 1971.

60. Kendall, B. *et al.* Uses of fetal electrocardiography. *American Journal of Nursing*, 64: 75-78, July, 1964.

61. Kerber, I. J. *et al.* Immunologic tests for pregnancy — a comparison. *Obstetrics and Gynecology*, 36: 37-43, July, 1970.

62. Khazan, A. F. et al. Biochemical studies of the fetus. V. Fetal pCO_2 and Apgar scores. *Obstetrics and Gynecology*, 38: 535-545, October, 1971.

63. Kim, M. H. *et al.* Rapid pregnancy urinary estrogen assays. A comparative study. *Obstetrics and Gynecology*, 37: 820-825. June, 1971.

64. Klaus, M. H. *et al.* Maternal attachment: Importance of the first postpartum days. *New England Journal of Medicine*, 286: 460-463, March 2, 1972.

65. Kopp, L. M. Ordeal or ideal — the second stage of labor. *American Journal of Nursing*, 71: 1140-1143, June, 1971.

66. Lamb, E. J. Prognosis for the infertile couple. *Fertility and Sterility*, 23: 320-325, May, 1972.

67. —————. Immunologic pregnancy tests — evaluation of Pregnosticon Dri-Dot and Pregnosticon Accuspheres. *Obstetrics and Gynecology*, 39: 665-672, May, 1972.

68. Lasater, C. Electronic monitoring of mother and fetus. *American Journal of Nursing*, 72: 728-730, April, 1972.

69. Leopold, G. R. Diagnostic ultrasound in detection of molar pregnancy. *Radiology*, 98: 171-176, January, 1971.

70. Lucey, J. F. The phototherapy in neonatal hyperbilirubinemia. *Seminars in Hematology*, 9: 127-135, April, 1972.

71. Mancini, R. E. and Andrada, J. A. Immunological factors in human male and female infertility.

In Samter, M., ed.). *Immunological Diseases*, 2d ed. Boston: Little, Brown and Co., 1971, pp. 1240-1256.

72. McCallin, P. F. *et al.* Gammaglobulin as prophylaxis against rubella-induced congenital anomalies. *Obstetrics and Gynecology*, 39: 185-189, February, 1972.

73. McLain, C. R. Hypertensive disorders of pregnancy. In Conn, Howard F. (ed.). *Current Therapy 1972*. Philadelphia: W. B. Saunders Co., 1972, pp. 738-741.

74. Mier, Thomas M., M.D. Personal communications.

75. Munsick, R. A. Air embolism and maternal death from therapeutic abortion. *Obstetrics and Gynecology*, 39: 688-690, May, 1972.

76. Nesbit, R. E. L. Abnormalities and diseases of the placenta and appendages. In Novak, Edmund R. and Woodruff, J. Donald. *Novak's Gynecologic and Obstetric Pathology*, 6th ed. Philadelphia: W. B. Saunders Co., 1967, pp. 484-522.

77. Neutel, C. I. and Buck, C. Effect of smoking during pregnancy on the risk of cancer in children. *Journal of National Cancer Institute*, 47: 59-64, July, 1971.

78. Neuwirth, R. S. A method of bilateral ovarian biopsy at laparoscopy in infertility and chronic anovulation. *Fertility and Sterility*, 23: 361-366, May, 1972.

79. Nitwowsky, H. M. Prenatal diagnosis of genetic abnormality. *American Journal of Nursing*, 71: 1551-1557, August, 1971.

80. Marshall, J. and Rowe, B. The effect of personal factors on the use of basal body temperature method of regulating births. *Fertility and Sterility*, 23: 417-421, June, 1972.

81. Novak, Edmund R. and Woodruff, J. Donald. Ectopic pregnancy. In *Novak's Gynecologic and Obstetric Pathology*, 6th ed. Philadelphia: W. B. Saunders Co., 1967.

82. Ostrow, J. D. The mechanism of bilirubin photodegradation. *Seminars in Hematology*, 9: 113-125, April, 1972.

83. O'Sullivan, J. V. The effects of legalized abortion in England. *Hospital Progress*, 52: 75-78, June, 1971.

84. Paul, R. H. *et al.* Clinical fetal monitoring. *Obstetrics and Gynecology*, 37: 779-784, May, 1971.

85. _____. A clinical fetal monitor. *Obstetrics and Gynecology*, 35: 161-168, February, 1970.

86. Peckman, C. H. Uterine bleeding during pregnancy. Factors relating to its incidence. *Obstetrics and Gynecology*, 39: 48-51, January, 1972.

87. Poppers, P. J. Obstetric anesthesia and analgesia. In Conn, Howard F. (ed.). *Current Therapy 1972*. Philadelphia: W. B. Saunders Co., 1972, pp. 741-749.

88. Powell, L. W. Clinical aspects of unconjugated hyperbilirubinemia. *Seminars in Hematology*, 9: 91-105, January, 1972.

89. Prescott, G. H., Magenis, R. E. and Buist, N. R. Amniocentesis for antenatal diagnosis of genetic disorders. *Postgraduate Medicine*, 51: 212-217, March, 1972.

90. Queenan, J. T. *et al.* Amniocentesis for prenatal diagnosis of erythroblastosis fetalis. *Obstetrics and Gynecology*, 25: 302-307, March, 1965.

91. _____. Intrauterine transfusion for erythroblastosis fetalis. *American Journal of Nursing*, 65: 68-72, August, 1965.

92. Ravitch, M. Omphalocele. *Surgical Clinics of North America*, 51: 1383-1386, December, 1971.

93. Robinson, D. E. *et al.* Ultrasonic visualization of placenta. *Medical Journal of Australia*, 2: 1062-1064, December 5, 1970.

94. Rodger, B. P. Therapeutic conversation and posthypnotic suggestion. *American Journal of Nursing*, 72: 714-718, April, 1972.

95. Schaffer, Alexander J. and Avery, M. E. *Diseases of the Newborn*, 3rd ed. Philadelphia: W. B. Saunders Co., 1971, pp. 554-557.

96. Schwarz, R. H. Fetal diagnosis and treatment. In Fitzpatrick, Elise, Reeder, Sharon R. and Mastroianni, Luigi. *Maternity Nursing*, 12th ed. Philadelphia: J. B. Lippincott Co., 1971, pp. 515-528.

97. Seward, E. M. Preventing postpartum psychosis. *American Journal of Nursing*, 72: 520-523, March, 1972.

98. Slatin, M. Why mothers bypass prenatal care. *American Journal of Nursing*, 71: 1388-1389, July, 1971.

99. Smyth, C. N. Ultrasonics. In Philipp, Elliot E. Barnes, Josephine and Newton, Michael. *Scientific Foundations of Obstetrics and Gynecology*. Philadelphia: F. A. Davis Co., 1970, pp. 678-690.

100. Steinberg, C. R. Fever and bacteremia associated with hypertonic saline abortion. *Obstetrics and Gynecology*, 39: 673-678, May, 1972.

101. Stewart, G. K. *et al.* Therapeutic abortion in California. Effects on septic abortion and maternal mortality. *Obstetrics and Gynecology*, 37: 510-514, April, 1971.

102. Sunderman, F. William *et al.* (eds.). *The Clinical Pathology of Infancy*. Springfield, Illinois: Charles C. Thomas Publishers, 1967, p. 353.

103. Sutnick, A. I. *et al.* Susceptibility to leukemia: Immunologic factors in Down's syndrome. *Journal of the National Cancer Institute*, 47: 923-934, November, 1971.

104. Swartz, D. P. and Patchell, R. D. Abortion. In Conn, Howard F. (ed.). *Current Therapy 1972*. Philadelphia: W. B. Saunders Co., 1972, pp. 729-732.

105. Swolin, K. *et al.* Laparoscopy vs hysterosalpingography in sterility investigations. A comparative study. *Fertility and Sterility*, 23: 270-273, April, 1972.

106. *Technical Methods and Procedures of the American Association of Blood Banks*, 5th ed. Chicago: American Association of Blood Banks, 1970.

107. Thaler, M. M. Clinical aspects of neonatal hyperbilirubinemia. *Seminars in Hematology*, 9: 107-112, April, 1972.

108. Thompson, Edward T. and Hayden, Adeline (eds.). *Standard Nomenclature of Diseases and Operations*, 5th ed. New York: McGraw-Hill Book Co., Inc., 1961, p. 382.

109. Tyson, J. E. and Felig, P. Medical aspects of diabetes in pregnancy and the diabetogenic effects of oral contraceptives. *Medical Clinics of North America*, 55: 947-959, July, 1971.

110. Vellay, Pierre. *Childbirth without pain.* New York: E. P. Dutton, Inc., 1960, p. 21.

111. Voegtli, Ottilia. *How to Use Temperature Rhythm.* Springfield, Illinois: Charles C. Thomas Publisher, 1966 (designed for lay readers.)

112. Waldron, K. W. *et al.* Cesarean section in the lateral position. *Obstetrics and Gynecology*, 37: 706-710, May, 1971.

113. Walker, T. A. *et al.* Tubal pregnancy complicating uterine twin pregnancy after ovulation induction therapy. *Surgical Clinics of North America*, 52: 425-428, April, 1972.

114. Williams, S. L. Phototherapy in hyperbilirubinemia. *American Journal of Nursing*, 71: 1307-1399, July, 1971.

Chapter XII
Endocrine and Metabolic Disorders

ENDOCRINE GLANDS

A. Origin of Terms:

1. acro (G) — extremity
2. crine (G) — to secrete
3. dema (G) — swelling
4. goiter (L) — throat
5. hormone (G) — to excite
6. physis (G) — growth
7. pituita (L) — phlegm
8. thyro (G) — shield
9. tropho (G) — nourishment

B. Anatomical Terms:

1. endocrine glands — ductless glands elaborating internal secretions which are absorbed directly into the blood stream and influence various body functions.
2. hormone — active principle of an internal secretion.
3. hypophysis, pituitary gland — small ovoid body situated in the hypophysial fossa of the sphenoid bone. It is composed of the adenohypophysis and neurohypophysis, each performing distinct functions. The adenohypophysis or anterior pituitary is known as the master endocrine gland because of its physiological effect upon the suprarenals, gonads, pancreas and thyroid.[38] Some important hormones of the adenohypophysis are
   a. adenocorticotrophic hormone (ACTH) affecting the adrenal cortex and combating inflammatory processes. (ACTH is essential to maintain life.)[99]
   b. follicle stimulating and luteinizing hormones regulating the reproductive cycle.
   c. growth hormones promoting normal bone development.
   d. prolactin stimulating the secretion of milk.
   e. thyrotrophic hormone evoking increased uptake of iodine by the thyroid.[24]
   The neurohypophysis is thought to be not a true endocrine but a depot for neurosecretions known as the antidiuretic hormone (ADH) containing vasopressin and oxytocin.[99]
4. parathyroids — two to four small glands, usually a pair attached to each thyroid lobe. They secrete a hormone which regulates the metabolism of calcium and phosphorus.[86]
5. suprarenals, adrenals — two glands, one on top of each kidney. They are composed of an inner medullary substance and an outer cortex. The medulla produces adrenalin and noradrenalin. The adrenal cortex forms the adrenocortical steroids known as the corticosteroids or corticoids. They include the glucocorticoids and mineralocorticoids. C-19 derivatives yield androgens and C-18 derivatives estrogens.[35]
   Adrenocortical steroids help to regulate sodium, potassium and chloride metabolism, the water balance and carbohydrate, protein and fat metabolism.[35]
6. thymus — endocrine gland secreting thymin, a hormone which inhibits neuromuscular transmission.[44]
7. thyroid — the gland consists of two large lateral lobes and a central isthmus. It produces the hormones, thyroxine and triiodothyronine, with different physiological properties.[54]

C. Diagnostic Terms:

1. acromegaly — disease characterized by enlarged features, particularly of the face and hands. This is the result of oversecretion of the pituitary growth hormone.[68, 24, 59, 22]
2. Addison's disease — primary adrenal cortical insufficiency, a chronic syndrome. Pigmentation is a dominant trait.[66, 35, 90]
3. adrenal apoplexy — adrenal infarction associated with hemorrhage. It is usually a complication of anticoagulation therapy or septicemia. Hypotension is present.[66, 35]

222

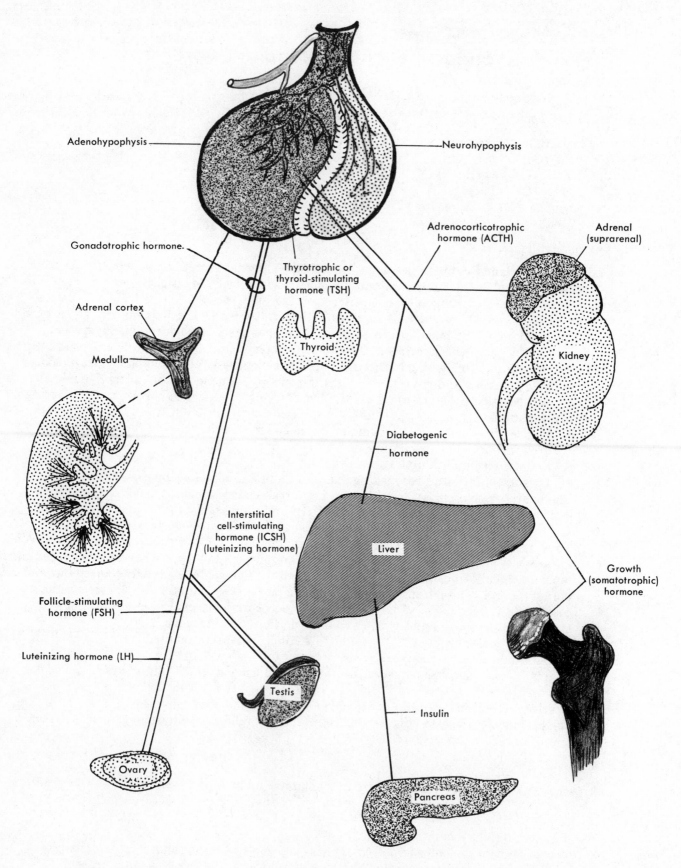

Adenohypophysis

Neurohypophysis

Gonadotrophic hormone.

Adrenocorticotrophic hormone (ACTH)

Adrenal (suprarenal)

Thyrotrophic or thyroid-stimulating hormone (TSH)

Adrenal cortex

Thyroid

Medulla

Kidney

Diabetogenic hormone

Interstitial cell-stimulating hormone (ICSH) (luteinizing hormone)

Liver

Growth (somatotrophic) hormone

Follicle-stimulating hormone (FSH)

Luteinizing hormone (LH)

Testis

Insulin

Ovary

Pancreas

Fig. 61 – Hormones of the adenohypophysis; direct and indirect effect on target organs.

4. adrenal crisis, Addisonian crisis — acute adenocortical insufficiency and a life-threatening event resulting from a lack of glucocorticoids, hyperkalemia and depletion of extracellular fluid during acute stress. Clinical manifestations are lassitude, headache, mental confusion, gastric upset, circulatory collapse, coma and death.[66, 35]

5. adrenal neoplasms:
   a. adenomas and adenocarcinomas — benign or malignant glandular tumors arising from the adrenal cortex. Oversecretion of androgen by the tumor may cause virilization in women and children; excess estrogen production by tumor may result in feminization in men.[1, 53, 83]
   b. neuroblastomas — tumors arising from the adrenal medulla. They are generally associated with metastases to bones.[1]
   c. pheochromocytomas — tumors usually arising from adrenal medulla and characterized by proxysmal hypertension.[1, 104, 9]

6. Conn's syndrome, primary aldosteronism — excessive secretion of aldosterone associated with pathology of adrenal cortex resulting in potassium depletion, sodium retention, extreme exhaustion, paresthesias, cardiac enlargement and increased CO_2 combining power.[66, 99]

7. Cushing's disease — syndrome attributed to the hyperproduction of cortisone and hydrocortisone by the adrenal cortex. Obesity, weakness and hypertension are typical manifestations.[66, 90, 27]

8. dwarfism, pituitary — congenital underdevelopment due to hyposecretion of the growth hormone.[24, 76]

9. giantism — abnormal growth, particularly of long bones before the closure of the epiphyseal lines. It is due to overproduction of the growth hormone of the anterior pituitary.

10. goiter — an enlargement of the thyroid gland. It may be classified as:
   a. nontoxic diffuse goiter
   b. toxic diffuse goiter
   c. nontoxic nodular goiter
   d. toxic nodular goiter.[26, 8]

11. hypercalcemic syndrome — abnormally high calcium levels of the blood seen in bone malignancies, endocrine and metabolic disorders such as multiple myeloma, acute adrenal insufficiency, hyperthyroidism, vitamin D intoxication, sarcoidosis and milk-alkali syndrome. It may be due to prolonged bed rest in osteoporosis, Paget's disease and other disorders.[94, 106, 96, 43]

12. hyperinsulinism due to islet cell tumor — condition marked by hypoglycemic episodes with a blood sugar below 30 or 40 mg per 100 ml, convulsions increasing in frequency and severity and eventually coma.[32]

13. hyperparathyroidism, primary — overproduction and overactivity of the parathyroid hormone present in hypercalcemia, osteitis fibrosa and tissue calcification.[7, 55, 56]

14. hyperthyroidism, thyrotoxicosis, exophthalmic goiter, Graves disease — thyrotoxic state currently considered an immunologic disorder. The antigen, probably of thyroid origin, is still unknown. Excessive hormone secretion increases oxygen consumption and thus accounts for the high metabolic rate. Clinical characteristics are goiter, protrusion of the eyeballs, tachycardia, tremors, emotional instability, sweating and weight loss.[97, 113, 26, 58]

15. hypoparathyroidism — abnormally decreased production of the parathyroid hormone causing hypocalcemia. It may be associated with reduced serum calcium and elevated serum phosphate levels.[7]

16. hypothyroidism — condition resulting from insufficiency of thyroid hormones in the blood.

17. myxedema — hypothyroidism causing lethargy, nonpitting edema, weakness and slow speech.

18. reactive hypoglycemia — a common hormonal disturbance initiated by an anxiety state which stimulates both increased consumption of carbohydrates and gastric emptying. This is followed by a high blood sugar which in turn accelerates insulin production and causes reactive hypoglycemia. It is also known as postprandial reactive hypoglycemia.

19. Simmond's disease — primary chronic pituitary insufficiency causing general debility.

20. tetany — hypofunction of the parathyroids, resulting in intermittent, tonic spasms due to calcium deficiency.

21. thymitis, autoimmune — autoimmune reaction in thymus, probably the basic thymus lesion in myasthenia gravis.[44]

22. thymotoxicosis — excessive secretion of thymin.[44]

23. thyroiditis — inflammation of the thyroid gland.
    a. acute thyroiditis — sudden onset of inflammatory process with local tenderness of thyroid.
    b. Hashimoto's thyroiditis, struma lymphomatosa — lymphoid goiter or lymphocytic thyroiditis, thought to be an autoimmune, hereditary disease and not as the name suggests an infectious or inflammatory disorder. It occurs almost exclusively in women. A medium sized, rubbery, firm goiter, low metabolism and hypothyroidism are common clinical findings.[70, 26]
    c. Riedel's struma — a rare chronic type of the old age group characterized by fibrotic changes and a wooden sensation in neck.[26]
    d. subacute thyroiditis — inflammation usually subsequent to viral infection in the respiratory tract indicative of an immunologic response to the virus.[47, 26]

24. thyroid neoplasms:
    a. adenomas — benign glandular tumors.
    b. carcinomas — malignant tumors, with subsequent metastases to cervical lymph nodes, the long bones and lungs.[58, 71, 88]

D. Operative Terms:

1. adrenalectomy — removal of adrenal gland or glands.[95, 74, 85]

2. cryohypophysectomy — one of several procedures which uses the stereotaxic trans-sphenoidal approach, achieves pituitary ablation (removal of hypophysis) by the application of a cryoprobe.[67, 103]

3. microneurosurgery of pituitary gland — microdissection of tumor under magnification and with intense illumination using a binocular surgical microscope.[92]
   Techniques are:
   a. Hardy's oronasal-transsphenoidal approach — entering the sphenoid sinus via nasal septum for removal of intrasellar tumor.[49, 92]
   b. Rand's transfrontal-transphenoidal approach — opening the sphenoid sinus through a frontal craniotomy for removal of tumor attached to optic chiasm.[92, 77, 40]

4. parathyroidectomy — removal of parathyroid tissue to control hyperparathyroidism.[108, 46]

5. thymectomy — removal of thymus gland.

6. thyroidectomy — removal of thyroid for persistent hyperthyroidism refractory to anti-thyroid therapy.

E. Symptomatic Terms:

1. exophthalmos — abnormal protrusion of the eyeballs.

2. hirsutism — excessive growth of hair.

3. hyperkinesia, hyperkinesis — hypermotility, abnormally increased motility.

4. malignant exophthalmos — excessive protrusion of the eyeballs which fails to respond to treatment and leads to loss of sight.

5. paroxysmal hypertension — sudden recurrence of high blood pressure after a remission. It may be caused by conditions of the adrenal gland.

6. postural hypertension — high blood pressure associated with changes in posture.
7. pressor effect — stimulating effect.
8. proptosis — forward displacement of the globes in the orbit, same as exophthalmos.
9. virilism — masculinization in women.
10. vitiligo — white patches on the skin of the hands and feet. They may be seen in hyperthyroidism.

METABOLIC DISEASES

A. Origin of Terms:

1. keton (G) — ketone
2. melano- (G) — black
3. meli, melit (G) — honey
4. metabole (G) — change
5. porphyr- (G) — purple
6. tophus (L) — porous stone

B. Diagnostic Terms:

1. acid-base imbalance — disturbance in acid-base balance of the blood concerned with carbon dioxide (carbonic acid) as the acid component and bicarbonate as the base component of the equation. As a result abnormal changes develop in the carbon dioxide tension (Pco_2) and hydrogen ion concentration (pH). Lungs and kidneys play major roles in:
   a. metabolic acidosis — primary alkali deficit characterized by a low pH and Pco_2. It occurs in Addison's disease, starvation, diarrhea, renal and liver diseases, overtreatment with acids, etc.
   b. metabolic alkalosis — primary alkali excess marked by increased pH and Pco_2. It is caused by excessive loss of acid, gastric suction, potassium deficit, Cushing's syndrome, overtreatment with alkaline salts, etc.
   c. respiratory acidosis — primary CO_2 excess, low pH and high Pco_2 indicative of impaired gaseous exchange and hypoventilation resulting in carbon dioxide retention. It may develop in overdepression of respiratory center, lung disease and heart failure.
   d. respiratory alkalosis — primary CO_2 deficit, high pH and low Pco_2 present in hyperventilation. It is seen in overstimulation of respiratory center, high altitudes, fever, hysteria and anxiety.[19, 96]
2. alkalosis — abnormal increase of alkalinity in the blood.
3. carcinoid syndrome, carcinoidosis — peculiar metabolic disorder characterized by flushing, diarrhea, dyspnea and valvular heart disease. The symptoms are related to an overproduction of serotonin by the malignant carcinoid tumor of the gastrointestinal tract, usually the terminal ileum. Metastases to the liver and adjacent lymphnodes may occur.[4, 107]
4. diabetes insipidus — metabolic disorder due to hyposecretion of the antidiuretic hormone of the pituitary gland. Its clinical manifestations are polydipsia and polyuria.[65]
5. diabetes mellitus — a chronic metabolic disease genetically determined and in its advanced stage clinically manifested in a nonstressed patient by fasting hyperglycemia, ketoacidosis, atherosclerotic and microvascular pathologic changes, protein breakdown and neuropathies.[31, 13, 33, 91, 30, 82, 42, 15, 3, 11, 109, 110, 23, 5, 57]
6. galactosemia — inborn error of carbohydrate metabolism resulting in an incapacity for metabolizing galactose. Consequently galactose blood levels increase abnormally and galactose may be present in the urine. The neonate is normal. Gastrointestinal disorders, ascites, cirrhosis, proteinuria, mental retardation and cataracts develop in infancy if galactose is not eliminated from the diet.[12]

7. gout, gouty arthritis — disorder of purine metabolism and recurrent form of arthritis manifested by an abnormal increase of uric acid in the blood, tophi, joint involvement and in severe cases uric acid nephrolithiasis or renal failure.[87]

8. lipidosis, pl. lipidoses — any disorder noted for abnormally increased lipid concentrations in tissues.
   According to Fredrickson metabolic lipid disorders comprise:
   a. abnormal plasma lipoprotein concentrations including
      (1) hyperlipoproteinemia — 5 types
      (2) hypolipoproteinemia — 4 disorders
   b. primary tissue lipid storage diseases.
   c. granulomatous diseases with lipid storage.
   d. xanthomas.
   e. adipose tissue disorders.[36, 112, 60, 37, 10, 63, 62]
   The complexity of the subject matter precludes the definition of terms.   For Frederickson's classic exposition of disorders of lipid metabolism see *Harrison's Principles of Internal Medicine*, 6th ed., 1970, pp. 629-639.

9. metabolic stone disease — nephrolithiasis classified according to etiology.   Kidney stones may form in hypercalcemia states, renal tubular syndromes, hyperuricemia, defective enzyme metabolism and other disorders.[101]

10. obesity — excess of adipose tissue which presents a potential risk to good health.   The metabolic factor causing obesity may be the steroid excess of glucocorticoids in Cushing's syndrome.   Since obese persons usually have hypertriglyceridemia and hypercholesterolemia they are more prone to develop atherosclerosis, hypertension and diabetes mellitus than nonobese persons.[39]

11. phenylketonuria — hereditary metabolic disorder causing mental retardation.   Phenylketone bodies are found in serum and urine.   The disease is due to an inborn error of amino acid metabolism.

12. porphyria — inborn faulty porphyrin metabolism resulting in porphyrinuria.
    a. congenital, erythropoietic type — porphyria characterized by skin lesions due to photosensitivity from porphyrin in subcutaneous tissues.
    b. hepatic intermittent acute type — porphyria noted for liver damage, brownish pigmentation of the skin and neurological symptoms.[93]

13. Wolman's disease — rare familial xanthomatosis characterized by punctuate calcium deposits throughout the enlarged adrenal glands, hepatosplenomegaly and visceral foam cells filled with triglyceride and cholesterol.   The disease is lethal.[84]

14. xanthomatosis — a widespread eruption of xanthomas on the skin and tendons.   The xanthomas are yellow, lipid-containing plaques which are usually associated with hyperlipoproteinemia.[36]

C. Symptomatic Terms:

1. exacerbation — aggravation of symptoms.
2. glycosuria — the presence of sugar in the urine.
3. hyperchloremia — excessive chloride concentration in the circulating blood.
4. hypercholesterolemia — excessive cholesterol concentration in the circulating blood.
5. hyperchylomicronemia — excessive chylomicron concentration in the circulating blood.
6. hyperglycemia — excessive sugar concentration in the circulating blood.
7. hyperkalemia — excessive potassium concentration in the circulating blood.
8. hypernatremia — excessive sodium concentration in the circulating blood.
9. hypertriglyceridemia — excessive triglyceride concentration in the circulating blood.
10. hyperuricemia — excessive uric acid concentration in the circulating blood.[87]
11. hyponatremia — abnormally low serum sodium level due to a disturbed ratio of water to sodium.[34]

12. ketosis — excess ketone bodies in the body fluids and tissues due to incomplete combustion of fatty acids which may result from a faulty or absent utilization of carbohydrates. Ketosis may produce severe acidosis. It develops in uncontrolled diabetes mellitus and starvation.[73]
13. Kussmaul breathing — classic manifestation in diabetic acidosis marked by unusually deep respirations associated with dyspnea. This type of breathing is due to an abnormally increased acid content of the blood resulting in continuous overstimulation of the respiratory center.
14. melanosis — black pigments deposited in body tissues.
15. polydipsia — excessive thirst.
16. polyphagia — overeating.
17. remission — symptoms decreased in severity.
18. steatorrhea — excess fecal fat due to malabsorption of lipids, enzyme deficiency of pancreas, or intestinal disease.[89]
19. tophi (sing. tophus) — sodium biurate deposits near a joint. Condition is peculiar to gout.

HORMONAL DISORDERS AND CYTOGENETICS

A. Origins of Terms:

1. acro- (G) — extremity
2. centre (G) — center
3. chroma (G) — color
4. cyto- (G) — cell
5. gamete (G) — spouse
6. gen (G) — to produce
7. idio- (G) — distinct
8. karyo- (G) — nucleus
9. mitos (G) — thread
10. mono- (G) — single
11. mutant (G) — to change
12. ovum (G) — egg
13. soma (G) — body
14. sperm (G) — seed
15. spermato (G) — to sow seed
16. syndrome (G) — running together

B. Cytogenetic Terms:[102, 98, 18, 29]

1. acrocentric — centromere located at one end.
2. autosome, autosomal chromosome — nonsex chromosome.
3. centromere — constriction in center of chromosome.
4. chromosomal aberration — abnormality of chromosomes.
   a. acquired — developed after birth as in chronic myeloid leukemia.
   b. congenital — present in the fertilized ovum as in mongolism.
   c. monosomy — pertaining to absence of one chromosome as in Turner's syndrome — XO.
   d. trisomy — chromosome found in triplicate as in mongolism.
5. chromatin — deoxyribonucleic acid, known as DNA, found in chromosomes and stainable by basic dyes.
6. chromosome — threadlike body of chromatin in cell nucleus. Chromosomes are bearers of hereditary substances, called genes. Normally the number of chromosomes for each species remains constant. At present chromosomes have become the prime target of genetic investigation.
7. cytogenetics — branch of science concerned with the origin and development of cells in heredity.
8. DNA - deoxyribonucleic acid — chromosomal material thought to transmit hereditary characteristics, currently subject to intense research.
9. dominant — pertaining to a gene which exerts its effect even in the presence of a contrasting or opposite gene.
10. equatorial plate — same as metaphase plate.
11. gamete — mature germ cell, sperm or ovum.
12. gene — basic unit of heredity found at a definite locus (place) on a particular chromosome. There may be thousands of genes to one DNA molecule.

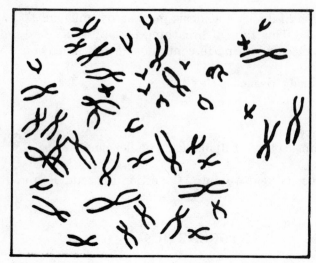

Fig. 62 – Chromosomes from a normal human male cell, grown in tissue culture and arrested at the metaphase.

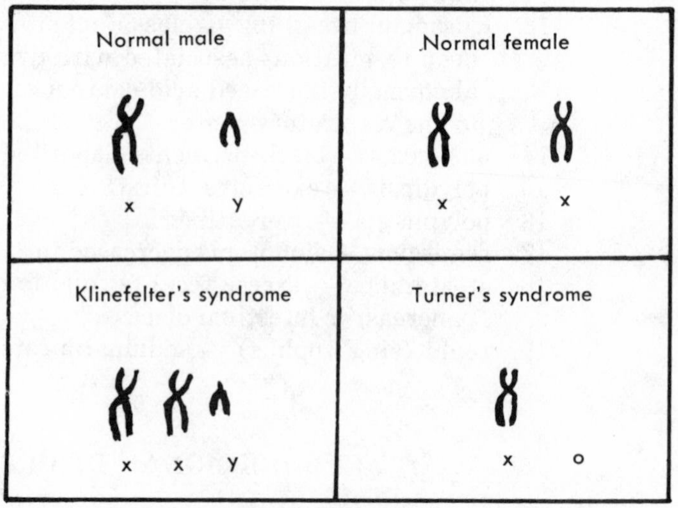

Normal male	Normal female
x y	x x
Klinefelter's syndrome	Turner's syndrome
x x Y	x o

Fig. 63 – Human sex chromosomes, normal pattern and chromosomal aberrations.

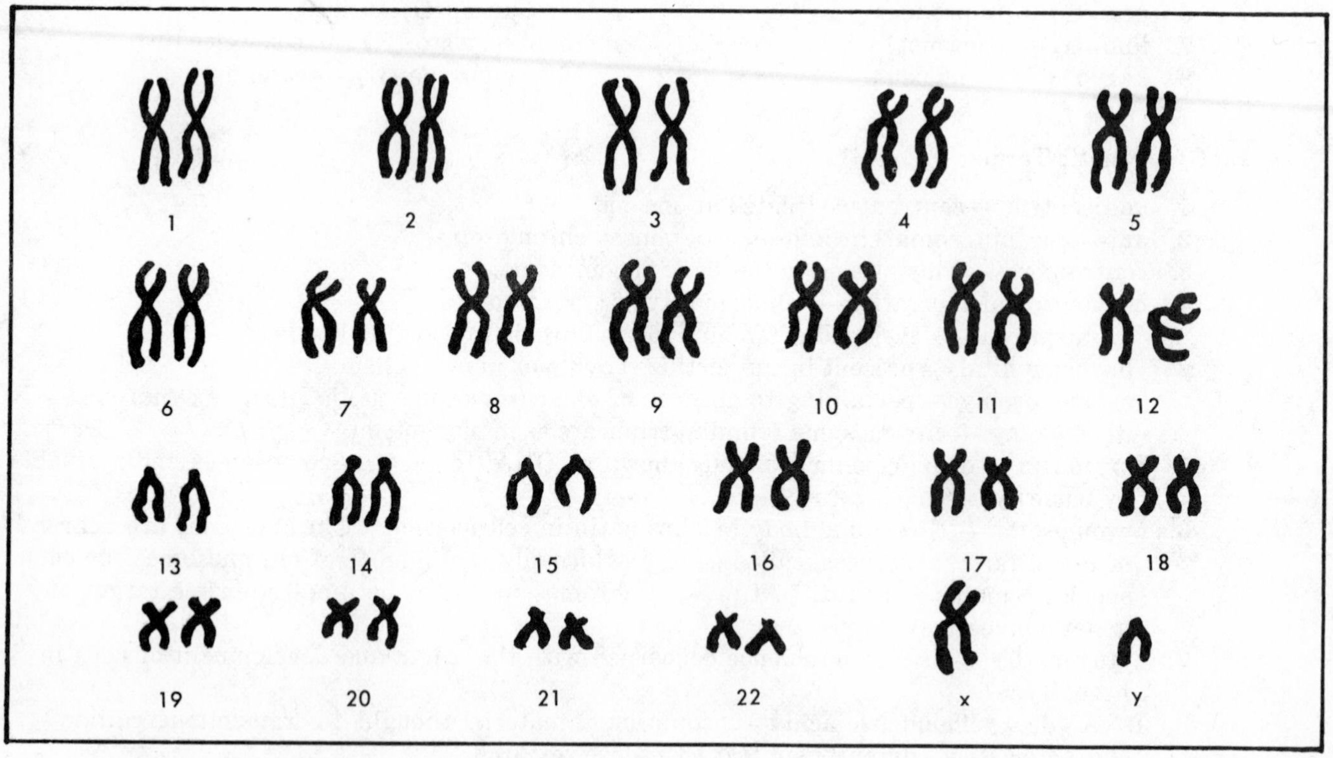

1	2	3	4	5
6	7	8	9	10	11	12
13	14	15	16	17	18
19	20	21	22	x	y

Fig. 64 – Karyotype or idiogram of a normal human male. It was constructed from fig. 62.

(Sister Leo Rita Volk, SSM. Cytogenetic Research Laboratory
St. Mary's Health Center, St. Louis, Missouri)

13. genotype — genetic constitution irrespective of external appearance.
14. idiogram — a diagram representing the karyotype (chromosome pattern) of the cells of an individual.
15. karyotype — a group of characteristics as form, number and size used to identify an individual's chromosomal pattern. A karyotype of a normal person has 46 chromosomes including 22 autosomal pairs and 2 sex chromosomes. They are arranged and numbered according to the 1961 International Classification System of Denver, Colorado. This is known as karyotyping.
16. metaphase — chromosomes lying on equatorial plate.
17. mitosis — process of cell division.
18. mutation — change occurring in genes.
19. phenotype — apparent type with visible characteristics which may be independent of genotype (hereditary type).
20. recessive — pertaining to a gene which is ineffective in the presence of contrasting or opposite genes.
21. sex chromosomes — those determining the sex of offspring; XX for female, XY for male.
22. X-chromosome — sex chromosome normally found in male and female.
23. Y-chromosome — sex chromosome present in male.

C. Diagnostic Terms:

1. Klinefelter's syndrome, seminiferous tubule dysgenesis — inherited disorder in which chromosomal aberration results in sterility due to defective embryonic development of the seminiferous tubules. The symptom complex comprises various degrees of
   a. aspermia or oligospermia — lack or scanty secretion of semen.
   b. eunuchoidism — sparsity of hair on face and body, female voice.
   c. gynecomastia — overdevelopment of the mammary glands in the male.
   d. hypoplasia of testes, hypogonadism — small, firm testes.
   Mental retardation and psychiatric disorders are common.[48, 75, 105]
2. Turner's syndrome, gonadal dysgenesis, ovarian dysgenesis — a complex inherited disorder caused by chromosomal aberration. Constant clinical signs are rudimentary ovaries composed of a fibrotic streak in each broad ligament and infertility. The classical syndrome includes different degrees of
   a. estrogen deficiency — inadequate secretion of female hormones.
   b. hypomastia — abnormally small breasts.
   c. malformations — structural defects such as dwarfism, shieldlike chest, webbed neck, coarctation of the aorta and others.
   d. true primary amenorrhea — absence of menses.[48, 69, 28]

Table 19
CYTOGENETIC STUDIES*

Chromosomal Findings	Normal Male	Normal Female	Klinefelter's Syndrome	Turner's Syndrome
Chromosome count	46	46	47	45
Chromosomal pattern	XY	XX	XXY	XO
Chromatin nuclear sex	Chromatin negative	Chromatin positive	Chromatin positive — genetic female	Chromatin negative — genetic male
Major clinical signs	Proper size and function	Proper size and function	Testicular hypoplasia Sterility	Ovarian hypoplasia Infertility

* Cf. Sir Eric Riches (ed.) *Modern Trends in Urology.* London: Butterworths, 1960, pp. 255-261. Other chromosomal patterns and chromatin nuclear sex have been reported, less frequently.

RADIOLOGY

A. Terms Related to Radiography:

1. radiogram of the soft tissues of the neck — method of demonstrating compression of the trachea and calcification within a thyroid neoplasm.[2, 14, 61]
2. radiogram of adrenals — method of obtaining radiological evidence of adrenal calcifications of tumors. Abdominal x-ray films, urography and planigraphy may be used.[1, 84]

B. Terms Related to Radiotherapy:

1. neuroblastomas of adrenal medulla — these tumors are considered radiosensitive and radiocurable.[9]
2. thyroid tumors — these neoplasms respond well to radiotherapy.[83]

CLINICAL LABORATORY

A. Terms Primarily Related to Endocrine Function Studies:

1. adrenal gland:
   a. adrenal cortex — outer portion of adrenal gland. The cortex produces many steroid hormones including 3 major groups:
      (1) steroids controlling the salt and water metabolism.
          Example — aldosterone.
      (2) steroids regulating the glucose metabolism and promoting gluconeogenesis.
          Example — hydrocortisone.
      (3) steroids affecting androgenic activity.
          Example — androsterone.
   b. adrenal medulla — inner portion of adrenal gland which secretes adrenalin (epine-phrin) and noradrenalin (norepinephrin).
   c. aldosterone — potent salt-retaining hormone of adrenal cortex which affects electrolyte balance.
   d. aldosterone in urine — quantitative measurement of aldosterone excreted in urine.
      Normal values
      urinary aldosterone level .... 2-23 micrograms in 24 hours.
      Increase in primary and secondary aldosteronism, nephrosis with edema, congestive heart failure with edema, hepatic cirrhosis with ascites and in the second and third trimesters of normal pregnancy.[25, 52]
   e. catecholamines in urine — determination of pressor amines, primarily the excretion of adrenalin and noradrenalin.
      Normal values — Method of DuToit
      adrenalin .... below 10 micrograms in 24 hour urine.
      noradrenalin .... below 100 micrograms in 24 hour urine.
      Increase in pheochromocytoma excretion in 24 hour urine 10-100 times more than normal.
      Results vary with physical exercise.[20, 25]
   f. corticoids — steroid hormones secreted by the adrenal cortex.
   g. 17-hydrocorticosteroids
      Normal values — Method of Porter-Silber
      17-OH corticoids in men.... urine ...... 5-15 milligrams in 24 hours.
      17-OH corticoids in women.. urine ...... 5-13 milligrams in 24 hours.
      17-OH corticoids in men.... blood ...... 9-28 micrograms in 100 ml.
      17-OH corticoids in women.. blood ...... 8-25 micrograms in 100 ml.
      Increase usually in Cushing's syndrome, in marked stress, acute pancreatitis and in eclampsia.
      Decrease in hypopituitarism and Addison's disease.[52]

h. 17-ketosteroids in urine — in men measurement of the metabolites of the adreno-cortical steroids, adrenal and gonadal androgens; in women and children primarily measurement of adrenal gland secretion. The levels of the 17-KS in urine aid in the detection of endocrine disorders.

Normal values — Method of Vestergaard

17-KS excretion in men.... urine ..... 8.0-15.0 milligrams in 24 hours.

17-KS excretion in women.. urine ..... 6.0-11.5 milligrams in 24 hours.

Increase in adrenocortical tumor especially if malignant, interstitial neoplasm of testes, adrenogenital syndrome and occasionally in Cushing's disease.

Decrease in Addison's disease and myxedema.[52]

i. Thorn ACTH test — an ACTH stimulation test which measures adrenocortical reserve. Eosinophil counts are done before and usually 4 hours following the administration of an adrenal stimulant.[84]

2. thyroid gland:

Tests have been developed to measure microquantities of iodine chemically and radiologically in order to determine thyroid function. The thyroid gland synthesizes iodine into thyroid hormones, primarily into thyroxine. Free iodine combines with a protein to form thyroglobulin which is stored in the thyroid gland. The thyroid hormone which circulates in the blood is loosely combined with serum protein.

a. protein-bound iodine PBI — test measures the amount of thyroid hormone circulating in the blood.

Normal values — Method of Barker

PBI .... 3.5-8 micrograms per 100 ml.

Increase in hyperthyroidism, acute thyroiditis, and some malignant neoplasms of thyroid gland.

Decrease in hypothyroidism, myxedema and cretinism.[16]

Other tests are presented in Chapter XX.

B. Terms Primarily Related to Metabolic Studies:

1. basal metabolic rate — measurement of number of calories needed for the support of basic metabolic functions such as respiration, circulation, body temperature in a resting individual. The normal range is from −10 to +10 per cent.

2. blood sugar level — concentration of glucose in the blood.

3. calcitonin — a polypeptide, probably a thyroid secretion which reduces both the calcium and phosphate levels of plasma.[73]

4. carbohydrate tolerance tests:

a. cortisone-glucose tolerance test — the administration of cortisone acetate prior to a standard glucose tolerance test to detect subclinical diabetes or predict diabetic risks in members of families of diabetics.[58]

b. glucose tolerance tests — the intravenous or oral administration of a measured glucose load to discover disorders of carbohydrate metabolism.

Normal values — the true blood sugar method

fasting blood sugar .... below 100 milligrams/100 ml.

peak level .... below 160 milligrams/100 ml.

two hour value .... below 120 milligrams/100 ml.

Diabetes mellitus

peak level .... above 160 milligrams/100 ml.

two hour value .... above 120 milligrams/100 ml.[79]

c. postprandial blood sugar determination — a screening procedure for the detection of diabetes mellitus. Blood to determine sugar content is drawn 2 hours after the patient started to eat a meal containing 50-100 gm of carbohydrates.

Normal value — the true blood sugar method

blood sugar .... below 100 milligrams/100 ml.

Increase in hyperglycemia

blood sugar .... above 100 milligrams/100 ml.

Decrease in hypoglycemia

blood sugar .... below 60 milligrams/100 ml.[79]

d. tolbutamide (orinase) tolerance tests — the intravenous or oral administration of tolbutamide sodium to determine the presence or absence of diabetes mellitus when the standard glucose tolerance test fails to provide relevant results. Other indications are (1) hepatic disease, as a means of distinguishing hepatogenic from insulin deficient carbohydrate abnormalities, (2) pancreatic disease and (3) insulin-secreting pancreatic islet cell tumors or insulomas.[58, 79, 111]

5. carbon dioxide combining power — a test for determining the acid-base balance in the blood. In health and with normal activity the acid waste products of metabolism exceed the basic. (See Table 20 for specific information.)

Table 20

SOME ESSENTIAL TESTS IN METABOLIC DISORDERS

Test	Normal Values[a]	Increased Values	Decreased Values
Blood Sugar—fasting Adults—Folin-Wu Adults—True Newborns—True	80-120 mg/100 ml 60-100 mg/100 ml 30- 50 mg/100 ml	Diabetes mellitus Hypoinsulinism Hyperpituitarism Hyperthyroidism	Insulin effect Hyperinsulinism Hypopituitarism Addison's disease Hypothyroidism
CO₂ capacity Adults Infants	53-70 vol. % or 24-32 mEq/L 40-55 vol. % or 18-25 mEq/L	Alkalosis Hypercortico-adrenalism Excessive alkali therapy Respiratory conditions	Acidosis Diabetes Nephritis Eclampsia Severe diarrhea

[a] Cf. Opal E. Hepler. *Manual of Clinical Laboratory Methods*, 4th ed. Springfield, Illinois: Charles C. Thomas, 1955, p. 296.

6. Congo-red test — intravenous dye test valuable in the diagnosis of secondary amyloidosis.

Normal value — Method of Unger

retention of Congo-red in serum exceeds 60% of dye.

Decrease under 20% retention is strongly suggestive of amyloidosis.[80]

7. 5-HIAA — simple test measuring the urinary excretion of 5-hydroxyindole acetic acid, a metabolic product of serotonin. A marked increase is diagnostic of metastatic carcinoid. Further confirmatory evidence is provided by elevated serotonin blood levels.

Normal values —Method of Sjoerdsma

5-HIAA .... 2 - 10 mg urinary excretion in 24 hours.

In metastatic carcinoidosis .... 50 - 600 mg urinary excretion in 24 hours.

Normal values

serotonin blood levels .... 0.1 - 0.3 μg (micrograms) per ml.

In metastatic carcinoidosis .... 0.5 - 3.0 μg (micrograms) per ml.[81, 4, 99]

8. glucose tolerance — according to Allen: the more sugar a healthy person takes, the more he utilizes. The reverse is true of the diabetic.

9. insulin resistance — tolerance to high daily dosage (200 units) due to obesity or to the development of antibodies which bind insulin.

10. insulin tolerance test — the intravenous administration of regular or crystalline insulin to detect the presence of insulin resistance in patients with a tentative diagnosis of acromegaly or Cushing's syndrome.

Normal value — return to pre-injection level within 90 to 120 minutes.

Increase — prolonged fall, sometimes associated with hypoglycemic symptoms, indicative of abnormal sensitivity to insulin.

Decrease — lesser fall suggestive of insulin resistance.[58, 79]

11. Kepler water test — chemical test for Addison's disease based on urinary volumes, blood and urine chlorides and urea nitrogen determination.

12. ketone bodies — acetone bodies, products of faulty metabolism in diabetic acidosis. Since sugar is not utilized normally in diabetes mellitus, excessive fat is mobilized and employed in energy production. Other clinical states characterized by faulty fat metabolism which result in ketoacidosis are starvation, prolonged diarrhea and vomiting, von Gierke's disease, etc.

In ketoacidosis ketone bodies accumulate in the blood (ketonemia) and are excreted in the urine (ketonuria).

Ketone body determination:

Normal value

no ketone bodies in blood and urine.

Ketoacidosis

serum ketone test (serum acetone test) .... above 2.0 mg/100 ml.

urine ketone test (Acetest or Ketostix) .... purple color reaction with diacetic acid 5 - 10 mg/100 ml.

13. lipids — a group of organic substances, mostly composed of carbon, hydrogen and some oxygen. Lipids may also contain nitrogen and phosphorus. They are soluble in hydrocarbon and ether and insoluble in water.

Normal values — serum lipids

total lipids .... 400 - 800 mg/100 ml.
cholesterol .... 115 - 340 mg/100 ml.
triglycerides .... 10 - 190 mg/100 ml.
phospholipids .... 150 - 380 mg/100 ml.
fatty acids .... 9 - 15 mM/liter.
neutral fat .... 0 - 200 mg/100 ml.
phospholipid-P .... 8 - 11 mg/100 ml.[25]

14. lipoproteins — lipids and proteins combined. Lipids alone cannot enter the circulation, but lipoproteins can be transported by the blood stream. They comprise:

a. alpha lipoproteins — tiny particles containing much protein. They do not predispose to atherosclerosis.

b. beta lipoproteins — particles very small, cholesterol content high predisposing to atherosclerosis.

c. pre-beta lipoproteins — particles are relatively large and appear to be active in the transport of triglycerides.

d. chylomicrons — large particles present in serum during digestion of fat-containing foods. They disappear from serum 12 hours after the meal.[51, 21, 41]

Table 21

SERUM TRIGLYCERIDES AND CHOLESTEROL IN HYPERLIPOPROTEINEMIAS[a]

Phenotypes	Some Lipids in Health and Disease	Appearance of Serum	Triglycerides mg/100 ml	Cholesterol mg/100 ml
. . .	Health	. . .	25- 150	150- 300
Type I	Hyperlipemia, fat induced Hyperglyceridemia Familial hyperchylomicron- emia	Lactescence (milky appearance)	1000-2000	250- 500
Type II	Hypercholesterolemia Hereditary xanthomatosis Essential familial choles- terolemia	. . .	150- 500	300-1800

Phenotypes	Some Lipids in Health and Disease	Appearance of Serum	Triglycerides mg/100 ml	Cholesterol mg/100 ml
Type III	Hyperglyceridemia Hyperlipemia, carbohydrate induced Hypercholesterolemia	Turbid	175-1500	200-1400
Type IV	Hyperglyceridemia, carbohydrate induced without hypercholesteremia	Turbid	175-1500	250- 500
Type V	Hyperglyceridemia, fat and carbohydrate induced	Turbid or milky	175-1500	300-1500

a Adapted from Israel Davidsohn and J. Bernard Henry. *Clinical Diagnosis by Laboratory Methods*, 14th ed. Philadelphia: W. B. Saunders Co., 1969, pp. 564-565.

15. metabolite — any product of metabolism, for example, the mineral metabolites: sodium, potassium and chloride which are profoundly influenced by the activity of the adrenal cortex.

   a. chloride salts are chiefly bound to sodium. In the gastric juice chlorides are present in the form of hydrochloride.
      Normal values — Method of Schales
      serum chloride . . . . 100 - 106 mEq/L.
      Increase in many conditions resulting from decreased excretion or increased intake.[20]

   b. potassium salts, as potassium chloride, phosphates and bicarbonates, are found within tissue cells, especially in muscle cells and blood plasma.
      Normal values — Method: Flame photometer
      serum potassium . . . . 3.5 - 5 mEq/L.
      Increase in Addison's disease.
      Decrease in Cushing's syndrome.[20]

   c. sodium salts, in the form of sodium chloride and sodium bicarbonate, are present in the blood plasma and extracellular fluids.
      Normal values — Method: Flame photometer
      serum sodium . . . . 136 - 145 mEq/L.
      Increase in Cushing's syndrome.
      Decrease in Addison's disease.

16. osmolality — solute concentration per unit of water, usually expressed in milliosmols per liter of a solution (mOsm/L).
   Normal values — serum osmolality . . . . 285 - 295 mOsm/L.

17. phenotype — the external expression of the genetic constitution of an organism.

18. transferrin — a glycoprotein which transports iron in plasma.

19. triglycerides — simple or neutral fats composed of 3 molecules of fatty acid that are esterified to glycerin.[73]

C. Terms Related to Cytogenetic Tests for Chromosomal Sex Determination:[29, 45]

1. biopsy of human skin — this is a microscopic examination of a small piece of epithelium to detect characteristic chromatin masses alongside the nuclear membrane in somatic cells. They are usually only found in females.

2. buccal or oral smear test, sex chromatin test, Barr test of nuclear sex — a stained smear of epithelial cells, scraped from the mucosa of the cheek, is studied under the microscope for chromatin bodies. Normally males are chromatin negative and females chromatin positive.

3. leukocyte cell smear from peripheral blood — a cytologic test for chromosomal sex differentiation. A small number of circulating neutrophils possess a characteristic drumstick chromatin attachment distinguishable from the remaining nucleus. This drumstick formation on the cell nucleus has not been found in males.

4. tissue culture of human cells — new method of culturing permits growth without chromosomal disorganization. Tissue is cultured in vitro to obtain sufficient mitoses. The culture is treated with colchicine to arrest mitosis in metaphase and with hypotonic saline to attain spreading of the chromosomes. Preparations are then squashed, stained and photographed under a microscope. The photomicrograph is enlarged and the chromosomes cut out and paired to make a karyotype.[17, 16]

ABBREVIATIONS

ACTH — adenocorticotrophic hormone
ADH — antidiuretic hormone
ATP — adenosine triphosphate
BEI — butonal extractable iodine
BMR — basal metabolic rate
CO_2 — carbon dioxide
CRF — corticotrophin releasing factor
CZI — crystalline zinc insulin
DOC — deoxycorticosterine
ECF — extracellular fluid
EFA — essential fatty acids
FBS — fasting blood sugar
FFA — free fatty acids
FSH — follicle stimulating hormone
FTI — free thyroxine index
GTT — glucose tolerance test
ICF — intracellular fluid

ICSH — interstitial cell stimulating hormone
IF — interstitial fluid
K — potassium
LATS — long-acting thyroid stimulator
LH — luteinizing hormone
MSH — melanocyte-stimulating hormone
NaCl — sodium chloride
NPH — neutral protein Hagedorn (insulin)
PBI — protein-bound iodine
PGH — pituitary growth hormone
PP — postprandial
PZI — protamine zinc insulin
17-KS — 17 ketosteroids
17-OH — 17 hydroxycorticoids
TSH — thyroid stimulating hormone
TTH — thyrotrophic hormone

ORAL READING PRACTICE

Hypothyroidism

Hypothyroidism is a functional disorder caused by insufficiency of the circulating thyroid hormones. Any biological, chemical or physical factors which reduce the hormone supply may result in thyroid failure.

In primary hypothyroid states the condition may be congenital as in **cretinism,** or acquired as in juvenile **myxedema** or adult myxedema. Surgical excision, atrophy or disease of the thyroid gland stop or lower hormone production and a lack of iodine in food seriously hampers hormone synthesis.

In secondary hypothyroid states the pituitary gland elaborates an inadequate amount of the thyroid stimulating hormone (TSH) which drastically reduces thyroid function. This deficit of **thyrotrophin (TSH)** occurs in **postpartum pituitary necrosis** or Sheehan's disease and primary chronic hypopituitarism or Simmond's syndrome. A total absence of TSH is seen in **hypophysectomized** patients.

The judicious use of replacement therapy with **thyroxine** or **triiodothyronine** in **thyroid** failure and a thyrotrophin preparation in pituitary failure is imperative to maintain relatively normal metabolic processes and overcome hypothyroidism.[6]

Table 22

SOME ENDOCRINE CONDITIONS AMENABLE TO SURGERY

Organs Involved	Diagnoses	Operations	Operative procedures
Adrenal gland	Adenoma of the adrenal cortex, unilateral, anterior to kidney	Unilateral adrenalectomy with excision of neoplasm	Abdominal approach with preliminary exploration of ovaries in the female followed by removal of neoplasm
Adrenal gland	Cushing's syndrome associated with (1) psychosis (2) multiple bone fracture (3) severe diabetes	Subtotal adrenalectomy Bilateral adrenalectomy	Removal of one adrenal gland Removal of adrenals by the subdiaphragmatic route, transthoracic or transabdominal approach
Adrenal glands	Metastatic cancer of the breast	Bilateral adrenalectomy	Excision of both adrenals
Parathyroid	Parathyroid adenoma Hyperparathyroidism	Excision of adenoma of parathyroid gland	Removal of neoplasm to prevent recurrent renal calculi
Thyroid gland	Solitary thyroid nodule of unknown nature	Surgical exploration	Tissue from thyroid nodule removed — frozen section made
Thyroid gland	Hyperthyroidism-exophthalmic goiter	Partial or subtotal thyroidectomy	Removal of part of thyroid gland
Thyroid gland	Papillary carcinoma with metastases to adjacent lymph nodes	Complete or total thyroidectomy with neck dissection	Excision of entire thyroid gland with dissection of the upper portion of neck
Thyroid gland	Postthyroidectomy hemorrhage	Thyroidotomy	Reopening of thyroid wound for removal of hematoma and control of hemorrhage
Thymus gland	Myasthenia gravis	Sternotomy Thymectomy	Splitting the sternum and removal of thymus gland

REFERENCES AND BIBLIOGRAPHY

1. Ackerman, Lauren V. and del Regato, Juan A. Tumors of the suprarenal gland. In *Cancer Diagnosis Treatment and Prognosis*, 4th ed. St. Louis: The C. V. Mosby Co., 1970, pp. 691-712.

2. —————. Tumors of the thyroid gland. *Ibid.*, pp. 377-395.

3. Albrink, M. and Davidson, P. C. Dietary therapy and prophylaxis of vascular disease in diabetes. *Medical Clinics of North America*, 55: 877-897, July, 1971.

4. Almy, T. P. Disorders of motility — the carcinoid syndrome. In Beeson, Paul B. and McDermott, Walsh (eds.). *Cecil Loeb Txtbook of Medicine*, 13th ed. Philadelphia: W. B. Saunders Co., 1971, pp. 1234-1258.

5. Arky, R. A. Hypoglycemia in diabetes mellitus. *Medical Clinics of North America*, 55: 919-930, July, 1971.

6. Asper, S. P. Physiological approach to correction of hypothothyroidism. *Archives of Internal Medicine*, 107: 112-120, January, 1961.

7. Aurbach, G. D. Parathyroid. In Beeson, Paul B. and McDermott, Walsh (eds.). *Cecil-Loeb Textbook of Medicine*, 13th ed. Philadelphia: W. B. Saunders Co., 1971, pp. 1846-1855.

8. Ayromlooi, J. Congenital goiter due to maternal ingestion of iodides. *Obstetrics and Gynecology*, 39: 818-822, June, 1972.

9. Baker, G. Pheochromocytoma without hypertension presenting as cardiomyopathy. *American Heart Journal*, 83: 688-693, May, 1972.

10. Barclay, M. et al. Lipoproteins in cancer patients. *Ca — A Cancer Journal for Clinicians*. 21: 202-212, May-June, 1971.

11. Barker, W. F. Peripheral vascular disease in diabetes. *Medical Clinics of North America*, 55: 1045-1055, July, 1971.

12. Beutler, E. Galactosemia. In Beeson, Paul B. and McDermott, Walsh (eds.). *Cecil-Loeb Textbook of Medicine*, 13th ed. Philadelphia: W. B. Saunders Co., 1971, pp. 1659-1661.

13. Bondy, P. K. Diabetes mellitus. In Beeson, Paul B. and McDermott, Walsh (eds.). *Cecil-Loeb Textbook of Medicine*, 13th ed. Philadelphia: W. B. Saunders Co., 1971, pp. 1639-1656.

14. Bradley, E. L. Angiothyrography. A clinically useful diagnostic procedure. *Archives of Surgery*, 104: 662-666, May, 1972.

15. Bressler, R. and Galloway, J. A. Insulin treatment of diabetes mellitus. *Medical Clinics of North America*, 55: 861-876, July, 1971.

16. Cervenka, J. Prenatal sex determination. *Obstetrics and Gynecology*, 37: 912-915, June, 1971.

17. *Chemistry chromosomes and congenital anomalies.* New York: The National Foundation.

18. Chusid, Joseph G. Congenital defects. In *Correlative Neuroanatomy & Functional Neurology*, 14th ed. Los Altos, California: Lange Medical Publications, 1970, pp. 291-294.

19. Cohn, C. and Kaplan, A. Blood chemistry. In Miller, Seward E. and Weller, John M. (eds.). *Textbook of Clinical Pathology*, 8th ed. Baltimore: The Williams & Wilkins Co., 1971, pp. 235-278.

20. Conn, R. B. Normal laboratory values of clinical importance. In Beeson, Paul B. and McDermott, Walsh (eds.). *Cecil-Loeb Textbook of Medicine*, 13th ed. Philadelphia: W. B. Saunders Co., 1971, pp. 1914-1923.

21. Cox, M. and Wear, R. F. Campbell's soup program to prevent atherosclerosis. *American Journal of Nursing*, 72: 253-259, February, 1972.

22. Cross, J. N. *et al.* Treatment of acromegaly by cryosurgery. *Lancet*, 1: 215-216, January, 1972.

23. Danowski, T. S. Nonketotic coma and diabetes mellitus. *Medical Clinics of North America*, 55: 913-918, July, 1971.

24. Daughaday, W. H. The adenohypophysis. In Williams, Robert H. (ed.). *Textbook of Endocrinology*, 4th ed. Philadelphia: W. B. Saunders Co., 1968, pp. 27-84.

25. Davidsohn, Israel and Henry, J. Bernard (eds.). Tables of normal values. In *Todd-Sanford Clinical Diagnosis by Laboratory Methods*, 14th ed. Philadelphia: W. B. Saunders Co., 1969, pp. 1263-1271.

26. DeGroot, L. J. Diseases of the thyroid. In Beeson, Paul B. and McDermott, Walsh (eds.). *Cecil-Loeb Textbook of Medicine*, 13th ed. Philadelphia: W. B. Saunders Co., 1971, pp. 1753-1780.

27. Demura, R. *et al.* Responses of plasma ACTH, GH, LH and 11-hydroxycorticosteroids to various stimuli in patients with Cushing's syndrome. *Journal of Clinical Endocrinology and Metabolism*, 34: 852-859, May, 1972.

28. Durowski, W. P. *et al.* Unilateral ovarian dysgenesis with prenatal virilization. *Obstetrics and Gynecology*, 39: 842-849, June, 1972.

29. Eggen, R. R. Cytogenetics. In Davidson, Israel and Henry, John B. (eds.). *Todd-Sanford Clinical Diagnosis by Laboratory Methods*. 14th ed. Philadelphia: W. B. Saunders Co., 1969, pp. 1208-1240.

30. Emmer, M. *et al.* Diabetes in association with other endocrine disorders. *Medical Clinics of North America*, 55: 1057-1064, July, 1971.

31. Fajans, S. S. What is diabetes? Definition, diagnosis and course. *Medical Clinics of North America*, 55: 793-805, July, 1971.

32. Fajans, S. S. and Thorn, G. W. Hyperinsulinism, hypoglycemia and glucagon secretion. In Wintrobe, Maxwell M. *et al.* (eds.). *Harrison's Principles of Internal Medicine*, 6th ed. New York: McGraw-Hill Book Co., pp. 542-549.

33. Felig, P. Pathophysiology of diabetes mellitus. *Medical Clinics of North America*, 55: 821-834, July, 1971.

34. Finkel, R. M. Hyponatremia. *Medical Clinics of North America*, 56: 645-650, May, 1972.

35. Forshaw, P. H. and Melmon, K. L. The adrenals. In Williams, Robert H. (ed.). *Textbook in Endocrinology*, 4th ed. Philadelphia: W. B. Saunders Co., 1968, pp. 287-403.

36. Frederickson, D. S. Disorders of lipid metabolism and xanthomatosis. In Wintrobe, Maxwell M. *et al.* (eds.). *Harrison's Principles of Internal Medicine*, 6th ed. New York: McGraw-Hill Book Co., pp. 629-639.

37. Frederickson, D. S. *et al.* The Dietary Management of Hyperlipoproteinemia — A Handbook for Physicians. Bethesda, Maryland: National Institute of Health, 1970.

38. Gardner, Ernest, Gray, Donald and O'Rahilly, Ronan. *Anatomy — A Regional Study of Human Structure*, 3rd ed. Philadelphia: W. B. Saunders Co., 1969, pp. 612-703.

39. Gastineau, C. F. Obesity: risks, causes, and treatments. *Medical Clinics of North America*, 56: 1021-1028, July, 1972.

40. Giancarlo, H. R. Effect of ultrasonic hypophysectomy on diabetic retinopathy. *Laryngoscope*, 81: 452-464, March, 1971.

41. Glomset, J. A. and Williams, R. H. Lipid metabolism and lipopathies. In Williams, Robert H. (ed.). *Textbook of Endocrinology*, 4th ed. Philadelphia: W. B. Saunders Co., 1968, pp. 1039-1117.

42. Goetz, F. C. Management of adult-onset diabetes. The impact of the University Group Diabetes Program. *Postgraduate Medicine*, 52: 63-68, July, 1972.

43. Goldsmith, R. S. Treatment of hypercalcemia. *Medical Clinics of North America*, 56: 951-960, July, 1972.

44. Goldstein, G. Myasthenia gravis and the thymus. In DeGraff, Arthur C. *Annual Review of Medicine*, vol. 22. Palo Altos, California: Annual Reviews, Inc., 1971, pp. 119-124.

45. Gordon, H. Disease in families. *Postgraduate Medicine*, 52: 56-58, July, 1972.

46. Gordon, H. E. Surgical management of secondary hyperparathyroidism. *Archives of Surgery*, 104: 520-526, April, 1972.

47. Greene, J. N. Subacute thyroiditis. *Journal of Internal Medicine*, 51: 97-108, July, 1971.

48. Grumbach, M. M. Gonads. In Beeson, Paul B. and McDermott, Walsh (eds.). *Cecil-Loeb Textbook of Medicine*, 13th ed. Philadelphia: W. B. Saunders Co., 1971, pp. 1799-1832.

49. Hardy, J. Transsphenoidal hypophysectomy. *Journal of Neurosurgery*, 34: 582-594, April, 1971.

50. Hayles, A. B. and Cloutier, M. D. Clinical hypothyroidism in the young — a second look. *Medical Clinics of North America*, 56: 871-884, July, 1972.

51. Henry, J. B. Clinical chemistry. In Davidsohn, Israel and Henry, John B. (eds.). *Todd-Sanford Clinical Diagnosis by Laboratory Methods*, 14th ed. Philadelphia: W. B. Saunders Co., 1969, pp. 487-600.

52. Henry, J. B. and Krieg, A. F. Endocrine measurements. In Davidsohn, Israel and Henry, John B. (eds.). *Todd-Sanford Clinical Diagnosis by Laboratory Methods*, 14th ed. Philadelphia: W. B. Saunders Co., 1969, pp. 601-644.

53. Hoffman, D. L. *et al.* Treatment of adrenocortical carcinoma with o, p' -DDD. *Medical Clinics of North America*, 56: 999-1012, July, 1972.

54. Ingbar, S. H. and Woeber, K. A. The thyroid gland. In Williams, Robert H. (ed.). *Textbook of Endocrinology*, 4th ed. Philadelphia: W. B. Saunders Co., 1968, pp. 105-286.

55. Johnson, W. J. Prevention and treatment of progressive secondary hyperparathyroidism in advanced renal failure. *Medical Clinics of North America*, 56: 961-975, July, 1972.

56. Kelly, T. R. *et al.* Primary hyperparathyroidism at a community hospital. *American Journal of Surgery*, 123: 573-576, May, 1972.

57. Kimball, C. P. Emotional and psychosocial aspects of diabetes mellitus. *Medical Clinics of North America*, 55: 1007-1018, July, 1971.

58. Kolb, F. O. Endocrine disorders. In Krupp, Marcus A. and Chatton, Milton J. *Current Diagnosis & Treatment*, 11th ed. Los Altos, California: Lange Medical Publications, 1972, pp. 596-689.

59. Kolodny, H. D. *et al.* Acromegaly treated with chlorpromazine. *New England Journal of Medicine*, 284: 819-822, April 15, 1971.

60. Koppers, L. E. *et al.* Lipid disturbances in endocrine disorders. *Medical Clinics of North America*, 56: 1013-1020, July, 1972.

61. Kuntz, C. H. *et al.* Selective arteriography of parathyroid adenomas. *Radiology*, 102: 29-36, January, 1972.

62. Kuo, P. T. Hyperlipidemia in atherosclerosis. Dietary and drug treatment. *Medical Clinics of North America*, 54: 657-669, May, 1970.

63. LaRosa, J. C. Hyperlipoproteinemia. II. Dietary management. *Postgraduate Medicine*, 52: 75-79, July, 1972.

64. Leaf, A. and Coggins, C. H. The neurohypophysis. In Williams, Robert H. (ed.). *Textbook of Endocrinology*, 4th ed. Philadelphia: W. B. Saunders Co., 1968, pp. 85-103.

65. Leaf, A. Posterior pituitary. In Beeson, Paul B. and McDermott, Walsh, (eds.). *Cecil-Loeb Textbook of Medicine*, 13th ed. Philadelphia: W. B. Saunders Co., 1971, pp. 1748-1752.

66. Liddle, G. W. Adrenal cortex. In Beeson, Paul B. and McDermott, Walsh, (eds.). *Cecil-Loeb Textbook of Medicine*, 13th ed. Philadelphia: W. B. Saunders Co., 1971, pp. 1780-1799.

67. Maddy, J. A. *et al.* Cryohypophysectomy in the management of advanced prostatic cancer. *Cancer*, 28: 322-328, August, 1971.

68. Males, J. L. and Townsend, J. L. Acromegaly: an analysis of 20 cases. *Southern Medical Journal*, 65: 321-324, March, 1972.

69. McDonough, P. G. *et al.* Gonadal dysgenesis with ovarian function. Clinical and cytogenetic findings in 6 patients. *Obstetrics and Gynecology*, 37: 868-872, June, 1971.

70. McConahey, W. M. Hashimoto's thyroiditis. *Medical Clinics of North America*, 56: 885-896, July, 1972.

71. McKenney, J. F. *et al.* The variable nature of the thyroid nodule. *Surgical Clinics of North America*, 52: 383-396, April, 1972.

72. Melmon, K. L. The endocrinologic manifestations of the carcinoid tumor. In Williams, Robert H. (ed.). *Textbook of Endocrinology*, 4th ed. Philadelphia: W. B. Saunders Co., 1968, pp. 1161-1180.

73. Miller, Benjamin F. and Keane, C. Brackman. *Encyclopedia and Dictionary of Medicine and Nursing*. Philadelphia: W. B. Saunders Co., 1972.

74. Murphy, G. P. *et al.* Hypophysectomy and adrenalectomy for disseminated prostatic carcinoma. *Journal of Urology*, 105: 815-825, June, 1971.

75. Nichols, G. L. *et al.* Klinefelter's syndrome in identical twins with 46 XX chromosome constitution. *American Journal of Medicine*, 52: 482-491, April, 1972.

76. Novak, L. P. Effect of HGH on body composition of hypopituitary dwarfs. *Mayo Clinic Proceedings*, 47: 241-246, April, 1972.

77. Onofrio, B. M. Current trends in pituitary surgery. *Medical Clinics of North America*, 56: 909-914, July, 1972.

78. Page, Lot B. and Culver, Perry J. (eds.). Thyroid function tests. In *A Syllabus of Laboratory Examinations in Clinical Diagnosis*, 2nd ed. Cambridge, Massachusetts: Harvard University Press, 1962, pp. 475-485.

79. —————. Diseases of carbohydrate metabolism. *Ibid.*, pp. 466-474.

80. —————. Laboratory evaluation of inflammation and necrosis. *Ibid.*, pp. 250-264 and p. 6.

81. —————. Examination of the urine. *Ibid.*, pp. 325-326.

82. Prout, T. E. A prospective view of the treatment of adult-onset diabetes. *Medical Clinics of North America*, 55: 1065-1075, July, 1971.

83. Qazi, Q. H. Genital changes in congenital virilizing adrenal hyperplasia. *Journal of Pediatrics*, 80: 653-654, April, 1972.

84. Queloz, J. M. *et al.* Wolman's disease. *Radiology*, 104: 357-359, August, 1972.

85. Raker, J. W. Surgery of the adrenal glands. In Welsh, Claude E. *et al.* (eds). *Advances in Surgery*, vol. 5. Chicago: Year Book Medical Publishers, Inc., 1971, pp. 129-144.

86. Rasmussen, H. The parathyroids. In Williams, Robert H. (eds.). *Textbook of Endocrinology*, 4th ed. Philadelphia: W. B. Saunders Co., 1968, pp. 847-965.

87. Rastegar, A. *et al.* The physiologic approach to hyperuricemia. *New England Journal of Medicine*, 286: 470-476, March 2, 1972.

88. Rayfield, E. J. *et al.* Small cell tumors of the thyroid. A clinicopathologic study. *Cancer*, 28: 1023-1030, October, 1971.

89. Rogers, A. I. Steatorrhea. *Postgraduate Medicine*, 50: 123-129, December, 1971.

90. Reichlin, S. Neuroendocrinology. In Williams, Robert H. (ed.). *Textbook of Endocrinology*, 4th ed. Philadelphia: W. B. Saunders Co., 1968, pp. 967-1016.

91. Rimoin, D. L. Inheritance in diabetes mellitus. *Medical Clinics of North America*, 55: 807-819, July, 1971.

92. Rhoton, A. L. Microneurosurgery of the pituitary gland. *Medical Clinics of North America*, 56: 915-930, July, 1972.

93. Schmid, R. Porphyria. In Beeson, Paul B. and McDermott, Walsh (eds.). *Cecil-Loeb Textbook of Medicine*, 13th ed. Philadelphia: W. B. Saunders Co., 1971, pp. 1704-1709.

94. Scholz, D. A. *et al.* Diagnostic considerations in hypercalcemic syndromes. *Medical Clinics of North America*, 56: 941-950, July, 1972.

95. Schoonees, R. *et al.* Bilateral adrenalectomy for advanced prostatic carcinoma. *Journal of Urology*, 108: 123-125, July, 1972.

96. Schwartz, W. B. Disorders of fluid, electrolyte and acid-base balance. In Beeson, Paul B. and McDermott, Walsh (eds.). *Cecil-Loeb Textbook of Medicine*, 13th ed. Philadelphia: W. B. Saunders Co., 1971, pp. 1618-1639.

97. Selenkow, H. A. and Sugbar, S. H. Diseases of the thyroid. In Wintrobe, Maxwell M. et al. (eds.). *Harrison's Principles of Internal Medicine*, 6th ed. New York: McGraw-Hill Book Co., pp. 444-465.

98. Seely, J. R. The role of chromosome analysis in practice. *Postgraduate Medicine*, 51: 174-180, April, 1972.

99. Sexton, Daniel L., M.D. Personal communications.

100. Sjoerdsma, A. The carcinoid syndrome. In Beeson, Paul B. and McDermott, Walsh (eds.). *Cecil Loeb Textbook of Medicine*, 13th ed. Philadelphia: W. B. Saunders Co., 1971, pp. 1837-1840.

101. Smith, L. H. The diagnosis and treatment of metabolic stone disease. *Medical Clinics of North America*, 56: 977-988, July, 1972.

102. Sohval, A. R. Human chromosome analysis. *American Journal of Medicine*, 31: 402-403, September, 1961.

103. Spodick, D. H. Cryohypophysectomy in diabetes. *Annals of Internal Medicine*, 73: 141-142, July, 1970.

104. Sullivan, J. M. Pheochromocytoma. *Archives of Surgery*, 104: 130-131, February, 1972.

105. Swanson, D. W. and Stipes, A. H. Psychiatric aspects of Klinefelter's syndrome. *American Journal of Psychiatry*, 126: 814-822, December, 1969.

106. Swinton, N. W. *et al.* Hypercalcemia and familial pheochromocytoma. *Annals of Internal Medicine*, 76: 455-458, March, 1972.

107. Teitelbaum, S. L. The carcinoid — a collective review. *American Journal of Surgery*, 123: 564-572, May, 1972.

108. Wang, C. A. Surgery of parathyroid glands. In Welsh, Claud E. *et al.* (eds.). *Advances in Surgery*, vol 5. Chicago: Year Book Medical Publishers, Inc., 1971, pp. 109-128.

109. Williamson, J. R. *et al.* Microvascular disease in diabetes. *Medical Clinics of North America*, 55: 847-860, July, 1971.

110. Winegrad, A. I. and Clements, R. S. Diabetic ketoacidosis. *Medical Clinics of North America*, 55: 899-911, July, 1971.

111. Wolfe, W. G. Insulinoma of the pancreas: Use of tolbutamide test, arteriography and selenium scan in modern diagnosis. *Archives of Surgery*, 104: 56-61, January, 1972.

112. World Health Organization. Classification of hyperlipidemias and hyperlipoproteinemias. *Circulation*, 45: 501-508, February, 1972.

113. Zellman, H. E. Hyperthyroidism. *Medical Clinics of North America*, 56: 717-724, May, 1972.

Chapter XIII

The Sense Organ of Vision

EYE

A. Origin of Terms:

1. choroid (G) — skin-like
2. converge (L) — incline
3. cornea (L) — horny
4. crystal (G) — clear ice
5. cyclo- (G) — circle
6. enucleate (L) — remove kernel
7. iris (G) — rainbow
8. kerato- (G) — horny
9. nystagmus (G) — nod
10. oculus (L) — eye
11. ophthalmo- (G) — eye
12. opsis (G) — sight
13. opto- (G) — vision
14. phakos (G) — lens
15. pyon (G) — pus
16. schisis (G) — division
17. sclera (G) — hard
18. uva (L) — grape
19. vitreous (L) — glassy
20. zonule (L) — tiny band

B. Anatomical Terms:[23, 83]

1. bulb of the eye — the globe or eyeball.
2. chambers of the eye:
   a. anterior chamber — space in front of the iris and back of the cornea.
   b. posterior chamber — space in back of the iris and in front of the lens.
3. coats of the eye:
   a. cornea — anterior transparent part of the outer tunic of the eye. The sclera is the posterior opaque part of the outer tunic. It is composed of dense fibrous tissue which has a protective function.
   b. retina — innermost light perceiving tunic, perceives and transmits the sensory impulses of light to the optic nerve.
   c. uvea, uveal tract — intermediate vascular tunic composed of the
      (1) choroid — which contains a layer of blood vessels and provides nutrition for the retina, lens and vitreous.
      (2) ciliary body — thickened part of the vascular tunic of the eye. Its circularly arranged processes secrete aqueous humor. The ciliary muscle regulates the shape of the lens.[23]
      (3) iris — anterior highly pigmented part of the uvea. The pupil is an opening in the center of the iris. Its size is controlled by a sphincter muscle and dilator muscle.
4. ciliary zonule — suspensory ligament of the lens attaching the ciliary body and contiguous retina to the lens capsule.
5. crystalline lens — a transparent biconvex body enclosed in a capsule and lying directly in back of the iris.
6. fovea — small depression in the macula adapted for most acute vision.[83]
7. fundus oculi — inner posterior portion of the eye which can be seen with an ophthalmoscope.
8. macula lutea — small avascular area of the retina around the fovea.[83]
9. orbit — bony cavity of the skull in which lies the eyeball.
10. vitreous body — a jelly-like, transparent mass which occupies the space behind the lens.

240

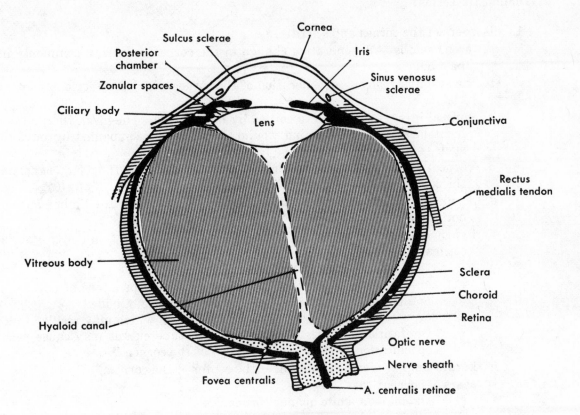

Fig. 65 — Horizontal section of eyeball through optic nerve.

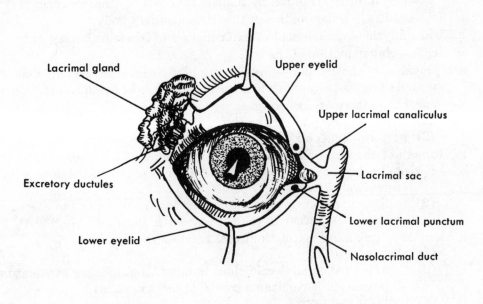

Fig. 66 — Lacrimal apparatus.

C. Diagnostic Terms:

1. disorders of the cornea and sclera:[52, 67]
   a. arcus senilis — degenerative change in the cornea occurring commonly in persons past 50.
   b. corneal dystrophy — degeneration of the cornea which may seriously interfere with vision.
   c. corneal injury — damage to cornea by foreign body, chemical, thermal or radiation burn, laceration, penetrating wound, frequently accompanied by intraocular damage such as traumatic cataract and iris prolapse.[53, 42]
   d. corneal ulcer — a form of superficial keratitis due to pathogenic organism entering the corneal epithelium.[54]
   e. dermoid — a skin-like tumor or cyst generally located at the limbus and involving both cornea and sclera.
   f. hypopyon — pus in anterior chamber in back of cornea; frequently associated with corneal ulcer.[54]
   g. keratitis — inflammation of the cornea.
      (1) superficial — inflammatory reaction consisting of a loss of corneal epithelium and ulcer formation due to infection from the outside.
      (2) deep — invasion of deep layers of the cornea which may result in its perforation. Interstitial keratitis due to syphilis or tuberculosis may cause permanent opacification (loss of transparency) of the cornea.[54]
   h. keratoconus — a conical bulging of the center of the cornea.
   i. scars of cornea:
      (1) leukoma — a white opaque cornea.
      (2) macula — opaque spot seen on cornea.
      (3) nebula — grayish opacity of cornea.
   j. scleritis — inflammation of the sclera.

2. disorders of the uveal tract:[68]
   a. choroidal hemorrhage — local bleeding of choroid which may be associated with vascular disorder, trauma, choroiditis, diabetes or other diseases.[54]
   b. iridocyclitis — inflammation of the iris and ciliary body.
   c. iridodialysis — detachment of outer margin of iris from ciliary body.
   d. iritis — inflammation of the iris.
   e. sympathetic ophthalmia — inflammation of uveal tract usually following perforating wound of opposite eye with incarceration or loss of uveal tissue.[39, 67]
   f. synechia — there are two kinds:
      (1) anterior synechia — adhesion of the iris to the cornea.
      (2) posterior synechia — adhesion of the iris to the lens.[68]
   g. tumors of the uveal tract — intraocular tumors of the choroid, iris or ciliary body.
      (1) nevi (sing. nevus), benign melanomas — pigmental lesions which usually do not interfere with vision.
      (2) malignant melanomas — pigmented lesions, usually unilateral, which lead to loss of vision and occur in the fifth or sixth decade of life.[54, 61, 26]
   h. uveitis — inflammation of the uveal tract caused by:
      (1) allergy
      (2) organisms such as Coccidioides immitis, Histoplasma capsulatum, Mycobacterium tuberculosis, Toxoplasma gondii, other organisms
      (3) irritants and toxins
      (4) connective tissue diseases.[54, 68]

3. disorders of the vitreous:
   a. infection of vitreous — bacterial, fungal or parasitic infection resulting in liquefaction, opacification and shrinkage of vitreous.[52]

b. vitreous detachment — vitreous detached from retina in one or both eyes. It may lead to retinal tear.[69]

c. vitreous hemorrhage — rare but serious disorder, usually caused by rupture of a retinal vessel and followed by sudden loss of vision.[52, 69]

4. disorders of the lens and intraocular pressure:

a. cataract — an opaque lens, congenital or acquired. Lenticular opacity is usually linked with the process of aging. Insoluble proteins may form in the lens and eventually lead to dehydration, lowered metabolism and tissue necrosis. In the cataractous lens sodium and calcium content tend to be increased and potassium, protein and ascorbic acid content decreased. Visual impairment is slowly progressive.[52, 62, 25, 21, 22]

b. ectopia lentis — displacement of the lens seen primarily in Marfan's syndrome in its congenital form. It also may be due to trauma.[52]

c. glaucoma — abnormal accumulation of aqueous humor within the eye resulting in increased intraocular pressure which, **untreated, leads to blindness.** Some types of glaucoma are:

(1) acute glaucoma — severe obstruction of aqueous humor drainage, sharp rise of intraocular tension, agonizing eye pain, dilated pupils, steamy cornae and ciliary injection.

(2) chronic glaucoma

(a) closed angle glaucoma — intermittent attacks of angle closure of anterior chamber, formation of adhesions in angle with attacks and gradual obliteration of angle requiring peripheral iridectomy, if unresponsive to medical therapy.

(b) open angle glaucoma — interference with aqueous outflow creating an elevated intraocular pressure. The open type is bilateral and if untreated leads slowly to visual impairment and cupping of optic disk.[55, 40, 34]

5. disorders of the retina:

a. atrophy and degeneration of retina — a reduction of visual acuity due to degenerative processes seen in the elderly.

b. detachment of the retina — separation from the choroid resulting in blindness if not relieved.[54, 35, 65]

c. edema of the retina — condition due to active hyperemia, generally resulting from trauma.[52]

d. diabetic retinopathy — condition characterized by pinpoint aneurysms, which may be caused by dilatation of capillaries.[70, 4]

e. hypertensive retinopathy — retinal changes resulting from persistently high diastolic blood pressure. This condition may occur in essential hypertension, renal arteriolar sclerosis, glomerulonephritis and the toxemias of pregnancy.[70]

f. macular degenerations — a group of degenerative disorders of the retina:

(1) circinate degeneration — rather common macular retinopathy, seen in older age groups. It is usually bilateral and characterized by a girdle of yellow white spots surrounding the macular area. The peripheral vision may be retained but the central vision is lost.[71, 54]

(2) cystic degeneration of macula — sharply delineated red, round cystic defect in macula. The wall of the fluid-filled cyst may rupture and a macular hole may result. If the fovea is involved, central vision is blurred.[52, 54, 15]

(3) disciform macular degeneration, Kuhnt Junius disease — a dark dome-shaped elevation in the macular area apparently containing extravasated blood from a retinal hemorrhage. Central vision is impaired or lost.[54, 71]

(4) retinoschisis — a separation of the sensory retina into two layers appearing as a shallow elevation of the peripheral retina. Usually vision is unaffected.[54, 71, 38, 8]

g. occlusion of central retinal artery — rare unilateral disorder due to thrombus, embolus or atheromatous plaque suddenly causing total loss of sight in the affected eye. It may occur in advanced age or during oral contraceptive therapy.[72]

h. occlusion of central retinal vein — thrombosis of the central retinal vein leading to sudden, painless loss of sight.[72]

i. retinal arteriolar sclerosis — a form of sclerosis due to hypertension characterized by copper-wire arterioles in the retina. In the advanced stage of the sclerotic process the arterioles resemble silver wire.[70, 54]

j. retinal atherosclerosis — obstructive changes in retinal vessels which may cause a sudden vascular accident in the retina.

k. retinal hemorrhage — moderate or massive bleeding from the retina.

l. retinitis pigmentosa — hereditary degenerative disease principally affecting the rod and cone layer of the retina. Ophthalmologic examination reveals spider-shaped pigment epithelium (tapetum). Night blindness is the dominant feature.[52, 71, 32]

m. retinoblastoma — malignant tumor arising from the retina, commonly seen in young children. It is hereditary.[51, 11, 66, 43]

n. retrolental fibrosplasia — bilateral, retinal disease in premature infants.[51]

6. disorders of the optic nerve:[52, 33]

a. optic atrophy — a destruction of the fibers of the optic nerve associated with loss of visual acuity.

b. optic coloboma — congenital defect in optic nerve resulting from imperfect closure of fetal cleft. Defects in choroid and retina may coexist. Visual impairment is common.[52, 33]

c. optic neuritis — inflammation of the optic nerve; may involve the sheaths of the nerve (optic perineuritis) or its main body.[33, 45]

d. papilledema, choked disk — edema of the papilla or optic nerve head usually due to increased intracranial pressure.[33]

e. papillitis — inflammation of the papilla or head of the optic nerve.

f. retrobulbar neuritis — optic neuritis in which nerve involvement occurs behind the optic disk and cannot be seen ophthalmoscopically. Visual acuity is seriously affected or entirely lost. Its most common cause is multiple sclerosis.[3, 45]

7. optic nerve tumors:

a. gliomas — glial tumors which may be derived from astrocytes of the optic nerve and are either solitary tumors or occur in von Recklinghausen's neurofibromatosis.[43]

b. meningiomas — usually orbital tumors arising in the sheath of the optic nerve. Secondary involvement may cocur.[43]

D. Operative Terms:

1. cataract surgery:[56, 73]

a. aspiration of cataract — removal of cataract by suction through a small limbal incision which does not need suture. Procedure may be used for young patients below 30 years of age.[73]

b. cryoextraction of cataract — application of the tip of the cryoextractor to the anterior surface of the lens until the cataract firmly adheres to the instrument. When the freezing process has extended for 2 to 3 mm into the lens substance, the probe with the lens frozen to it is lifted out.[73, 17, 2]

c. enzymatic zonulysis (or zonulolysis) — instillation of chrymotrypsin, a fibrinolytic enzyme, into the anterior chamber to resolve the ciliary zonules and thus facilitate the removal of the cataractous lens. The procedure is used in the 20-50 year age group in whom the zonules are tough, making cataract extraction difficult.[73]

    d. extracapsular extraction — incision into anterior capsule in order to express the opaque lens.[56, 5]

    e. intracapsular extraction — removal of entire lens in its capsule; method of choice especially for senile cataracts.[56]

    f. linear extraction — surgical procedure used for persons under the age of 35 since in that age group the nucleus of the lens is soft. It is also an emergency operation in severe glaucoma secondary to swelling of the cataractous lens.

2. discission of lens — needling or breaking up of the lens with a knife needle; indicated in congenital cataracts in children and adults under the age of 35. Several needlings may be necessary.

3. enucleation — removal of the eyeball indicated in penetrating injuries, malignant tumors of the eye and as an emergency measure in threatened sympathetic ophthalmia.[64]

4. evisceration — removal of contents of eyeball but leaving the sclera and cornea.

5. glaucoma operations — surgical procedures for highly increased intraocular pressure, irreducible by miotics.[74, 56]

    a. in acute glaucoma

        (1) basal iridectomy — partial excision of the peripheral (basal) portion of the iris.

        (2) iridencleisis — iris inclusion operation.

    b. in chronic glaucoma

        (1) peripheral iridotomy — incision into iris to keep the iris angle open and drain aqueous humor into Schlemm's canal.

        (2) complete iridectomy — removal of iris; rarely done.

    c. in secondary glaucoma

        (1) keratocentesis — paracentesis of cornea.

        (2) cyclodialysis — surgical procedure to promote the escape of aqueous humor in aphakic glaucoma.[39]

        (3) cyclodiathermy — application of high frequency electric current to ciliary body.

    d. in infantile glaucoma

        goniotomy — incision across anterior chamber for establishing normal aqueous outflow through regular channels.[74]

6. iridectomy — excision of iris, either partial or complete.

7. keratoplasty, corneal graft, corneal transplant — surgical replacement of a section of an opaque cornea with normal, transparent cornea to restore vision.

    a. lamellar keratoplasty — using part thickness corneal transplant.[47]

    b. penetrating keratoplasty — using full thickness corneal transplant.[50]

8. photocoagulation, ocular — generation and emission of light of appropriate intensity and at a given distance to stimulate the coagulation of tissue in microseconds.[6, 75]

9. photocoagulation, laser (ocular) — light amplification by emission of radiation using

    a. argon laser beam — a blue-green light which is effectively absorbed by red hemoglobin, choroid and pigment epithelium and has been used with success in the treatment of diabetic retinopathy and senile macular degeneration.[10, 84, 36]

    b. krypton laser — emission of yellow light, used to treat chorioretinal and ophthalmic vascular disorders.[19]

    c. ruby laser — emission of red light; current clinical research.

    d. xenon laser — emission of red light; current clinical research.

10. repair of retinal detachment — surgical reattachment of the retina to the choroid. It may be accomplished by

    a. cryopexy of sclera — application of a supercooled probe to the sclera to produce a chorioretinal scar with minimal damage to the sclera.[75]

    b. laser photocoagulation — procedure for mending small retinal tears. A laser beam is directed through the dilated pupil to produce a chorioretinal inflammatory reaction which seals the small tear.[75]

c. scleral buckling operation — removal of strip of sclera near the retinal separation, drainage of subretinal fluid, placement of implant and tightening of sutures around implant to buckle the sclera.[75]

Research to detect sutureless scleral buckling materials is now in progress.[9]

11. vitrectomy — removal of vitreous for the control of fibrotic overgrowth in severe intraocular trauma.[13]

E. Symptomatic Terms:[57, 58]

1. amaurosis fugax — fleeting blindness manifested by transient monocular blindness and binocular blurring. It may result from transient embolization of retinal arterioles and suggest pending stroke.[49]

2. amblyopia — dimness of vision in one eye that is normal on ophthalmoscopic examination.[51]

3. amblyopia ex anopsia — diminished visual acuity in one eye not due to organic eye disease. It is known as the "lazy eye".

4. ametropia — optic defect or refractive error which does not permit parallel light rays to fall exactly on the retina.

5. anisometropia — inequality in refractive power of right and left eye.

6. Argyll-Robertson pupil — absence of light reflex without change in the contractile power of the pupil, a reliable sign of syphilis of the central nervous system.

7. astigmatism — images are warped and distorted due to irregular corneal curvature which prevents clear focusing of light.

8. binocular blindness — blind in both eyes.

9. binocular vision — ability to focus both eyes on one object and fuse the two images produced into one.

10. color blindness — reduced ability to distinguish between colors.

11. diplopia — double vision.

12. emmetropia — normal vision, no refractive error.

13. enophthalmos — recession of the eyeball into the orbit.

14. exophthalmos, exophthalmus — protrusion of the eyeball in hyperthyroidism and orbital space-taking lesions.[29, 27, 80]

15. hypermetropia, hyperopia — farsightedness, parallel rays of light from a distant object.

16. hyphemia — blood in the anterior chamber in front of the iris.

17. leukokoria, white pupil — white pupillary reflex referred to as amaurotic cat's eye, suggesting the presence of a sight destroying condition such as a retinablastoma, curable in its early phase.[51]

18. malignant exophthalmos, progressive proptosis — increasing forward displacement of the eyeball in Graves' disease causing severe ocular symptoms such as fullness of eyelids, lacrimation, epiphora, corneal ulcerations, chemosis and edema of conjunctiva.[41]

19. monocular blindness — blind in one eye.

20. myopia — nearsightedness; parallel rays from a distant object are focused in front of the retina; a refractive error.

21. nyctalopia — night blindness.[51]

22. nystagmus — constant involuntary movement of the eyeballs. It may be due to a disease of the central nervous system.

23. photophobia — marked intolerance to light.

24. presbyopia — gradual loss of accommodation, a common condition in persons past middle age.

25. scotoma — a blind spot in the vision.

ACCESSORY ORGANS OF VISION

A. Origin of Terms:

1. blepharo- (G) — eyelid
2. canaliculus (L) — small canal
3. cantho- (G) — angle
4. cilia (L) — eyelashes
5. dacryo- (G) — tear
6. dacryoaden (G) — tear gland
7. dacryocyst (G) — tear sac
8. fissure, fissura (L) — cleft, slit
9. fornix (L) — arch
10. junctus (L) — joined
11. lacrima (L) — tear
12. oblique (L) — slanting
13. palpebra (L) — eyelid
14. rectus (L) — straight

B. Anatomical Terms:[83, 7, 76]

1. canthus (pl. canthi) — the lateral or medial angles at both ends of the palpebral fissures (slits between the eyelids).
2. cilia, eyelashes — rows of hairs at the free margin of the eyelids.
3. conjunctiva (pl. conjunctivae) — mucous membrane that lines the deep surface of the eyelid and is reflected over the front of the eyeball. It is divided into a
   a. bulbar conjunctiva — colorless, transparent portion covering the anterior part of the globe.
   b. palpebral conjunctiva — lining the posterior or deep surface of the lids.
4. fornix (pl. fornices) conjunctivae — angle between palpebral and bulbar conjunctivae.
5. lacrimal apparatus:
   a. lacrimal gland — tear gland; its orbital part lies in the lacrimal fossa of the upper, outer part of the orbit, its palpebral part in the upper eyelid.
   b. lacrimal ducts — tear ducts extending from gland to superior conjunctival fornix.
   c. lacrimal canaliculi — one canaliculus (canal) for each eyelid to conduct tears from lacrimal punctum to lacrimal sac.
   d. lacrimal puncta (sing. punctum) — minute openings, the beginning of the canaliculi.
   e. lacrimal sac — tear sac situated in lacrimal groove on medial wall of orbit.
   f. nasolacrimal duct — duct draining lacrimal sac and opening into inferior nasal meatus.
6. ocular muscles — muscles controlling the movements of the eyeball.
   a. two oblique muscles (two obliqui).
   b. four rectus muscles (four recti).
7. palpebral fissure — opening between the eyelids.
8. tarsal glands — secretory follicles in the tarsal plate.
9. tarsal plate — supporting connective tissue of the eyelid.

C. Diagnostic Terms:

1. disorders of the eyelid.[52, 76]
   a. blepharitis — inflammation of the eyelid.
   b. blepharoptosis — drooping of the upper eyelid, congenital or acquired.[12]
   c. chalazion (pl. chalazia) — a true granuloma of the eye appearing as a painless swelling at the tarsus.
   d. ectropion — outward turning of the margin of the eyelid.
   e. entropion — inward turning of the margin of the eyelid.
   f. hordeolum (pl. hordeola)
      (1) external hordeolum — pyogenic infection of a sebaceous gland at the margin of the lid.
      (2) internal hordeolum — purulent infection of a sebaceous gland embedded in the conjunctiva of the eyelid.
   g. tumors of the lid — congenital or acquired: dermoids, fibromas, hemangiomas and carcinomas.

248

2. disorders of the conjunctiva:[54]
   a. conjunctivitis — inflammation of the conjunctiva associated with pain, edema, hyperemia, exudation and infiltration. There are many forms of conjunctivitis.[24]
   b. ophthalmia neonatorum, gonococcal conjunctivitis of the newborn — the conjunctival sac of the infant is filled with pus containing gonococci.
   c. pterygium — a membrane of conjunctival tissue which extends like a wing from the limbus toward the center of the cornea.
   d. trachoma — chronic inflammation of the conjunctivae followed by granulation, capillary infiltration of the cornea (pannus) and blindness. The etiological agent is the virus of trachoma.
3. disorders of the lacrimal apparatus:[52, 54, 76]
   a. acute dacryoadenitis — unilateral or bilateral inflammation of the lacrimal gland. It is frequently seen in children as a complication of measles and parotitis (mumps).
   b. chronic dacryoadenitis — a chronic, painless swelling of the lacrimal glands showing no signs of acute inflammation.
   c. dacryocystitis — an acute or chronic inflammation of the lacrimal sac, usually due to nasolacrimal stenosis.
   d. lacrimal abscess — localized accumulation of pus in lacrimal gland.
4. disorders of ocular motility:[33, 52]
   a. ophthalmoplegia externa, external ophthalmoplegia — paralysis of extraocular muscles causing restriction or loss of eye movements.[52, 31]
   b. ophthalmoplegia interna, internal ophthalmoplegia — paralysis of the fibers of the third nerve causing paralysis of the iris sphincter and ciliary muscle.[52, 33]
   c. strabismus, squint — condition in which the optic axes fail to be directed toward the same object.
     (1) convergent squint or esotropia — the eyes are directed toward the medial line.
     (2) divergent squint or exotropia — the eyes are turned laterally (outwards).[51]

D. Operative Terms:

1. blepharectomy — excision of lesion of an eyelid.
2. blepharoplasty — plastic repair of an eyelid.[7, 20]
3. blepharorrhaphy — suture of a lacerated or injured eyelid.
4. dacryoadenectomy — removal of a lacrimal gland.
5. dacryocystectomy — removal of the lacrimal sac.
6. dacryocystorhinostomy — surgical creation of an opening into the nose for the tears.[7]
7. repair of strabismus — surgical correction by advancement, recession, resection, tucking or tenotomy of any one or more of the ocular muscles.[77]
8. tarsorrhaphy — surgical closure of an eyelid.

E. Symptomatic Terms:

1. blepharedema — puffy, swollen, edematous eyelids.[60]
2. chemosis — conjunctival swelling near the cornea.
3. epiphora — overflow of tears, often due to lacrimal duct obstruction.
4. hyperemia — congestion.
5. lacrimation — secretion of tears.
6. pannus — newly formed capillaries covering the cornea like a film.

RADIOLOGY

A. Terms Related to Diagnosis:

1. distention dacryocystography — forceful injection of contrast medium into canaliculus during x-ray exposure to outline the nasolacrimal duct system in distended state. Direct x-ray magnification aids in the detection of the obstructive lesion.[46]

2. orbital arteriography — serial angiograms of the orbital arteries primarily via the ophthalmic branch of the internal carotid artery and secondarily via branches of the external carotid artery. The technique is used to detect arterial malformation or arteriovenous fistula of orbital vessels.[81]

3. orbital tomography — tomographic sections of the orbit delineating its extent, size and relation to adjoining structures.[48]

4. orbital venography — procedure of choice in the diagnosis of space-occupying lesions. The frontal vein approach is preferred.[28]

5. orbitography — useful diagnostic procedure for localization of retrobulbar tumors before visual damage has become irreparable.[37, 27, 30, 14, 18]

    a. negative contrast orbitography, orbital pneumotomography — radiographic visualization of the orbit using air or oxygen as contrast medium. It is indicated primarily when tumors of the optic nerve are suspected.[37]

    b. positive contrast orbitography — radiographic visualization of the orbit using water soluble preparations as contrast media. Retrobulbar lesions may be found in the muscle cone of the superior rectus.[37]

B. Terms Related to Therapy:

1. irradiation in bilateral retinoblastoma — enucleation of the more affected eye; radiotherapy to the less affected eye to preserve some degree of vision.[1]

2. irradiation in unilateral retinoblastoma — enucleation of eye and part of optic nerve; postoperative radiotherapy determined by histologic study.

3. irradiation in early epidermoid carcinoma of the conjunctiva — radium therapy may be able to eradicate the lesion.[1]

CLINICAL LABORATORY

A. Terms Related to Bacteriological Studies[78]

1. epithelial inclusion bodies — bodies found in conjunctival diseases, such as inclusion blennorrhea of the newborn, some adult forms of diffuse, follicular conjunctivitis and in trachoma. Epithelial scrapings stained with Giemsa's or Wright's stain reveal the inclusion bodies.

2. epithelial scrapings from the cornea or conjunctiva — procedure used for identifying the etiological organism of bacterial conjunctivitis or keratitis. A thin layer of epithelial cells is removed with a spatula or scalpel. The scrapings are transferred to two or more slides and stained; one by Gram's method, the other with Giemsa's or Wright's stain. These methods permit the identification of the predominant organism as well as eosinophils and epithelial inclusion bodies. Since pathogenic organisms are freely present in epithelial cells before they appear in secretions, the study of scrapings offers a valuable aid to early diagnosis.

3. etiological organisms in conjunctival disease, commonly seen —

    a. Diplococcus pneumoniae   d. Streptococcus

    b. Neisseria gonorrhoeae   e. Virus of trachoma and others.[78]

    c. Staphylococcus

B. Terms Related Primarily to Functional Testing:

1. accommodation — ability to see at various distances due to the contraction and relaxation of the ciliary muscle. The focusing power is measurable.

2. contact lenses — small corneal lenses which fit directly on the eyeball under the eyelids, medically used to correct vision in keratoconus (cone-shaped cornea) and other eye conditions.

3. corneal sensitivity — the examiner touches the corneas with a cotton fiber to determine whether each cornea is normally sensitive.

4. dark adaptation — ability of retina to adjust to low levels of illumination.

5. diopter — unit of measurement of refractive power or strength of lenses.

6. electroretinography — the recording of retinal action currents. Procedure aids in the detection of degenerative disorders of the retina.

7. electrotonography — aqueous outflow study based on change in intraocular pressure following the application of an electronic tonometer to the eye for four minute period. Low pressure reading obtained from a electronic scale and recorded by an automatic writer suggest the presence of glaucoma.[79]

8. fluorescein angiography — ophthalmoscopy following intravenous fluorescein injection for detecting subtle vascular conditions of macular lesions.[79]

9. fluorescein funduscopy — intravenous injection of fluorescein followed by fundus examination. Arterial, arteriovenous and venous phase of retinal blood flow are recorded by rapid serial photography.[59]

10. gonioscopy — examination of the iris angle of the eye using an optical instrument. Obstruction of the filtration angle may occur in glaucoma.[79]

11. keratometry — measurement of the curves of the cornea with a keratometer.

12. major amblyoscopy — test for evaluating the sensory status of the eyes. Procedure is also used in orthoptic study before and after strabismus surgery.[79]

13. ocular stereophotography — three dimensional photographing to detect fundus lesions of the eye by means of the indirect ophthalmoscopic principle. Photographing is done at a known magnification, exposure and depth effect to determine progression or retrogression of lesions over a period of time.[16]

14. ophthalmodynamometry — measurement of the pressure in the central retinal arteries for indirectly evaluating the blood flow in the carotid arteries.[82, 79]

15. ophthalmoscopy — examination of the eye grounds (fundi) with an ophthalmoscope.

16. orthoptic training — a program of scientifically planned exercises for promoting or restoring the normal coordination of the eyes.[63]

17. perimetry — instrumental measurement of field of vision.

18. probing of lacrimal drainage system — establishing drainage of obstructed system after unsuccessful irrigation. A metal probe is passed through the upper or lower punctum and canaliculus, into the lacrimal (tear) sac, nasolacrimal duct and nose.[79]

19. retinoscopy — light beam test for detecting refractive errors.

20. scotometry — examining the central visual field for areas of decreased sensitivity and mapping out blind spots (scotomas) on a special chart.[59]

21. slit lamp biomicroscopy — use of a combination of slit lamp and biomicroscope for intense illumination and high magnification of the eyeball or lids. Layers of cornea and lens are clearly visualized and pathologic processes such as opacities are detected with accuracy.[59, 79]

22. tonometry — determination of intraocular pressure by a tonometer; e.g. that of Schiotz.

23. visual acuity — determination of the minimum cognizable under standard conditions of illumination using the Snellen chart or one of its modifications.

24. ultrasonography, ophthalmic — use of ultrasonic waves as a diagnostic aid in evaluating some pathologic eye lesions since certain structures, as for example the cornea, lens and chambers, produce echoes that are clearly identifiable.[59]

ABBREVIATIONS

A. General:

Accom. — accommodation
anisometr. — anisometropia
AgNO₃ — silver nitrate
Astigm. — astigmatism
c. gl. — with correction (with glasses)
cx — cylinder axis
cyl — cylindrical lens
Em — emmetropia
EOM — extraocular movements
EPF — exophthalmos producing factor
EPS — exophthalmos producing substance
HM — hand motion
IOP — intraocular pressure

KW — Keith-Wagner (ophthalmoscopic findings)
LP or PL — light perception
Mix. Astig. — mixed astigmatism
Myop. — myopia
OD or RE — right eye (oculus dexter)
Ophth. or Oph. — ophthalmology
OS or LE — left eye (oculus sinister)
OU — each eye (oculus uterque)
s. gl. — without correction (without glasses)
ST — esotropia
TU or T — intraocular tension
VA — visual acuity
VC — acuity of color vision
VF — visual field
XT — exotropia

B. Organizations:

NINDB — National Institute of Neurological Diseases and Blindness

NSPB — National Society for the Prevention of Blindness

ORAL READING PRACTICE

Glaucoma

Glaucoma is a disease of the eye characterized by an elevated intraocular pressure. Normally, the internal pressure of the eye is about 18-22mm Hg, a pressure higher than that of the other organs. The maintenance of a normal intraocular pressure depends primarily on the amount of **aqueous humor** present in the eye. The formation of aqueous humor and its elimination is a continuous process. If the production and absorption are in perfect balance, all is well, but if there is a disturbance of balance, the eye is seriously affected.

The **ciliary** processes form the aqueous humor which passes through the pupil space to the anterior chamber. It leaves through the **canal of Schlemm** and is picked up by the aqueous veins which contain a mixture of blood and aqueous. In most cases of glaucoma the elevated intraocular pressure results from interference with the elimination of aqueous humor, although increased rate of production may be the source of the imbalance.

Ophthalmologists distinguish two main types: primary and secondary glaucoma. Secondary glaucoma is related to various eye conditions which bring about marked fluctuations and elevations in the intraocular pressure; for example, **iritis** and **iridocyclitis**, intraocular **neoplasms,** dislocation of the lens, central vein **occlusion** and trauma.

The clinical picture is variable depending on the degree of elevation and gradual or abrupt onset. The patient with acute glaucoma may experience a sudden increase in pain which tends to be extreme and associated with nausea and vomiting. The cornea may look steamy and the conjunctiva **edematous.**

In chronic simple glaucoma no pain is present and visual loss proceeds insidiously. Treatment consists of the judicious use of **miotics** which sometimes constrict the pupil so effectively that the aqueous humor can escape. If no alleviation can be achieved, operative intervention becomes imperative. Various forms of surgical drainage, such as **iridectomy, iridencleisis, sclerectomy, cyclodialysis** or **goniotomy,** are indicated. The same operations are performed for acute simple glaucoma.

In secondary glaucoma, resulting from obstruction of the **central retinal** vein, **enucleation** of the eye may be necessary. **Cyclodiathermy** tends to relieve pain, but, if unsuccessful, **retrobulbar** injection of alcohol is sometimes employed to combat the condition.[40, 34, 55, 44]

Table 23

SOME EYE CONDITIONS AMENABLE TO SURGERY

Organs Involved	Diagnosis	Operations	Operative Procedures
Eyeball	Penetrating wound of eyeball	Enucleation of eyeball	Removal of eyeball
Eyeball	Malignant exophthalmos with infiltrative ophthalmopathy due to Graves' disease	Orbital decompression of the proptosed globe	Transantral ethmoid approach Differential decompression by slitting the periosteum in posterio-anterior direction Creation of nasoantral window for drainage
Retina Uvea Iris Conjunctiva	Retinoblastoma Malignant melanoma Epidermoid carcinoma	Evisceration of eyeball	Removal of the eyeball and as much as possible of the optic nerve
Retina Choroid Sclera	Detachment of retina	Scleral buckling operation	Diathermy to sclera and choroid; release of subretinal fluid Inward buckling of treated area and insertion of silicone implant; firm contact of choroid with retina reestablished
Retina Choroid Sclera	Detachment of retina	Cryopexy	Application of freezing probe to sclera to promote formation of chorioretinal scar and thus fusion
Cornea	Corneal scar Keratoconus	Keratoplasty lamellar transplant or penetrating transplant	Replacement of opaque cornea with transparent cornea using part thickness or full thickness corneal graft
Vitreous Cornea	Small foreign body in vitreous	Haab giant magnet technique Keratotomy	Foreign body dislodged by magnet and removed through corneal incision

Organs Involved	Diagnosis	Operations	Operative Procedures
Cornea Iris Vitreous	Glaucoma acute, primary	Keratocentesis Peripheral iridectomy Cyclodialysis	Paracentesis of cornea Surgical removal of part of iris Surgical communication between the anterior chamber and suprachoroidal space
Crystalline lens Iris	Cataract congenital senile	Discission Peripheral iridectomy Intracapsular extraction of cataract	Needling of lens Approach to cataract by removal of iris Excision of cataract within it capsule
Crystalline lens	Cataract	Intracapsular cryoextraction of cataract	Tip of cryoextractor applied to anterior surface of lens Freezing of lens substance Frozen lens lifted out on cryoextractor
Iris	Cyst of iris	Electrolysis	Insertion of an electrolysis needle in the center of cyst to induce shrinkage
Ocular muscle	Strabismus	Recession of ocular muscle	Correction of defect by drawing muscle backward
Eyelid	Laceration of eyelid Hordeolum Blepharoptosis	Blepharorrhaphy Blepharotomy Repair of eyelid	Suture of eyelid Incision with drainage of meibomian gland Surgical correction of ptosis
Lacrimal sac	Abscess of lacrimal sac	Dacryocystotomy	Incision and drainage of tear duct
Lacrimal gland	Retention cyst of lacrimal gland	Dacryoadenectomy	Removal of tear gland
Lacrimonasal duct	Stenosis of lacri- monasal duct	Dacryocystorhinostomy	Fistulization of lacrimal sac into nasal cavity

REFERENCES AND BIBLIOGRAPHY

1. Ackerman, Lauren V. and del Regato, Juan A. Cancer of the eye. In *Cancer Diagnosis Treatment and Prognosis*, 4th ed. St. Louis: The C. V. Mosby Co., 1970, pp. 956-977.
2. Amoils, S. P. *et al.* A new method of cryoextraction. *Archives of Ophthalmology*, 86: 674-678, December, 1971.
3. Armaly, M. F. Selective perimetry for glaucomatous defects in ocular hypertension. *Archives of Ophthalmology*, 87: 518-524, May, 1972.
4. Balodimos, M. C. Treatment of diabetic retinopathy. Pituitary ablation and retinal photocoagulation. *Medical Clinics of North America*, 55: 989-999, July, 1971.
5. Baloglow, P. Cataract extraction after filtering operations. *Archives of Ophthalmology*, 88: 12-15, July, 1972.
6. Blair, C. J. *et al.* Photocoagulation of the macula and papillomacular bundle in the human. *Archives of Ophthalmology*, 88: 167-171, August, 1972.
7. Bonuik, M. Eyelids, lacrimal apparatus and conjunctiva. *Archives of Ophthalmology*, 88: 91-105, July, 1972.
8. Byer, N. E. Spontaneous regression of senile retinoschisis. *Archives of Ophthalmology*, 88: 207-209, August, 1972.
9. Calabria, G. A. *et al.* Further experience with sutureless scleral buckling materials. II. Cyanoacrylate tissue adhesive. *Archives of Ophthalmology*, 86: 82-87, July, 1971.
10. Chapman, W. E. Argon lasers in photocoagulation therapy. *Postgraduate Medicine*, 49: 45-46, June, 1971.

254

11. Cleasby, G. W. Bilateral retinoblastoma. *Archives of Ophthalmology*, 88: 88-90, July, 1972.
12. Cohen, H. B. Congenital ptosis. *Archives of Ophthalmology*, 87: 161-163, February, 1972.
13. Coles, W. H. *et al.* Vitrectomy in intraocular trauma. *Archives of Ophthalmology*, 87: 621-628, June, 1972.
14. Dayton, G. O. Surgery of the orbit. *The Radiologic Clinics of North America*, 10: 11-20, April, 1972.
15. Dobbie, J. G. The aging macula. *Postgraduate Medicine*, 51: 140-145, April, 1972.
16. Donaldson, David L. Abstract of Thomas E. Andert Memorial Lecture. St. Louis University School of Medicine, December 3, 1971.
17. Durham, D. G. A hazard of cryoextraction. *Archives of Ophthalmology*, 87: 117-118, February, 1972.
18. Erkonen W. and Dolan, K. D. Ocular foreign body localization. *The Radiologic Clinics of North America*, 10: 101-114, April, 1972.
19. Esperance, F. A. Clinical photocoagulation with the krypton laser. *Archives of Ophthalmology*, 87: 693-700, June, 1972.
20. Fox, S. A. Upper lid reconstruction. *Archives of Ophthalmology*, 88: 46-48, July, 1972.
21. Fraunfelder, F. T. Electric cataracts. I. Sequential changes, unusual and prognoatic findings. *Archives of Ophthalmology*, 87: 179-183, February, 1972.
22. _____. Electric cataracts. II. Ultrastructural lens changes. *Archives of Ophthalmology*, 87: 184-195, February, 1972.
23. Gardner, Ernest, Gray, Donald and O'Rahilly, Ronan. *Anatomy — A Regional Study of Human Structure*, 3rd ed. Philadelphia: W. B. Saunders Co., 1969, pp. 644-667.
24. Goldstein, J. H. Keratoconjunctivitis sicca. *Postgraduate Medicine*, 51: 154-160, February, 1972.
25. Jeffe, N. S. The lens. *Archives of Ophthalmology*, 87: 453-486, April, 1972.
26. Hager, W. S. *et al.* The diagnosis of malignant melanoma of the ciliary body or choroid. Use of the radioactive phosphorus uptake test. *Southern Medical Journal*, 65: 49-54, January, 1972.
27. Hanafee, W. N. Clinical diagnosis of orbital tumors. *The Radiologic Clinics of North America*, 10: 3-10, April, 1972.
28. _____. Orbital venography. *The Radiologic Clinics of North America*, 10: 63-83. April, 1972.
29. Hartweg, J. H. *et al.* Unilateral exophthalmos. *Plastic and Reconstructive Surgery*, 49: 576-578, May, 1972.
30. Harwood, Nash, D. C. Optic gliomas and pediatric neuroradiology. *The Radiologic Clinics of North America*, 10: 83-100, April, 1972.
31. Koerner, F. Chronic progressive external ophthalmoplegia. *Archives of Ophthalmology*, 88: 155-166, August, 1972.
32. Krill, A. E. *et al.* Fluorescein angiography in retinitis pigmentosa. *American Journal of Ophthalmology*, 69: 826-835, May, 1970.
33. Laties, A. M. Neurophthalmology. In Scheie, Harold G. and Albert, Daniel M. *Adler's Textbook of Ophthalmology*, 8th ed. Philadelphia: W. B. Saunders Co., 1969, pp. 291-337.

34. Levene, R. A new concept of malignant glaucoma. *Archives of Ophthalmology*, 87: 497-506, May, 1972.
35. Lincoff, H. and Gieser, R. Finding the retinal hole. *Archives of Ophthalmology*, 85: 565-569, May, 1971.
36. Little, H. L. *et al.* Argon laser slit lamp retinal photocoagulation. *Transactions American Academy of Ophthalmology and Otolaryngology*, 74: 85-97, January, 1970.
37. Lombardi, G. Orbitography. In Newton, T. H. and Potts, D. G. *Radiology of the Skull and Brain*. St. Louis: The C. V. Mosby Co., 1971, pp. 559-567.
38. Manschot, W. A. Pathology of hereditary juvenile retinoschisis. *Archives of Ophthalmology*, 88: 131-138, August, 1972.
39. Mattis, Robert D., M.D. Personal communications.
40. O'Grady, R. B. Glaucoma. *Postgraduate Medicine*, 51: 69-72, March, 1972.
41. Ogura, J., Wessler, S. and Avioli, L. V. Surgical approach to the ophthalmopathy of Graves' disease. *Journal of American Medical Association*, 216: 1627-1631, June 7, 1971.
42. Rabb, M. F. Acute corneal injuries: classification and management. *Surgical Clinics of North America*, 52: 107-114, February, 1972.
43. Russel, D. S. and Rubinstein, L. J. *Pathology of Tumors of the Nervous System*, 3rd ed. Baltimore: The Williams and Wilkins Co., 1971, pp. 222-233.
44. Rutkowski, P. C. *et al.* Mydriasis and increased intraocular pressure 1. Pupillographic studies 2. Iris fluorescein studies. *Archives of Ophthalmology*, 87: 21-24, January, 1972.
45. Percy, A. K. *et al.* Optic neuritis and multiple sclerosis. *Archives of Ophthalmology*, 87: 135-139, February, 1972.
46. T. H. and Coin, C. G. Dacryocystography. *The Radiologic Clinics of North America*, 10: 129-142, April, 1972.
47. Polack, F. M. Lamellar keratoplasty. *Archives of Ophthalmology*, 86: 293-300, September, 1971..
48. Potter, G. D. Tomography of the orbit. *The Radiologic Clinics of North America*, 10: 21-38, April, 1972.
49. Sacks, J. G. Neuro-ophthalmologic signs of extracranial cerebrovascular insufficiency. *Postgraduate Medicine*, 52: 115-119, July, 1972.
50. Saleeby, S. S. Keratoplasty. *Archives of Ophthalmology*, 87: 538-539, May, 1972.
51. Schaffer, D. B. Pediatric ophthalmology. In Scheie, Harold G. and Albert, Daniel M. *Adler's Textbook of Ophthalmology*, 8th ed. Philadelphia: W. B. Saunders Co., 1969, pp. 105-182.
52. Scheie, Harold G. and Albert, Daniel M. Ophthalmic entities. In *Adler's Textbook of Ophthalmology*, 8th ed. Philadelphia: W. B. Saunders Co., 1969, pp. 1-38.
53. _____. Ocular injuries. Abrasions and superficial lacerations of the cornea. *Ibid.*, pp. 361-380.
54. _____. Medical ophthalmology. *Ibid.*, pp. 183-290.

55. _____. Glaucoma: classification of glaucoma, primary and secondary glaucoma. *Ibid.*, pp. 336-360.

56. _____. Principles of ocular surgery. *Ibid.*, pp. 381-397.

57. _____. Symptomatology of eye diseases. *Ibid.*, pp. 398-407.

58. _____. Optical defects of the eye. *Ibid.*, pp. 441-451.

59. _____. Special examinations of the eye. *Ibid.*, pp. 419-440.

60. Shehadi, S. I. Reducing the eyelid edema and ecchymosis that occur after corrective rhinoplasty. *Plastic and Reconstructive Surgery*, 49: 508-511, May, 1972.

61. Shields, J. A. *et al.* Melanocytoma of the choroid clinically simulating a malignant melanoma. *Archives of Ophthalmology*, 87: 396-400, April, 1972.

62. Shoch, D. E. Cataract and aphakia. *Postgraduate Medicine*, 51: 166-170, May, 1972.

63. Smith, P. *et al.* Selected ophthalmologic and orthoptic measurements in families. *Archives of Ophthalmology*, 87: 278-282, March, 1972.

64. Soll, D. B. Enucleation surgery. *Archives of Ophthalmology*, 87: 196-197, February, 1972.

65. Tasman, W. Retinal detachment secondary to proliferative diabetic retinopathy. *Archives of Ophthalmology*, 87: 286-289, March, 1972.

66. Tolentino, F. L. Cryotherapy of retinoblastoma. *Archives of Ophthalmology*, 87: 52-55, January, 1971.

67. Vaughan, Daniel, Asbury, Taylor and Cook, Robert. Cornea and sclera. In *General Ophthalmology*, 6th ed. Los Altos, California: Lange Medical Publications, 1971, pp. 74-91.

68. _____. Uveal tract — specific types of uveitis. *Ibid.*, pp. 92-101.

69. _____. Vitreous detachment — vitreous hemorrhage. *Ibid.*, pp. 126-127.

70. _____. Ocular disorders associated with systemic disorders. *Ibid.*, pp. 231-257.

71. _____. Degenerative diseases involving the retina. *Ibid.*, pp. 104-108.

72. _____. Vascular diseases of the retina. *Ibid.*, pp. 108-110.

73. _____. Lens — cataract surgery. *Ibid.*, pp. 116-125.

74. _____. Surgical procedures used in the treatment of the glaucomas. *Ibid.*, pp. 207-211.

75. _____. Retinal detachment — treatment. *Ibid.*, pp. 110-112.

76. _____. Lids and lacrimal apparatus. *Ibid.*, pp. 46-73.

77. _____. Surgical correction of strabismus. *Ibid.*, pp. 182-183.

78. _____. Bacteriologic and microscopic examination. *Ibid.*, p. 37.

79. _____. Special examinations by the ophthalmologist. *Ibid.*, pp. 21-35.

80. Veirs, E. R. and Cunningham, R. D. Considerations in the management of dysthyroid eye disease. *Surgical Clinics of North America*, 52: 353-358, April, 1972.

81. Vignaud, J. *et al.* Orbital arteriography. The *Radiologic Clinics of North America*, 10: 39-61, April, 1972.

82. Werff, T. J. The pressure measured in ophthalmodynamometry. *Archives of Ophthalmology*, 87: 290-292. March, 1972.

83. Yanoff, M. Anatomy of the human eye. In Scheie, Harold G. and Albert, Daniel M. *Adler's Textbook of Ophthalmology*, 8th ed. Philadelphia: W. B. Saunders Co., 1969, pp. 39-73.

84. Zweng, H. C. *et al.* Argon laser photocoagulation of diabetic retinopathy. *Archives of Ophthalmology*, 86: 395-400, October, 1971.

Chapter XIV
The Sense Organ of Hearing

EAR

A. Origin of Terms:

1. acoustic (G) — hearing
2. aditus (L) — approach, entrance
3. auditio (L) — hearing
4. auricle (L) — ear
5. cochlea (G) — snail
6. labyrinth (G) — maze

7. myringa (L) — eardrum
8. ossicle (L) — little bone
9. ot, oto (G) — ear
10. salpingo (G) — tube, trumpet
11. tympano (G) — eardrum
12. vestibule (L) — antechamber

B. Anatomical terms:[16, 42]

1. external ear — division of ear consisting of the auricle and the external auditory canal or meatus.
   a. auricle, pinna — the external ear, made up chiefly of elastic fibrocartilage which is shaped to catch the sound waves.
   b. cerumen — ear wax, formed by the ceruminous glands of the skin lining the meatus.
   c. external auditory meatus — ear passage, composed of a cartilaginous and a bony part.
   d. helix — outer folded margin of the auricle.
2. middle ear, tympanic cavity — division of ear containing the ossicles for the conduction of air-borne sound waves.
   a. auditory tube, eustachian tube, pharyngotympanic tube — channel of communication between pharynx and middle ear.
   b. orifices of the tympanic cavity:
      (1) aditus ad antrum — opening to the mastoid antrum.
      (2) fenestra cochleae, fenestra rotunda — round window facing the internal ear.
      (3) fenestra vestibuli, fenestra ovalis — oval window in which the stapes lodges.
      (4) orifice from the external auditory meatus into the middle ear. It is closed by the tympanic membrane or eardrum.
      (5) opening into auditory tube.
   c. ossicles of the tympanic cavity — three tiny bones: malleus (hammer), incus (anvil) and stapes (stirrup). They transmit vibrations to the internal ear.
3. inner ear[16] — division of ear composed of a number of fluid-filled spaces and the membranous labyrinth which lies within the bony (osseous) labyrinth. The perilymphatic space of the bony labyrinth contains the cochlea, vestibule and semicircular canals. Because of the complexity of the structures, only a few basic facts are given here.
   a. cochlea — spiral tube possessing a bony core, the modiolus which contains the spiral ganglion and transmits the cochlear nerve. It is the essential organ of hearing.
   b. vestibular apparatus — the utricle and semicircular ducts which are concerned with the maintenance of the equilibrium.
   c. vestibulocochlear nerve, eighth cranial nerve, formerly acoustic or auditory nerve — nerve comprising two distinct fiber sets.
      (1) cochlear branch — fibers distributed to the hair cells of the spiral organ. They are concerned with hearing.
      (2) vestibular branch — fibers distributed to portions of the utricle, saccule, and semicircular ducts. They aid in maintaining body balance.[16]

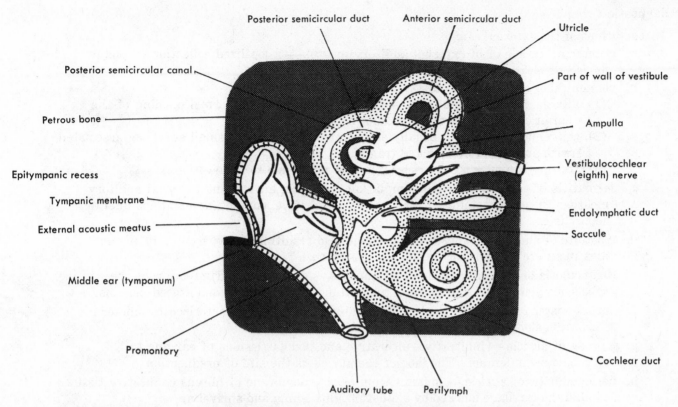

Posterior semicircular duct

Anterior semicircular duct

Utricle

Posterior semicircular canal

Part of wall of vestibule

Petrous bone

Ampulla

Epitympanic recess

Vestibulocochlear (eighth) nerve

Tympanic membrane

External acoustic meatus

Endolymphatic duct

Saccule

Middle ear (tympanum)

Promontory

Cochlear duct

Auditory tube

Perilymph

Fig. 67 – Schematic section through middle and internal ear.

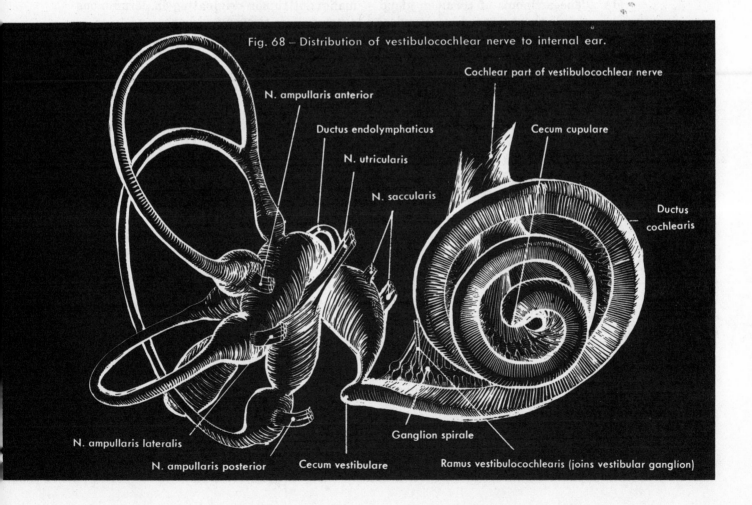

Fig. 68 – Distribution of vestibulocochlear nerve to internal ear.

N. ampullaris anterior

Cochlear part of vestibulocochlear nerve

Ductus endolymphaticus

Cecum cupulare

N. utricularis

N. saccularis

Ductus cochlearis

N. ampullaris lateralis

Ganglion spirale

N. ampullaris posterior

Cecum vestibulare

Ramus vestibulocochlearis (joins vestibular ganglion)

C. Diagnostic Terms:

1. conditions of the external ear:
    a. abscess of auricle or of external auditory meatus — a localized collection of pus of auricle or meatus.
    b. congenital or acquired defects —
        (1) atresia of external auditory meatus — absence of the normal opening of the ear or closure of the external auditory meatus.[28]
        (2) congenital microtia — usually a deformed or misplaced, small aural tag associated with absence of meatus and tragus.[28, 5]
        (3) traumatic avulsion of auricle — loss of pinna due to injury.[5]
    c. dermatitis of external ear — inflammation of skin of auricle and external auditory meatus. Types encountered: dry, moist, exfoliative, contact, eczematous, allergic, seborrheic.
    d. frostbite of auricle — exposure to extreme cold resulting in hyperemia, blanching and, in severe cases, in ulceration and gangrene.
    e. furunculosis of the external auditory meatus — usually a mild infection of the sebaceous glands and hair follicles which tends to develop in debilitated persons.
    f. herpes zoster of auricle — acute inflammatory condition characterized by blister formation along the distribution of the sensory nerve.
    g. leprosy of auricle — infiltrative, ulcerative and nodular lesions of ear due to Mycobacterium leprae. The lobe of the auricle is the site of predilection.
    h. perichondritis of auricle — inflammation of the membrane of fibrous connective tissue around the cartilage marked by exudation, thickening and shriveling.
    i. tumors of external auditory canal —
        (1) adenocarcinoma of cerumen gland — malignant tumor originating in ceruminous glands characterized by a tendency to invade soft tissues and bones and to recur after surgical removal.[2]
        (2) aural polyp — benign tumor on a pedicle which may occlude the external auditory canal and thus interfere with sound conduction.
        (3) cerumen gland adenoma — benign tumor originating in ceruminous glands.[2]

2. conditions of the tympanic membrane:
    a. injury of tympanic membrane, for example, blow on the ear, violent sneezing with closed nostrils.
    b. myringitis, tympanitis — inflammation of the eardrum.
    c. perforation of tympanic membrane — hole in eardrum, if small will heal without treatment, if large may require tympanoplasty.
    d. rupture of tympanic membrane — condition usually due to trauma, for example, direct injury to ear.
    e. tumors — rare disorders which may be endotheliomatous, fibromatous, angiomatous or show other histologic patterns.[14, 11]
    f. tympanosclerosis — involvement of mucous membrane of middle ear or drum by sclerosis of exudate with fixation of the ossicles and drum, diffuse calcification and thickening of the mucosa lining the cavity.[3, 60]

3. conditions of the middle ear:
    a. aerotitis media, barotitis media, aural barotrauma — painful condition caused by atmospheric pressure changes in middle ear chiefly during ascent and descent of air travel or experienced on descent by navy divers.[12, 15]
    b. cholesteatoma — a globular pearly mass covered with a thin shell of epidermis and connective tissue. It usually forms following middle ear infection and is nature's way of arresting suppuration. Pseudocholesteatomas are common.
    c. congenital ossicular malformation — abnormality of ossicles which causes impaired hearing of the conductive type and may respond to surgical correction.[44]

    d. dislocation of ossicles — condition usually due to head injury which damages the eardrum, dislocates the ossicular chain thus causing a conductive type of hearing loss. Surgical repair is recommended.[44]

    e. fracture of temporal bone — usually concurrent middle ear involvement signaled by the presence of blood and cerebrospinal fluid, vertigo, sensorineural or conductive hearing loss and paralysis of the facial nerve.[44]

    f. glomus jugulare — a minute tumor of chemoreceptor cells arising from the jugular bulb in the middle ear. It may cause episodes of dizziness, nystagmus, blackouts and paralysis of vocal cords.[3, 46]

    g. mastoiditis — infection of the middle ear which has extended to the antrum and mastoid cells. Mastoiditis may be acute, subacute, chronic and recurrent.[68, 7, 10]

    h. middle ear effusion — acute or chronic presence of fluid in middle ear generally without infection.
        (1) secretory otitis media, mucoid otitis media, glucotitis — thick, cloudy, viscous exudate in middle ear containing cells and mucous strands.[39, 45, 62]
        (2) serous otitis media — thin, clear amber fluid in middle ear.[45, 19, 10, 22, 12]
        (3) serous otitis media with hemotympanum — serum and blood in middle ear space resulting from temporal bone fracture, tumor or blood disorder.[39, 23, 12]

    i. otitis media — inflammation of the middle ear. Common types encountered are:
        (1) acute suppurative otitis media — marked by intense congestion of mucosa of middle ear, blockage of eustachian tube, serous exudate which becomes infected and rupture of the eardrum. Bacterial invaders are Staphylococcus aureus, Diplococcus pneumoniae, Streptococcus pyogenes, Hemophilus influenzae and others.[44]
        (2) chronic, suppurative otitis media — characterized by continuation of middle ear infection resulting in protracted suppuration.

    j. salpingitis of eustachian tube — inflammation of the auditory tube. It may be acute or chronic.

  4. conditions of the inner ear:
    a. acoustic neuroma — benign tumor of the eighth cranial nerve affecting more the vestibular branch than the cochlear branch of the nerve and causing vertigo, tinnitus and hearing impairment.[13, 36]

    b. labyrinthitis — inflammation of the labyrinth, usually secondary to acute or chronic suppurative otitis media with or without cholesteatoma or to acute upper respiratory infection.[48]

    c. Menière's disease, endolymphatic hydrops — neurologic disorder in its classic form exhibiting a triad symptom complex:
        (1) explosive attacks of true vertigo
        (2) fluctuating hearing loss of the sensorineural type
        (3) tinnitus.
    Dizziness, ataxia and a feeling of fullness in the ear are usually present. Remissions may last years.[37, 34, 40, 51]

    d. otosclerosis recently termed otospongiosis — newly formed spongy bone replacing the hard bone of the labyrinth. It may result in conduction deafness with fixation of the stapes and stapedial footplate followed later by nerve degeneration resulting in mixed deafness.[47, 32]

    e. vestibular neuronitis — sudden vestibular failure in one ear without hearing impairment or tinnitus, apparently due to viral infection or a demyelinating reaction to infection.[37]

  5. hearing loss:
    a. Two basic types are recognized.
        (1) conductive hearing loss — impairment of hearing resulting from obstruction of sound waves which do not reach the inner ear. The interference may be due

to impacted cerumen, exudate, blockage of external auditory canal or eustachian tube, otosclerosis or other causes.[47] Otitis media of some type is the most common cause of conductive hearing loss.[3]

    (2) sensorineural hearing loss — inability of the cochlear division of the eighth cranial nerve to transmit electric impulses to the brain or of the hair cells of the organ of Corti to change sound to electric energy. Dysfunction may be due to neural degeneration of the organ of Corti, alterations in endolymph, cochlear conductive disorder or other causes.[3]

  b. Conductive or sensorineural hearing loss or both may be found in the following types:

    (1) congenital deafness — loss of hearing from birth.[6]

    (2) hysterical deafness — simulated hearing loss associated with neurotic behavior and emotional instability, thus psychogenic in nature.

    (3) Mondini's deafness — genetic deafness due to aplastic changes in the osseous and membranous labyrinth.[41, 6]

    (4) noise deafness, industrial hearing loss, occupational hearing loss — impairment or loss of hearing induced by constant noise, explosions or blows to the head. It disappears in a quiet environment if neural damage is in its early phase.[63]

    (5) sudden hearing loss, spontaneous hearing loss — usually an abrupt onset of sensorineural loss of hearing in one ear due to viral infection, vascular accident, trauma, shrinkage of organ of Corti or other causes. Bilateral sudden hearing loss is uncommon.[17, 18]

6. otogenic complications:

  a. brain abscess — a sequela of chronic suppuration of the ear, often an otitis media.[59, 49, 66]

  b. lateral sinus phlebitis or thrombosis — usually the result of direct contact with infected mastoid cells. In thrombosis the clot may occlude the sinus.[59, 51]

  c. otitic meningitis — inflammation of meninges following ear infection.[38, 49, 66]

  d. petrositis — inflammation of the petrous portion of the temporal bone.[38, 49, 66]

D. Operative Terms:

1. microsurgery of ear — the use of a high power binocular dissecting microscope with built-in illumination in ear operations.[50, 69]

2. the external ear:

  a. amputation of the aural deformity (microtia) — excision of microtia, proper surgical revision of existing malformation as a foundation for a prosthesis and prosthetic reconstruction of pinna.[5, 28]

  b. correction of meatal atresia — most difficult reconstructive procedure of the ear performed under high power magnification using a binocular dissecting microscope. It should only be attempted in the presence of bilateral atresia.[55]

  c. otoplasty — correction of deformed pinna.[3]

  d. otoscopy with magnification — inspection of the auditory canal and eardrum for diagnosis or for removal of polyp or granulation tissue followed by microscopic study.[25]

  e. pneumatic otoscopy — inspection of the ear using an otoscope with an attachment for stimulating variations in air pressure that put the eardrum in motion. It provides a valuable aid in the differential diagnosis of fluid ear, cholesteatoma, labyrinthine fistula and other ear conditions.[25]

3. the middle ear:

  a. catheterization of auditory tube — removing exudate with catheter and inflating middle ear.

  b. mastoid antrotomy — surgical opening of mastoid antrum, usually done for children with middle ear infection.

  c. mastoidectomy, radical — removal of all diseased tissue in mastoid antrum and tympanic cavity and conversion of both into one dry cavity which communicates with the external ear. An operating microscope is used.[65, 49]

d. myringotomy, tympanotomy — opening of the eardrum in area which tends to heal readliy, to avoid spontaneous rupture at a site which rarely closes.

e. myringoplasty — surgical repair of tympanic membrane by tissue grafts.[53]

f. paracentesis tympani — surgical puncture of the eardrum for evacuation of fluid from middle ear.

g. stapedectomy — removal of stapes, reestablishing connection between incus and oval window by interposition of prosthesis and tissue or inert cover over oval window.[20, 24, 9, 33]

h. tympanoplasty — reconstruction surgery of the sound conducting parts of the middle ear using skin graft or vein or fascia or perichondrium and an operating microscope.[21, 54, 57, 64, 4]

i. tympanotomy, exploratory — exploration of middle ear through tympanomeatal approach.

4. the inner ear:

a. decompression of endolymphatic sac — removal of bone around the sac for improvement of vascularization so that endolymph can escape to cerebrospinal fluid system.[3, 34]

b. labyrinthectomy — total destruction of labyrinth with or without removal of Scarpa's ganglion for intractable vertigo.[56]

E. Symptomatic Terms:

1. anacusis — sound perception as such completely lost.
2. auditory agnosia — sound perception at end organ intact, but comprehension of sound lost centrally.
3. aural discharge — drainage from ear.
4. impacted cerumen — dried ear wax.
5. nystagmus — involuntary rhythmic movements in one eye or both which may be horizontal, rotary, vertical, circulatory, oblique or mixed type. They commonly occur in vestibular disease.[51]
6. otalgia — pains in ear, severe earache.
7. otorrhagia — bleeding from the ear.
8. otorrhea — purulent drainage from the ear.
9. paracusis of Willis — ability of person with conductive hearing loss to hear better in the presence of noise.
10. presbycusis — impaired hearing which is part of the aging process.
11. tinnitus — ringing in the ears.
12. vertigo — illusion of movement of individual in relation to his environment. The patient feels that he himself is spinning (subjective type) or the objects are whirling about him (objective type).[48, 37]

a. central vertigo — present in disorders of vestibular nuclei, cerebellum or brainstem, characterized by slow onset, prolonged duration and absence of hearing impairment or tinnitus.[51, 37]

b. peripheral vertigo — present in disorders of vestibular nerve and semicircular canals. It is episodic and explosive, marked by sudden, violent attack lasting minutes to hours and usually accompanied by tinnitus and impaired hearing.[36, 48]

RADIOLOGY

A. Terms Related to Diagnosis:

1. polytomography — a new technique of obtaining multiple serial section views of the ear which are of diagnostic value in middle and inner ear disorders such as pure cochlear otosclerosis, Menière's disease and others. It is also helpful in detecting the site of facial nerve injury by cholesteatoma or bullet in stylomastoid foramen.[32, 25, 56, 67]
2. radiogram of skull — x-ray examination to detect temporal bone or basal skull fractures which cause cochlear or vestibular damage or to locate brain tumors which encroach on the auditory center or interfere with the neural pathway of the 8th cranial nerve.

3. stereoscopic examination — radiographic examination producing an impression of the third dimension.
4. stereoscopic views of mastoids — exact views of both mastoids may be obtained by stereograms.
5. ultrasonography — use of ultrasonic technique for detecting the presence of fluid in the middle ear space.   No echo returns in the absence of fluid in normal ears; but echoes do return in fluid-filled ears.[1]

B. Terms Related to Therapy:

ultrasonic irradiation — ultrasound energy for round window irradiation in the treatment of Menière's disease.[29]

CLINICAL LABORATORY

A. Terms Related to the Laboratory Diagnosis of Ear Conditions:

1. direct smears and cultures from middle ear secretions — tests to determine predominating organisms.   Common bacterial invaders are in
    a. aural furunculosis — Staphylococcus of low virulence.
    b. suppurative otitis media:
       (1) Diplococcus pneumoniae
       (2) Staphylococcus, albus or aureus
       (3) Streptococcus pyogenes, others.[44]
2. spinal fluid examination and blood cultures — tests to detect complications such as otitic meningitis or bacteremia.

B. Terms Related to Functional Tests of Cochlear Apparatus:

1. audiometry — measurement of hearing for the purpose of accurately evaluating the extent and nature of hearing impairment.[26]
2. audiometric test — a quantitative measurement of hearing loss.   Results are plotted according to an established normal on an audiogram which is a graphic representation of a patient's threshold of hearing at different frequencies and intensities.
3. electrocochleography — new method of testing hearing particularly in infants one to six months old.[4]
4. electrodermal audiometry — measurement detects how the electrical conductivity of the skin is modified by sound.[26]
5. electroencephalic audiometry — measurement shows how the electrical activity of the brain is modified by sound.[26]
6. impedance audiometry — collective term which describes the various measurements taken with an impedance bridge.[26, 25]
    a. maximum compliance (C_m) — procedure measures compliance at air pressure maximum.
    b. stapedius reflex threshold — technic measures compliance versus sound level in opposite ear.
    c. tympanogram — procedure measures compliance versus air pressure.[26, 30]
7. speech audiometry — valuable aid in clinical audiology.   The patient's functioning in his environment is estimated by a speech discrimination score.[31]
8. stereoaudiometry — term refers to audiometric procedures which seek to determine the efficiency of binaural hearing.[61]
9. tone decay test — valuable special auditory test which demonstrates the phenomenon of tone decay.[31, 35]
10. tuning fork tests — means for determining the type of hearing impairment in relation to sound conduction and sound perception.   The Rhine test, Schwabach test and Weber test are commonly used.[31]

C. Terms Related to Functional Tests of the Vestibular Apparatus:

1. caloric test — procedure which conveys information of the functional capacity of each labyrinth and the presence of horizontal and rotary nystagmus.[25]
2. electronystagmogram — a record of eye movements by electric tracing induced by caloric or positional stimulation.[3, 8, 58]
3. Romberg test — procedure which tests body balance when eyes are closed and feet together side by side.

ABBREVIATIONS

ABLB — alternate binaural loudness balance
AC — air conduction
AC and BC — air and bone conduction
AD — right ear (auris dextra)
as — left ear (auris sinistra)
BC — bone conduction
CM — cochlear microphonics
ENG — electronystagmogram
ENT — ear, nose and throat
EP — endocochlear potential
ERA — evoked response audiometry

ETF — eustachian tubal function
HD — hearing distance
MACS — mastoid air cell system
Oto. — otology
SAL — sensorineural acuity level
SEM — scanning electron microscopy
SISI — short increment sensitivity index
stereo. — stereogram
VASC — visual-auditory screening test for children

ORAL READING PRACTICE

Otitic Meningitis

Acute or chronic suppurative otitis media may be followed by **intracranial** complications such as **thrombophlebitis** of the **lateral sinus, extra** or **intradural** abscess, **labyrinthitis,** facial paralysis and others.

Meningitis is one of the most serious **sequelae** of ear infections. Its incidence is higher in small children than in adults because of the intimate relation of the middle ear to the middle cranial fossa in early life. Symptoms may develop slowly or there may be an abrupt onset of the disease without **prodromal** manifestations. A chill occasionally signals the beginning of the acute phase. With the cerebral invasion of **pathogenic** organisms the cardinal symptoms make their appearance: a constantly high fever, a headache progressively becoming worse to the point of being excruciating, and vertigo, particularly in the presence of **labyrinthine** involvement. As the disease progresses **prostration** increases, convulsions occur, particularly in children, and the patient becomes very irritable, exhibiting marked personality changes. **Delirium** simulates **maniacal** attacks in extreme cases. In infants the large fontanelle is bulging, but there is no pulsation. The Kernig's sign is positive as evidenced by pain and reflex contraction in the hamstring muscles when the examiner attempts to extend the leg after flexing the thigh upon the body. Muscular rigidity of back and neck and retraction of the head are characteristic manifestations. In addition, the patient suffers from **photophobia, hyperesthesia** at touch and **opisthotonos.** If treatment remains ineffectual, progressive drowsiness and coma develop, the deep reflexes disappear and the prognosis is poor.

Spinal fluid findings clinch the diagnosis. The fluid appears cloudy and purulent and the pressure is increased. The cell count is high in **lymphocytes** and **polymorphonuclear** leukocytes. The protein content of the spinal fluid markedly rises while the sugar drops. An excessively high protein is usually associated with **ventricular blockage** and signals a fatal outcome.

Smear and culture findings generally indicate that the bacterial invaders, causing the ear infection, are the same as those of the **otogenic** complication in the brain.

The Streptococcus pyogenes and **Diplococcus pneumoniae** are the common etiological agents of diffuse purulent meningitis, while **Neisseria meningitidis,** a very pyogenic diplococcus, provokes epidemic cerebrospinal meningitis.

The best treatment is prophylactic. Antibiotic therapy and the establishment of adequate drainage of the suppurative focus in the ear have lowered the incidence of otitic meningitis within the last two decades. Once the disease has developed, vigorous treatment must be instituted to combat the infection, prevent ventricular blocking and maintain electrolyte balance and nutrition.[38, 66]

Table 24

SOME EAR CONDITIONS AMENABLE TO SURGERY

Organs Involved	Diagnoses	Operations	Operative Procedures
Ear	Carcinoma of ear	Amputation of ear Otoplasty	Removal of ear Plastic repair of ear
External auditory meatus	Foreign body in external auditory meatus Papilloma	Otoscopy with removal of foreign body Excision of papilloma	Endoscopic examination of external auditory meatus for removal of foreign body or lesion
Middle ear	Otitis media acute serous	Paracentesis tympani Myringotomy	Puncture of eardrum and evacuation of fluid from middle ear Incision of eardrum and drainage of middle ear
Middle ear	Perforation of eardrum chronic	Myringoplasty	Reconstruction of eardrum
Middle ear Mastoid	Otitis media acute Mastoiditis acute	Complete mastoidectomy	Scooping out and obliterating of infected air cells Removal of diseased mastoid process
Middle ear Mastoid	Otitis media chronic suppurative Mastoiditis chronic suppurative or recurrent	Radical mastoidectomy or modified radical mastoidectomy Repair of middle ear Tympanoplasty	Endaural approach to temporal bone and thorough removal of diseased tissues Surgical creation of a new cavity composed of healthy mastoid tissue, the tympanum and external auditory canal.*
Mastoid	Mastoiditis chronic perforation of pars tensa	Tympanoplasty with or without mastoidectomy	Closure of perforation by skin graft or vein or fascia or perichondrium
Middle ear	Otosclerosis conductive deafness with fixation of stapes	Stapes mobilization operation Stapedioplasty	Surgical opening and loosening of stapedial foot plate Removal of stapes and insertion of delicate prosthesis to replace stapes

Organs Involved	Diagnoses	Operations	Operative Procedures
(Cont'd)		Vein plug stapedioplasty	Removal of entire stapes, insertion of vein plug, creation of an arthroplasty for intact sound conduction
		Fenestration operation of oval window	Removal of stapes and foot plate, creation of a new oval window, and replacement of stapes
Internal ear	Menière's disease 1. unilateral	Labyrinthectomy	Endaural or postaural approach to inner ear
		Exenteration of air cells	Removal of air cells
		Avulsion of endolymphatic labyrinth	Destruction of membranous labyrinth
	2. bilateral	Ultrasonic surgery	Selective destruction of osseous vestibular labyrinth by ultrasonic waves avoiding bombardment of cochlea
Vestibulocochlear nerve	Acoustic neuroma	Excision of neoplasm	Removal of neoplasm which involved some area of the neural passageway of hearing

REFERENCES AND BIBLIOGRAPHY

1. Abramson, D. H. and Abramson, A. L. Ultrasonics in Otolaryngology. *Archives of Otolaryngology*, 96: 146-150, August, 1972.

2. Althaus, S. R. and Ross, J. A. T. Cerumen gland neoplasia. *Archives of Otolaryngology*, 92: 40-42, July, 1970.

3. Aylward, Howard, J., M.D. Personal communications.

4. Bryce, D. P. What is new in surgery — Otorhinolaryngology. *Surgery, Gynecology & Obstetrics*, 134: 271-274, February, 1972.

5. Bulbulian, A. H. Prosthesis for microtia and other deformities of the ear. In Paparella, Michael M., Hohmann, Albert and Huff, John S. *Clinical Otology — An International Symposium*. St. Louis: The C. V. Mosby Co., 1971, pp. 83-93.

6. Burnam, J. A. and Hudson, W. R. Reconstructive surgery for congenital hearing loss. *Southern Medical Journal*, 64: 1460-1464, December, 1971.

7. Carithers, H. A. Acute otitis media and acute mastoiditis. In Conn, Howard F. (ed.). *Current Therapy 1972*. Philadelphia: W. B. Saunders Co., 1972, pp. 115-116.

8. Coats, A. C. Central electronystagmography. *Archives of Otolaryngology*, 92: 43-53, July, 1970.

9. Cody, D. T. Complications of stapedectomy. In Paparella, Michael M., Hohmann, Albert and Huff, John S. *Clinical Otology. An International Symposium*. St. Louis: The C. V. Mosby Co., 1971, pp. 53-74.

10. Deatch, W. W. Ear nose & throat. In Krupp, Marcus A., Chatton, Milton J. and Margen, Sheldon. *Current Diagnosis & Treatment*, 11th ed. Los Altos, California: Lange Medical Publications. 1972. pp. 85-91.

11. DeWeese, D. D. Primary intratympanic meningioma. *Archives of Otolaryngology*, 96: 45-51, July, 1972.

12. Duvall, A. J. Fluid ear. *Postgraduate Medicine*, 52: 79-83, August, 1972.

13. Fishman, R. A. Intracranial tumors. In Beeson, Paul B. and McDermott, Walsh, (eds.). *Cecil-Loeb Textbook of Medicine*, 13th ed. Philadelphia: W. B. Saunders Co., 1971, pp. 273-281.

14. Freedman, S. I. *et al.* Cavernous angiomas of tympanic membrane. *Archives of Otolaryngology*, 96: 158-160, August, 1972.

15. Freeman, P. and Edmonds, C. Inner ear barotrauma. *Archives of Otolaryngology*, 95: 556-563, June, 1972.

16. Gardner, Ernest, Gray, Donald and O'Rahilly, Ronan. *Anatomy — A Regional Study of Human Structure*, 3rd ed. Philadelphia: W. B. Saunders Co., 1969, pp. 631-643.

17. Glasscock, M. E. *et al.* Sudden loss of hearing: a medical emergency. *Southern Medical Journal*, 64: 1485-1489, December, 1971.

18. Goodwin, M. R. *et al.* Effects of intense electrical stimulation on hearing. *Archives of Otolaryngology*, 95: 570-573, June, 1972.

19. Gottschalk, G. H. Serous otitis — A conservative approach to treatment. *Archives of Otolaryngology*, 96: 110-116, August, 1972.

20. Guilford, F. R. Technics of stapedectomy. In Paparella, Michael M., Hohmann, Albert and Huff, John S. *Clinical Otology — An International Symposium*. St. Louis: The C. V. Mosby Co., 1971, pp. 46-52.

21. _____. Current tympanoplasty trends, I. *Ibid.*, pp. 128-136.

266

22. Gunderson, T. *et al.* The middle ear mucosa in serous otitis media. *Archives of Otolaryngology,* 96: 40-44, July, 1972.

23. Hiraide, F. and Paparella, M. M. Vascular changes in middle ear effusions. *Archives of Otolaryngology.* 96, 45-51, July, 1972.

24. House, H. P. Stapes surgery for otosclerosis. In Paparella, Michael M., Hohmann, Albert and Huff, John S. *Clinical Otology — An International Symposium.* St. Louis: The C. V. Mosby Co., 1971, pp. 43-45.

25. Huff, J. S. Preoperative principles and preparation. In Paparella, Michael M., Hohmann, Albert and Huff, John S. *Clinical Otology — An International Symposium.* St. Louis: The C. V. Mosby Co., 1971, pp. 13-18.

26. Jerger, J. F. Suggested nomenclature for impedance audiometry. *Archives of Otolaryngology,* 96: 1-3, July, 1972.

27. Kalbian, V. V. Deafness following oral use of neomycin. *Southern Medical Journal,* 65: 499-500. April, 1972.

28. Konigsmark, B. W. *et al.* Recessive microtia, meatal atresia and hearing loss. *Archives of Otolaryngology,* 96: 105-109, August, 1972.

29. Kossoff, G. Safety factors of the ultrasonic round window irradiation technique. *Archives of Otolaryngology,* 96: 113-116, August, 1972.

30. Lassman, F. M. Current trends in audiology. In Paparella, Michael M., Hohmann, Albert and Huff, John S. *Clinical Otology — An International Symposium.* St. Louis: The C. V. Mosby Co., 1971, pp. 27-33.

31. Linnell, C. Practical clinical audiology. In Paparella, Michael M., Hohmann, Albert and Huff, John S. *Clinical Otology — An International Symposium.* St. Louis: The C. V. Mosby Co., 1971, pp. 19-26.

32. Linthicum, F. H. Diagnosis of cochlear otosclerosis. *Archives of Otolaryngology,* 95: 564-569, June, 1972.

33. _____. Histological evidence of the causes of failure in stapes surgery. *Annals of Otology,* 80: 67-77, January. 1971.

34. McLaurin, J. W. Menière's disease. In Conn, H. F. (ed.) *Current Therapy 1972.* Philadelphia: W. B. Saunders Co., 1972, pp. 666-670.

35. Morales-Garcia, C. *et al.* Tone decay test in neuro-otological diagnosis. *Archives of Otolaryngology,* 96: 231-247, September, 1972.

36. Nelson, J. R. Episodic vertigo. In Conn, H. F. (ed.). *Current Therapy 1972.* Philadelphia: W. B. Saunders Co., 1972, pp. 663-665.

37. _____. Vertigo — Menière's disease — vestibular neuronitis. In Beeson, Paul B. and McDermott, Walsh (eds.). *Cecil-Loeb Textbook of Medicine,* 13th ed. Philadelphia: W. B. Saunders Co., 1971, pp. 163-167.

38. Palva, T., Palva A. and Karja, J. Fatal meningitis in a case of otosclerosis operated upon bilaterally. *Archives of Otolaryngology,* 96: 130-137, August, 1972.

39. Paparella, M. M. and Jurgens, G. L. Middle ear fluid problems. In Paparella, Michael M., Hohmann, Albert and Huff, John S. *Clinical Otology — An International Symposium.* St. Louis: The C. V. Mosby Co., 1971, pp. 146-155.

40. Paparella, M. M. The dizzy patient. *Postgraduate Medicine,* 52: 97-102, August, 1972.

41. Paparella, M. M. and Fakhyr, M. E. Mondini's deafness. *Archives of Otolaryngology,* 95: 134-140, February, 1972.

42. Pratt, Lindsay L. Applied anatomy. In Ryan, Robert E., Ogura, Joseph H., Biller, Hugh F. and Pratt, Lindsay L. *Synopsis of Ear, Nose and Throat Diseases,* 3rd ed. St. Louis: The C. V. Mosby Co., 1970, pp. 3-18.

43. _____. Diseases of the external ear. *Ibid.,* pp. 28-34.

44. _____. Diseases of the middle ear space. *Ibid.,* pp. 35-41.

45. _____. Fluid in the middle ear. *Ibid.,* pp. 42-44.

46. _____. Tumors involving the middle ear. *Ibid.,* pp. 60-61.

47. _____. Common causes of hearing loss. *Ibid.,* pp. 72-78.

48. _____. Labyrinthitis. *Ibid.,* pp. 89-90.

49. _____. Diseases of the mastoid process. *Ibid.,* pp. 49-59.

50. _____. Microsurgery of the ear. *Ibid.,* pp. 79-85.

51. Resch, J. A. Neurologic aspects of vestibular disease. In Paparella, Michael M., Hohmann, Albert and Huff, John S. *Clinical Otology — An International Symposium.* St. Louis: The C. V. Mosby Co., 1971, pp. 167-170.

52. Schuknecht, H. F. Sensorineural hearing loss — pathologic types and manifestations. In Paparella, Michael M., Hohmann, Albert and Huff, John S. *Clinical Otology — An International Symposium.* St. Louis: The C. V. Mosby Co., 1971, pp. 177-190.

53. _____. Mastoidectomy and myringoplasty for chronic otitis media and mastoiditis. *Ibid.,* pp. 197-199.

54. _____. Current tympanoplasty trends, II. *Ibid.,* pp. 137-139.

55. Shambaugh, G. E. Congenital atresia — surgical considerations. In Paparella, Michael M., Hohmann, Albert and Huff, John S. *Clinical Otology — An International Symposium.* St. Louis: The C. V. Mosby Co., 1971, pp. 95-97.

56. _____. Medical management of vertigo. *Ibid.,* pp. 171-173.

57. Siedentop, K. H., Hamilton, L. R. and Osenar, S. B. Predictability of tympanoplasty results. *Archives of Otolaryngology,* 95: 146-150, February, 1972.

58. Spooner, T. R. and Goode, R. L. The hyperthermic electronystagmogram in multiple sclerosis. *Archives of Laryngology,* 95: 543-546, June, 1972.

59. Swartz, M. N. Parameningeal infections. In Beeson, Paul B. and McDermott, Walsh (eds.). *Cecil-Loeb Textbook of Medicine,* 13th ed. Philadelphia: W. B. Saunders Co., 1971, pp. 223-228.

60. Teatini, G. Dealing with tympanosclerosis. In Paparella, Michael M., Hohmann, Albert and Huff, John S. *Clinical Otology — An International Symposium.* St. Louis: The C. V. Mosby Co., 1971, pp. 140-143.

61. _____. Stereoaudiometry. *Ibid.,* pp. 34-39.

62. Tos, M. and Bak-Pedersen, K. The pathogenesis of chronic secretory otitis media. *Archives of Otolaryngology,* 95: 511-521, June, 1972.

63. Ward, W. D. Noise-induced deafness — practical considerations. In Paparella, Michael M. Hohmann, Albert and Huff, John S. *Clinical Otology — An International Symposium.* St. Louis: The C. V. Mosby Co., 1971, pp. 191-196.

64. Wehrs, R. E. Homograft tympanic membrane in tymanoplasty. *Archives of Otolaryngology,* 93: 132-139, February, 1971.

65. Williams, H. L. Anatomic principles in mastoid surgery. In Paparella, Michael M. Hohmann, Albert and Huff, John S. *Clinical Otology — An International Symposium.* St. Louis: The C. V. Mosby Co., 1971, pp. 109-119.

66. Wolfowitz, B. L. Otogenic intracranial complications. *Archives of Otolaryngology.* 96: 220-222, September, 1972.

67. Wright, J. W. and Taylor, C. E. Facial nerve abnormalities revealed by polytomography. *Archives of Otolaryngology,* 95: 426-430, May, 1972.

68. Zoller, H. Acute mastoiditis and its complications: a changing trend. *Southern Medical Journal,* 65: 477-480, April, 1972.

69. Yasargil, M. G. Intracranial microsurgery. *Clinical Neurosurgery. Proceedings of the Congress of Neurological Surgeons.* Baltimore: The Williams & Wilkins Co., 1970, pp. 250-256.

Chapter XV
Systemic Disorders

INFECTIOUS DISEASES

A. Origin of Terms:

1. ameba (G) — change
2. bacillus (L) — rod
3. bacterio- (G) — rod
4. coccus (G) — berry
5. gon, gono- (G) — offspring
6. histo- (G) — tissue
7. inoculate (L) — to engraft
8. myco- (G) — fungus
9. protozoon (G) — first animal
10. pseudopod (G) — false foot
11. saprophyte (G) — rotten plant
12. spirochete (G) — coiled hair
13. staphylo- (G) — little grape
14. strepto- (G) — twisted
15. treponema (G) — turned thread
16. virus (L) — poison
17. zoster (G) — girdle

B. Some Basic Terms:

1. acid-fast bacilli — organisms that resist acid-alcohol decolorization after they have been stained with a special dye (carbofuchsin).
2. aerobes — organisms requiring oxygen for growth.
3. agglutination — clumping of bacteria (or blood cells) following mixture with antisera.
4. allergen — substance capable of bringing about a hypersensitive state when introduced into the body.
5. allergy — state of hypersensitivity in which a person experiences certain symptoms upon coming in contact with an allergen.
6. anaerobes — organisms capable of growing in the absence of atmospheric oxygen.
7. antigen — substance that will cause the body to form antibodies.[34, 48]
8. antiseptic — substance that prevents bacterial growth.
9. antitoxin — immune serum that prevents the deleterious action of a toxin.
10. contagious — communicable.
11. culture medium — a milieu which promotes the growth of bacteria.
12. direct contact — spread of disease from person to person.
13. exudate — fluid or blood elements that have escaped into body cavities or tissues.
14. fungus (pl. fungi) — a vegetable, unicellular organism that feeds upon organic matter.
15. gram-negative — pertaining to bacteria which do not retain the Gram stain (crystal violet) following suitable decolorization.
16. gram-positive — pertaining to bacteria which retain the Gram stain after suitable decolorization.
17. hypersensitivity — exaggerated sensitivity to an infective, chemical or other agent, such as an extreme allergic reaction to a foreign protein. Hypersensitivity may be of the
    a. immediate type — occurring within 1-30 minutes, e.g. anaphylactic shock
    b. delayed type — developing gradually within 24-48 hours or longer, e.g. tuberculin reaction.
    c. subacute delayed type, Arthus reaction — developing within 4 to 10 hours; characterized by a marked infiltration of small vessels with polymorphonuclear leukocytes, local edema and bleeding without thrombus formation.[2]
18. immunity — resistance to disease, either natural or acquired.
19. inoculation — the process of introducing pathogenic organisms.
20. microorganism — a plant or animal only recognized under microscopic vision.
21. molds — plants belonging to a division of organisms known as fungi.
22. mycology — the study or science of fungi.

23. nucleus — functional center of a cell.
24. parasite — a plant or animal that exists on or within another and derives nourishment from its host.
25. pathogenic — disease producing.
26. putrefaction — decomposition of organic material.
27. pyogenic — pus forming.
28. saprophyte — an organism which grows on dead matter.
29. sensitivity (drug related) — ability of infective organism to respond to the bacteriostatic or bacteriocidal action of an antibiotic or other agent.
30. susecptibility — ability to acquire an infection following exposure to pathogenic organisms.
31. virus (pl. viruses) — infectious agent of protein-coated nucleic acid and submicroscopic size, depending completely on the cells of its host.[37]
    Current research efforts focus on viruses as possible causes of cancer. Trentin and others have shown that several serotypes of adenovirus are oncogenic producing sarcoma in hamsters.[11]
32. yeast — unicellular organism which usually reproduces by budding.

C. Terms Pertaining to Infections Due to Viruses:

1. adenoviral infections — 31 serotypes of DNA bearing adenovirus, transmitted by person-to-person contact and capable of latency in lymphoid tissue. Adenoviruses may cause epidemic outbreaks of
   a. acute respiratory disease (ARD) — severe grippe-like respiratory infection involving the pharynx, larynx, bronchi and nasal mucosa and characterized by fever, sore throat, hoarseness, cough, headache and malaise.
   b. febrile pharyngitis — inflammation of pharynx with exudate, enlarged cervical lymph nodes and fever.
   c. keratoconjunctivitis, epidemic (EKC) — serious eye infection with corneal infiltrates and follicular conjunctival lesions. Epidemics may be initiated in clinics by contaminated eye drops.
   d. pharyngoconjunctival fever — severe type of pharyngitis associated with acute follicular conjunctivitis, usually lasting 5 days.
   e. pneumonia, adenoviral — highly fatal bronchopneumonia in infants, with sore throat, cough, prostration and high fever.[33, 16]
2. chickenpox, varicella — acute infectious disease, characterized by sudden onset, mild fever and skin eruption. The prognosis is good.
3. cytomegalovirus infections — common viral infections occurring congenitally or in acquired forms in newborn, child or adult, with or without symptoms, as local or systemic disorders. Infected cells are oversize and contain intranuclear and cytoplasmic inclusion bodies. Viremia and viruria clinch the diagnosis.[38, 29]
   a. cytomegalic inclusion disease, salivary gland virus disease — systemic disorder with cytomegalovirus present in salivary glands, liver, spleen and other viscera. In adults the disease is usually associated with the terminal phase of leukemia, malignancy or other chronic debilitating diseases.
   b. cytomegalovirus postperfusion and posttransfusion syndromes — the clinical picture resembles that of infectious mononucleosis, but the heterophil antibody is negative.[35, 36, 24]
4. German measles, rubella — mildly contagious disease with catarrhal symptoms and a rash resembling measles.[15, 32]
5. herpes simplex, herpes febrilis, fever blisters — acute infectious condition of the skin or mucous membranes, marked by vesicular lesions which may become infected. Condition is primary or recurrent.
6. herpes zoster — a viral disease affecting primarily one or more dorsal root ganglia or extramedullary cranial nerve ganglia. It is characterized by a vesicular eruption in the skin or mucous membrane along the course of the peripheral nerves which arise in the affected ganglia.

7. infectious hepatitis, viral hepatitis — disease associated with jaundice, liver damage and leukopenia.[28, 43]
8. infectious mononucleosis — disease thought to be of viral origin. It exhibits a characteristic lymphocytosis and irregular clinical pattern. Glandular swelling and throat symptoms may be present. The condition is seen in children and young adults.[44]
9. influenza — acute febrile disease due to the influenza virus, A, B or C. It is generally characterized by respiratory symptoms and joint pains. It may occur in epidemic or even pandemic form.
10. measles, rubeola — highly communicable disease, clinically manifested by Koplik spots of the buccal mucosa, a rash and catarrhal symptoms.[40]
11. mumps, infectious parotitis — virus disease of the salivary glands, which tends to involve other organs, especially the testes and ovaries.
12. parrot fever, psittacosis — acute infectious disease, marked by fever, headache and early lung involvement, cough, delirium and prostration. It is transmitted through contact with infected birds or through laboratory infection.
13. rabies, hydrophobia — acute encephalitis which causes paralysis, delirium and convulsions.
14. smallpox, variola — communicable disease, characterized by a rash which changes from macules, papules, vesicles, pustules to scabs.

D. Terms Pertaining to Infections Due to Cocci:*

1. erysipelas — acute febrile, inflammatory disease marked by localized skin lesions which tend to migrate. The infection is due to the Streptococcus pyogenes.
2. furunculosis — a condition resulting from boils generally caused by Staphylococcus aureus.
3. gonorrhea — a specific infection which usually has its inception in the urethra and attacks the genital mucous membrane. The infection may also affect the conjunctiva and joints. The etiological agent is Neisseria gonorrhoeae (gonococcus).[8]
4. meningitis — inflammation of meninges. The epidemic form is caused by Neisseria meningitidis.

E. Terms Pertaining to Infections Due to Bacilli:

1. bacillary dysentery, shigellosis — acute infection marked by diarrhea, tenesmus, fever and, in severe cases, mucus and blood in stool. Prognosis tends to be serious in infants and debilitated aged individuals. The disease is caused by various species of Shigella.[7]
2. diphtheria — an acute infection, generally associated with fever and the formation of a grayish membrane in the throat from which the Klebs-Loeffler bacillus can be cultured.
3. food poisoning — disease characterized by an abrupt onset of gastrointestinal symptoms caused by food intoxication or infection.
   a. botulism — true food poisoning, a fatal, afebrile condition, marked by weakness, constipation, headache and forms of paralysis. The intoxication is due to the botulinus bacillus (Clostridium botulinum).[23]
   b. Staphylococcus intoxication — a poisoning associated with more or less violent and abrupt onset of nausea, vomiting and prostration. Severe diarrhea may occur.
   c. Salmonella infection, salmonellosis — condition causing typhoid and paratyphoid fevers.[41]
4. undulant fever, brucellosis — a general infection characterized by intermittent or continuous fever, headache, chills and profuse perspiration. The etiological agents are three species of Brucella.

F. Terms Pertaining to Infections Due to Fungi and Yeasts:

1. actinomycosis — chronic ray fungus disease characterized by multiple abscesses which form draining sinuses. Lesions occur in face, neck, lungs, abdomen, the latter being highly fatal.

---

* Infections due to cocci are so numerous that it has only been possible to give one example of the most important pathogenic organisms.

2. aspergillosis — infection with Aspergillus which attacks the lungs, skin, external ear, nasal sinuses, meninges and bones. It is mainly found among agricultural workers and pigeon feeders.[55]

3. blastomycosis — mycotic infection either limited to subcutaneous tissue or disseminated throughout the lungs or multiple body systems. It is prevalent in Illinois, Tennessee, Louisiana and North Carolina.

4. candidiasis — acute or subacute fungus infection which causes thrush, glossitis, vaginitis, onychia and pneumonitis. It is also seen in patients receiving chemotherapy.

5. coccidioidomycosis — either a primary, acute infection of the lungs, lymph nodes or skin with a favorable prognosis or a generalized infection including the meninges that is prone to be fatal. It is prevalent in southwestern United States.[53]

6. cryptococcosis — a very serious mycotic infection forming multiple abscesses and lesions of skin, subcutaneous tissue, lungs and meninges. The etiological agent is the Crytococcus neoformans.

7. histoplasmosis — mycotic disease caused by Histoplasma capsulatum which produces benign pulmonary lesions and rarely attacks the reticuloendothelial system. It is prevalent in Missouri, Central Mississippi, and other parts of the United States.[26]

8. mycology — the study of science of fungi.

9. mycosis (pl. mycoses) — any fungus disease.

10. nocardiosis — infection chiefly caused by Nocardia asteroides, either localized in the lungs or disseminated through multiple systems: skin, subcutaneous tissue, brain and others.

G. Terms Pertaining to Infections Due to Spirochetes:

1. relapsing fever — a contagious disease marked by intermittent attacks of fever.

2. venereal syphilis — infectious, relapsing disease which is characterized by a primary lesion or hard chancre. It is followed by a secondary skin eruption with typical reddish brown, coppery spots, periods of latency and systemic late lesions in the central nervous and cardiovascular systems.[9, 10, 51]

H. Terms Pertaining to Infections Due to Protozoa:

1. amebic dysentery, amebiasis — a parasitic infection marked by diarrhea, pain and fever. It is caused by the protozoan Entamoeba histolytica.[17]

2. malaria — disease due to the presence and multiplication of parasites in the blood. It is manifested by splenomegaly, anemia and sweating.
   There are four types:
   a. quotidian — paroxysms occur every 24 hours due to daily sporulation.
   b. tertian — paroxysms occur every 48 hours.
   c. quartan — paroxysms occur every 72 hours and are accompanied by seizures.
   d. falciparum — paroxysms usually occur between 24-48 hours; causes cerebral vascular occlusion. It has highest mortality of malaria.[50]

IMMUNOLOGICAL DISEASES

A. Origin of Terms:

1. ana (G) — without
2. auto (G) — self
3. fluorescent (L) — to flow
4. histos (G) — tissue, web
5. immune (L) — safe, exempt
6. lysis (G) — dissolution
7. phoresis (G) — a carrying in
8. phylaxis (G) — protection

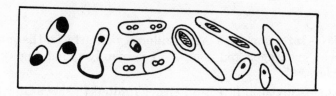

Fig. 69 – Bacilli. Rod-shaped or club-shaped organisms.

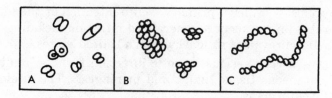

Fig. 70 – Cocci. Spherical or oval organisms. A. Diplococci (in pairs); B. Staphylococci (in clusters); C. Streptococci (in chains).

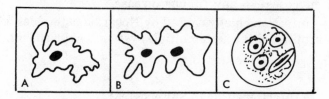

Fig. 71 – Amebae. Unicellular animal organisms, capable of changing form by throwing out foot-like processes (pseudopodia) which help them to move about and obtain nourishment. A. Ameba; B. Ameba dividing; C. Cyst of Entamoeba histolytica.

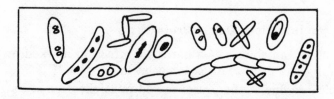

Fig. 72 – Salmonella and Shigella. Simple, non-spore forming rods, often joined end-to-end.

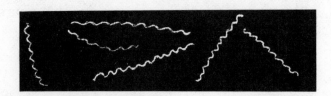

Fig. 73 – Treponema pallidum. Coiled, virulent organisms containing 8 to 14 spirals.

B. Some Basic Terms:

1. anaphylaxis — excessive hypersensitivity to foreign protein or other substance, clinically manifested by edema of larynx, bronchospasm, hypoxia, respiratory distress, hypotension and vascular collapse.[3]

2. autoantibodies — antibodies elicited by an individual's own antigens.

3. autohemolysins — antibodies acting on the corpuscles of an individual's own blood.[56]

4. autoimmune diseases — immunologic disorders in which the patient's own tissues produce antigenic stimuli. By using the fluorescein antibody technique, the presence of autoimmunity has been detected in certain cases of
   chronic thyroiditis
   disseminated lupus erythematosus
   rheumatoid arthritis
   viral hepatitis
   poliomyelitis and other diseases.[20, 1, 27]
   Recent studies indicate that antigen-antibody complexes play a significant role in diseases of hypersensitivity and in delayed hypersensitivity.
   Infectious diseases have also been targets of immunological research. Investigations have led to the preparation of labeled antisera for the identification of Streptococci, Staphylococci, Entamoeba coli, Proteus and other pathogenic agents.

5. autoimmunization — the production of antibodies or other immunological responses to antigens in an individual without any artificial intervention.

6. cytotoxicity — the destruction of cells by autoantibodies as seen in acquired hemolytic anemia and other diseases.

7. fluorescein — a red crystalline powder used for diagnostic purposes.

8. fluorescence — luminescence of a substance when exposed to short wave rays.

9. histocompatibility — tissue compatibility between a recipient and donor based on immunologic identity or similarity of tissues necessary for successful transplantation.[45, 56]

10. immune response — formation of antibodies due to a specific stimulus.[56]

11. immunohematology — branch of hematology dealing with antigen-antibody reactions and their effects on the blood.

12. immunoelectrophoresis — procedure employed to separate and identify multiple protein components. In the test use is made of physiochemical and immunologic specificity.[56, 14]

13. immunogen — one of a group of substances capable of stimulating an immune response or initiating a certain degree of active immunity under favorable conditions. Its effects may be detrimental or beneficial.[4]

14. immunogenicity — the ability of an immunogen to evoke an immune response,[4, 67] or the ability of an antigen to stimulate antibody formation.
    Immunogenicity is the same as antigenicity.[56]

15. immunoglobulin concentration — the amount of serum protein components determined by immunoelectrophoresis for establishing the presence or absence of elevated or depressed immunoglobulin levels. Thus an exaggerated susceptibility to infection or antibody deficiency may be detected. The immunoglobulins so far discovered are
    Immunoglobulin G — IgG — yG-globulin
    Immunoglobulin A — IgA — yA-globulin
    Immunoglobulin M — IgM — yM-globulin
    Immunoglobulin D — IgD — yD-globulin
    Immunoglobulin E — IgE — yE-globulin.[20]

16. immunology — the medical science which is concerned primarily with immunity or resistance to disease of the human being. In its practical aspects it deals with methods of diagnosing or preventing disease or influencing its course by serotherapy and vaccination.

17. immunopathology — the study of disorders or diseases resulting from antigen-antibody reactions or alterations produced by immunologic responses.[56]

18. immunosuppressive therapy — treatment instituted to suppress all immune responses and thus prevent the rejection of a graft.[56]

19. rejection phenomenon — reaction to graft based on the formation of antibodies directed against the donated tissue or organ.[56]

20. transplantation immunity — immune responses to transplanting organs depending on the histocompatibility of the type of graft.

    a. allograft, homograft — tissue or organ from one individual is transferred to another individual of the same species.

    b. autograft — tissue or organ is transplanted from one part of the body to another in the same individual.

    c. isograft — tissue or organ is transplanted from one identical twin to another. Histocompatibility exists in its most complete form.

    d. xenograft, heterograft — tissue or organ from donor from one species is implanted in recipient from another species.[45] Grafts between species are subject to intense medical research.[6, 19, 46]

DISEASES OF CONNECTIVE TISSUE

A. Origin of Terms:

1. colla (G) — glue
2. erythema (G) — redness
3. lupus (L) — wolf, meaning destructive
4. sclera, sclero (G) — hard

B. Anatomical Terms:

1. collagen — a substance present between the fibers of connective tissue throughout the body.

2. collagen diseases — a group of diseases in which the connective tissues have undergone pathological changes. The prognosis is fatal.

3. connective tissue — a variety of tissues composed of widely spaced cells between which intercellular material is deposited. This intercellular substance offers the distinguishing mark of the specific connective tissue; for example, mineral salts are located in the interspaces of bone and are responsible for its hardness, while for blood the intercellular substance is liquid. Other variations of connective tissue are areolar, adipose, fibrous, cartilage and lymphoid tissues.

C. Diagnostic Terms:

1. dermatomyositis — a disease of unknown etiology. It is characterized by an insidious onset, and subsequent dermatitis and widespread degeneration of the skeletal muscles.[54]

2. disseminated lupus erythematosus — collagenous disease which affects the synovial and serous membranes and vascular system. It is clinically recognized by a typical butterfly lesion on the bridge of the nose and on the cheeks. The prognosis is usually fatal.[31]

3. Marfan's syndrome, arachnodactyly — hereditary disorder of a connective tissue element resulting in skeletal, ocular and cardiovascular abnormalities. Clinical features are spidery fingers, disproportionately long limbs, funnel chest, lax, redundant ligaments, ectopia lentis (displaced lens) with impaired vision. Hemodynamic stress on the media of the aorta may lead to dissecting aortic aneurysm. Other disorders may be present.[5]

4. polyarteritis, periarteritis nodosa — a systemic disease, characterized by the presence of nodules along the course of the muscular arteries.

5. scleroderma — chronic disease causing a leathery induration of the skin, progressive atrophy and pigmentation. Systemic involvement of the mucous membranes, musculoskeletal, vascular and digestive systems may lead to a fatal prognosis.

Table 25

IMPORTANT LABORATORY TESTS FOR INFECTIOUS DISEASES

A. VIRAL DISEASES[a,b,c]

Diseases	Etiological Agent	Tests for Diagnosis
Acute respiratory disease Conjunctivitis Keratoconjunctivitis Pharyngitis	Adenovirus type 4 and 7, others type 3, others type 8, also 3 and 7a	Virus isolation from throat and conjunctival swabs or washings Complement fixation Neutralization Hemagglutination inhibition
Bronchitis Bronchiolitis Coryza Pneumonia	Respiratory syncytial virus	Complement fixation Neutralization Hemagglutination inhibition
Classical influenza Acute bronchitis Common cold Croup	Myxovirus Influenza A, B, C Parainfluenza 1, 2, 3, 4	Virus isolation from throat washings and sputum Complement fixation Hemagglutination inhibition
Mumps (parotitis) Orchitis Encephalitis	Mumps virus	Virus isolation from saliva, mouth washings, spinal fluid and/or testicular tissue
Conjunctivitis Coryza Pharyngitis Pleurodynia Aseptic meningitis Diarrhea neonatorum	Picornavirus Coxsackie A virus types 1-24 Coxsackie B virus types 1-20 ECHO virus types 1-28	Tests available but impractical
Poliomyelitis	Poliovirus types 1, 2, 3	Virus isolation from feces Complement fixation Neutralization
Chickenpox (varicella) Herpes zoster	Varicella virus	Complement fixation Neutralization Fluorescent antibody
Cytomegalic inclusion disease CMV induced postperfusion and posttransfusion syndromes	Cytomegalovirus CMV	Virus isolation from culture of peripheral leukocytes, urine and pharyngeal washings Complement fixation Indirect immunofluorescence
Infectious mononucleosis	Epstein-Barr virus EBV	Virus identification from lymphoid cells Complement fixation Indirect immunofluorescence Immunoglobulins IgM and IgG

Diseases	Etiological Agent	Tests for Diagnosis
German measles (rubella)	Rubella virus	Virus isolation from blood Complement fixation Neutralization Fluorescent antibody
Measles (rubeola)	Rubeola virus	Virus isolation from blood Complement fixation Neutralization Hemagglutination inhibition
Psittacosis (ornithosis)	Bedsonia virus	Virus isolation from sputum, throat swabs or washings Complement fixation Neutralization Fluorescent antibody

B. BACTERIAL DISEASES[d,e]

Disease	Etiology of Disease	Tests for Diagnosis
Abscesses	Staphylococcus aureus	Microscopic: Smears and cultures from infected lesions
Bacterial endocarditis	Streptococcus various kinds	Microscopic: Blood culture
Erysipelas	Streptococcus pyogenes (hemolyticus)	Microscopic: Smears and cultures of material obtained from nasal orifices
Gonococcal infections	Neisseria gonorrhoeae (gonococcus)	Microscopic: Smears and cultures from secretions Kolmer complement fixation test for gonorrhea
Meningococcal meningitis	Neisseria meningitidis (meningococcus)	Microscopic: Smears and cultures from nasopharynx, spinal fluid and blood
Pneumonia	Diplococcus pneumoniae	Microscopic: Typing and culturing of sputum; blood culture Animal inoculation of sputum
Scarlet fever	Streptococcus pyogenes (hemolyticus)	Skin tests: Dick test: Intradermal injection of dilute scarlet fever streptococcus toxin Schultz-Charlton test, the Rash Extinction Test for Scarlet Fever: Intradermal injection of convalescent scarlet fever serum
Genitourinary infections	Streptococcus faecalis (enterococci)	Microscopic: Smears and cultures
Genitourinary infections	Enterobacter group Escherichia group Klebsiella Proteus group Pseudomonas aeruginosa	Microscopic: Smears and cultures

Disease	Etiology of Disease	Tests for Diagnosis or Susceptibility
Bacillary dysentery	Shigella dysenteriae Shigella flexneri	Serologic: Agglutination test Microscopic: Culture from stool
Diphtheria	Corynebacterium diphtheriae (Klebs-Loeffler bacillus)	Microscopic: Culture from throat or larynx Schick test: Intradermal injection of diluted diphtheria toxin
Food poisoning (botulism)	Clostridium botulinum	Animal inoculation for toxin in suspected food
Gas gangrene	Clostridium perfringens (Welchii)	Microscopic: Anaerobic culture from lesion
Influenzal meningitis in children	Hemophilus influenzae usually type B	Microscopic: Cultures from mouth or nose Typing of organism
Leprosy (Hansen's disease)	Mycobacterium leprae (leprosy or Hansen's bacillus)	Microscopic: Smear and culture from cutaneous skin lesions — nodules, plaques, ulcers Animal inoculation
Tuberculosis, pulmonary and extrapulmonary	Mycobacterium tuberculosis (tubercle bacillus)	Microscopic: Smear and culture from sputum, gastric, and bronchial washings, drainage and tuberculous lesions from organs Animal inoculation of material Tuberculin tests — Mantoux, Tine, Heaf
Tularemia	Pasteurella tularensis (bacterium tularense)	Serologic: Agglutination test Animal inoculation of material Skin test for tularemia
Typhoid fever Paratyphoid fever Food infection	Salmonella typhi Salmonella paratyphi - A, B or C	Microscopic: Culture from stool and urine Serologic: Widal reaction agglutination of bacilli
Undulant fever (brucellosis)	Brucella melitensis abortus suis	Serologic: Agglutination test for undulant fever
Whooping cough (pertussis)	Bordetella pertussis (pertussis bacillus)	Microscopic: Culture on cough plate Skin test

C. MYCOTIC DISEASES[f]

Disease	Etiology of Disease	Tests for Diagnosis
Actinomycosis	Actinomyces	Microscopic: Direct smears or cultures from sinuses, sputum Animal inoculation
Blastomycosis	Blastomyces	Microscopic: Direct smears or culture from abscesses, sputum Animal inoculation

Disease	Etiology of Disease	Tests for Diagnosis
Candidiasis	Candida albicans (Monilia)	Microscopic: Direct smears and cultures from skin and nail scrapings, sputum, material from vagina
Coccidioido-mycosis	Coccidioides immitis	Microscopic: Direct smears or culture from sputum, gastric content, pleural fluid, abscesses Animal inoculation Skin test
Histoplasmosis	Histoplasma capsulatum	Microscopic: Direct smears or culture of bone marrow, lymph nodes Animal inoculation Skin tests — Tine and intradermal
Nocardiosis	Nocardia asteroides and related species	Microscopic: Cultures from sputum, lung abscesses, brain abscesses, skin or other lesions

D. SPIROCHETAL AND PROTOZOAL DISEASES[d,g]

Disease	Etiology of Disease	Tests for Diagnosis
Syphilis	Treponema pallidum	Serologic: Wasserman, Kahn, Kolmer, VDRL and RPCF Dark field examination of scraping from chancre and TPI
Amebic dysentery	Entamoeba histolytica	Microscopic: Examination of fresh stools
Malaria Malignant cerebral malaria	Plasmodium vivax malariae falciparum	Microscopic: Examination of blood smears
Toxoplasmosis	Toxoplasma gondii	Serologic: Sabin-Feldman dye test Complement fixation Agglutination Fluorescence Skin test

[a] M. Schaeffer. Diagnosis of viral and rickettsial infections. In Miller, Seward E. and Weller, John M. *Textbook of Clinical Pathology*, 8th ed. Baltimore: The Williams and Wilkins Co., 1971, pp. 345-366.

[b] E. Jawetz, J. L. Melinick and E. A. Adelberg. Isolation of viruses from clinical specimens — Serologic diagnosis of virus infections. In *Review of Medical Microbiology*, 9th ed. Los Altos, California: Lange Medical Publications, 1970, pp. 301-330.

[c] _____. Adenovirus group — Picornavirus group — Paramyxovirus group. *Ibid.*, pp. 345-404.

[d] _____. Pyogenic cocci — Gram-positive bacilli — myobacteria — Spirochetes and other spiral microorganisms. *Ibid.*, pp. 161-226.

[e] T. Hamilton, B. W. Hamilton. Diagnosis of bacterial infections. In Miller, Seward E. and Weller, John M. *Textbook of Clinical Pathology*, 8th ed. Baltimore: The Williams & Wilkins Co., 1971, pp. 367-415.

[f] A. L. McQuown. Diagnosis of mycological infections. *Ibid.*, pp. 416-432.

[g] S. E. Miller. Diagnosis of parasitological infections. *Ibid.*, pp. 433-476.

CLINICAL LABORATORY

A. Terms Related to Hematologic and Serologic Tests:

1. infectious mononucleosis
   a. sheep cell differential test — a specific and qualitative test based on the fact that anti-sheep agglutinins in infectious mononucleosis are completely removed with beef cells and are incompletely or not removed with Forssman antigen (guinea pig or horse kidney).[21]
   b. spot test for infectious mononucleosis, Monospot — a complete one-minute differential slide test for the detection of the specific heterophile antibodies associated with infectious mononucleosis.
      Negative test — the agglutination pattern is stronger on the right side of the slide (II).
      Positive test — the agglutination pattern is stronger on the left side of the slide (I).
      If no agglutination appears on either side of the slide or if agglutination is equal on both sides of the slide (I-II), the test is negative.
      The basic principles of absorption in the Monospot slide test are comparable to those laid down by Davidsohn in the sheep agglutinin differential test.[21]

2. lupus erythematosus
   a. anti-DNP, antinucleoprotein — the most typical antinuclear antibody (ANA) which causes the LE-cell phenomenon and is present in untreated systemic lupus erythematosus (SLE).[21] Antinuclear factors may also be found in rheumatoid arthritis, other connective tissue diseases and disseminated malignancies.
   b. LE-cell — large granulocyte containing purplish stainable inclusions (Wright stain) thinly rimmed with cytoplasm. The nucleus is pushed aside.
   c. LE-cell factor, LE-serum factor — one of several autoantibodies reacting against nucleoprotein to transform nuclei into homogenous globular bodies which are then phagocytized by intact granulocytes to form typical LE-cells.[21]
   d. LE-cell phenomenon — the presence of the LE serum factor (antinucleoprotein factor) causing an agglutination reaction between antigen-treated particles and the serum containing antinuclear globulins.
   e. LE-test — rapid slide test for antinucleoprotein factors associated with systemic lupus erythematosus. The test specimen is compared with control serums.
      Negative test — no agglutination
      Positive test — any degree of agglutination of the latex particles.

3. rheumatoid arthritis —
   a. rheumatoid factor — protein belonging to a family of antibodies which evolved in response to antigenic stimulation by an altered immunoglobulin. Consequently they are antiglobulins.[57]
   b. tests for rheumatoid factor — they utilize the ability of antiglobulins to agglutinate cells coated with 7S immunoglobulin. Examples are:
      (1) bentonite flocculation test — pooled human gammaglobulin is used as antigen for coating particles.[57]
      (2) latex fixation test — pooled human gammaglobulin is adsorbed to standard latex particles.
      (3) Rheumanosticon — a rapid slide test for the detection of the rheumatoid factor, performed on serum or whole blood. The rheumatoid factor reacts with the coating material causing a visible agglutination of the inert latex particles.
         Negative end point — the mixture remains milky with no visible flocculation as demonstrated by the negative control.
         Positive end point — coarse agglutinated flocs are present as demonstrated by the positive control.

C. **Terms Related to Serological and Immunological Tests:**

1. antibody labeling with fluorescein — a histochemical technique for identifying antigen and antibody within tissues.
   a. direct immunofluorescent staining — sensitive serological test in which the specific antibody is labeled with fluorescein and the fluorescing antigen-antibody complex viewed in the tissues.
   b. indirect immunofluorescent method — procedure in which fluorescein-labeled anti-human globulin is employed in the detection of unlabeled antibody in human tissues. Since plasma cells show marked fluorescence, they are thought to be antibody-producing cells.
   Examples: Immunofluorescent skin test in systemic lupus erythematosus and rheumatoid factor by indirect immunofluorescence.[14, 57]
2. complement fixation (CF) test — antigen-antibody reaction requiring a complement for the union of antigen and antibody.[47]
3. hemagglutination inhibition (HI) test — the detection of the presence of specific antibodies capable of inhibiting agglutination of red cells by agents such as viruses.
4. immunofluorescence — the tagging of antibodies with a fluorescent dye in order to detect or localize antigen-antibody combinations.[56]
5. neutralization test — detection of the presence of antibodies capable of inactivating an infective agent, thus rendering it noninfective or neutral.

D. **Terms Related to Tests for Syphilis:**

1. darkfield illumination — test of choice for the detection of primary or secondary syphilis by identifying Treponema pallidum in a smear of a suspected lesion.[25]
2. fluorescent treponemal antibody (FTA) test — indirect immunological test based on a reaction between a treponemal antigen and the specific antispirochetal antibody in the syphilitic serum of the patient. Treponemas coated with fluorescent antibodies are seen under the ultraviolet microscope.[12]
3. fluorescent treponemal antibody-absorption test — of greater sensitivity and specificity for syphilis than the FTA test. Fluorescein tagged antihuman globulin is used as the reaction indicator and the reaction is visualized with an ultraviolet microscope.[22, 30, 47]
4. Kahn test — a flocculation test for syphilis, using a nontreponemal antigen, usually cardiolipin, an extract of beef heart.
5. Kolmer test — a modification of the Wasserman complement fixation test. The antigen used is nonspecific, that is, not derived from Treponema pallidum.
6. Reiter protein complement-fixation test (RPCF) — a new reliable test for syphilis. It is essentially Kolmer's technique using Reiter's protein antigen prepared from Treponema pallidum.
7. Venereal Disease Research Laboratory — a flocculation test for syphilis which is widely accepted.[47, 56]
8. Wasserman test — original complement fixation test for syphilis, a rather complex procedure. The antigen used is nontreponemal.

ABBREVIATIONS

AD — adenovirus
ALG — antilymphocytic globulin
ALS — antilymphocytic serum
ANA — antinuclear antibodies
APC — adenoidal-pharyngeal-conjunctival
ARD — acute respiratory disease
BFP — biological false positive (reaction)
CFT — complement fixation test
FA — fluorescent antibody
FTA — fluorescent treponemal antibody
FTA-ABS — fluorescent treponemal antibody-absorption

LE — lupus erythematosus
RPCF — Reiter protein complement fixation
RPR — rapid plasma reagin
SLE — systemic lupus erythematosus
STS — serological test for syphilis
TPI — Treponema pallidum immobilization test
va — variety
VD — venereal disease
VDG — venereal disease gonorrhea
VDRL — venereal disease research laboratory

ORAL READING PRACTICE
Herpes Zoster

Herpes zoster, zoster or shingles is an infectious disease caused by the zoster **virus.** It is characterized by vesicular lesions which follow the course of a **peripheral nerve** in a band-like fashion. Prior to the eruption, the patient may experience pain for several days without other symptoms. Once the **erythema** and **vesicles** appear in a typical **zoniform** distribution, the diagnosis is readily made. In the beginning, the eruption exhibits slightly edematous, fairly well-defined erythematous, oval or round areas on which vesicles form in groups. Generally, sensory changes along the path of the affected **neural zones** are associated with the eruption. Pain precedes, accompanies and follows the appearance of the skin lesion. It varies in duration and intensity from slight, brief **hyperesthesia** to **paroxysmal** attacks of pain or persistent, excruciating **neuralgia.** Similar to other nerve root involvements, the pain is especially agonizing at night and is intensified by motion. In rare cases it has led to drug addiction and even suicide. **Paresthesia** of the skin may be brought on by touching the affected area or it may develop spontaneously. In addition, the patient may develop tender, enlarged lymph nodes, rheumatic pains and general **malaise.**[49]

Although the characteristic feature of the disease is the skin eruption, herpes zoster is essentially an inflammation of one or more posterior root ganglia. The rash is confined to the dermal segment supplied by the sensory nerve arising from the involved posterior (sensory) root ganglion. The **neurotropic virus** destroys the ganglion cells and fibers. These changes result in a degeneration of the corresponding peripheral nerve.

One of the most painful forms of herpes is **Zoster ophthalmicus,** caused by a viral infection of the **trigeminal nerve.** This may lead to **corneal ulceration, keratitis, iritis, conjunctivitis** and **edema** of the **eyelids.**

Zoster oticus results from an inflammation of the vestibulocochlear nerve and is associated with deafness, **vertigo, tinnitus** and severe pain.[49]

REFERENCES AND BIBLIOGRAPHY

1. Allgood, J. W. and Chaplin, H. Idiopathic acquired autoimmune hemolytic anemia. *American Journal of Medicine.* 43: 254-273, August, 1967.

2. Austen, F. K. Consequence of the immune response. In Wintrobe, Maxwell M. (ed.). *Harrison's Principles of Internal Medicine*, 6th ed. New York: McGraw Hill Book Co., 1970, p. 347.

3. _____. Disorders due to hypersensitivity and altered immune response. In Wintrobe, Maxwell M. (ed.). *Harrison's Principles of Internal Medicine*, 6th ed. New York: McGraw Hill Book Co., 1970, pp. 346-347.

4. _____. Initiation of the immune response. In Wintrobe, Maxwell M. (ed.). *Harrison's Principles of Internal Medicine*, 6th ed. New York: McGraw Hill Book Co., 1970, p. 342.

5. Bearn, A. G. The Marfan syndrome. In Beeson, Paul B. and McDermott, Walsh (eds.). *Cecil-Loeb Textbook of Medicine*, 13th ed. Philadelphia: W. B. Saunders Co., 1971, pp. 1711-1712.

6. Billingham, R. E. The immunobiology of tissue transplantation. In Samter, Max (ed.). *Immunological Diseases*, 2d ed. Boston: Little, Brown and Co., 1971, pp. 265-268.

7. Beachman, P. S. Shiga bacillus dysentery. *Journal of Infectious Diseases*, 122: 232-233, September, 1970.

8. Brown, W. J. Trends and status of gonorrhea in the United States. *Journal of Infectious Diseases*, 123: 682-687, June, 1971.

9. _____. Status and control of syphilis in the United States. *Journal of Infectious Diseases*, 124: 428-432, October, 1971.

10. _____. Acquired syphilis — drugs and blood tests. *American Journal of Nursing*, 71: 713-715, April, 1971.

11. Burden, Kenneth L. and Williams, Robert P. Viral diseases primarily involving the respiratory tract or parotid glands. In *Microbiology*, 6th ed. New York: The Macmillan Co., 1968, p. 730.

12. _____. Bacteriological and serological diagnosis. In *Microbiology*, 6th ed. New York: The Macmillan Co., 1968, pp. 578-579.

13. Burnham, T. K. The immunofluorescent "Band" test for lupus erythematosus. *Archives of Dermatology*, 103: 24-31, January, 1971.

14. Caperton, E. M. et al. Immunofluorescent skin test in systemic lupus erythematosus. *Journal of American Medical Association*, 222: 935-937, November 20, 1972.

15. Chang, T. W. Strategy of rubella vaccination. *Journal of Infectious Diseases*, 123: 224-225, February, 1971.

16. Connor, J. D. Etiologic role of adenoviral infection to pertussis syndrome. *New England Journal of Medicine*, 283: 390-394, August 20, 1970.

17. Conrad, M. E. Hematologic manifestations of parasitic infections. *Seminars in Hematology*, 8: 267-303, July, 1971.

18. Criep, L. H. The immune response. In Criep, Leo H. *Dermatologic Allergy: Immunology, Diagnosis, Management.* Philadelphia: W. B. Saunders Co., 1967, pp. 101-102.

19. _____. Transplantation immunity. In Criep, Leo H. *Dermatologic Allergy: Immunology, Diagnosis, Management.* Philadelphia: W. B. Saunders Co., 1967, pp. 400-406.

20. Davidsohn, Israel and Henry, John B. (eds.). *Todd-Sanford Clinical Diagnosis by Laboratory Methods*, 14th ed. Philadelphia: W. B. Saunders Co., 1969, pp. 530, 536-537.

21. _____. Infectious mononucleosis — lupus erythematosus. *Ibid.*, pp. 284-323.

22. Deacon, W. E. *et al.* Fluorescent treponemal antibody-absorption test for syphilis. *Journal of American Medical Association*, 198: 156-160, November 7, 1966.

23. Donadio, J. A. Diagnosis and treatment of botulism. *Journal of Infectious Diseases.* 124:108-113, July, 1971.

24. Foster, K. M. and Jack, L. A. A prospective study of the role of cytomegalovirus in posttransfusion mononucleosis. *New England Journal of Medicine*, 280: 1311-1315, June 12, 1969.

25. Foster, M. T. Diagnosis and treatment of venereal disease. *Postgraduate Medicine*, 50: 66-73, July, 1971.

26. Furcolow, M. L. Histoplasmosis. In Samter, Max (ed.). *Immunological Diseases*, 2d ed. Boston: Little, Brown and Co., 1971, pp. 644-651.

27. Gardner, F. H. Idiopathic thrombocytopenia purpura. In Samter, Max (ed.). *Immunological Diseases*, 2d ed. Boston: Little, Brown and Co., 1971, pp. 1111-1124.

28. Garibaldi, R. A. *et al.* Viral hepatitis: Morbidity trends. *Journal of Infectious Diseases*, 122: 234-235, September, 1970.

29. Hanshaw, J. B. Congenital cytomegalovirus infection: A fifteen year perspective. *Journal of Infectious Diseases*, 123: 555-561, May, 1971.

30. Hardy, P. H. and Nell, E. Characteristics of fluorescein labelled antiglobulin preparations that may affect the fluorescent treponemal antibody-absorption test. *American Journal of Clinical Pathology*, 56: 181-186, August, 1971.

31. Holman, H. R. Systemic lupus erythematosus. In Samter, Max (ed.). *Immunological Diseases*, 2d ed. Boston: Little, Brown and Co., 1971, pp. 995-1013.

32. Horstmann, D. M. Rubella: The challenge of its control. *Journal of Infectious Diseases*, 123: 640-654, June, 1971.

33. Jackson, G. C. Adenoviral infections of the respiratory tract. In Beeson, Paul B. and McDermott. Walsh (eds.). *Cecil Loeb Textbook of Medicine.* Philadelphia: W. B. Saunders Co., 1971, pp. 364-365.

34. Jawetz, E., Melinick, J. L. and Adelberg, E. A. Antigens and antibodies. In *Review of Medical Microbiology*, 9th ed. Los Altos, California: Lange Medical Publications, 1970, pp. 135-149.

35. Kantor, G. L. and Goldberg, L. S. Cytomegalovirus-induced postperfusion syndrome. *Seminars in Hematology*, 8: 261-266, July, 1971.

36. Kantor, G. L. *et al.* Cytomegalovirus infection associated with cardiopulmonary bypass. *Archives of Internal Medicine*, 125: 488-492, March, 1970.

37. Kilbourne, E. D. Introduction to viral diseases. In Beeson, Paul B. and McDermott, Walsh (eds.). *Cecil-Loeb Textbook of Medicine*, 13th ed. Phil-adelphia: W. B. Saunders Co., 1971, pp. 357-358.

38. _____. Cytomegalovirus infections. In Beeson, Paul B. and McDermott, Walsh (eds.). *Cecil-Loeb Textbook of Medicine*, 13th ed. Philadelphia: W. B. Saunders Co., 1971, pp. 466-467.

39. Laboratory aids in infectious mononucleosis. *Bulletin of Laboratory Medicine.* 9, No. 8, 1960.

40. Landrigan, P. J. Current status of measles in the United States — 1970. *Journal of Infectious Diseases*, 124: 620-621, December, 1971.

41. Loewenstein, M. S. *et al.* Salmonellosis associated with turtles. *Journal of Infectious Diseases*, 124: 433, October, 1971.

42. Logan, W. S. *et al.* Chronic cutaneous herpes simplex. *Archives of Dermatology*, 103, 606, June, 1971.

43. Malacarne, P. Infectious hepatitis: A possible mitogenic factor. *Journal of Infectious Diseases*, 123: 213-215, February, 1971.

44. McCollum, R. W. Infectious mononucleosis and the Epstein-Barr virus. *Journal of Infectious Diseases*, 121: 347, March, 1970.

45. Merrill, J. P. Transplantation — immunological considerations. In Wintrobe, Maxwell M. (ed.). *Harrison's Principles of Internal Medicine*, 6th ed. New York: McGraw Hill Book Co., 1970, pp. 357.

46. _____. Allograft rejection. In Samter, Max (ed.). *Immunological Diseases*, 2d ed. Boston: Little, Brown and Co., 1971, pp. 483-496.

47. Miller, Seward E. and Weller, John M. *A Textbook of Clinical Pathology.* 8th ed. Baltimore: The Williams and Wilkins Co., 1971, pp. 404-407.

48. Minden, P. and Farr, R. S. Antigen-antibody reactions and their measurements. In Samter, Max (ed.) *Immunological Diseases*, 2d ed. Boston: Little, Brown and Co., 1971, pp. 179-197.

49. Murrell, T. W. Herpes zoster. In Conn, Howard F., (ed.). *Current Therapy.* Philadelphia: W. B. Saunders Co., 1972, pp. 639-640.

50. Neva, F. A. and Sheagren, J. N. Malaria: host-defense mechanisms and complications. *Annals of Internal Medicine*, 73: 295-306, August, 1970.

51. Dlansky, S. Syphilis. In Samter, Max (ed.). *Immunological Diseases*, 2d ed. Boston: Little, Brown and Co., 1971, pp. 735-742.

52. Page, Lot B. and Culver, Perry J. *Syllabus of Laboratory Examinations in Clinical Diagnosis*, 2d ed. Cambridge, Massachusetts: Harvard University Press, 1960, pp. 183-184.

53. Pappagianis, D. Coccidioidomycosis. In Samter, Max (ed.). *Immunological Diseases*, 2d ed. Boston: Little, Brown and Co., 1971, pp. 652-661.

54. Pearson, C. M. Polymyositis and dermatomyositis. In Samter, Max (ed.). *Immunological Diseases*, 2d ed. Boston: Little, Brown and Co., 1971, pp. 1039-1051.

55. Pepys, J. Pulmonary aspergillosis, farmer's lung and related diseases. In Samter, Max (ed.). *Immunological Diseases*, 2d ed. Boston: Little, Brown and Co., 1971, pp. 693-713.

56. Tucker, Eugene, M.D. Personal communications.

57. Vardiman, J. *et al.* Localization of rheumatoid factor by direct immunofluorescence. *Laboratory Medicine*, 3: 39-40, November, 1972.

Chapter XVI

Geriatrics and Psychogeriatrics

ORIENTATION

A. Origin of Terms:

1. arcus (L) — bow, arch
2. asthenia (G) — weakness
3. chalasis (G) — a slackening
4. geras (G) — old age
5. geron (G) — old man
6. presbys (G) — old
7. rhytis (G) — wrinkle
8. senilis (L) — old
9. senium (L) — old age
10. senescere (L) — to grow old

B. General Terms:

1. geriatrician — specialist in diseases of old age.
2. geriatrics — branch of medical science concerned with the diseases of old age and their treatment.
3. gerontologist — scientist who studies the process of aging in its biological, mental and socioeconomic implications.
4. gerontology — the scientific study of all facets of aging including branches of science which contribute to an understanding of older adults such as physiology, psychology, sociology and public health.
5. podiatrist — specialist concerned with the diagnosis and treatment of defects, injuries and diseases of the feet. Older adults are in particular need of the services of a podiatrist.
6. presbyatrics, presbytiatrics — the medical treatment of the aging.
7. psychogerontology — science that deals with the mental and emotional life of older persons, their ideation, memory and level of consciousness.
8. senescence — the declining years of life or a normal process of growing old.
9. senility — old age with its mental and physical infirmities.

SOME PHYSICAL DISORDERS OF OLDER ADULTS*

A. Diagnostic Terms:

1. cranial arteritis, giant cell arteritis, arteritis of the aged — a panarteritis of older adults primarily involving the temporal arteries ophthalmic and retinal arteries and clinically noted for a boring headache, scalp tenderness; pain, blanching and occasionally gangrene of the tongue probably due to lingual arteritis; peripheral neuropathy and sudden blindness.[2]
2. osteitis deformans, Paget's disease of bone — a skeletal disorder characterized by decalcification, marked bone destruction and rapid bone repair, architectural abnormality of new bone, increased vascularity and fibrosis. Striking features are its intensification with advancing years, fracture proneness and the frequency of a coexisting osteogenic sarcoma.[39, 14, 9]
3. polymyalgia rheumatica — a special type of muscular rheumatism seen more frequently in older women than men, clinically manifested by pain and stiffness in back, shoulder, neck and occasionally in pelvic girdle.[2]

---

*The disorders presented occur more frequently in older age groups than in younger ones.

4. progeria of adult, Werner's syndrome — premature aging including early graying, baldness, sparse eyebrows, fine wrinkles around mouth, taut skin, beaked nose, spindly extremities, keratoses and ulcers of extremities. In addition diabetes mellitus, arteriosclerosis and bilateral cataracts are usually present. This rare syndrome is thought to be genetically transmitted.[38]

5. senile macular degeneration — a degenerative process initially noted by a disturbance of pigmentation in the macula, associated with abnormal foveal reflex and leading to visual loss in the aging.[36]

6. senile osteoporosis — a disorder of protein metabolism seen in the aging marked by increased porosity of bone which is especially pronounced in the spine and pelvis and leads to spontaneous fractures, deformities and collapse of vertebrae with reduction of the person's height.[14, 9, 31]

7. senile purpura — hemorrhagic disorder characterized by easy bruising and purple extravasations chiefly on arms and legs of aging skin.[22]

8. senile sebaceous adenomas — benign lesions, typically appearing on the face of elderly persons as pearly oval papules with a central depression.[5, 42, 16, 25]

B. Operative Terms:

1. blepharoplasty for blepharochalasis — plastic repair of redundant eyelids.[23, 35, 30, 15]

2. dermabrasion and excision of
   a. furrowed brows — application of dermabrader to frown furrows and removal of skin over furrowed area.
   b. perioral wrinkles — application of dermabrader to each vertical lip line for elimination of wrinkles around the mouth.[29, 23]

3. face-lift operation — reconstructive plastic surgery of the face, the art of surgical sculpture applied to the human face to restore function, remove the marks of time and correct defects.[29, 23, 1, 7]

4. rhytidectomy — surgical removal of subcutaneous fat pads and superfluous skin to eliminate wrinkles.[3, 23, 29, 15]

5. rhytidoplasty — surgical elimination of wrinkles achieved by removal of excess skin and tightening of remaining skin to restore youthful appearance.[23, 20] A dermal fat graft is inserted in the following forms of repair:
   a. glabellar rhytidoplasty — operative procedure for removing the vertical furrows between the eyebrows.[4]
   b. cervicofacial rhytidoplasty — surgical correction of wrinkles of the neck and face.[29, 20]

C. Symptomatic Terms:

1. arcus senilis, gerontoxon — white or grayish opaque ring just within the sclerocorneal junction of the eye, seen in elderly persons.[36]

2. blepharochalasis — relaxed, baggy eyelids; redundancy may interfere with vision.

3. geroderma — atrophic, thinned and wrinkled skin of old age.[36]

4. gerontopia, senopia — second sight.

5. presbyacusia, presbycusis — impaired perception and discrimination of sounds seen in the aging.

6. presbyopia — defective vision resulting from changes in accommodation in the aging process.

7. senile pruritus — itching of brittle, dry skin of the aged leading to scratching followed by excoriations and eczematoid changes.[5]

8. senile tremor — generally an intention tremor, rarely a constant tremor of senescent persons.

SOME MENTAL DISORDERS OF OLDER ADULTS

A. Diagnostic Terms:

1. Alzheimer's disease — a degenerative disorder beginning in the fifth or sixth decade of life, pathologically characterized by cortical atrophy, loss of nerve cells, senile plaques in gray matter and neurofibrillar degeneration. The onset of the dementia is insidious. The patient loses interest in social contacts, becomes anxious, depressed, disoriented; aphasia, agnosia and apraxia develop; the gait shows a hesitant shuffle and incapacitating flexion contractures mark the terminal decerebrate phase of life.[34, 24, 13, 32]

2. chronic brain syndrome — permanent damage to brain tissue leading to cerebral insufficiency and deterioration of cognitive faculties. It is usually associated with advanced cerebral atherosclerosis in the aging.[12]

3. Pick's disease — progressive dementia due to severe cortical atrophy of frontal and/or temporal lobes. The presence of Pick bodies in cortical neurons clinches the diagnosis. Characteristically there is relative retention of concrete learned material and of personal orientation.[40, 24, 13, 32]

4. senile psychoses — inclusive term concerned with a variety of states from mild senescent mental disorders to the extreme deterioration of senile dementia. Kolb refers to the following clinical types.[19, 28]
   a. delirium and confusion — a psychotic reaction to fever, dehydration, surgery and other somatic states. The aged is disoriented, bewildered, hallucinating and wandering about aimlessly.[26, 21]
   b. depression and agitation — psychotic state characterized by egocentric behavior, melancholy, intense agitation, defective memory and mental decline.[41, 17, 8]
   c. paranoia — a common psychotic reaction of senescence in which delusions of persecution tend to predominate.
   d. presbyophrenia, Wernicke's syndrome — mental disorder found in older individuals who previously had a dynamic personality. The presbyophrenic patient is constantly busy in an unproductive or destructive way, he is out of touch with reality, very forgetful, covering up his memory lapses with confabulations.[19, 11]
   e. senile dementia — irreversible deterioration of cognitive faculties.[18]

B. Symptomatic Terms:

1. agnosia — sensory inability to recognize objects.
2. apraxia — total disability to execute purposeful movements although muscle strength, coordination and sensibility appear intact.
3. confabulation — making up tales to fill in memory gaps. The patient is not construing deliberate falsehoods but believes his fantasies to be true.
4. depression — morbid sadness, melancholy, dejection out of proportion with loss or injury endured; frequently observed in the aged.
5. regression — return to infantile patterns of reacting, seen in senile psychosis, severe illness and under other circumstances.

ABBREVIATIONS

AAHA — American Association of Homes for the Aging
AARP — American Association of Retired persons
ANHA — American Nursing Home Association
AOA — Administration on Aging
HUD — Housing and Urban Development
NCOA — National Council on the Aging
VISTA — Volunteers in Service to America
WHCoA — White House Conference on Aging

ORAL READING PRACTICE
ATHEROSCLEROTIC OCCLUSIVE DISEASE OF THE DESCENDING AORTA AND ITS MAIN BRANCHES

Despite variable pathological features **atherosclerotic occlusive** disease exhibits a distinctive pattern especially as to the extent and location of the occlusion. No matter where the **obliterative** process occurs the lesion is generally **segmental** in nature and well localized.[6] It is significant that a comparatively normal **patent lumen** exists **proximal** and **distal** to the obstructed segment. Confirmatory evidence of these characteristic findings is provided by **arteriography** which is of primary importance in diagnostic evaluation.

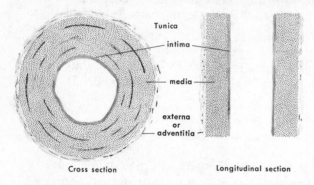

Tunica

intima

media

externa
or
adventitia

Cross section   Longitudinal section

Fig. 74 – Normal artery, arterial coats and lumen.

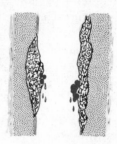

Fig. 77 – Atheromatous plaques in intima, capillary bleeding and early mural thrombosis.

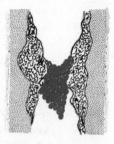

Fig. 79 – Rupture of ulcerated intimal plaque, mural thrombosis and occlusion.

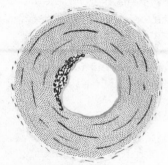

Fig. 75 – Early atherosclerosis.

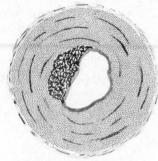

Fig. 76 – Advanced atherosclerosis.

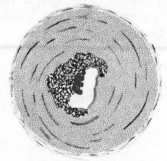

Fig. 78 – For advanced artherosclerosis.

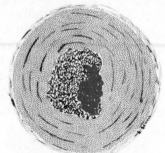

Fig. 80 – Thrombosis and occlusion.

As in occlusive vascular disease of the heart and brain the pathological lesions consist of **intimal atheromatous plaques** with or without **thrombus** formation.[33, 27] Their typical location is the bifurcation of arteries where they produce arterial obstruction followed by **arterial** insufficiency of the parts distal to the occlusive process. The segmental localization of the **atheromatous** lesions permits a direct surgical attack for restoring the circulation in the major blood vessels. Three basic operative procedures are currently advocated: **thromboendarterectomy, excision** and **graft** replacement and graft bypass.[6] Severe coexisting **cardiac** and **cerebral** disease as well as far advanced senescence are considered contraindications, but elderly persons, otherwise in fair health, are thought to be good candidates for surgical intervention. Low risk patients with **compensated heart disease, diabetes mellitus** and **hypertension** are also advised to undergo surgery.

The most common types of **atherosclerotic vascular** disease apart from **coronary** or cerebral involvement are **aortoiliac** and **femoropopliteal** occlusions and occlusions of the **renal** artery.

Aortoiliac Occlusions

The **aortic bifurcation occlusion syndrome** or Leriche's syndrome is also known as chronic **aortoiliac thrombosis.** This progressive atheromatous occlusive disease of the abdominal aorta is seen chiefly in males of middle age or advancing years.[6]

Symptoms are those of **ischemia** including coldness, intermittent **claudication, paresthesias** and muscular **atrophy** of the lower extremities. **Peripheral** pulses of the **femoral, popliteal** and **pedal** regions tend to be markedly decreased to the point of being barely palpable or completely absent. **Ischemic** changes may eventually produce **pregangrenous** or gangrenous lesions of the feet. Another significant feature is a soft blowing **systolic murmur** heard over the abdomen.

The **pathological** picture usually reveals atheromatous mural lesions of considerable extent with relatively uninvolved proximal and distal arterial segments adjoining the occlusion.

Angiographic studies are imperative, since they provide **visualization** of the entire arterial tree below the area where the **contrast medium** is injected into the aorta at the level of the twelfth **lumbar vertebra.** This method not only demonstrates aortoiliac occlusion, but also an associated superficial **femoral** artery occlusion, should it be present. If surgery is indicated both occlusions can be corrected in one operation. In the presence of minimal **medial** and **adventitial** mural lesions which are well localized, a thromboendarterectomy will be the method of choice. Extensive obstructive lesions are usually treated by excision with graft replacement. Aged individuals seem to get best results from **bypass** grafts.[6] Since normal circulation is restored and followed by symptomatic relief, surgical intervention has proven highly satisfactory.

Femoropopliteal Occlusions

The atherosclerotic obstruction in the femoropopliteal region tends to be discrete, locally confined to a segment and framed on either side by comparatively normal arterial lumen. There may be extensive involvement of the superficial femoral artery with **patency** of the popliteal artery. Sometimes the occlusive lesion is diffuse and spreads to the small arteries of the calf making surgery impossible. Principal manifestations are intermittent **claudication** and **peripheral** ischemia. **Radiographic** visualization should not be restricted to the femoropopliteal arteries but include the iliacs and abdominal aorta to insure that no discrete lesions remain undetected. The operation of choice is femoropopliteal reconstruction which is achieved by removing the **saphenous** vein from the knee to the **saphenofemoral** junction. The obstruction is bypassed by an **autogenous** graft of the saphenous vein. Since distal **pulsatile** blood flow is restored and symptoms are relieved, the objectives of the surgical attack are accomplished.[6]

Occlusions of the Renal Artery

When atherosclerotic renal artery occlusion is associated with hypertension it requires **anti-hypertensive** therapy. The occlusive process may occur **unilaterally** or **bilaterally.** **Aortography** permits visualization of the renal arteries and their occlusive lesions. The normal circulation to the kidney may be restored by a bypass graft.

Results of Vascular Surgery

De Bakey and Crawford, prominent **cardiovascular** surgeons, reported gratifying results in 1221 patients who had undergone surgery for aortoiliac and femoropopliteal occlusions despite the fact that many if not most of them were of advanced age.[6]

Vascular occlusion presents a major health problem in senescence. Its onset and insidious continuance is part of physiological aging. It assumes pathological dimensions only after months or years of undetected progress. It must be emphasized that modern vascular surgery can provide relief for aging patients with atherosclerotic occlusive disease.

REFERENCES AND BIBLIOGRAPHY

1. Baker, T. J. and Gordon, H. L. The temporal face lift. *Plastic and Reconstructive Surgery,* 47: 313-315, April, 1971.
2. Beeson, P. B. Cranial arteritis and polymyalgia rheumatica. In Beeson, Paul B. and McDermott, Walsh, (eds.). *Cecil-Loeb Textbook of Medicine.* Philadelphia: W. B. Saunders Co., 1971, pp. 837-838.
3. Carlin. G. A. and Gurdin, M. M. Ancillary procedures for the aging face and neck. *Surgical Clinics of North America,* 51: 371-386, April, 1971.
4. Castanares, S. Forehead wrinkles, glabellar frown and ptosis of the eyebrows. *Plastic and Reconstructive Surgery,* 34: 406, 1964.
5. Conrad, A. H. Dermatologic disorders. In Cowdry, E. V. and Steinberg, F. U. (eds.). *The Care*

of the Geriatric Patient, 4th ed. St. Louis: The C. V. Mosby Co., 1971, pp. 59-70.

6. DeBakey, M. E. and Crawford, E. S. Atherosclerotic occlusive vascular disease. *Modern Concepts of Cardiovascular Disease*, 29: 571-576, January, 1960.

7. Epstein, E. Dermatologic surgery in aging skin. *Geriatrics*, 26: 94-99, March, 1971.

8. Fisher, H. K. and Dlin, B. M. Man's determination of his time of illness or death. Anniversary reactions and emotional deadlines. *Geriatrics*, 26: 89-94, July, 1971.

9. Forsyth, B. T. Arthritis and bone disease. In Cowdry, E. V. and Steinberg, F. U. (eds.). *The Care of the Geriatric Patient*, 4th ed. St. Louis: The C. V. Mosby Co., 1971, pp. 16-23.

10. Frenay, Sister Agnes C. and Pierce, Gloria L. The climate of care of a geriatric patient. *American Journal of Nursing*, 72: 1747-1750, September, 1971.

11. Garner, H. H. The older patient: A confrontation problem-solving. *Postgraduate Medicine*, 49: 202-208, February, 1971.

12. Goldfarb, A. I. Geriatric psychiatry. In Freedman, Alfred M. and Kaplan, Harold I. (eds.) *Comprehensive Textbook of Psychiatry*. Baltimore: The Williams & Wilkins Co., 1967, pp. 1564-1587.

13. Hardin, W. B. and O'Leary, J. L. Senile dementia. In Cowdry, E. V. and Steinberg, F. U. (eds.). *The Care of the Geriatric Patient*, 4th ed. St. Louis: The C. V. Mosby Co., 1971, pp. 314-316.

14. Heaney, R. P. Diseases of the bone. In Beeson, Paul B. and McDermott, Walsh, (eds.). *Cecil-Loeb Textbook of Medicine*. Philadelphia: W. B. Saunders Co., 1971, pp. 1856-1882.

15. Hurwitz, Arlene. About faces. *American Journal of Nursing*, 71: 2168-2171, November, 1971.

16. Jackson, R. Solar and senile skin: changes caused by aging and habitual exposure to the sun. *Geriatrics*, 27: 106-112, August, 1972.

17. Kastenbaum, R. *et al.* Premature death and self-injurious behavior in old age. *Geriatrics*, 26: 71-81, July, 1971.

18. Kinsbourne, M. Diagnosis of cognitive deficit in the aged. *Postgraduate Medicine*, 50: 191-194, October, 1971.

19. Kolb, Lawrence C. *Modern Clinical Psychiatry*, 8th ed. Philadelphia: W. B. Saunders Co., 1973, pp. 183-195.

20. Loeb, R. Earlobe tailoring during facial rhytidoplasties. *Plastic and Reconstructive Surgery*, 49: 485-489, May, 1972.

21. Lyon, G. G. Stimulation through remotivation. *American Journal of Nursing*, 71: 982-986, May, 1971.

22. Maekawa, T. Hematologic diseases. In Cowdry, E. S. and Steinberg, F. U. (eds.). *The Care of the Geritaric Patient*. St. Louis. The C. V. Mosby Co., 1971, pp. 112-125.

23. McDowell, F. Plastic surgery. In Cowdry, E. V. and Steinberg, F. U. (eds.). *The Care of the Geriatric Patient*, 4th ed. St. Louis: C. V. Mosby Co., 1971, pp. 236-249.

24. McHugh, P. R. Dementia. In Beeson, Paul B. and McDermott, Walsh (eds.). *Cecil-Loeb Textbook of Medicine*. Philadelphia: W. B. Saunders Co., 1971, pp. 102-107.

25. Morgan, R. J. Allergic skin problems in older individuals. *Geriatrics*, 25: 146-157, September, 1970.

26. Moses, D. Assessing behavior in the elderly. *Nursing Clinics of North America*, 7: 225-234, June, 1972.

27. Netter, Frank H. and Yonkman, Frederick F. (eds.). Pathologic changes in coronary artery disease. In *A Compilation of Paintings on the Normal and Pathologic Anatomy and Physiology, Embryology and Diseases of the Heart*, vol. 5. The Ciba Collection of Medical Illustrations, 1969, pp. 214-217.

28. Ozonoff, M. B. *et al.* Intracranial calcification. In Newton, T. H. and Potts, D. G. *Radiology of the Skull and Brain*. St. Louis: The C. V. Mosby Co., 1971, pp. 823-873.

29. Pickrell, K. L. Reconstructive plastic surgery of the face. *Clinical Symposia*, 19: 71-99, July-August-September, 1967.

30. Rees, T. D. and Guy, C. L. Patient selection and techniques in blepharoplasty and rhytidoplasty. *Surgical Clinics of North America*, 51: 353-370, April, 1971.

31. Riggs, B. L. et al. Treatment for postmenopausal and senile osteoporosis. *Medical Clinics of North America*, 56: 989-998 July, 1972.

32. Robbins, Stanley L. Alzheimer's disease — Pick's disease. In *Pathology*, 3rd ed. Philadelphia: W. B. Saunders Co., 1967, p. 1429.

33. _____. Atherosclerosis — etiology and pathogenesis. *Ibid.*, pp. 573-578.

34. Rosenstock, H. A. Characteristics of Alzheimer's presenile dementia. *Geriatrics*, 26, 145, November, 1971.

35. Safian, J. A late report on an early operation for "baggy eyelids". *Plastic and Reconstructive Surgery*, 48: 347-348, October, 1971.

36. Scheie, Harold G. and Albert, Daniel M. Degenerative diseases and ocular changes of aging. In *Adler's Textbook of Ophthalmology*, 8th ed. Philadelphia: W. B. Saunders Co., 1969, pp. 274-290.

37. _____. Optical defects in the eye. *Ibid.*, pp. 441-451.

38. Tannenbaum, M. H. Werner's syndrome — Progeria of the adult. *Archives of Internal Medicine*, 116: 499-504, October, 1965.

39. Wilner, D. and Sherman, R. Bone sarcoma associated with Paget's disease. *Ca-A Cancer Journal for Clinicians*, 16: 238-240, November-December, 1966.

40. Wisniewski, H. M. *et al.* Pick's disease. A clinical and ultrastructural study. *Archives of Neurology*, 26: 97-108, February, 1972.

41. Wolff, K. The treatment of the depressed and suicidal geriatric patient. *Geriatrics*, 26: 65-69, July, 1971.

42. Zakon, S. J. Skin diseases of the aged. *Postgraduate Medicine*, 49: 206-209, January, 1971.

PART II

SUPPLEMENTARY TERMS

Chapter XVII
Selected Terms Pertaining to Oncology

ORIENTATION

A. Origin of Terms:

1. astro- (G) — star
2. benign (L) — mild
3. carcino- (G) — cancer
4. ependyma (G) — wrap
5. glia (G) — glue
6. kerato- (G) — horny
7. malignant (L) — of bad kind
8. medulla (L) — marrow
9. oma (G) — tumor
10. onco (G) — mass
11. plakia (G) — plate
12. plasia (G) — a molding
13. proliferate (L) — to bear offspring
14. sarco (G) — flesh
15. scirrhous (G) — hard
16. tumor (G) — swelling

B. Terms Used in Oncology:

1. anaplasia — alteration in tissue cells frequently accompanied by malignant behavior.[36]
2. autonomy — disregard by the malignant tumor for normal limitations of growth.[36]
3. behavior of tumor — a biological interpretation indicating the potentialities of a new growth; for example; its ability to spread its histological appearance, cellular proliferation (rapid cell division) and others.[34]
4. benign — mild, not malignant, not recurrent.
5. cachexia — a progressive state of malnutrition, emaciation, debilitation and anemia.[39, 16]
6. cancer — a group of malignant diseases characterized by uncontrolled cell growth.
7. carcinoembryonic antigen (CEA) — a cancer-specific antigen and glycoprotein found in malignant endodermal layers of tissue, in the fetal mucosa of the colon and in the plasma of patients with cancer of the gastrointestinal tract. The test is invaluable in studying the course of the disease. After complete excision of the malignant lesion the high CEA level returns to normal. When cancer growth recurs the CEA level again becomes elevated. The new antigen is also referred to as neoplastic or tumor-associated antigen.[33, 22, 13, 31]
8. carcinogenic agent — an agent capable of inducing a carcinoma.
9. carcinoid, argentaffinoma — tumor, found in intestine and derived from argentaffin cells. Contains a large amount of serotonin and may metastasize.[37, 23]
10. carcinolysis — destruction of cancer cells.
11. carcinoma — malignant neoplasm which arises from epithelial tissue.[1, 35, 27]
12. carcinoma in situ — a true malignant tumor of squamous or glandular epithelium in which **no invasion** of underlying or adjacent structures has occurred. Lesions may remain in situ (position) for an indefinite period, even years, before they become invasive.[1, 9]
13. dedifferentiation — alterations toward decreased specialization of tissue.[7]
14. differentiation — specialization of a tissue or organ to perform a particular function. It is accompanied by characteristic morphologic alterations simulating parent tissue.
15. dyskeratosis — premature keratinization of epidermal cells due to a defect in keratin formation. It may be benign or malignant.
16. embryonal, embryonic — pertaining to an embryo, also to marked immaturity.
17. erythroplakia — well defined red patches with a velvety appearance and often tiny ulcers which may signal a malignant change in the mucous membrane.[5]
18. functioning tumor — term usually refers to neoplasm of endocrine derivation which synthesizes and releases hormones into the bloodstream and may cause some endocrine dysfunction. In a broader sense any well-differentiated neoplasm capable of forming the product of the normal parent cell, may be considered a functional tumor.[1, 2]

19. hyperplasia — abnormal cell growth with increase in size. Expressed more scientifically: cellular proliferation in excess of normal, **not** progressive (as in neoplasia) but reaching an equilibrium.[34]

20. implantation — the spontaneous passage of tumor cells to a new site with subsequent growth.[1, 2]

21. invasion — the act of invading or infiltrating and destroying the surrounding tissue.

22. leukoplakia — a keratin producing condition of the mucous membrane showing dyskeratosis and characterized by well-defined white patches which may be precancerous or cancerous lesions.[5]

23. malignant — virulent, pertaining to the invasive, metastatic properties of a new growth.

24. medullary — marrow-like; term used in oncology in reference to soft tumors.

25. metastasis formation — development of secondary centers of neoplastic growth at some distance from the primary tumor.[2, 14, 42]

26. metastasize — to disseminate or spread via lymphatics or blood stream; term used in relation to malignant tumors.[17, 19, 20, 6]

27. neoplasm — an actively growing tissue composed of cells which have undergone an abnormal type of irreversible differentiation. The new growth is useless and progressive.

28. papilloma — benign growth which resembles in its histological structure that of the parent epithelium from which it is derived. Some skin papillomas are wart-like growths derived from squamous epithelium. Papillomas arising from the larynx, tongue, urinary bladder or ureter are usually composed of transitional epithelium and tend to undergo malignant changes.[21, 18]

29. papillomatosis — the presence of multiple papillomata.

30. polyp — a nonspecific term signifying a tissue growth of mucous membrane which may be an inflammatory lesion or a true tumor. There are two kinds:
    a. pedunculated polyp — a mass of tissue attached to an organ by a freely movable, narrow stalk or pedicle.
    b. sessile polyp — a mass of tissue attached by a broad base.

31. polyposis — the presence of multiple polyps usually in the gastrointestinal tract. Multiple polyps show a definite tendency to undergo malignant transformation.[18, 28]

32. sarcoma — a malignant connective tissue tumor.[1]

33. scirrhous — hard; term used in oncology to designate a hard tumor.

34. specific viral oncogenes — tumor producing hereditary units of viral origin which have their locus on chromosomes and are capable of reproduction. They may be included in the tissues of a healthy host in a state of repression in which they cause no harm. The period of repression may last months, years or a lifetime. For no apparent reason or for a known possible cause these embryonal genes may undergo malignant transformation and multiply rapidly. Excessive proliferation and disorderly cell growth are indicative of the process of derepression resulting in active oncogenesis or tumor formation.[26, 24, 12]

C. Some Terms Related to Cancer Surgery:

1. autologous marrow infusion — the administration of the patient's own stored marrow to prevent suppression of bone marrow function and hasten hemopoietic recovery during potentially toxic antineoplastic therapy.[10, 40]

2. carcinoid surgery — choice of operation depending on size, location, metastatic lesions and the presence of single or multiple tumors.[15]
    a. bowel resection — partial removal of small intestine, local mesentery and lymph nodes with ileal, jejunal or duodenal carcinoids.
    b. right hemicolectomy — removal of right hemicolon, local mesentery and lymph nodes for appendiceal carcinoid with metastases.
    c. simple appendectomy — removal of appendix with appendiceal carcinoid.
    d. subtotal gastric resection — partial removal of stomach including gastric carcinoids.[38]

3. hemipelvectomy — removal of malignant pelvic structures and head of femur.[11]

4. pelvic exenteration — removal of pelvic viscera including reproductive organs, lymph nodes, rectum and bladder and construction of an ileal conduit or other type of ureteral anastomoses. It is done for advanced metastatic cancer.[11]

5. perfusion in the treatment of cancer — direct injection of an antineoplastic agent into the vascular bed of an isolated malignant lesion using a pump oxygenator to provide extracorporeal oxygenation and circulation regionally. Because the area of tumor is isolated (by tourniquet on an extremity, for example) the antineoplastic agent does not get into the general circulation except by "leaking" in small amounts. This method permits the administration of high concentrations of cancerocidal agents and simultaneously reduces the risk of systemic toxic effects on normal tissues, such as the bone marrow.[4, 3]

Table 26

CLASSIFICATION OF SOME COMMON NEOPLASMS

Histological Derivation	Benign Neoplasms	Malignant Neoplasms[a]	Site of Predilection
Epithelial tissue (a) Covering epithelium	Squamous cell papilloma — a benign neoplasm composed of squamous epithelial cells, flat and pavement-like in appearance	Carcinomas:[a,b] Epidermoid carcinoma Squamous cell carcinoma — a malignant neoplasm of squamous epithelial cells	Skin, buccal mucosa, tongue, salivary gland, lip, larynx, bladder, others
		Basal cell carcinoma — a malignant neoplasm, frequently forming a rodent ulcer and destructive by invasion, rarely by metastasis	Skin, especially face: canthus of eye, tip of nose, chin, lip, others
(b) Glandular epithelium	Adenoma — a benign neoplasm arising from glands	Adenocarcinoma — a malignant neoplasm composed of glandular epithelium and characterized by many variations of anaplasia and metastases	Breast, bronchi, digestive tract, especially stomach and rectosigmoid, endocrine glands, others
	Cystadenoma — a cystic neoplasm arising from glandular epithelium (a) serous type — uni or multilocular serous cyst composed of epithelial and connective tissue (b) pseudomucinous type — a cystic neoplasm in which the lining epithelium produces mucus	Cystadenocarcinoma — a cystic, malignant new growth of glandular epithelium (a) serous type — (rare) frequently bilateral loculations characteristic; cyst containing a transudate (b) pseudomucinous type — malignant changes, cells undergoing stratification; implants on peritoneal surface characteristic of neoplasm: fluid of cyst viscid in nature	Ovary, salivary gland, breast, thyroid Ovary Ovary

Histological Derivation	*Benign Neoplasms*	*Malignant Neoplasms*[a]	*Site of Predilection*
Embryonal tissue		Choriocarcinoma — a highly malignant tumor of chorionic epithelium; early metastasis common	Uterus, testes, mediastinum
	Testicular adenoma — a glandular tumor derived from germinal epithelium, extremely rare[c]	Embryonal carcinoma of testis — a malignant new growth of germinal epithelium[c]	Testes
	Teratoma, mature — a mixed tumor composed of any type of embryonic and adult tissue, as teeth, hair, bone, cartilage, others	Malignant teratoma, immature — a mixed tumor malignant in one or the other tissue elements	Testes, ovaries, retroperitoneal and sacrococcygeal regions
Connective tissue		**Sarcomas:**[d]	
	Chondroma — a benign neoplasm composed of cartilaginous elements	Chondrosarcoma — a malignant neoplasm of cartilaginous elements usually arising from the end of long bones	Bones: femur, humerus, endolarynx, maxillary sinus, nasal fossa, others
	Lipoma — a benign neoplasm composed of adipose tissue (fat)	Liposarcoma — a sarcoma composed of adipose tissue	Neck, shoulder, back, gluteal region, thigh, others
	Fibroma, fibroid — a benign neoplasm of smooth muscle tissue	Fibrosarcoma — a sarcoma composed of fibrous tissue	Extremities, head, neck, breast, others
	Leiomyoma — a benign neoplasm of smooth muscle tissue	Leiomyosarcoma — a malignant neoplasm of smooth muscle tissue	Uterus, endometrium, vulva, bladder, small intestine, esophagus, stomach, others
	Osteoid osteoma — benign tumor derived from osteoblastic tissue	Osteosarcoma, Osteogenic sarcoma — a malignant tumor of osteoblastic or osseous tissue	Long bones, especially femur, humerus, fibula, also bones of pelvis, others
		Ewing's sarcoma — a malignant tumor of endothelial tissue; early and wide metastases to other bones	Femur, tibia, fibula, humerus, mandible, pelvic bones, others
	Giant cell tumor of bone — neoplasm arising from connective tissue of the marrow of the epiphyses	Malignant giant cell tumor — malignant alterations of giant cells and metastases *very rare*	Femur, radius, tibia, ulna, ribs, vertebrae, fibula, others
Reticuloendothelial tissue		Multiple myeloma, Plasma cell myeloma — malignant tumors derived from plasma cells of bone marrow	Flat bones, ribs, vertebrae, pelvis, skull, others

Histological Derivation	Benign Neoplasms	Malignant Neoplasms[d,e]	Site of Predilection
Cont'd		Reticulum cell sarcoma — a malignant neoplasm — composed of reticulum cells	Lymph nodes, spleen
		Lymphosarcoma — a highly malignant sarcoma composed of lymphoid tissue	Lymph nodes, thymus, spleen, others
Vascular tissue	Angioma Hemangioma — a tumor of blood vessels	Angiosarcoma Hemangiosarcoma — a malignant blood vessel tumor	Blood vessels, subcutaneous tissues, muscles, others
	Lymphangioma — a tumor of the lymphatic vessels	Lymphangiosarcoma — a sarcoma of the lymphatic vessels	Lymphatic vessels, neck, others
Nerve tissue or other tissue found in nervous system		Glioma group — primary intracranial tumors composed of glial tissues. Various types of cells are present[f,g,h]	Brain
		(a) Astrocytoma — a neoplasm of glial tissue containing star-shaped cells or astrocytes[f,g]	Cerebral hemisphere, brain stem
		(b) Ependymoma — a neoplasm of the lining of the ventricles	Ventricles of the brain
		(c) Glioblastoma multiforme — most malignant form of gliomas, highly invasive and destructive	Cerebrum, cerebellum, brain stem, spinal cord
		(d) Oligodendroglioma — a relatively rare, slowly growing glioma with areas of calcification[h,f]	White matter of the frontal lobe
		Medulloblastoma — a malignant tumor composed of medullary or neuroepithelium	Cerebellum
	Meningioma — a benign tumor arising from the meninges; a common tumor	Meningosarcoma — a sarcoma of the meninges; very rare type	Meninges, cerebral hemisphere, optic chiasm
Nerve tissue	Ganglioneuroma	Ganglioneuroblastoma — malignant ganglioneuroma composed of ganglionic cells and neuroblasts	Mediastinum, retroperitoneum
	Neurofibroma — a tumor of peripheral nerve sheaths	Neurofibrosarcoma — a malignant neoplasm of peripheral nerve sheath	Peripheral nerves, hand, mediastinum, ureter, others

Histological Derivation	Benign Neoplasms	Malignant Neoplasms	Site of Predilection
Pigment-forming tissue	Nevus — pigmented mole of developmental origin	Malignant melanoma — a malignant pigmented tumor[i,j]	Skin, eye, extremities

[a] Lauren V. Ackerman and Juan A. del Regato. Pathology of cancer. In *Cancer — Diagnosis, Treatment and Prognosis*, 4th ed. St. Louis: The C. V. Mosby Co., 1970, pp. 33-68.

[b] A. C. Ritchie. The classification, morphology and behavior of tumors. In Florey, Lord, (ed.) *General Pathology*, 4th ed. Philadelphia: W. B. Saunders Co., 1970, pp. 668-719.

[c] Stanley L. Robbins. Testicular tumors. In *Pathology*, 3rd ed. Philadelphia: W. B. Saunders Co., 1967, pp. 1086-1091.

[d] _____. Osteogenic tumors, chondroma series, giant cell series, angioma series, multiple myeloma. *Ibid.*, pp. 1341-1355.

[e] _____. Tumors of blood vessels and lymphatic channels. *Ibid.*, pp. 608-615.

[f] Dorothy S. Russell and L. J. Rubinstein. *Pathology of Tumors of the Nervous System*, 3rd ed. Baltimore: The Williams and Wilkins Co., 1971.

[g] E. A. Kahn and E. C. Crosby. Gliomas of the cerebral hemispheres. In Kahn, E. A. *et al. Correlative Neurosurgery*, 2d ed. Springfield, Illinois: Charles C. Thomas, Publisher, 1969, pp. 44-67.

[h] Eugene F. Tucker, M.D. Personal communications.

[i] Anthony N. Domonkos. Pigmented nevi and tumors. *In Andrews' Diseases of the Skin — Clinical Dermatology*, 6th ed. Philadelphia: W. B. Saunders Co., 1971, pp. 803-822.

[j] Poole, W. L. Modern therapeutic approach to malignant melanoma. *Southern Medical Journal*, 64: 1449-1451, December, 1971.

ORAL READING PRACTICE

Neoplasms

Oncology is the science or study of tumors. A **neoplasm** or tumor is a new growth of tissue which may distort the size and appearance of the organ. It serves no useful purpose since it adds nothing to the further development or repair of the organ.

Tumors may be divided into **benign** and **malignant** neoplasms. Typical benign tumors are generally encapsulated by connective tissue, not invasive, and slow-growing. They never metastasize. However, they may cause serious dysfunctions if they encroach on vital organs, obstruct the circulation or air passages and compress nerves. Microscopically, the pattern of benign neoplasms is orderly and well organized.[1, 36, 34]

In contradistinction, typical malignant tumors have no capsule, are **invasive**, progressively growing, metastasize and endanger physical well-being and even life. Their microscopic pattern exhibits disorder. Benign tumors may persist for years and then, without apparent cause, undergo malignant changes.

Another method of classifying tumors is based on their histological derivation. The majority of tumors arise from **epithelial** and **connective** tissues, others from **hemopoietic, vascular** and nerve tissue and still others are of mixed origin.[1, 36, 34]

The actual cause of tumor formation is unknown although experimental investigations have established a few theories which merit attention.

1. The **embryonic theory** maintains that cells which should have produced tissue cease to develop prematurely in the embryo and are included in the growing tissue after birth. Such embryonic remnants are responsible for malignancies, especially the sarcomas. According to this theory, the classification of neoplasms is related to the degree of maturity of the tumor cells. Benign tumors are composed of mature cells, while malignant tumors approach more closely the embryonic character of tissue.

Convincing as the embryonic theory seems to be, it is no longer tenable. The differences of the **histological** components of tumors outweigh the similarities to embryonic tissue in neoplasms. Most authorities in **pathology** accept the view that tumors arise from adult cells and in the **neoplastic** process develop characteristics which differ considerably from those of the embryonic stage of tissue development.[34]

The **biochemical theory** assumes that certain biophysical and biochemical changes in the environment of the cells cause the cells to develop neoplastic properties.[8]

The **virus theory** asserts that **viruses** are an integral part of the malignant transformation of cells. This concept has met with disfavor on the ground that cancer is not of infectious origin. Opponents argue that tumors cannot be transmitted from person to person or other contact infection. It is an established fact that malignant neoplasms may be induced by **hormones, carcinogenic chemicals, ionizing radiation** and other factors.[24] Despite opposition the **viral etiology** of cancer continues to be the subject of intensive research.

A working **hypothesis** is expressed by Gross who assumes that **latent oncogenic viruses** may be present in normal healthy hosts. Prompted by certain **trigger stimuli** these inactive, but potentially **oncogenic viruses** may change into **formidable pathogens,** accelerate the multiplication of cells and develop malignant tumors, lymphomas or leukemia.[24]

Gross further comments that an inactive **oncogenic virus** could be suspected on the basis of the individual's family history of tumors or leukemia among grandparents, parents and siblings. This assumption does not imply that all descendants would necessarily harbor an oncogenic agent nor would it mean that all who carry oncogenic viruses would develop cancer or leukemia. Tumor producing viruses appear to be well adapted to their **carrier hosts** and become activated only on occasions.[24]

A new view of cancer viruses has gained wide acceptance within the past decade. Temin of the University of Wisconsin presented convincing evidence that in cells invaded by **cancer-inducing RNA viruses, DNA is synthesized** from the **viral RNA template.** The discovery of an **enzyme,** the **RNA dependent polymerase,** gives further support to the presence of viruses in cancer cells.[12, 43, 32, 36]

Robert Huebner of the **viral carcinogenesis** group of the National Cancer Institute at Bethesda, Maryland, confirms the presence of the RNA dependent polymerase in oncogenic viruses.[26]

The Huebner-Todaro **hypothesis** implies that "the occurrence of most cancer is a natural biological event determined by **spontaneous** and/or **induced derepression** of an **endogenous specific viral oncogene.** Viewed in this way ultimate control of cancer will therefore very likely depend on delineation of the factors responsible for **derepression** of virus expression and of the nature of the **repressors** involved."[26]

The **genetic theory** which offers evidence that heredity influences **susceptibility** to neoplastic reactions, is linked to the viral theory through extensive research confirming the possible transmission of the C-type RNA virus from parent to offspring.[26, 24]

For several decades the familial occurrence of cancer has been sporadically pointed up in medical literature.[18, 28, 29] It may well be that current advances in **viral carcinogenesis** provide the answer.

The unraveling of further **genetic data** and their implications in the clinical field should prove to be a most fascinating adventure and become a major benefit to mankind.

REFERENCES AND BIBLIOGRAPHY

1. Ackerman, Lauren V. and del Regato, Juan A. Pathology of cancer. In *Cancer — Diagnosis, Treatment and Prognosis,* 4th ed. St. Louis: The C. V. Mosby Co., 1970, pp. 33-68.

2. Ackerman, L. V. and Rosai, J. The pathology of tumors. Part five: Functioning tumors, spread of cancer. The radiotherapist and pathologist. *Ca — A Cancer Journal for Clinicians,* 22: 41-54, January-February, 1972.

3. Arcangeli, N. C. *et al.* A reappraisal of intra-arterial chemotherapy. Results obtained in 145 patients with head and neck cancer treated during 1963-1966 with intra-arterial chemotherapy followed by radical radiotherapy. *Cancer,* 26: 577-582, September, 1970.

4. Baker, C. G. Evaluating new antineoplastic agents. *Ca — A Cancer Journal for Clinicians,* 22: 99-101, March-April, 1972.

5. Baker, H. W. Diagnosis of oral cancer. Part one. *Ca — A Cancer Journal for Clinicians*, 22: 31-39, January-February, 1972.

6. Barrie, J. R. *et al.* Cervical nodal metastases of unknown origin. *Ca — Cancer Journal for Clinicians*, 21: 112-119, March-April, 1971.

7. Berenblum, I. The nature of tumor growth. In Florey, Lord (ed.). *General Pathology*, 4th ed. Philadelphia: W. B. Saunders Co., 1970, pp. 668-719.

8. —————. The epidemology of cancer. *Ibid.*, pp. 720-743.

9. Bridger, G. P. *et al.* Carcinoma in *situ* involving the laryngeal mucous glands. *Archives of Otolaryngology*, 94: 389-400, November, 1971.

10. Buckner. C. D. *et al.* High-dose cyclophosphamide therapy for malignant disease. Toxicity, tumor response and the effects of stored autologous marrow. *Cancer*, 29: 357-365, February, 1972.

11. Butcher, H. R. Surgery of cancer. In Ackerman, Lauren V. and del Regato, Juan A. *Cancer — Diagnosis, Treatment and Prognosis*. St. Louis: The C. V. Mosby Co., 1970, pp. 69-73.

12. Chedd, G. Fishing for viruses in cancer cells. *Ca — A Cancer Journal for Clinicians*, 21: 36-38, January-February, 1971.

13. Collins, J. J. and Black, P. H. Specificity of the carcinoembryonic antigen (CEA). *New England Journal of Medicine*, 285: 175-177, July 15, 1971.

14. Creasman, W. T. and Lukeman, J. Role of the fallopian tube in dissemination of malignant cells in corpus cancer. *Cancer*, 29: 456-457, February, 1972.

15. Crowder, B. L., Judd, E. S. and Dockerty, M. B. Gastrointestinal carcinoids and the carcinoid syndrome: Clinical characteristics and therapy. *Ca — A Cancer Journal for Clinicians*, 18: 212-218, July-August, 1968.

16. DeWys, W. Working conference on anorexia and cachexia of neoplastic disease. *Ca — A Cancer Journal for Clinicians*, 21: 72-76, January-February, 1971.

17. Diddle, A. W. Carcinoma of the cervix uteri with metastases to the neck. *Cancer*, 29: 453-455, February, 1972.

18. Falor, W. H. Chromosomes in noninvasive papillary carcinoma of the bladder. *Journal of the American Medical Association*, 216: 791-794, May 3, 1971.

19. Francis, K. C. The role of amputation in the treatment of metastatic bone cancer. *Clinical Orthopaedics and Related Research*, 73: 61-63, November-December, 1970.

20. Chose, M. K. *et al.* Functioning primary thyroid carcinoma and metastases producing hyperthyroidism. *Journal of Clinical Endocrinology and Metabolism*, 33: 639-646, October, 1971.

21. Gibb, A. G. *et al.* Papilloma of the trachea. *Journal of Laryngology and Otology*, 85, 1205-1207, November, 1971.

22. Gold, P., Krupey, J. and Ansari, H. Position of the carcinoembryonic antigen of the human digestive system in ultrastructure of tumor cell surface. *Journal of the National Cancer Institute*, 45: 219-225, August, 1970.

23. Gordon, D. L. *et al.* Carcinoid of the pancreas. *American Journal of Medicine*, 51: 412-425, September, 1971.

24. Gross, L. Viral etiology of cancer, leukemia and allied diseases. *Ca — A Cancer Journal for Clinicians*, 20: 242-247, July-August, 1970.

25. Hansen, Hobart R., M.D. Personal communications.

26. Huebner, R. J. and Todaro, G. J. Oncogenes of RNA tumor viruses as determinants of cancer. *Proceedings of the National Academy of Sciences*, 64: 1087-1092, 1969.

27. Johnson, D. E., Hogan, J. M. and Ayala, A. G. Transional cell carcinoma of the prostate. A clinical morphological study. *Cancer*, 29: 287-293, February, 1972.

28. Kennedy, B. W. *et al.* Familial multiple polyposis; a "curable" disease. *Wisconsin Medical Journal*, 70: 230-231, November, 1971.

29. Lynch, H. T. *et al.* Hereditary factors in cancer. Study of two large midwestern kindred. *Archives of Internal Medicine*, 117: 206-212, February, 1966.

30. Lynch, H. T. A family study of adenocarcinoma of the colon and multiple primary cancer. *Surgery Gynecology & Obstetrics*, 134: 781-786, May, 1972.

31. Moore, T. L. *et al.* Carcinoembryonic antigen (CEA) in bowel disease. *Journal of American Medical Association*, 222: 944-947, November 20, 1972.

32. Morton, D. L. *et al.* Cancer excerpt: Immunologic and virus studies with human sarcomas. *Ca — A Cancer Journal for Clinicians*, 20: 102-105, March-April, 1970.

33. Reynoso, G. *et al.* Carcinoembryonic antigen in patients with different cancers. *Journal of American Medical Association*, 220: 361-365, April 17, 1972.

34. Ritchie, A. C. The classification of morphology and behavior of tumors. In Florey, Lord (ed.). *General Pathology*, 4th ed. Philadelphia: W. B. Saunders Co., 1970, pp. 668-719.

35. Sanfelippo, M. P. Factors in the prognosis of adenocarcinoma of the colon and rectum. *Archives of Surgery*, 104: 401-406, April, 1972.

36. Shimkin, M. B. Cancer research. In Ackerman, Lauren V. and del Regato, Juan A. *Cancer — Diagnosis, Treatment and Prognosis*, 4th ed. St. Louis: The C. V. Mosby Co., 1970, pp. 14-32.

37. Soga, J. *et al.* Pathologic analysis of carcinoids. Histologic reevaluation of 62 cases. *Cancer*, 28: 990-998, October, 1971.

38. —————. Argentaffin cell adenocarcinoma of the stomach: an atypical carcinoid? *Cancer*, 28: 999-1003, October, 1971.

39. Theologides, A. Pathogenesis of cachexia in cancer. *Cancer*, 29: 484-488, February, 1972.

40. Thomas, E. D. *et al.* Isogenic marrow grafting in man. *Experimental Hematology*, 21: 16-18, 1971.

41. Tucker, Eugene, M.D. Personal communications.

42. Viola, M. V. When to hospitalize for metastatic carcinoma. *Ca — A Cancer Journal for Clinicians*, 21: 47-57, January-February, 1971.

43. Watson, James D. A geneticist's view of cancer. In *Molecular Biology of the Gene*, 2d ed. New York: W. A. Benjamin, Inc., 1970, pp. 588-628.

Chapter XVIII
Selected Terms Pertaining to Anesthesiology

GENERAL ANESTHESIA

A. Origin of Terms:

1. algesia (G) — sense of pain
2. basis (G) — base
3. conscious (L) — aware
4. esthesia (G) — sensation
5. ether (G) — air
6. ignis (L) — fire
7. narcose (G) — stupor
8. sedation (L) — quieting, calming

B. General Terms:

1. analeptics — stimulants of central nervous system, for example, coramine and caffeine.
2. analgesia — loss of normal sense of pain.
3. analgesics — drugs which relieve pain.
4. anesthesia — inability to feel.
   a. general anesthesia — state of unconsciousness accompanied by varying degrees of muscular relaxation and freedom from physical pain.
   b. local anesthesia — absence of sensation and, consequently, of pain in a part of the body; consciousness retained.
5. anesthesiologist — a physician who specializes in anesthesiology.
6. anesthesiology — the science and study of anesthesia.
7. anesthetic — an agent producing insensibility to pain.
8. anesthetist — a professional person, not necessarily a physician, who is qualified to administer anesthesia.
9. ataraxics — drugs exerting a calming effect, used for premedication as antianxiety agents and relaxants.
10. basal anesthesia — anesthesia providing a state of unconsciousness (narcosis) which usually lacks sufficient depth to permit major surgery.[44]
11. controlled breathing — respiratory rate and depth regulated by the intermittent pressure on a reservoir bag of the anesthetic machine.[44, 45, 55]
12. hyperventilation — excessive respiration (or movement of air in and out of the lungs) causing an abnormal loss of carbon dioxide from the blood.
13. hypoxia — a reduction of oxygen supply to the body tissues.
14. lid reflex — tapping of the eyelid to evoke its immediate closure; the lid reflex is a guide to determine the depth of anesthesia. It is lost in the stage of surgical anesthesia.[44]
15. inhalational therapy — administration of inhalant gases such as oxygen or carbon dioxide to relieve oxygen want or stimulate respiration.
16. neuroleptanalgesics — potent analgesics and tranquilizers producing detached quiescence and somnolence, used for premedication and general anesthesia or as adjuncts to other anesthetic agents.
17. neuromuscular blocking agents, skeletal muscle relaxants — drugs which serve as adjuncts to general anesthesia by producing muscular relaxation thus reducing the need for deep levels of anesthesia.[44]
    a. competitive (stabilizing) blocking agents — relaxants which inhibit transmission of motor nerve impulses at the myoneural junction, e.g. curare and gallamine triethiodide (Flaxedil Triethiodide). Paniuronium bromide is a recently released competitive blocking neuromuscular agent which is longer acting and does not possess histamine or ganglionic blocking properties.[44]
    b. depolarizing agents — relaxants which block motor nerve impulses at the myoneural junction, e.g. succinylcholine chloride (Anectine Chloride) and decamethonium bromide (Syncurine). Depolarizing agents mimic the action of acetylcholine at the nerve-muscle junction causing a discharge of the end-plate potential.[28, 7, 47]

18. preanesthetic medication, premedication — a combination of drugs including opium derivatives, barbiturates, tranquilizers, ataraxics, neuroleptanalgesics and the belladonna group in the preanesthetic preparation. Their function is:
   a. to induce psychic depression and relaxation
   b. to reduce reflex activity and metabolic rate
   c. to decrease nausea and vomiting
   d. to protect cardiovascular stability
   e. to minimize mucus production
   f. to prevent convulsive reactions.
   Less anesthetic is needed and anesthesia is achieved more rapidly. Type and dosage of premedicants must be tailored to the individual patient's needs.[53, 36, 42]

19. transient global amnesia — syndrome characterized by an abrupt loss of memory which is self-limited, not recurrent nor associated with severe damage of the central nervous system. It occurs in the postanesthetic period and lasts less than 24 hours.[19]

20. vasoconstrictors — drugs causing a constriction of the blood vessels. They are used in combination with local anesthetics to produce a vasoconstriction locally, thus preventing the anesthetic from being carried away from the site of injection.

C. Terms Related to Stages of Anesthesia:

1. stage of analgesia — period from first inhalations of anesthetic to beginning of loss of consciousness. The patient is awake, his sensorium is clear, his reflexes continue to be active, but he is insensitive to surface pain.

2. stage of delirium — period from loss of consciousness to beginning of surgical anesthesia. There is depression of the cerebral cortex and loss of control of higher centers. Reflexes tend to be exaggerated, struggling, excitement, incoordination and disorientation may occur. This stage is often absent in children.

3. stage of surgical anesthesia — period from second stage to cessation of spontaneous respiration. This stage is subdivided into 4 planes.
   a. the first plane — muscle tone is unchanged and eyeball movements continue when the lids are raised. The pupil reacts to light.
   b. the second plane — smaller muscles throughout the body lose their tone and ocular movements cease. The pupils are centrally fixed.
   c. the third plane — muscular relaxation throughout the body includes large muscles. The corneal reflexes are abolished. Respiration becomes diaphragmatic.
   d. the fourth plane — the relaxation of large muscles and loss of reflexes are complete. The pupils are widely dilated. Diaphragmatic activity is decreased.

4. stage of toxicity — period from onset of apnea to circulatory failure. Respiratory movement ceases, the depression of the cardiovascular system increases and the blood pressure drops rapidly. If artificial respiration is instituted, the condition may be reversible.[8, 37, 54]

D. Terms Related to Methods of General Anesthesia:

1. endotracheal anesthesia — introduction of a catheter into the trachea for the purpose of conducting the anesthetic mixture directly from the apparatus to the lungs. This may be achieved by oral or nasal intubation. The catheter is then attached to a closed or semiclosed inhaler. In present day practice this form of inhalation anesthesia is the method of choice for most major operations since it permits a patent airway, the aspiration of secretions, the use of positive pressure, controlled breathing and adequate ventilation.[37, 54, 38]

2. inhalation anesthesia — general anesthesia produced by the inhalation of vaporized liquids or gases.   Several methods are used.
   a. the closed method — a technic in which the patient rebreathes the anesthetic mixture, contained in a special apparatus.   This apparatus is composed of a tight fitting mouth or nose mask or tube, a rebreathing bag and a device permitting the absorption of carbon dioxide.[44]
   b. the open method — a liquid anesthetic drug dropped on a gauze mask which covers the patient's nose and mouth and permits the inhalation of the vaporized drug.
   c. the semiclosed method — a technic which differs from the closed method by the use of an exhalation valve which allows partial rebreathing and carbon dioxide removal with soda lime.[37, 54, 26, 27, 13, 46, 32, 20, 4, 22]
3. intravenous anesthesia — the intravenous administration of drugs for basal narcosis. A stage of unconsciousness is produced, but analgesia and muscular relaxation may prove unsatisfactory.[39]
4. rectal anesthesia — the rectal administration of drugs to produce basal anesthesia.   The reflexes are partially abolished and a hypnotic state is present.   Pentothal, Avertin and Ether have been used for this purpose.

E. Terms Related to Dissociative Anesthesia:

1. dissociative anesthesia — selective blocking of pain conduction and perception, leaving those parts of the central nervous system which do not participate in pain transmission and perception, free from the depressant effects of drugs.   The profound analgesia induced by this type of anesthesia is associated with somnolence in which the patient appears to be disconnected from his environment.[10, 49, 11, 52]
2. neuroleptanalgesia, neuroleptanesthesia — a balanced highly effective anesthetic state for control of well-defined pain during surgery resulting from the depression of certain corticothalamic systems.   It may be used as sole anesthesia or as adjunct to local, regional or general anesthesia.   Neuroleptanalgesia is a type of dissociative anesthesia.[23, 43]

LOCAL AND REGIONAL ANESTHESIA

A. Origin of Terms:

1. acus (L) — needle
2. cauda (L) — tail
3. conduct (L) — to lead
4. dura (L) — hard
5. filter (L) — to strain through
6. hypno (G) — sleep
7. segment (L) — portion
8. pressor (L) — to press
9. punctura (L) — puncture
10. vas, vaso (L) — vessel

B. Terms Related to Methods of Local Anesthesia:

1. acupuncture anesthesia — insertion of stainless steel acupuncture needles at carefully selected points identified as the most effective for anesthesia of a particular operation. The needles are connected to a direct current battery source for electral stimulation. Instead of electricity the acupuncturist may manipulate the needles in an up-and-down, plus twirling motion, for twenty minutes to produce anesthesia.   The advantages of Chinese acupuncture are:
   a. absolute safety of the anesthesia
   b. effective anesthetic for debilitated patients
   c. patient conscious and alert during entire procedure
   d. adequate anesthesia for prolonged surgery
   e. no interruption of food and fluid intake
   f. no postoperative nausea, vomiting, low blood pressure or respiratory complications.[16, 1, 24]
2. caudal or sacral anesthesia — a method of epidural anesthesia in which the anesthetic solution is injected into the sacral canal.[18, 48, 25]

3. conduction anesthesia — term including various forms of local anesthesia: direct nerve block, epidural block, spinal anesthesia and infiltration anesthesia.[41, 31]

4. epidural block — spinal nerves blocked as they pass through the epidural space.[41, 18]

5. infiltration anesthesia — injection of a dilute anesthetic agent under the skin to anesthetize the nerve endings and nerve fibers.[41]

6. intravenous regional anesthesia — a method of producing analgesia in the extremities using lidocaine (or other drug) as regional anesthetic to act at the main nerve trunks.[40, 50]

7. nerve and field block — insensibility of a local area achieved by:
   a. direct nerve block — injection of an anesthetic solution into easily accessible nerves, as those of the extremities.
   b. field block — anesthetic solution deposited around the nerve at the point of its terminal branches.[41, 12]

8. spinal anesthesia — anesthesia produced by the injection of a local anesthetic solution into the subarachnoid space of the lumbar region to block the roots of the spinal nerves. Tetracaine, procaine and lidocaine are frequently used.[41, 19]

9. subarachnoid alcohol block — injection of absolute ethyl alcohol (hypobaric alcohol about 0.8 ml) in any interspace of the spinal cord. The alcohol floats to the top, bathes the nerve roots and destroys the pain fibers.[15]

10. surface or topical anesthesia — direct application of an anesthetic drug to a mucous membrane to produce insensibility to the nerve endings. Cocaine and viscous lidocaine are used for surface anesthetics.[41]

ABBREVIATIONS

A. General:

ACh — acetylcholine
Anes. — anesthesiology
$CHCl_3$ — chloroform
C_{10} — decamethonium
C_3H_6 — cyclopropane
C_2H_4 — ethylene
C_2H_5Cl — ethyl chloride
C_2HCl_3 — trichloroethylene (Trilene)
CO_2 — carbon dioxide
dTC — d-tubocurarine
HCl — hydrochloride

He — helium
NLA — neuroleptanalgesia
N_2O — nitrous oxide
NR — non-rebreathing
NT — nasotracheal
O_2 — oxygen
OD — open drop
OT — orotracheal
Pent. — pentothal
SC — semiclosed
Vin. — vinyl ether (Vinethene)

B. Standard Pharmacology Texts:

NF — The National Formulary
ND — New Drugs
PDR — Physicians' Desk Reference

USD — The Dispensary of the United States of America
USP — United States Pharmacopeia

ORAL READING PRACTICE

Induced Hypothermia

The value of local **hypothermia** was recognized a century ago by Larrey, surgeon general of Napoleon's army. It was his custom to pack the soldiers' injured extremities in ice to control shock and pain. In 1939 Temple Fay used hypothermia as a **palliative** measure for patients suffering from **malignancies**. This treatment he abandoned since it proved to be no cure for cancer.[21]

Interest in hypothermia was revived when Bigelow and his associates published their investigation. They found that progressive body cooling lowers the **metabolic** requirements of the patient. They also found that shivering neutralizes the benefit obtained by hypothermia since it increases the oxygen requirement.[57]

Further research led from the application of these physiological findings to the regime of anesthesia used during **intracardiac** surgery. Prior to 1950 the high oxygen requirement of the heart and brain and the continuous flow of blood through the cardiac chambers had presented insurmountable barriers to direct vision surgery of the heart. The development of safe techniques employing hypothermia and **extracorporeal circulation** removed these barriers and opened a new era in the correction of cardiovascular defects.[58, 59, 3, 29, 14]

The **anesthesiologist** who uses hypothermia is primarily concerned with reducing the patient's oxygen requirement, for it results in **hypometabolism** and a diminished need for anesthesia. At present surface cooling and blood cooling are widely accepted methods of hypothermia.[57, 3]

Zeavin, Virtue and Swan of the University of Colorado advocate **immersion cooling,** a form of surface cooling, to lower the temperature of the body surface. Following the **induction** of anesthesia, the patient is immersed in ice water. His temperature continues to fall an additional 50% after he is removed from the ice bath. For example, if during the immersion his temperature was lowered 10°C (centigrade), it will fall another 5° after immersion has been discontinued.

Another widely accepted technique is surface cooling which can be used under controlled conditions. After the patient is anesthetized and an **endotracheal** tube has been inserted, it is possible to lower his body temperature gradually by wrapping the patient in an ice cold blanket or placing him on a water mattress through which ice water circulates. Continuous recording of the **esophageal** temperature by a special recorder keeps the anesthesiologist informed of changes in body temperature. Light anesthesia is generally an adequate means of preventing shivering. **Muscle relaxants** and tranquilizers have also been used as adjuncts.[44]

With hypothermia of the body to 28°C, it is possible to perform **inflow occlusion** by obstructing the **inferior** and **superior venae cavae** and to operate within the heart for a period of eight minutes.

The limitations with respect to time prevented the repair of many acquired and **congenital cardiac defects** and led to the development of the heart-lung machine which extends this time to several hours. The temperature of the patient is controlled during **cardiopulmonary bypass** by the use of a heat exchanger in the **extracorporeal circuit** allowing body temperature to be varied as needed by surgical requirements.[44, 59]

In the past the heart-lung machine was usually primed with cold blood which induced body cooling. Presently cold intravenous fluids are used for priming and lowering the body temperature.

Hypothermia frequently results in **ventricular fibrillation** at a temperature below 25°C. This ineffective type of muscular contraction of the heart must be converted by **electrical defibrillation** to a state of cardiac **asystole** whereupon the normal pacemaker will usually become operative and restore an effective output of blood from the heart.

Cardiac massage is employed to propel blood to the vital organs during **ventricular asystole** (arrest) or ventricular fibrillation until conversion to an effectively beating heart is accomplished.

With the use of the pump oxygenator cardiac massage is unnecessary as the vital organs are being perfused. In all other situations of **cardiac arrest** or ventricular fibrillation cardiac massage is a life-supporting emergency measure.[44]

In the late sixties induced hypothermia fell into disrepute because of the risk of **cardiac arrhythmias** complicating the extreme lowering of body temperature. Many anesthesiologists abandoned the procedure in favor of **normothermia.**[9, 50, 33, 51, 5] By introducing effective safety measures in the anesthetic program, Mohri and colleagues stimulated renewed interest in hypothermia in the early seventies.[34] They advocated surface cooling with ice bags, a short period of cardiopulmonary bypass before **circulatory arrest** and **bypass resuscitation** and rewarming for cardiac surgery in neonates and infants. Obviously it is left to the discerning judgment of the anesthesiologist if hypothermia or normothermia should be the method of choice.[35, 2, 17, 1]

Table 27

CLASSIFICATION OF GENERAL ANESTHETICS

Anesthetic Agents	Systemic Effects

A. Volatile substances, administered by inhalation
  1. *Liquids* producing vapors:
    Chloroform ....USP
    Compound 469 (Forane)......Experimental
    Ether ....USP
    Ethyl chloride ....USP
    Halothane (Fluothane) ....USP
    Methoxyflurane (Penthrane) ....ND
    Trichloroethylene (Trilene) ....USP
    Vinyl ether (Vinethene) ....USP
 	
  2. *Gases:*
    Cyclopropane ....USP
    Ethylene ....USP
    Nitrous oxide ....USP
	A. Chemical substances and depressants of central nervous system; surgically useful because they are complete anesthetics providing
	
	  1. analgesia
	
	  2. suppression of reflex activity
	
	  3. muscular relaxation
	
	  4. loss of consciousness

B. Nonvolatile substances administered intravenously or rectally
  1. Ultrashort acting Barbiturates
    Methohexital (Brevital) ....USP
    Thiamylal (Surital) ....USP
    Thiopental (Pentothal) ....USP
 	
  2. Derivative of Ethyl Alcohol
    Tribromoethanol (Avertin) ....USP
    Solution Avertin in Amylene hydrate
	B. Basal narcotics, medullary depressants and incomplete anesthetics; surgically useful as adjuncts to other anesthetics. They produce
	  1. unconsciousness
	
	  2. inadequate control of reflex activity
	
	  3. unsatisfactory muscular relaxation
	
	  4. hypnosis and amnesia (following Avertin)

C. Nonvolatile substances administered intravenously or intramuscularly
 	
  1. Neuroleptics and Nonbarbiturates
    Ketamine CI-581 (Ketalar)
    Droperidol (Inapsine)
 	
  2. Neuroleptic and Potent Narcotic
    Analgesic
    Innovar (Droperidol and Fentanyl)
	C. Shortacting anesthetics, depressants of certain corticothalamic systems; useful as sole anesthetic and as adjunct to conventional anesthesia. They produce
	  1. profound analgesia
	
	  2. amnesia
	
	  3. increased cardiovascular activity
	
	  4. unsatisfactory muscular relaxation

REFERENCES AND BIBLIOGRAPHY

1. Armstrong, M. E. Acupuncture. *American Journal of Nursing*, 72: 1582-1588, September, 1972.
2. Barratt-Boyes, B. G. *et al.* Intracardiac surgery in neonates and infants using deep hypothermia with surface cooling and limited cardiopulmonary bypass. *Circulation,* (Suppl. I) 43: 25-30, May, 1971.
3. Benazon, D. Hypothermia. In Seurr, Cyril and Feldman, Stanley (eds.). *Scientific Foundations of Anaesthesia.* Philadelphia: F. A. Davis, Co., 1970, pp. 265-277.
4. Blake, D. A. *et al.* Qualitative analysis of halothane metabolites in man. *Anesthesiology,* 36: 152-154, February, 1972.
5. Brickman, R. D. *et al.* Circulatory arrest during profound hypothermia. *Archives of Surgery,* 103: 259-264, August, 1971.
6. Brielmaier, Charles R., M.D. Personal communications.
7. Cohen, E. N. Uptake, distribution and elimination of the muscle relaxants. In Seurr, Cyril and Feldman, Stanley (eds.). *Scientific Foundations of Anaesthesia.* Philadelphia: F. A. Davis Co., 1970, pp. 350-356.
8. Cohen, P. J. and Dripps, R. D. Signs and stages of anesthesia. In Goodman. Louis S. and Gilman, Alfred (eds.). *The Pharmacological Basis of Therapeutics,* 4th ed. New York: The Macmillan Co., 1970, pp. 49-55.
9. Cooley, D. A. *et al.* Ischemic contracture of the heart: "Stone heart". *American Journal of Cardiology,* 29: 575-577, April, 1972.
10. Corssen, G. Changing concepts in pain control during surgery: Dissociative anesthesia with CI-581. *Anesthesia and Analgesia . . . Current Researches,* 47: 746-758, November-December, 1968.
11. Corssen, G. *et al.* Ketamine in the anesthetic management of asthmatic patients. *Anesthesia and*

Analgesia . . . Current Researches, 51: 588-596, July-August, 1972.

12. Covino, B. G. Local anesthesia. *New England Journal of Medicine*, 286: 1035-1042, May 11, 1972.

13. Cromwell, T. H. *et al.* The cardiovascular effects of compound 469 (forane) during spontaneous ventilation and CO_2 challenge in man. *Anesthesiology*, 35: 17-25, July, 1971.

14. Dalton, B. Anesthesia for cardiac surgery. *Anesthesiology*, 36: 521-522, May, 1972.

15. Derrick, W. S. Subarachnoid alcohol block in the control of pain. *Ca — A Cancer Journal for Clinicians*, 21: 248-251, July-August, 1971.

16. Diamond, E. G. Acupuncture anesthesia. Western medicne and Chinese traditional medicine. *Journal of American Medical Association*, 218: 1558-1563, December 6, 1971.

17. Dillard, D. H. *et al.* Correction of heart disease in infancy utilizing deep hypothermia and total circulatory arrest. *Journal of Thoracic and Cardiovascular Surgery*, 61: 64-69, January, 1971.

18. Doughty, A. The relief of pain in labour. In Wylie, W. D. and Churchill-Davidson, H. C. (eds.). *A Practice of Anesthesia*, 3rd ed. Chicago: Year Book Medical Publishers, Inc., 1972, pp. 1403-1441.

19. Dykes, M. H. *et al.* Transient global amnesia following spinal anesthesia. *Anesthesiology*, 36: 615-617, June, 1972.

20. Fourcade, H. E. *et al.* The ventilatory effects of forane, a new inhaled anesthetic. *Anesthesiology*, 35: 26-31, July, 1971.

21. Frenay, Sr. Agnes Clare. Balanced anesthesia and induced hypothermia. *American Journal of Nursing*, 55: 1245-1247, October, 1955.

22. Galbert, M. W. Use of halothane in a balanced technic for cesarean section. *Anesthesia and Analgesia . . . Current Researches*, 51: 701-704, September-October, 1972.

23. Garfield, J. M. *et al.* A comparison of psychologic responses to ketamine and thiopental-nitrous oxide-halothane anesthesia. *Anesthesiology*, 36: 329-338, April, 1972.

24. Greene, N. M. This is no humbug — or is it? *Anesthesiology*, 36: 101-102, February, 1972.

25. Greiss, F. Obstetric anesthesia. *American Journal of Nursing*, 71: 67-69, January, 1971.

26. Hickey, R. F. The effects of ether, halothane and forane on apneic thresholds in man. *Anesthesiology*, 35: 32-37, July, 1971.

27. Homi, J. *et al.* A new anesthetic agent — forane: Preliminary observations in man. *Anesthesia and Analgesia . . . Current Researches*, 51: 439-447, May-June, 1972.

28. Koelle, G. B. Neuromuscular blocking agents. In Goodman, Louis S. and Gilman, Alfred (eds.). *The Pharmacological Basis of Therapeutics*, 4th ed. New York: The Macmillan Co., 1970, pp. 601-619.

29. Levitsky, S. *et al.* Cardiovascular surgical emergencies in the first year of life. *Surgical Clinics of North America*, 52: 61-75, February, 1972.

30. Liu, C. K. and Lee, J. Y. Cardiac arrhythmias in anesthesia and in acute myocardial infarction. *International Anesthesiology Clinics*, 10: 67-79, Spring, 1972.

31. Lund, P. C. The hazards and acute emergencies of conduction anesthesia. *International Anesthesiology Clinics*, 10: 153-187, Spring, 1972.

32. Miller, R. D. Comparative neuromuscular effects of forane and halothane alone and in combination with d-tubocurarine in man. *Anesthesiology*, 35: 38-42, July, 1971.

33. Moffitt, E. A. *et al.* Normothermia versus hypothermia for whole-body perfusion: Effects on myocardial and body metabolism. *Anesthesia and Analgesia . . . Current Researches*, 50: 505-516, July-August, 1971.

34. Mohri, H. *et al.* Method of surface-induced deep hypothermia for open-heart surgery in infants. *Journal of Thoracic Cardiovascular Surgery*, 58: 262-270, August, 1969.

35. Mohri, A. et al. Deep hypothermia combined with cardiopulmonary bypass for cardiac surgery in neonates and infants. *Journal of Thoracic and Cardiovascular Surgery*, 64: 422-429, September, 1972.

36. O'Neill, A. A. Premedication for ketamine anesthesia. Phase I: The classic drugs. *Anesthesia and Analgesia . . . Current Researches*, 51: 475-482, May-June, 1972.

37. Price, H. L. and Dripps, R. D. General anesthetics II. Volatile anesthetics: Diethyl ether, divinyl ether, chloroform, halothane, methoxyflurane and other halogenated anesthetics. In Goodman, Louis S. and Gilman, Alfred (eds.). *The Pharmacological Basis of Therapeutics*, 4th ed. New York: Macmillan Co., 1970, pp. 79-92.

38. _____. General anesthetics I. Gas anesthetics: Nitrous oxide, ethylene and cyclopropane. *Ibid.*, pp. 71-78.

39. _____. General anesthetics III. Intravenous anesthetics. *Ibid.*, pp. 93-97.

40. Raj, P. P. *et al.* Site of action of intravenous regional anesthesia. *Anesthesia and Analgesia . . . Current Researches*, 51: 776-786, September-October, 1972.

41. Ritchie, J. M., Cohen, P. J. and Dripps, R. D. Local anesthetics. In Goodman, Louis S. and Gilman, Alfred (eds.). *The Pharmacological Basis of Therapeutics*, 4th ed. New York: The Macmillan Co., 1970, pp. 371-401.

42. Sadove, M. S. et al. Anesthesia in the acute surgical emergency. *Surgical Clinics of North America*, 52: 47-60, February, 1972.

43. Sadove, M. S. *et al.* Clinical study of droperidol in the prevention of the side effects of ketamine anesthesia: a progress report. *Anesthesia and Analgesia . . . Current Researches*, 50: 526-532, July-August, 1971.

44. Schweiss, John F., M.D. Personal communications.

45. Spencer, G. T. Artificial respiration. In Wylie, W. D. and Churchill-Davidson, H. C. (eds.). *A Practice of Anaesthesia*, 3rd ed. Chicago: Year Book Medical Publishers, Inc. 1972, pp. 452-503.

46. Stevens, W. C. *et al.* The cardiovascular effects of a new inhalation anesthetic, forane, in human volunteers at constant arterial carbon dioxide tension. *Anesthesiology*, 35: 8-16, July, 1971.

47. Thomas, E. T. and Dobkin, A. B. Untoward effects of muscle relaxant drugs. *International Anesthesiology Clinics*, 10: 207-225, Spring, 1972.

48. Touloukian, R. J. *et al.* Caudal anesthesia for neonatal anoperineal and rectal operations. *Anes-*

306

thesia and Analgesia . . . Current Researches, 50: 565-568, July-August, 1971.

49. Trudnowski, R. J. *et al.* Neuroleptanalgesia for patients with kidney malfunction. *Anesthesia and Analgesia . . . Current Researches, 50:* 679-684, July-August, 1971.

50. Tucker, G. T. and Boas, R. A. Pharmakinetic aspects of intravenous regional anesthesia. *Anesthesiology,* 34: 538-549, June, 1971.

51. Weygandt, G. R. The effects of citrated blood and hypothermia on acid-base balance during cardiopulmonary bypass. *Anesthesiology,* 36: 268-277. May, 1972.

52. Winters, W. D. Epilepsy and anesthesia with ketamine. *Anesthesiology,* 36: April, 1972.

53. Wollman, H. and Dripps, R. D. Preanesthetic medication. In Goodman, Louis S. and Gilman, Alfred (eds.). *The Pharmacological Basis of Therapeutics,* 4th ed. New York: The Macmillan Co., 1970, pp. 56-59.

54. _____. Uptake distribution, elimination and administration of inhalational anesthetics. *Ibid.,* pp. 60-70.

55. Wylie, W. D. and Churchill-Davidson, H. C. (eds.). The mechanics of respiration: controlled respiration. In *A Practice of Anesthesia,* 3rd ed. Chicago: Year Book Medical Publishers, Inc. 1972, pp. 49-77.

56. _____. The mechanics of respiration — respiratory movements in anaesthesia. *Ibid.,* pp. 49-77.

57. _____. Hypothermia. Methods of lowering the body temperature in man. *Ibid.,* pp. 1273-1297.

58. _____. Anesthesia and cardiac disease. *Ibid.,* pp. 652-690.

59. _____. The extracorporeal circulation. *Ibid.,* pp. 691-715.

Chapter XIX
Selected Terms Pertaining to Physical Therapy

ORIENTATION

A. Origin of Terms:

1. manus (L) — hand
2. physio- (G) — nature
3. physical (L) — natural
4. therapy (G) — treatment

B. General Terms:

1. physiatrist — a physician who specializes in physical medicine and rehabilitation.[24]
2. physical agents — active forces such as water, radiant energy, massage, exercise, electricity and ultrasound energy.[24]
3. physical medicine — that branch of medical science which uses physical agents in the diagnosis and management of disease.[24]
4. physical therapist — a professional person qualified to provide physical therapy in areas such as: direct patient care, consultation, supervision, teaching, administration, research and community service.[38]
5. physical therapy — a profession which uses knowledge and skills pertaining to physical therapy in caring for individuals disabled by disease and injury. The primary focus is on the functional restoration of patients affected with skeletal, neuromuscular, cardiovascular and pulmonary disorders.
6. physical therapy assistant — a skilled technical worker who administers physical therapy treatments under the supervision of a physical therapist.[38]
7. prosthetist — a person who designs and fits prostheses.
8. rehabilitation — a treatment process designed to help physically handicapped individuals make maximal use of residual capacities and to enable them to obtain optimal satisfaction and usefulness in terms of themselves, their families and their community.[24, 40, 48, 12, 49]

PHYSICAL THERAPY PROCEDURES AND RELATED TESTS

A. Origin of Terms:

1. actino (G) — ray
2. cryo, crymo (G) — cold
3. electro (G) — amber
4. helio (G) — sun
5. hydro (G) — water
6. insulate (L) — to make
7. ion (G) — going
8. mechano (G) — machine
9. meter (G) — measure
10. oscillation (L) — swinging
11. phoresis (G) — to carry, to bear
12. photo (G) — light
13. polar (G) — axis, pole
14. radio (L) — ray
15. thermo (G) — heat

B. Terms Related to Physical Therapy Procedures:

1. electrotherapy — the use of electrical currents in the treatment of disease. Included are general terms and terms related to procedures:
   a. anode — positive pole of a direct current.
   b. cathode — negative pole of a direct current.
   c. condenser — a device for storing electricity.

    d. conductor — a substance capable of transmitting heat or electricity.

    e. diathermy — the therapeutic use of high frequency currents to generate deep heat within parts of the body. Types of diathermy include the autotherm, microtherm and shortwave units.[26]

    f. electric current — a stream of electrons flowing along a conductor.

        (1) alternating current — an intermittent, asymmetrical current obtained from the secondary winding of an induction coil, also known as faradic current.

        (2) direct current — a unidirectional current with distinct polarity, also called constant or galvanic current.[41]

    g. ion — a moving particle carrying an electrical charge.

    h. iontophoresis — the introduction of medicinal ions into the tissues by means of a direct current.[44]

    i. polarity — pertains to a direct current with positive and negative poles.

    j. ultrasonics — the use of sound waves, considerably above the range of hearing, for therapeutic purposes.[17]

        (1) phonophoresis — the introduction of medicinal ions, such as hydrocortisone, into the tissues by means of ultrasound.[15]

        (2) ultrasound — a form of acoustic vibration occurring at frequencies too high to be perceived by the human ear.[41, 17]

2. hydrotherapy — the use of water in its various forms: liquid, solid and vapor.[53]

    a. Archimedes' principle — a body fully or partially immersed in a liquid experiences an upward thrust equal to the weight of the liquid which it displaces.[51]

    b. contrast bath — the use of hot and cold water alternately.

    c. cryotherapy, crymotherapy — the use of cold, especially cold packs, immersion in ice water, or ice massage.[33]

    d. underwater exercise — immersion of the patient in water, tank or pool, to permit free active motion, relaxation and full abduction of the extremities, and sometimes gait training.

    e. whirlpool — a treatment which offers temperature control in combination with the mechanical effects of water in motion.[53]

3. massage — manipulation of the soft tissues of the body most effectively performed with the hands, and administered to produce effects on the nervous and muscular systems and the local and general circulation of the blood and lymph.[3, 21]

    a. effleurage — superficial or deep stroking movements.

    b. friction — deep circular or rolling movements.

    c. petrissage — kneading or compression movements.

    d. tapotement — percussion movements including cupping, hacking, clapping, tapping and beating.[41]

    e. vibratory — frequently performed with a mechanical device especially to increase bronchial drainage.[3, 21]

4. radiation therapy — the therapeutic use of radiant energy, especially infrared and ultraviolet rays.

    a. infrared — an invisible form of radiant energy, ranging from about 7000 A° to 140000 A° in the electromagnetic spectrum, and producing heat on absorption.[38]

    b. ultraviolet — an invisible form of radiant energy ranging from about 136 A° to 4000 A° and producing chemical actions on absorption.[38]

        Related terms are:

        (1) cold quartz — a type of ultraviolet lamp used for local irradiation.

        (2) cosine angle law — a law which indicates that the intensity is greatest when the surface to be treated is at a right angle to the lamp.[38]

        (3) electromagnetic spectrum (EMS) — a graphic representation of the various waves of radiant energy in ascending order of length.

        (4) erythema — a latent inflammatory reaction caused by a chemical action which takes place in the skin.

        (5) heliotherapy — exposure of the body to sunlight or solar radiation.

 (6) inverse square law — a law which states that the intensity of radiation from any source varies inversely with the square of the distance from the source.

 (7) minimal erythematous dose — irradiation sufficient to cause slight reddening of the skin.[41]

 (8) suberythematous dose — irradiation insufficient to cause slight reddening of the skin.[41]

 (9) third-degree erythematous dose — irradiation sufficient to cause edema and blister formation.[41]

5. therapeutic exercise — exercise concerned with bodily movement and designed to maintain or restore normal function. This includes:

 a. muscle contraction
  (1) concentric — when a muscle is contracted from the extended to the shortened position.[28]
  (2) eccentric — in contracting, the muscle lengthens as it contracts.
  (3) isokinetic — there is maximal contraction throughout the range of motion.[51, 40]
  (4) isometric — contraction of the muscle without movement of the joint, also known as muscle setting.[40, 29]
  (5) isotonic — exercise in which a part is moved by muscle contraction.[28, 40]

 b. types of exercise
  (1) active — purposeful voluntary motion.[28]
  (2) active assistive — a combination of voluntary motion and the use of an external force.[28]
  (3) active resistive — voluntary muscle contraction against resistance.[29]
  (4) passive — exercise administered by a therapist or by an external force without assistance from the patient.[10]
  (5) progressive resistive — exercise in which resistance is progressively increased, also known as DeLorme exercise.[10]

 c. exercises for specific conditions
  (1) breathing — a system of exercises for patients with chronic obstructive pulmonary disease (COPD).[39]
  (2) Buerger-Allen — a system of exercises designed for patients with peripheral vascular disease.[28]
  (3) Codman's — stooping exercises for patients with shoulder conditions.[28]
  (4) coordination — exercises designed for patients with minimal cerebral dysfunction.[4, 11]
  (5) Frenkel — special exercises used in treating patients with ataxia.[28]
  (6) Guthrie-Smith — assistive exercises in which parts of the body (or the entire body) are supported by slings and springs.[28]
  (7) postural drainage — a procedure which includes positioning, massage, coughing and breathing exercises for patients with chronic obstructive pulmonary disease (COPD).[39]
  (8) prepartum and postpartum — exercises (including posture, relaxation and breathing) employed during pregnancy, the three stages of labor, and following delivery.
  (9) Williams — exercises for chronic low back pain designed to strengthen the abdominal and gluteal muscles, and to stretch the erector spinae and hip flexors.[28]

 d. systems of exercise
  (1) Bobath — a method of exercise used to inhibit abnormal postural reflexes and facilitate normal postural reflexes.[4]
  (2) Brunnstrom — a method of exercise which after eliciting synergies on a reflex basis, attempts to establish voluntary control of the synergies.[5, 37]
  (3) proprioceptive neuromuscular facilitation (PNF) — a system of exercise using spiral and diagonal movement patterns.[22, 50]

(4) Rood — system of exercise concerned with the interaction of somatic, autonomic and psychic factors and their role in regulating motor behavior.[45, 38]

(5) Temple Fay — system of exercise stressing reflex and developmental therapy as an approach to patient care.[35, 38]

e. terms related to therapeutic exercise

(1) orthetics — the systematic pursuit of straightening or correcting. It deals with exoskeletal devices to limit or assist motion of any given segment of the body.[41]

(2) prosthetics — deals with the addition or application of an artificial device to replace partially or totally missing extremities or organs.[41]

6. thermotherapy — the treatment of disease using various forms of heat.[42]

a. conduction — heat transferred from a warmer object to a cooler one when both objects are in contact.

b. convection — heat exchange between a surface and a fluid moving adjacent to the surface.

c. hydrocollator packs — local hot packs which employ silica gel as the heat-retaining agent.[14]

d. paraffin packs — the use of hot paraffin for therapeutic purposes.[14]

C. Terms Related to Tests and Measurements

1. activities of daily living — a test which serves to outline as accurately as possible how a patient functions in everyday life — in other words, how many daily activities he can perform in his own home and in connection with his work.[41, 25]

2. electrotesting — the use of electrical currents to test the reaction of muscles and motor nerves.[6, 19] This includes:

a. chronaxie — the minimum time required for a current twice the strength of rheobase to elicit a muscle contraction.

b. electromyography — the amplification and recording, both visually and audibly, of minute electrical potentials generated by muscle contractions. Electromyograms are valuable in the study of neuromuscular disorders.[13, 36, 40]

c. reaction of degeneration — the reaction of a muscle to galvanic but not faradic current.

d. rheobase — the minimal intensity of current required to elicit muscle contraction.

e. strength duration curve — the graphic representation of current strength and duration required to elicit a minimal muscle contraction.[51]

3. gait analysis — methods used to detect deviations in gait resulting from pain, weakness, incoordination or deformities.[9]

4. goniometry — testing the range of joint motion with the aid of a goniometer.[7, 30]

5. manual muscle testing — an important tool used to determine the extent and degree of muscle weakness resulting from disuse, injury or disease.[9]

6. perceptual motor testing — testing for perceptual motor skills: a response or family of responses in which receptor, effector and feedback processes show a high degree of spatial and temporal organization.[8, 9]

7. posture evaluation — evaluating the position in which various parts of the body are held while sitting, walking and lying.[41]

ABBREVIATIONS

A° — angstrom unit
AC — alternating current
ACC — anode closing contraction
ADL — activities of daily living
ADP — adenosine diphosphate
AE — above elbow
AK — above knee
AOC — anode closing contraction
APRL — Army Prosthetic Research Laboratory

APTA — American Physical Therapy Association
ATP — adenosine triphosphate
BE — below elbow
BK — below knee
C — centigrade
CCC — cathode closing contraction
COC — cathode opening contraction
COPD — chronic obstructive pulmonary disease
DC — direct current

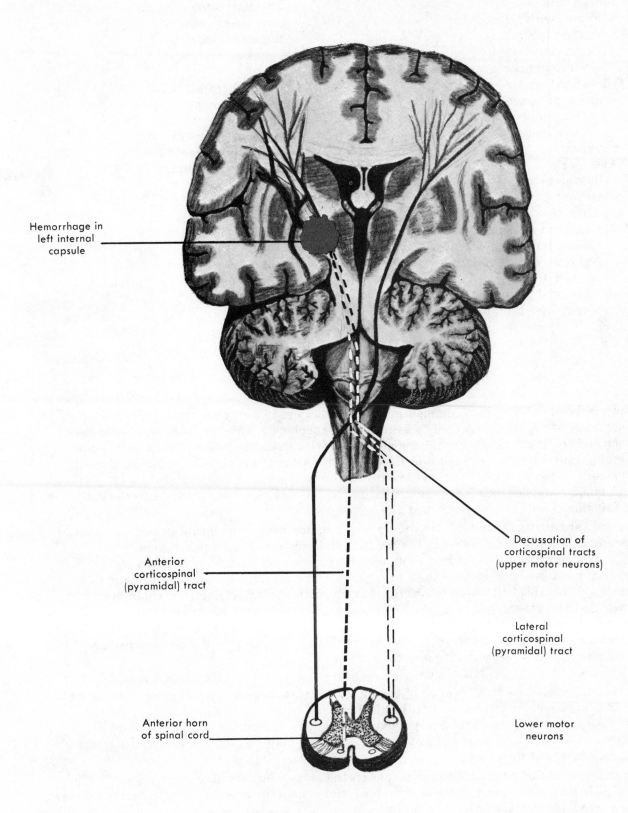

Hemorrhage in
left internal
capsule

Decussation of
corticospinal tracts
(upper motor neurons)

Anterior
corticospinal
(pyramidal) tract

Lateral
corticospinal
(pyramidal) tract

Anterior horn
of spinal cord

Lower motor
neurons

Fig. 81 — Cerebral hemorrhage in the left internal capsule resulting in right-sided hemiplegia because of the crossing (decussation) of the corticospinal (pyramidal) tracts in the medulla oblongata.

DTR — deep tendon reflex
EMF — electromotive force
EMG — electromyogram,
    electromyograph
EMS — electromagnetic spectrum
F — fahrenheit
FAD — flavin adenine dinucleotide
IPPB — intermittent positive
    pressure breathing
IR — infrared
KJ — knee jerk
LOM — limitation of motion
LPT — licensed physical therapist
MA — milliampere
MED — minimal erythemal dose
MFT — muscle function test
NRA — National Rehabilitation
    Association
OT — occupational therapist,
    occupational therapy

PFT — pulmonary function test
PNF — proprioceptive neuro-
    muscular facilitation
PRE — progressive resistive
    exercise
PT — physical therapist
    physical therapy
R — resistance
RD — reaction of degeneration
ROM — range of motion
SACH — solid ankle cushion heel
SED — suberythemal dose
SOS — surgical orthopedic splinting
US — ultrasound
UV — ultraviolet
V — volt
W — watt
WHO — World Health Organization

ORAL READING PRACTICE

Hemiplegia

Hemiplegia is one of the most common muscular disorders of central origin. When the paralysis occurs suddenly, it is referred to as stroke or **apoplexy**. The involvement affects the **corticobulbar** and **corticospinal fibers**. Motor neurons, with cell bodies located in the **cortex** and **axons** extending into the cord, are known as upper motor neurons in contradistinction to those in the **anterior horn** of the cord which extend toward the muscles and are called lower motor neurons. A similar division exists for the cranial nerves in regions where their nerve nuclei perform a function corresponding to that of the spinal cord.[1, 4]

A **cerebral thrombosis** tends to devitalize an upper motor neuron resulting in its degeneration all the way from the thrombotic lesion to the cord. The lower motor neuron remains uninvolved. Following the initial period of shock, the muscles respond to **reflex arcs** mediated by the cord. Since these reflexes tend to be exaggerated, the muscles of the hemiplegic patient become spastic. This **spasticity** may interfere seriously with the exercise of the **voluntary** muscle power that the patient has regained. Drugs and therapies have been tried to overcome the unfortunate handicap and, in extreme cases, surgical intervention has been imperative. It consists of a **transection** of the motor nerve to the extremity, resulting in **flaccid musculature**, which is preferred to the incapacitating spasticity.[32]

Hemiplegia which occurs suddenly is usually due to involvement of the **internal capsule** resulting from a rupture of a small branch of the middle **cerebral artery**. An occlusion of the main trunk affects a large portion of the **cerebral hemisphere** and causes contralateral hemiplegia. Small infarcts may produce transient and permanent paralysis. Since the advent of **angiography**, there has been sufficient evidence that the **vascular occlusion** may involve the **cervical** segment of the internal **carotid** artery.

It is a well known fact that hemiplegia occurs on the side opposite to the brain injury. The reason for this is that about ninety per cent of upper motor neurons cross over to the contralateral side at the level of the medulla oblongata.[18]

With adequate rehabilitation the majority of patients who survive a stroke can literally be put back on their feet and return to normal living with little or no **residual damage** depending on the extent of their **cerebrovascular accident**.[27, 31, 5, 2, 49]

Chapter edited by Sister Mary Imelda Pingel SS.M., professor and chairman of the Department of Physical Therapy, St. Louis University.

REFERENCES AND BIBLIOGRAPHY

1. Alpert, S. *et al.* Absence of electromyographic evidence of lower motor neuron involvement in hemiplegic patients. *Archives of Physical Medicine and Rehabilitation*, 52: 178-181, April, 1971.

2. Basmajian, J. V. Neuromuscular facilitation techniques. *Archives of Physical Medicine and Rehabilitation*, 52: 40-42, January, 1971.

3. Beard, Gertrude and Wood, Elizabeth C. *Massage: Principles and Techniques*, Philadelphia: W. B. Saunders Co., 1964, pp. 4-8.

4. Bobath, Berta. *Abnormal Postural Reflex Activity Caused by Brain Lesions*, 2nd ed. London: William Heinemann Medical Books Limited, 1971, pp. 103-104.

5. Brunnstrom, Signe. *Movement Therapy in Hemiplegia*, New York: Harper and Row Publishers, 1970.

6. Chusid, Joseph G. Electromyography. In *Correlative Neuroanatomy and Functional Neurology*, 14th ed. Los Altos, California: Lange Medical Publications, 1970, pp. 247-250.

7. Cole, T. M. Goniometry: the measurement of joint motion. In Krusen, Frank H. Kottke, Frederic J. and Ellwood, Paul M. (eds.). *Physical Medicine and Rehabilitation*, 2nd ed. Philadelphia: W. B. Saunders Co., 1971, pp. 40-57.

8. Cross, Kenneth, D. Role of practice in perceptual-motor learning. In *Proceedings Exploratory and Analytical Survey of Therapeutic Exercise* (NUSTEP). Baltimore: The Waverly Press, Inc., 1966, pp. 487-510.

9. Daniels, Lucille and Worthingham, Catherine. *Muscle Testing: Technique of Manual Examination*, 3rd ed. Philadelphia: W. B. Saunders Co., 1972, pp. 8-9.

10. Darling, R. C. Exercise. In Downey, John A. and Darling, Robert C. (eds.). *Physiological Basis of Rehabilitation*. Philadelphia: W. B. Saunders Co., 1971, pp. 167-183.

11. DeHaven, G. E. and Murdock, J. B. Coordination exercises for children with minimal cerebral dysfunction, *Physical Therapy*, 50: 337-343, March, 1970.

12. Fordyce, W. E. Psychological assessment and management. In Krusen, Frank H., Kottke, Frederick J. and Ellwood, Paul M. (eds.). *Physical Medicine and Rehabilitation*, 2nd ed. Philadelphia: W. B. Saunders Co., 1971, pp. 168-195.

13. Forward, E. Patient evaluation with an audio-electromyogram monitor: "The muscle whistler." *Physical Therapy*, 52: 402-403, April, 1972.

14. Greenberg, R. S. The effects of hot packs and exercise on local blood flow. *Physical Therapy*, 52: 273-278, March, 1972.

15. Griffin, J. E. and Touchstone, J. C. Low-intensity phonophoresis of cortisol in swine. *Physical Therapy*, 48: 1336-1344, December, 1968.

16. Halberstam, J. L. Avoidance conditioning of water responses in elderly brain damaged patients. *Archives of Physical Medicine and Rehabilitation*, 52: 318-327, July, 1971.

17. Inaba, M. K. *et al.* Ultrasound in treatment of painful shoulders in patients with hemiplegia. *Physical Therapy*, 52: 737-742, July, 1972.

18. Jebson, R. H. *et al.* Function of normal hand in stroke patients. *Archives of Physical Medicine and Rehabilitation*, 52: 170-174, April, 1971.

19. Johnson, E. W. Electrodiagnosis. In Krusen, Frank H., Kottke, Frederic J. and Ellwood, Paul M. (eds.). *Physical Medicine and Rehabilitation*, 2nd ed. Philadelphia: W. B. Saunders Co., 1971, pp. 222-256.

20. Kamon, E. Electromyographic kinesiology of jumping. *Archives of Physical Medicine and Rehabilitation*, 52: 152-157, April, 1971.

21. Knapp, M. E. Massage. In Krusen Frank H., Kottke, Frederic J. and Ellwood, Paul M. (eds.). *Physical Medicine and Rehabilitation*, 2nd ed. Philadelphia: W. B. Saunders Co., 1971, pp. 381-384.

22. Knott, Margaret and Voss, Dorothy E. *Proprioceptive Neuromuscular Facilitation*, 2nd ed. New York: Hoeber Medical Division. Harper and Row, Publishers, 1968.

23. Kottke, F. J. Therapeutic exercise. In Krusen, Frank H., Kottke, Frederic J. and Ellwood, Paul M. (eds.). *Physical Medicine and Rehabilitation*, 2nd ed. Philadelphia: W. B. Saunders Co., 1971, pp. 385-482.

24. Krusen, F. H. The scope of physical medicine and rehabilitation. In Krusen, Frank H., Kottke, Frederic J. and Ellwood, Paul M. (eds.). *Physical Medicine and Rehabilitation*, 2nd ed. Philadelphia: W. B. Saunders Co., 1971, pp. 1-13.

25. Laubenthal, K. N. *et al.* A quantitative analysis of knee motion during activities of daily living. *Physical Therapy*, 52: 34-42, January, 1972.

26. Lehmann, J. F. Diathermy. In Krusen, Frank H., Kottke, Frederic J. and Ellwood, Paul M. (eds.). *Physical Medicine and Rehabilitation*, 2nd ed. Philadelphia: W. B. Saunders Co., 1971, pp. 273-345.

27. Levenson, C. Rehabilitation of the stroke hemiplegia patient. In Krusen, Frank H., Kottke, Frederic J. and Ellwood, Paul M. (eds.). *Physical Medicine and Rehabilitation*, 2nd ed. Philadelphia: W. B. Saunders Co., 1971, pp. 521-553.

28. Licht, S. Other exercises. In Licht, Sidney and Johnson, Ernest W. (eds.). *Therapeutic Exercise*, 2nd ed. Baltimore: Waverly Press Inc., 1969, pp. 912-921.

29. Moore, J. C. Active resistive stretch and isometric exercise in strengthening wrist flexion in normal adults. *Archives of Physical Medicine and Rehabilitation*, 52: 264-269, July, 1971.

30. Moore, M. L. Clinical assessment of joint motion. In Licht, Sidney and Johnson, Ernest W. (eds.). *Therapeutic Exercise*, 2nd ed. Baltimore, Waverly Press Inc., 1969, pp. 128-162g.

31. Moskowitz, E. *et al.* Long-term followup of the poststroke patient. *Archives of Physical Medicine and Rehabilitation*, 53: 167-172, April, 1972.

32. Norton, B. J. *et al.* An approach to the objective measurement of spasticity. *Physical Therapy*, 52: 15-25, January, 1972.

33. Olson, J. E. and Stravino, V. D. A review of cryotherapy. *Physical Therapy*, 52: 840-853, August, 1972.

34. Olson, V. L. *et al.* The maximum torque generated by the eccentric, isometric and concentric contractions of the hip abductor muscles. *Physical Therapy*, 52: 149-158, February, 1972.

314

35. Page, D. Neuromuscular reflex therapy as an approach to patient care. In *Proceedings Exploratory and Analytical Survey of Therapeutic Exercise* (NUSTEP), Baltimore: The Waverly Press, Inc., 1966, pp. 816-837.
36. Payton, O. D. Electromyographic evidence of the acquisition of a motor skill. A pilot study. *Physical Therapy*, 52: 261-266, March, 1972.
37. Perry, E. Principles and techniques of the Brunnstrom approach to the treatment of hemiplegia. In *Exploratory and Analytical Survey of Therapeutic Exercise* (NUSTEP). Baltimore: The Waverly Press, Inc., 1967, pp. 789-815.
38. Pingel, Sister Mary Imelda, *Personal communications*.
39. Plumstead, A. J. A modified slant board and vibrator for independent bronchial drainage. *Physical Therapy*, 52: 178-180, February, 1972.
40. Rosentswieg, J. *et al.* Comparison of isometric, isotonic and isokinetic exercises by electromyography. *Archives of Physical Medicine and Rehabilitation*, 53: 249-260, June, 1972.
41. Rusk, Howard A. *Rehabilitation Medicine*, 3rd ed. St. Louis: The C. V. Mosby Co., 1971.
42. Stillwell, G. K. Therapeutic heat and cold. In Krusen, Frank H., Kottke, Frederick J. and Ellwood, Paul M. (eds.). *Physical Medicine and Rehabilitation*, 2nd ed. Philadelphia: W. B. Saunders Co., pp. 259-272.
43. _____. Ultraviolet therapy. *Ibid.*, pp. 363-373.
44. _____. Electrical stimulation and iontophoresis. *Ibid.*, pp. 374-380.
45. Stockmeyer, S. A. An interpretation of the approach of Rood to the treatment of neuromuscular dysfunction. In *Exploratory and Analytical Survey of Therapeutic Exercise* (NUSTEP). Baltimore: The Waverly Press, Inc., 1967, pp. 900-956.
46. Stoner, E. K. Care of the amputee. In Krusen, Frank H., Kottke, Frederic J. and Ellwood, Paul M. (eds.). *Physical Medicine and Rehabilitation*, 2nd ed. Philadelphia: W. B. Saunders Co., 1971, pp. 97-144.
47. Tanigawa, M. C. Comparison of the hold-reflex procedure and passive mobilization on increasing muscle length. *Physical Therapy*, 52: 725-735, July, 1972.
48. Taylor, R. B. Clinical study of ultraviolet in various skin conditions. *Physical Therapy*, 52: 279-282, March, 1972.
49. Thetford, W. N. and Schucman H. Motivational factors and adaptive behavior. In Downy, John A. and Darling, Robert C. (eds.). *Physiological Basis of Rehabilitation*. Philadelphia: W. B. Saunders Co., 1971, pp. 353-371.
50. Voss, D. E. Proprioceptive neuromuscular facilitation. In *Exploratory and Analytical Survey of Therapeutic Exercise* (NUSTEP). Baltimore: The Waverly Press, Inc., 1967, pp. 839-889.
51. Wells, Katharine F. *Kinesiology: The Scientific Basis of Human Motion*, 5th ed. Philadelphia: W. B. Saunders Co., 1971, pp. 389-408.
52. Zausmer, E. Bronchial drainage: evidence supporting the procedures. *Physical Therapy*, 48: 586-591, June, 1968.
53. Zislis, J. M. Hydrotherapy. In Krusen, Frank H., Kottke, Frederic J. and Ellwood, Paul M. (eds.). *Physical Medicine and Rehabilitation*, 2nd ed. Philadelphia: W. B. Saunders Co., 1971, pp. 346-362.

Chapter XX
Selected Terms Pertaining to Nuclear Medicine

ORIENTATION

A. Origin of Terms:

1. atom (G) — indivisible
2. dense (L) — dense, compact
3. fission (L) — cleft, split
4. ion (G) — going
5. iso (G) — equal
6. kinetic (G) — movable
7. proto- (G) — first
8. tope (G) — place
9. tele- (G) — distant
10. scintilla (L) — spark

B. General Terms Related to Nuclear Medicine.

1. activated water — water contaminated by ionizing radiation.
2. activation analysis — a method for identifying and measuring the chemical elements in a sample to be analyzed. The sample is first made radioactive by bombardment with neutrons, charged particles, or other nuclear radiation. The newly radioactive atoms in the sample give off characteristic nuclear radiations that can identify the atoms and indicate their quantity. Activation analysis is frequently more sensitive than chemical analysis. It is being used more and more in research.[43, 3, 10]
3. acute exposure — a brief, intense radiation exposure in contradistinction to prolonged or chronic exposure.
4. alpha particle — a positively charged helium nucleus characterized by poorly penetrating but strongly ionizing radiation.
5. atom — smallest unit of any element which consists of a central nucleus and outer orbital electrons. The nucleus is composed of protons and neutrons except that of the hydrogen atom which has no neutrons.
    a. electrons — negatively charged particles revolving around the nucleus.
    b. neutrons — electrically neutral particles present in the nucleus of an atom.
    c. protons — positively charged particles present in the nucleus of an atom.
6. atomic weight — relative weight of an atom compared to that of one oxygen atom which is 16.
7. background radiation — the radiation of man's natural environment, consisting of that which comes from cosmic rays and from the naturally radioactive elements of the earth, including that from within man's body. The term may also mean radiation extraneous to an experiment.[43]
8. beta particle — nuclear particle which is more penetrating and less ionizing than an alpha particle. The effect of beta particles is moderately destructive and usually limited to the first few millimeters of tissue.
9. body burden — the amount of radioactive material present in the body of man or animals.[43]
10. bone seeker — a radionuclide that tends to lodge in the bones when it is introduced into the body. Example: strontium-90, which behaves chemically like calcium.[43]
11. byproduct material — in atomic energy law, any radioactive material (except source or fissionable material) obtained in the process of producing or using source or fissionable material. Includes fission products and many other radioisotopes produced in nuclear reactors.[43]
12. contamination, radioactive — the spread of radioactivity to places where it can have adverse effects on persons, experiments and equipment.
13. counter — a device for making radiation measurements or counting ionizing events. The term is used loosely as a synonym of detector.

14. curie — the unit for measuring the activity of all radioactive substances, or the quantity of radioactive material which undergoes 3.7×10^{10} disintegrations per second.

15. cyclotron — a particle accelerator in which charged particles receive repeated synchronized accelerations of "kicks" by electrical fields as the particles spiral outward from their source. The particles are kept in the spiral by a powerful magnet.[43] Cyclotrons are a valuable source of radionuclides for medical diagnosis and research.[40, 41]

16. decay, radioactive — diminished activity of a radioactive substance in the course of time.

17. decontamination — the removal of harmful radioactive material from persons, equipment, instruments, rooms and the like. Some articles may be decontaminated by thorough washing with detergents or other chemicals.[59]

18. dose (clinical radionuclides) — the amount of radionuclides for diagnostic evaluation known as tracer dose or for treatment referred to as therapeutic dose.[26, 54]

19. dosimeter — an instrument for measuring the dose of radiation.

20. external hazards — exposure to ionizing radiation from radioactive sources outside the body.

21. film badge — photographic, dental size x-ray film worn on the person for detecting radiation exposure.

22. gamma ray — short wave length electromagnetic radiation of nuclear origin. Gamma rays are more dangerous than alpha and beta particles as external radiation because of their high penetrability.[59]

23. Geiger-Müller counter — a sensitive radiation detector composed of a tube filled with gas and a scaler. It is used to measure beta radiation.[23, 31]

24. half-life, biological — the time required for a biological system, such as a man or an animal, to eliminate, by natural processes, half the amount of a substance which has entered it. The radioactive half-life is a factor in the biologic half-life.

25. half-life, radioactive — time required for a radioactive substance to lose 50 percent of its activity by decay.[25]

    For example:

    Radiophosphorus — ^{32}P has a half-life of 14 days. This means that a quantity of ^{32}P having a radioactivity of

    250.0 mCi (millicuries) on a certain day will have an activity of
    125.0 mCi (millicuries) 14 days later and
    62.5 mCi (millicuries) 28 days later.

26. health physics (radiobiology) — a branch of physics which deals with the protection of personnel from the hazards of ionizing radiation.[43]

27. internal hazards — those caused by exposure to ionizing radiation from radioactive substances deposited inside the body.

28. ion — an atomic particle, charged atom or chemically bound group of atoms.

29. ionization — the process of producing ions.

30. isotopes — atoms having the same number of protons (atomic number) but differing by their atomic weight.

31. labeled compound — a compound composed in part of a radionuclide. For example:

    Sodium radioiodide .... $Na^{131}I$
    Radiocobalt B_{12} .... $^{60}CoB_{12}$
    Chromic radiophosphate .... $Cr^{32}PO_4$

32. mass number — the sum of the neutrons and protons in a nucleus. The mass number of uranium-235 is 235. It is the nearest whole number to the atom's actual atomic weight.

33. maximum permissible concentration — that amount of radioactive material in air, water, and foodstuffs which competent authorities have established as the maximum that would not create undue risk to human health. (See also radioactivity concentration guide.)[43]

34. maximum permissible dose — that dose of ionizing radiation which competent authorities have established as the maximum that can be absorbed without undue risk to human health. (See also radiation protection guide.)[43]

35. median lethal dose (MLD, LD$_{50}$) — radiation dose which kills, in a given period, 50 per cent of a large group of animals or other organisms.[59]

36. microcurie (nuclear medicine) — unit for measuring the energy of a radionuclide in a tracer dose.   One microcurie is one millionth of a curie.[59]

37. millicurie (nuclear medicine) — unit for measuring the energy of a radionuclide in a therapeutic dose.   One millicurie equals a thousand microcuries.[59]

38. monitoring — area monitoring, a procedure for determining the amount of radioactive contamination present in a certain locality.   In personnel monitoring, individuals are monitored; namely, their breath, excreta, clothing and the like in order to detect health hazards and provide environmental safety.[46]

39. nuclear fission — the splitting of a heavy nucleus into two or more nuclei, resulting in nuclear conversion and the release of powerful energy.[25]

40. nuclear numbers:[51]

    Symbol
    a. atomic number   Z — number of protons in the nucleus of an atom.
    b. neutron number   N — number of neutrons in the nucleus of an atom.
    c. mass number   A — sum of neutrons and protons in the nucleus of an atom.
    $$A = Z + N.$$

41. nucleon — an essential part of a nucleus, synonym for protons or neutrons.

42. nucleus of an atom — central part of atom containing protons, or positively charged particles, and neutrons, or neutral particles.

43. nuclide — term denoting all nuclear species of chemical elements, both stable and unstable. It is used synonymously with isotope.

44. overexposure to radiation — excessive contamination by radiant energy which has deleterious effects on a person's health.   In massive overexposure symptoms of radiation injury develop in hours, days or weeks; in chronic overexposure to small amounts of radiation, within months or years.

45. photon — a discrete quantity of electromagnetic energy.   Photons have momentum but no mass or electrical charge.[43]

46. positron — a free positively charged electron.

47. proton — an elementary particle with a single positive electrical charge and a mass approximately 1847 times that of the electron.   The atomic number of an atom is equal to the number of protons in its nucleus.[43]

48. radiation — the propagation of energy through matter or space in the form of waves. In atomic physics the term has been extended to include fast-moving particles (alpha and beta rays, free neutrons, etc.).   Gamma rays and x-rays, of particular interest in atomic physics, are electromagnetic radiation in which energy is propagated in packets called photons.[43]

49. radiation protection guide — the total amounts of ionizing radiation dose over certain periods of time which may safely be permitted to exposed industrial groups.   These standards, established by the Federal Radiation Council, are equivalent to what was formerly called the "maximum permissible exposure."[43, 45, 31, 46]

50. radiation protection procedures — techniques used to safeguard patients and personnel from external and internal exposure.   Principles of safety are concerned with:
    a. **time** — the shorter the period of exposure the less dangerous the radiation dose.
    b. **distance** — the further away from the radioactive substance, the less radiation received.   Distance is a more important factor than time, and it varies inversely as the **square** of the distance.
    c. **shielding** — the denser the material between the individual and radioactive material, the less is the radiation hazard.   Protection from internal exposure is achieved by avoiding ingestion, inhalation and direct contact with radioactive materials.[24, 43, 46, 31]

51. radioactive tracer — radioisotope clinically used in minute amounts for labeling cells or tissues in diagnostic testing.[54]

52. radioactivity — the spontaneous decay or disintegration of an unstable atomic nucleus, accompanied by the emission of radiation.

53. radioassay — quantitative analysis of substances using radionuclide tracer techniques to detect minute quantities not easily measured by other means. Competitive protein binding (CPB) methods are frequently employed.[26]

54. radioautograph, autoradiograph — record of radiation from radioactive material in an object, made by placing its surface in close proximity to a photographic emulsion.[59] By this technique differences in cell function are discernible.

55. radiobiology — a branch of biology dealing with the effects of radiation on biologic systems.

56. radioimmunoassay — a radioassay of antigenic substances, usually protein-containing molecules such as the adrenocorticotrophic hormone (ACTH), glucagon, insulin and the growth hormone (HGH).[26]

57. radioisotopes — chemical elements that have been made radioactive by bombardment with neutrons in an atomic pile or cyclotron. Some occur in nature. By giving off radiation, they provide a valuable means for diagnosis and treatment. Radioisotopes differ from their nonradioactive partners by their atomic weight.

    For example:
    Potassium, the stable isotope has an atomic weight of 39.
    Radiopotassium, the unstable isotope has an atomic weight of 42.[59]

58. radionuclides, radioactive nuclides — comprehensive terms including isobars, isomers, isotones and isotopes that exist for a measurable length of time and differ by atomic weight, atomic number and energy state. The term radioisotope has become obsolete and radionuclide is the accepted term.[52]

    a. isobars — atoms have the same mass number (A), but have different atomic numbers (Z) and neutron numbers (N).

    b. isomers — atoms have the same atomic numbers (Z) and the same mass numbers (A) but differ in nuclear energy states.

    c. isotones — atoms have the same number of neutrons in the nucleus (N) but differ in atomic numbers (Z) and number of mass particles (A).

    d. isotopes — atoms have the same atomic numbers (Z), different numbers of mass particles (A) and therefore different number of nuclear neutrons (N).[51]

59. radionuclidic imaging devices — currently 3 kinds of instruments are in common use:

    a. Anger camera, scintillation camera, gamma camera — an instrument for presenting images of the distribution of radioactivity in any organ or part of the body. Its greatest assets are speed and sensitivity, which are of particular significance in dynamic function studies.[2]

    b. autofluoroscope, digital autofluoroscope — a device for producing pictures of the distribution of gamma-emitting radionuclides within organs. It is capable of concentrating on areas of special importance, which increases the value of dynamic function studies.[6]

    c. rectilinear scanner — the conventional scanner and a moving detector of radioactivity in selected areas of the body which is useful for static studies.[23]

60. reactor — a device by means of which a fission chain reaction can be initiated, maintained and controlled. Its essential component is a core with fissionable fuel. It usually has a moderator, a reflector, shielding, and control mechanisms.[10, 43]

61. relative biological effectiveness (RBE) — the relative effectiveness of a given kind of ionizing radiation in producing a biological response as compared with gamma rays.

62. scaler — an electronic instrument for counting radiation-induced pulses from Geiger counters and other radiation detectors.[43]

63. scan — image of the deposit of a radionuclide.

    a. photoscan — the pattern of radioactivity presented on x-ray film by a photorecorder.

    b. scintillation scan — image made by a scintillation counter to determine the size of a tumor, goiter or other involvement and to locate aberrant, metastatic lesions.

64. scanning (nuclear medicine) — method of mapping out the deposition of a radionuclide in an organ using a rectilinear scanning device.[26]

65. scintillation counter — a highly sensitive detector for measuring ionizing radiation capable of counting scintillations (light flashes) induced by radiation in certain materials.[23, 31]

66. scintiphotography, gammaphotography — the use of the Anger scintillation camera for obtaining photographs of the distribution of gamma-emitting radionuclides in living subjects.[49]
    Scintiphotography may be employed for:
    a. dynamic studies portraying rapidly changing images as the visualization of blood flow, vascular filling, or of ventilation.
    b. static studies requiring highly technical performance of individual images (views) and comparability of tracer concentration in related organs, for example: the intensity of radioactivity concentration in the spleen and marrow compared with that in the liver, in order to demonstrate portal-systemic shunting of venous blood flow after surgery.[49, 23]

67. teletherapy with ^{60}Co — treatment using shielded units which emit radiocobalt gamma rays from a distance. An effective dose permits the internal bombardment of deep seated tumors, a small dose suffices for surface lesions, and rotation allows the selection of irradiation patterns.[43]

68. tracer — an element or compound that has been made radioactive so that it can be easily followed (traced) in biological and industrial processes. Radiation emitted by the radioisotope pinpoints its location.[45, 26]

69. waste, radioactive — equipment and materials (from nuclear operations) which are radioactive and for which there is no further use. Wastes are generally referred to as high-level (having radioactivity concentrations of hundreds to thousands of curies per gallon or cubic foot), low-level (in the range of 1 microcurie per gallon or cubic foot, and intermediate (between these extremes).

70. whole body counter — a device used to identify and measure the radiation in the body (body burden) of humans and animals; uses heavy shielding to keep out background radiation and ultrasensitive scintillation detectors and electronic equipment.

NUCLEAR MEDICINE

A. Terms Related to Radionuclide Scanning:

1. bone marrow scanning — delineation of areas of active bone marrow to detect abnormal expansion of bone marrow and areas of bone marrow destruction. Scanning agents commonly used are:
   a. iron-52 or 59 — ^{52}Fe or ^{59}Fe
   b. technetium-99m sulfur colloid — ^{99m}Tc S colloid.
   The procedure is of diagnostic value in polycythemia, multiple myeloma and other disorders.[69]

2. bone scanning — scintillation scanning following the intravenous injection of a tracer dose of
   a. fluorine-18 — ^{18}F as sodium fluoride
   b. strontium-85 or 87 — ^{85}Sr or ^{87}Sr as strontium nitrate or citrate
   c. technetium-99m — ^{99m}Tc as technetium polyphosphate.[26]
   These radionuclides localize in actively metabolizing bone. The procedure is valuable in the detection of metastases to osseous tissue.[52, 8]

3. brain scanning — radionuclide uptake study of the brain to detect benign or malignant brain lesions. Radionuclides of choice are:
   a. technetium-99m — ^{99m}Tc pertechnetate
   b. indium-113m — ^{113m}In
   c. ytterbium-169 — ^{169}Yb.[52, 47, 8, 55, 61, 39]

4. central nervous system (CNS) scans (other than brain scans) — radionuclide images obtained by cisternography, myelography and ventriculography using a radio-pharmaceutical for labeling.[16, 9]

    a. radionuclide cisternography — a radionuclide is injected intrathecally for diagnostic evaluation. Scans of cisterns using albumin I-131 are valuable in delineating obstructive, nonobstructive or *ex vacuo* types of hydrocephalus.[18, 20, 14, 47, 42] They also aid in determining the point of leak in a persistent or intermittent cerebrospinal fluid (CSF) fistula, that may be manifested by CSF otorrhea or rhinorrhea.[18]

    b. radionuclide myelography — a labeled compound, usually albumin I-131 or albumin Tc 99m, is injected by lumbar puncture. The radionuclide ascends the pathways of the cerebrospinal fluid (CSF) via cervical subarachnoid space showing symmetrical distribution in the Sylvian fissure and reaching the lateral surface of the cerebral hemispheres. Scans taken at definite intervals demonstrate the flow pattern of CSF and subarachnoid cysts that communicate with the CSF pathway.[18]

    c. radionuclide ventriculography — a tagged albumin tracer is injected into both lateral ventricles or into a neurosurgical shunt to demonstrate the patency of the ventricular-vascular communication.[18, 14]

5. kidney scanning, renal scanning — diagnostic aid in the detection of abnormal shape, size and location of kidneys as well as certain renal diseases and space-occupying lesions. Radionuclidic tracers with high concentrations in viable renal tissue and renal tubules are:

    a. mercury-197 or 203 — ^{197}Hg or ^{203}Hg (chlormerodrin)

    b. technetium-99m — ^{99m}Tc pertechnetate

    c. ytterbium-169 — ^{169}Yb.[52, 12, 50, 30, 53, 8]

6. liver scanning, hepatic scanning — method of assessing liver damage, hepatomegaly, tumors and liver abscess. Several radiopharmaceuticals are used for labeling:

    a. gold-198 colloid — ^{198}Au colloid

    b. indium-113m colloid — ^{113m}In colloid

    c. technetium-99m sulfur colloid — ^{99m}Tc S colloid

    d. iodine-131 aggregated albumin — ^{131}I AA.[64]

7. lung scanning, pulmonary scanning — there are 2 kinds:[33]

    a. inhalation scan — lung scan in which the air passages are scanned for defects in ventilation. The radionuclide for labeling is usually xenon-133 — ^{133}Xe.[26, 28, 21] The procedure is complementary to perfusion scans which in turn supplement pulmonary function studies.

    b. perfusion scan — lung scan in which the pulmonary circulation is visualized. It is a valuable procedure in the detection of lung cancer and emboli and in the evaluation of therapy. Scanning agents used are

        (1) iodine-131 macroaggragated albumin — $^{131}IMAA$

        (2) indium-113 iron hydroxide — ^{113}In FeOH.[26, 52, 8]

8. lymph node scanning — intralymphatic injection of a colloid:

    a. gold-198 colloid — ^{198}Au

    b. technetium-99m sulfur colloid — ^{99m}Tc.

The patency of the lymphatic chains can be determined since the lymph nodes act as a filter to the colloid.[52, 63]

Staging of lymphoma cases: Hodgkin's granuloma, lymphoblastoma and others may be achieved by serial imaging 2 to 4 days following the injection of gallium-67 — ^{67}Ga (gallium citrate).[52, 8, 62]

9. mediastinal scanning — radionuclide studies of the heart and great vessels.

    a. cardiac blood pool scanning — delineation of cardiac blood pool and comparison of scanning image with radiographic image. Heart scans aid in the detection of cardiac hypertrophy, pericardial effusion and mediastinal lesions.[26] Radionuclides used for scanning are:

(1) iodinated I-131 — albumin ^{131}I

(2) iodipamide sodium I-131 — iodipamide Na ^{131}I

(3) indium-113m — ^{113m}In

(4) technetium-99m serum albumin — ^{99m}Tc HSA.[26, 15]

  b. radionuclide cardiac angiography — injection of small volume of short-lived radionuclide into a major vessel to detect altered flow dynamics in valvular heart disease.[4, 38, 22, 7]

10. pancreatic scanning — aid in the diagnosis of cancer of the pancreas using seleno-methionine-75 (^{75}Se) for labeling and scintillation scanning for the detection of space-occupying lesions.[52]

11. placental scanning, radionuclide placentography — technique used for delineating the position of the placenta as an aid to the diagnosis of placenta previa, the management of bleeding in the third trimester and safe performance of amniocentesis. It is important that maternal and fetal radiation exposure is kept at a minimum. Safe scanning agents are:

  a. technetium-99m — ^{99m}Tc HSA

  b. indium-113m transferrin — ^{113m}In transferrin.[32, 53, 34]

12. splenic scanning — useful technique in differential diagnosis of left upper quadrant pathology and in assessing abnormal position, enlargement or absence of the spleen. Effective radionuclide labels are:

  a. mercurihydroxypropane — ^{197}Hg MHP

  b. sodium chromate — Na$_2$ ^{51}CrO$_4$[11, 32]

B. Terms Related to Radionuclides in Diagnostic Tests:

1. blood and circulation studies:

  a. blood volume — sum total of red cell volume and plasma volume using sodium radio-chromate (Na$_2$^{51}CrO$_4$) or radioiodinated serum albumin (RISA) for labeling.

Normal ranges	Na$_2$^{51}CrO$_4$	RISA
total red cell volume	25-30 ml/kg	30-38 ml/kg.
total plasma volume	30-45 ml/kg	39-44 ml/kg.
total blood volume	55-75 ml/kg	69-82 ml/kg.[65,1, 66]

Findings are valuable in the diagnosis of polycythemia vera and management of fluid balance after surgery and severe burns.

  b. iron studies — they include

   (1) incorporation of iron (^{59}Fe) into red blood cells which in normal subjects is 60 to 80 per cent of the dose administered in 7 to 10 days.[65, 69]

   (2) plasma iron clearance — iron (^{59}Fe) disappearance half time in plasma which is normally 60 to 120 minutes,[69, 65]

   (3) serum iron-binding capacity, Irosorb-59 — simple, accurate test for the detection of iron deficiency anemias. Since the patient does not receive a radioisotope, the test can be used for all age groups without any hazard of radioactivity.[65, 69]

  c. red cell sequestration, RBC sequestration — measurement of rate of accumulation of chromium-51 (^{51}Cr) tagged red cells in spleen, liver and precordium by scintillation counting. The test aids in the diagnosis of hypersplenism due to any cause.[65, 17]

  d. red cell survival — determination of the rate of disappearance of labeled erythrocytes from the circulating blood. Chromium-51 (^{51}Cr) is usually the tagging agent.
Normal rate of RBC disappearance from the circulation is 28 to 32 days.
Decreased rate of cell survival is present in hemolytic anemias.[65, 69]

e. red cell volume — determination of absolute volume of chromium-51 labeled red cells in the circulating blood. The test is valuable in distinguishing polycythemia vera from other forms of polycythemia.[26]

2. clot formation studies:

   a. fibrinogen uptake test [125]I — detection of thrombi in their formative stage by locating the vascular lesion where fibrinogen is being utilized.[26, 13, 35]

   b. fibrinogen uptake test [131]I — (same as above except for the tracer ^{131}I).[26]

3. gastrointestinal studies:

   a. fat absorption test — measurement of fat digestion and absorption with radioiodine labeled triolein and oleic acid, useful in distinguishing malabsorption syndromes.

   b. GI blood loss determination — measurement of gastrointestinal bleeding by using chromium-51 (^{51}Cr) tagged red cells. They are normally absorbed into the digestive tract and are almost completely recovered in a 6 day stool collection. The test is of value in the detection of chronic and intermittent GI bleeding.[65]
   Normal ranges
   average daily blood loss in feces..0.3 — 2.8 ml.
   Increased amount indicates enteric blood loss.[65]

   c. GI protein loss determination — measurement of albumin leakage into the gastrointestinal tract using intravenous injection of chromium-51 (^{51}Cr) labeled albumin.
   Normal ranges
   average daily protein loss in feces…less than 1% of injected material.
   Increased amount suggests protein losing gastrointestinal disorder.

   d. vitamin B_{12} absorption test, method of Schilling — determination of vitamin B_{12} absorption as aid in diagnosis of pernicious anemia and malabsorption of B_{12} due to other causes. Using cobalt 57, 58 or 60 as a tracer, the amount of B_{12} absorbed is indirectly measured by determining the per cent of the test dose that is excreted in the urine in 24 hours. Since the pathophysiology of pernicious anemia is the inability to absorb vitamin B_{12}, the urinary excretion in these patients is low (less than 10 per cent). If a potent intrinsic factor is administered with the test dose B_{12}, it will permit absorption of B_{12} from the intestine in pernicious anemia, but will not increase the absorption of B_{12} in the presence of malabsorption due to diseases other than pernicious anemia.[26, 56]

4. renal studies:

   a. chlormerodrin Hg-197 uptake test — relative rates of accumulation of mercury-197 in the kidney may be used to determine renal blood flow and tubular function. Test results aid in screening hypertensive patients for unilateral kidney diseases.[48, 70]

   b. renal clearance test — recording the time it takes for the radioactive tracer to disappear in the blood and urine following intravenous infusion. The radionuclides of choice to detect clearance values are:
   (1) iodohippurate I-131 — OIH-[131]I
   (2) diatrizoate sodium I-131 — DIZ-[131]I.[58]

5. thyroid studies:

   a. Group of tests providing an accurate estimate of thyroid function:
   (1) competitive protein binding T-4, Murphy-Pattee technique, T-4 MP — determination of an unknown quantity of thyroxine by measuring the displacement of radionuclide-tagged thyroxine from its specific binding globulin. The tagged thyroxine will be released in proportion to the level of untagged thyroxine present.[26, 29]
   (2) TBI, thyroxine binding index — a test of thyroid function based on thyroxine binding globulin levels in patient's serum. A major problem is that the use of the contraceptive pill has become so prevalent that it interferes with the clinical interpretation of the test by elevating the level of the thyroxine binding globulin (TBG) similar to pregnancy.[26]

NUCLIDES ARE ATOMS OF AN ELEMENT DISTINGUISHABLE BY THEIR WEIGHT

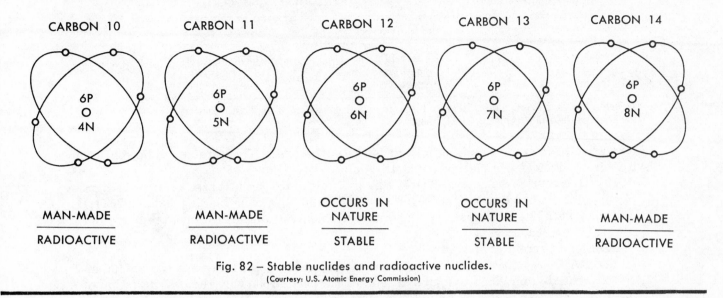

CARBON 10	CARBON 11	CARBON 12	CARBON 13	CARBON 14
6P 4N	6P 5N	6P 6N	6P 7N	6P 8N
MAN-MADE	MAN-MADE	OCCURS IN NATURE	OCCURS IN NATURE	MAN-MADE
RADIOACTIVE	RADIOACTIVE	STABLE	STABLE	RADIOACTIVE

Fig. 82 – Stable nuclides and radioactive nuclides.
(Courtesy: U.S. Atomic Energy Commission)

RADIOACTIVE IODINE — ^{131}I

FOR DIAGNOSING AND TREATING THYROID GLAND DISORDERS

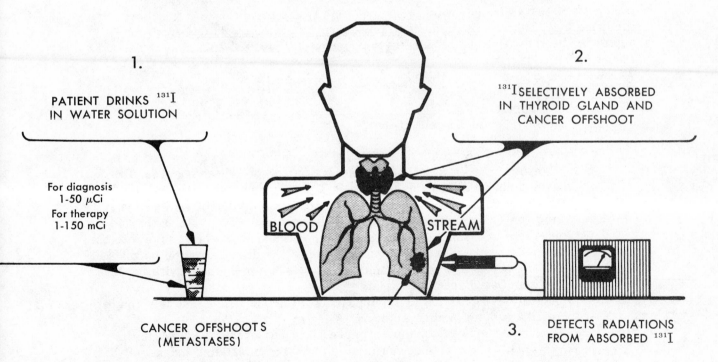

1.

PATIENT DRINKS ^{131}I IN WATER SOLUTION

For diagnosis
1-50 μCi
For therapy
1-150 mCi

2.

^{131}I SELECTIVELY ABSORBED IN THYROID GLAND AND CANCER OFFSHOOT

BLOOD STREAM

CANCER OFFSHOOTS (METASTASES)

3. DETECTS RADIATIONS FROM ABSORBED ^{131}I

MEDICAL ACTION:

1. DIAGNOSIS AND TREATMENT OF HYPERTHYROIDISM
2. LOCATION OF THYROID CANCER OFFSHOOTS (METASTASES)
3. LOCATION OF THYROID CANCER AND METASTASES

Fig. 83 – Radioiodine and the thyroid gland.   (Courtesy: U.S. Atomic Energy Commission)

Table 28

INTERPRETATION OF THYROXINE BINDING INDEX (TBI)[a]

Index Ranges	Thyroid Function	Erythrocyte Uptake
Normal	euthyroid	0.86 - 1.20
Increase	hypothyroid	1.20 or greater
Decrease	hyperthyroid	less than 0.86

[a] George E. Thoma. Diagnostic procedures for the estimation of thyroid function. *Southern Medical Journal*, 53: 410, April, 1960.

Alternative tests are T-3 resin uptake and T-3 sponge test. They are not to be confused with serum levels of circulating triiodothyronine (T-3).[26, 65]

(3) free thyroxine index (FTI) — this is a calculated result based on measuring the total thyroxine binding level (T-4 MP) and thyroxine binding index (TBI). The FTI eliminates errors of interpretation due to medications, pregnancy or other causes.[26]

b. Additional thyroid studies are:

(1) RAIU, radioactive iodine uptake determination — test measures the ability of the thyroid gland to trap and retain the nuclide following the oral ingestion of a ^{131}I tracer dose. A scintillation detector is used to determine the percentage of ^{131}I thyroidal uptake at some convenient time, usually 6 and 24 hours after the administration of the tracer dose.[26, 65, 29]

Table 29

RADIOIODINE UPTAKE OF THYROID GLAND[a]

Values	6 Hour Range	24 Hour Range
Normal	3 - 10%	10 - 30%
Increase	greater than 10%	greater than 30%
Decrease	less than 10%	less than 30%

[a] John A. Gantz, M.D. Personal communications.

(2) T-3 serum level — determination of triiodothyronine (T-3) concentration in human serum. An elevated T-3 serum level in the presence of normal T-4 (thyroxine) concentration may indicate T-3 thyrotoxicosis.[57, 67, 44]

(3) T-3 suppression test — measurement of the thyroidal uptake of radioiodine following the oral administration of triiodothyronine (T-3). In euthyroid patients there is usually a suppression of the second thyroidal uptake into the hypothyroidal range. In thyrotoxicosis it does not drop below the normal range. The test is useful in distinguishing neurotic individuals with borderline uptake from true hyperthyroidism.[26, 65, 27]

(4) T-4 by column — separation of organic from inorganic iodine. It is a rough index of T-4 protein binding ability.[26, 37]

(5) TBG, thyroxine binding globulin serum level — measurement of circulating levels of TBG. It is not to be confused with thyroxine binding index (TBI).[26, 37]

(6) TRF, thyrotropin releasing factor, TRH, thyrotropin releasing hormone serum level — measurement of TRF (or TRH) released from hypothalamus. It regulates release of thyrotropin from pituitary and is influenced by levels of serum thyroxine.[26, 37]

(7) TSH, thyroid stimulating hormone serum level — measurement of circulating levels of TSH. It is a valuable diagnostic aid in hypothyroidism in addition to the evaluation of pituitary function.[26]

(8) TSH thyroid stimulation test — a radioiodine measurement of thyroid gland following the parenteral injection of thyroid stimulating hormone (TSH). The test aids in the differential diagnosis of primary hypothyroidism in which a diseased thyroid fails to respond to TSH. In secondary hypothyroidism the thyroid gland will begin to function after a TSH injection since the gland is simply dormant rather than diseased.

A summary of radionuclides used in diagnostic evaluation is presented.

Table 30

RADIONUCLIDES IN DIAGNOSIS

Radionuclide	Labeled Tracer Nuclides	Diagnostic Tests	Clinical Use

Iodine-131
^{131}I
	Radioactive:
	  Sodium Iodide or
	    Potassium Iodide
	  Triiodothyronine
		Thyroidal ^{131}I
		  uptake
		Red cell uptake
		  determination
			Thyroid disease
			
			Thyroid disease

	Iodinated Human Serum
	    Albumin
		Circulation time and
		  blood volume deter-
		  mination, localiza-
		  tion of tumors and
		  cardiac output
			Vascular and
			Cardiac disease
			Neoplasms

	Cholografin	Mediastinal scanning
		  heart and aorta
		  (blood pool delin-
		  eation)
			Pericardial effu-
			  sion
			Cardiomegaly
			Aortic aneurysm
			Mediastinal lesion

	Macroaggregated Albumin	Lung scanning	Pulmonary lesion

	Iodo Triolein and
	    Oleic Acid
		Fat absorption
		  studies
			Pancreatitis
			Sprue
			Biliary obstruc-
			  tion

	Iodo Pyracet (Diodrast)
	    or
	  Diprotriozate (Miokon)
		Renogram for kidney
		  function measure-
		  ments
			Renal disease

	Sodium Iodohippurate
	    (Hippuran)
		Renocystogram	Kidney and bladder
			  diseases

Iodine-125
^{125}I
	Radioactive:
	  Sodium Iodide or
	    Potassium Iodide
		Thyroidal ^{125}I uptake
		Thyroidal scanning
			Thyroid disease

Sodium-24
 	
^{24}NA
	Radioactive Sodium
	  Chloride
		Blood circulation
		  studies
		Radiocardiograms
		  for cardiac output
		  measurement deter-
		  mination of sodium
		  space and of total
		  exchangeable sodium
			Arterial constric-
			  tion
			Heart disease
			
			Electrolyte
			  balance

Phosphorus-32
 	
^{32}P
	Radioactive Sodium
	  Phosphate
		Localization of
		  tumors and red cell
		  survival studies
			Neoplasms
			Hemolytic disease

Chromium-51
 	
^{51}Cr
	Radioactive Sodium
	  Chromate
		Red cell mass and
		  survival studies
		Spleen scanning
			Hemolytic disease

Radionuclide	Labeled Tracer Nuclides	Diagnostic Tests	Clinical Use
Iron-52 or 59 ^{52}Fe ^{59}Fe	Radioactive Ferrous Citrate	Determination of iron metabolism and storage in body for evaluating hematopoiesis Bone marrow scanning	Iron deficiency Hemolytic anemias Hematopoietic disorder
Cobalt-57 or 60 ^{57}Co ^{60}Co	Radioactive Cyanocobalamine B$_{12}$	Determination of intestinal absorption of vitamin B$_{12}$	Pernicious anemia Sprue
Gold-198 ^{198}Au	Radioiodinated Rose Bengal Radioactive Colloidal Gold	Hepatic scanning Hepatic scanning Bone marrow scanning	Liver disease Hepatic lesion Liver disease Hematopoietic disorder
Mercury-197 ^{197}Hg	Radioactive: Chlormerodrin Mercurihydroxypropane (MHP) labeled erythrocytes	Brain scanning Renal Scanning Spleen scanning	Brain lesion Kidney disease and lesion Hematopoietic disorder
Mercury-203 ^{203}Hg	Radioactive Chlormerodrin	Brain scanning Renal scanning	Brain lesion Kidney disease and lesion
Selenium-75 ^{75}Se	Radioactive Selenium Methionine	Pancreatic function and scanning	Diseases of pancreas
Strontium-85 ^{85}Sr	Radioactive: Strontium Nitrate or Strontium Chloride	Bone scanning Joint scanning	Bone neoplasms Rheumatoid arthritis
Technetium-99m ^{99m}Tc	Radioactive Technetium-99m Pertechnetate Human Serum Albumin Sulfur Colloid	Brain scanning Mediastinal scanning heart and aorta (blood pool delineation) Placental scanning Liver scanning Bone marrow scanning	Brain lesion Pericardial effusion Cardiomegaly Arotic aneurysm Mediastinal lesion Placenta previa Hepatomegaly, liver disease and lesion Delineation of active marrow Hematopoietic disorder

Radionuclide	Labeled Tracer Nuclides	Diagnostic Tests	Clinical Use

Indium-113m
 	
^{113m}In
	Radioactive Indium-113m
	  Chelate
	  Transferrin
	
	Iron Hydroxide
	
	Colloid
		Brain scanning
		Mediastinal scanning
		  heart and aorta
		    (blood pool delin-
		    eation)
		
		Lung scanning
		
		Liver scanning
			Brain lesion
			Pericardial effu-
			  sion
			Cardiomegaly
			Aortic aneurysm
			Mediastinal lesion
			Pulmonary embolism
			Lung cancer
			Hepatomegaly,
			  liver disease and
			  lesion

B. Terms Related to Radionuclides in Therapy:

In nuclear medicine radionuclides are primarily used for tracer studies and their significance in diagnostic evaluation has been firmly established. In contradistinction the application of radionuclides to treatment is more restricted and less gratifying in its scope than it is in regard to diagnosis. In the past research efforts have been principally directed toward the conquest of malignancies. Experience proves that radionuclides in the treatment of carcinomas serve as palliative agents, with some potential for prolonging life and a low capacity for inhibiting or destroying malignant growth.[37, 5, 19]

In addition, the possible carcinogenic properties of radioactive drugs constitute a limiting factor, particularly in the management of young patients. Current therapeutic uses of radionuclides are presented in Table 31.

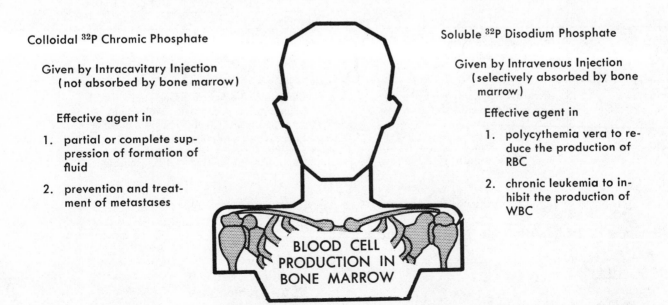

RADIOACTIVE PHOSPHORUS-32 THERAPY

In Form of

Colloidal ^{32}P Chromic Phosphate

Given by Intracavitary Injection
(not absorbed by bone marrow)

Effective agent in

1. partial or complete suppression of formation of
   fluid

2. prevention and treat-
   ment of metastases

Soluble ^{32}P Disodium Phosphate

Given by Intravenous Injection
(selectively absorbed by bone
marrow)

Effective agent in

1. polycythemia vera to reduce the production of
   RBC

2. chronic leukemia to inhibit the production of
   WBC

BLOOD CELL
PRODUCTION IN
BONE MARROW

Fig. 84 – Important therapeutic uses of radioactive phosphorus.

Table 31

RADIONUCLIDES IN TREATMENT[a]

Radionuclide	Method	Clinical Use
Cobalt-60 ^{60}Co	Intracavitary insertion of radiocobalt rods, pellets or beads Interstitial use of radio-cobalt needles, sutures or wires External high energy irradiation by telecobalt unit	Cancer of uterine cervix, larynx, nasopharynx, bladder Cancer of breast and other malignancies Various cancers
Phosphorus-32 ^{32}P	Intravenous administration of disodium phosphate Intracavitary infusion of colloidal chromic phosphate	Polycythemia vera and chronic leukemia; selected cases of multiple myeloma, lymphosarcoma and Hodgkin's disease Malignant pleural and peritoneal effusions
Gold-198 ^{198}Au	Intracavitary infusion of colloidal radiogold for irradiation of closed serous cavities Intravenous infusion of colloidal radiogold Interstitial injection of ^{198}Au Interstitial therapy with radiogold seeds and wires	Palliative therapy by reducing fluid accumulation in ascites or pleural effusion associated with malignant metastic involvement Chronic leukemia Carcinoma of cervix and prostate Carcinoma of buccal mucosa, lip and tongue
Iodine-131 ^{131}I	Oral administration of sodium radioiodine	Selected cases of hyperthyroidism, thyroid cancer, angina pectoris and heart failure
Strontium-90 ^{90}Sr	Use of radiostrontium on ophthalmic applicators	Lesions of the eye, removal of benign small tumors
Cesium-137 ^{137}Cs	External irradiation by tele-therapy unit	Selected cases of cancer
Iridium-192 ^{192}Ir	Interstitial use of radio-iridium seeds and wires	Selected cases of cancer
Yttrium-90 ^{90}Y	Intracavitary administration of colloidal radioyttrium	Ascites and effusions associated with malignant metastatic involvement; hepatomegaly, splenomegaly, chronic leukemia and polycythemia

[a] Cf. *Manual on Use of Radioisotopes in Hospitals*, 2nd ed.   Chicago: American Hospital Association, 1967.

ABBREVIATIONS

A. Symbols of Radionuclides in Nuclear Medicine:

^{111}Ag — radiosilver

^{72}As, ^{74}As — radioarsenic

^{198}Au — radiogold

^{57}Co, ^{60}Co — radiocobalt

^{51}Cr — radiochromium

^{137}Cs — radiocesium

^{61}Cu, ^{64}Cu — radiocopper

^{18}F — radiofluorine

^{52}Fe, ^{59}Fe — radioiron
^{67}Ga — radiogallium
^{197}Hg, ^{203}Hg — radiomercury
^{113m}In — radioindium
^{125}I, ^{131}I — radioiodine
^{192}Ir — radioiridium
^{42}K — radiopotassium
^{52}Mn — radiomagnesium
^{24}Na — radiosodium

^{32}P — radiophosphorus
^{86}Rb — radiorubidium
^{35}S — radiosulfur
^{85}Sr, ^{87}Sr — radiostrontium
^{99m}Tc — radiotechnetium
^{169}Yb — radioytterbium
* — radioactive (*Au — radiogold)
^{90}Y — radioyttrium

B. Symbols of Tests and Miscellaneous:

A — mass number
B/K — bladder kidney (scan ratio)
^{57}Co or ^{60}Co B$_{12}$ — radiocobalt labeled vitamin B$_{12}$
CPB — competitive protein binding
CPM — count per minute
EOB — end of bombardment
FTI — free thyroxine index
FUT — fibrinogen uptake test
GM — Geiger-Müller (counter)
HEG — high energy gamma
IHSA — iodinated human serum albumin
^{131}IHSA — radioiodinated human serum albumin
LD$_{50}$ — median lethal dose
MAA — macroaggregated albumin
MHP — mercuryhydroxypropane
MLD — median lethal dose
MPC — maximum permissible concentration

MPL — maximum permissible level or limit
N — neutron
PBI-131 — protein bound radioiodine
PIT — plasma iron turnover rate
RAIU — radioactive iodine uptake
RBE — relative biological effectiveness
REG — radiation exposure guide
RISA — radioiodinated human serum albumin
TBG — thyroxine binding globulin
TBI — thyroxine binding index
TBP — thyroxine binding protein
TBPA — thyroxine binding prealbumin
T-4 MP — T-4 Murphy-Pattee test
TRF — thyrotropin releasing factor
TRH — thyrotropin releasing hormone
TSH — thyrotropin
Z — atomic number

C. Scientific Organizations:

ACR — American College of Radiology
AEC — Atomic Energy Commission
ARRS — American Roentgen Ray Society
ARRT — American Registry of Radiologic Technologists
FASRT — Fellow of American Society of Radiologic Technologists
FRC — Federal Radiation Council

HP Soc. — Health Physics Society
ICRP — International Commission on Radiological Protection
NCRP — National Commission on Radiation Protection
RSNA — Radiological Society of North America
SNM — Society of Nuclear Medicine

D. Multiples of Curie Units:[26]

1 Ci	curie		1 curie
1 mCi	millicurie		10^{-3} curie
1 µCi	microcurie		10^{-6} curie
1 nCi	nanocurie		10^{-9} curie
1 pCi	picocurie		10^{-12} curie

E. Other Units of Measurements:

Bev — 1 billion electron volts

E — energy in ergs

erg — 1 unit of work

ev — 1 electron volt

Kev, keV — 1 thousand electron
volts

Mev, MeV — 1 million electron volts

r — roentgen

RAD, rad — radiation absorbed dose,
100 ergs/gm tissue

REM, rem — roentgen equivalent, man

REP, rep — roentgen equivalent,
physical

F. Symbols of Useful Landmarks:

AM — auditory meatus

CM — costal margin

G — glabella

I — inion

IC — iliac crest

N — nose

SN — sternal notch

SP — symphysis pubis

TC — thyroid cartilage

U — umbilicus

XP — xiphoid process

ORAL READING PRACTICE

The Thyroid Gland and Radioiodine

The avidity of the thyroid for iodine is an interesting and unique characteristic of this endocrine gland. It is the basis of many thyroid function studies and the medical treatment of many thyroid diseases.

With the development of nuclear reactors as a part of the atomic weapons program, radionuclides became abundantly available as byproducts. Investigations proved that many of these are useful in clinical medicine.

Nuclides are varieties of a chemical element that differ in their atomic weights, but possess the same chemical properties. Some elements are available as both stable and **radioactive nuclides,** for example:

Iodine-127, the stable element with an atomic weight of 127

Iodine-131, one of the **radionuclides** with an atomic weight of 131.

The latter is a widely used radionuclide of iodine and is generally the one implied by the term **radioiodine.**

The value of radioiodine (^{131}I) in the diagnosis and treatment of **hyperthyroidism** and in thyroid cancer therapy was established within the past decades. ^{131}I does not differ chemically from iodine, but differs physically in that it emits beta particles and gamma rays. Since the beta particles penetrate only 2 mm of tissue, they are almost all absorbed within the gland. On the other hand, about 90 per cent of the gamma rays escape and can be accurately measured outside the body with a radiation detector such as a **scintillation counter.**[37]

^{131}I has a half-life of eight days. This means that every eight days its radioactivity is reduced to half the intensity present eight days previously. The half-life is of clinical importance since the nuclide must exert its effect not too long, to avoid excessive radiation damage, nor too short to insure adequate results.[5, 37]

When a radioiodine uptake study is ordered, the patient receives a callibrated dose of ^{131}I either in a capsule or in a solution. The tracer dose ranges from 5-25 **microcuries** (μCi), while therapeutic doses are measured in **millicuries** (1mCi = 1000 μCi). After oral administration radioiodine is rapidly absorbed from the gastrointestinal tract and selectively picked up by thyroid tissue. Within 4 to 6 hours the gland has become the depot for about one-fourth of the nuclide ingested. In 24 hours thyroid function can be estimated by the amount of radioiodine retained. The thyroidal uptake of ^{131}I by the normal gland in 24 hours is 15-40 per cent of the tracer dose. In hyperthyroidism it is 50-100 per cent.[26, 65]

Currently T-4 **competitive protein binding,** Murphy-Pattee technique, together with thyroxine binding index and their calculated results, the free thyroxine index have gained wide acceptance and are thought to yield reliable evaluation of thyroid function.[26]

REFERENCES AND BIBLIOGRAPHY

1. Albert, S. N. Blood volume. In Blahd, William H. *Nuclear Medicine*, 2nd ed. New York: McGraw-Hill Book Co., 1971, pp. 593-619.

2. Anger, H. O. Scintillation cameras. In Blahd, William H. *Nuclear Medicine*, 2nd ed. New York: McGraw-Hill Book Co., 1971, pp. 53-64.

3. Anspaugh, L. R. and Robinson, W. L. Trace elements in biology and medicine. In Lawrence, John H. (ed.). *Recent Advances in Nuclear Medicine*. New York: Grune & Stratton, 1971, pp. 63-138.

4. Ashburn, W. *et al.* Radioisotope cardiac angiography. In Blahd, William H. *Nuclear Medicine*, 2nd ed. New York: McGraw-Hill Book Co., 1971, pp. 509-513.

5. Beierwaltes, W. H. Present status of radioiodine therapy of thyroid disease. In Lawrence, John H. (ed.). *Recent Advances in Nuclear Medicine*. New York: Grune & Stratton, 1971, pp. 19-38.

6. Bender, M. A. The autofluoroscope. In Blahd, William H. *Nuclear Medicine*, 2nd ed. New York: McGraw-Hill Book Co., 1971, pp. 64-71.

7. Bennett, K. R. *et al.* Correlation of myocardial ^{42}K uptake with coronary arteriography. *Radiology*, 102: 117-124, January, 1972.

8. Benua, R. Diagnostic nuclear medicine today and tomorrow. *Medical Clinics of North America*, 55: 545-560, May, 1971.

9. Bercaw, B. L. and Greer, H. Transport of intrathecal ^{131}RISA in benign intracranial hypertension. *Neurology*, 20: 787-790, August, 1970.

10. Bethard, W. F. The nuclear reactor in nuclear medicine. In Blahd, William H. *Nuclear Medicine*, 2nd ed. New York: McGraw-Hill Book Co., 1971, pp. 660-676.

11. Blahd, William H. Spleen scanning. In *Nuclear Medicine*, 2nd ed. New York: McGraw-Hill Book Co., 1971, pp. 439-444.

12. Braunstein, P. *et al.* Scintiscan evaluation of prominent renal columns. *Radiology*, 103: 103-106, July, 1972.

13. Browse, N. L. The ^{125}I fibrinogen uptake test. *Archives of Surgery*, 104: 160-163, February, 1972.

14. Chiro, G. D. *et al.* Radioisotope encephalocisternography and encephaloventriculography. *Journal of Neurosurgery*, 36: 127-132, February, 1972.

15. Cohen, M. B. Cardiac blood pool scanning. In Blahd, William H. *Nuclear Medicine*, 2nd ed. New York: McGraw-Hill Book Co., 1971, pp. 513-516.

16. Conway, J. J. and Vollert, J. M. The accuracy of radionuclide imaging in detecting pediatric dural fluid collections. *Radiology*, 105: 77-84, October 1972.

17. Cooper, R. M. *et al.* Platelet survival and sequestration patterns in thrombocytogenic disorders. *Radiology*, 102: 89-100, January, 1972.

18. DeChiro, G. and Ashburn, W. L. Radioisotope cisternography, ventriculography and myelography. In Blahd, William H. *Nuclear Medicine*, 2nd ed. New York: McGraw-Hill Book Co., 1971, pp. 277-312.

19. Dollinger, M. R. Management of recurrent malignant effusions. *Ca — A Cancer Journal of Clinicians*, 22: 138-147, May-June, 1972.

20. Donaghy, R. H. What's new in neurologic surgery. *Surgery Gynecology & Obstetrics*, 134: 269-271, February, 1972.

21. Effman, E. L. *et al.* ^{133}Xe studies of collateral ventilation and air trapping following endobronchial occlusion. *Radiology*, 105: 85-92, October, 1972.

22. Enright, L. P. *et al.* Acute intracardiac volume changes demonstrated with radioisotopic angiocardiography. *Journal of Thoracic and Cardiovascular Surgery*, 64: 136-141, July, 1972.

23. Feitelberg, S. and Gross, W. Radiation detectors: principles of operation. In Quimby, Edith H. *et al. Radioactive Nuclides in Medicine and Biology*, 3rd ed. Philadelphia: Lea & Febiger, 1970, pp. 185-200.

24. ――――――. Use of radiation detector in health protection. *Ibid.*, pp. 346-351.

25. Fields, Theodore and Seed, Linden (eds.). *Clinical Use of Radioisotopes*, 2d ed. Chicago: The Year Book Publishers, Inc., 1961, pp. 391-399.

26. Gantz, John A., M.D. Personal communications.

27. Gharib, H. and Wahner, H. W. Clinical experience with assays for triiodothyronine. *Medical Clinics of North America*, 56: 861-870, July, 1972.

28. Goodrich, J. K. *et al.* Xenon-133 measurement of regional ventilation. *Radiology*, 103: 611-620, June, 1972.

29. Gorman, C. A. Some problems in thyroid diagnosis. *Medical Clinics of North America*, 56: 841-848, July, 1972.

30. Hayes, M. *et al.* Radionuclide procedures in predicting early renal transplant rejection. *Radiology*, 103: 627-631, June, 1972.

31. Heslep, J. M. Principles of radiation safety. In Blahd, William H. *Nuclear Medicine*, 2nd ed. New York: McGraw-Hill Book Co., 1971, pp. 156-171.

32. Hutchinson, D. L. Placental localization with radioisotopes. In Blahd, William H. *Nuclear Medicine*, 2nd ed. New York: McGraw-Hill Book Co., 1971, pp. 517-520.

33. Jones, R. H. *et al.* Radionuclide quantitation of lung function in patients with pulmonary disorders. *Surgery*, 70: 891-903, October, 1971.

34. Johnson, P. M. *et al.* Placental imaging with ^{113m}In. Results in 100 patients. *Radiology*, 103: 359-364, May, 1972.

35. Kakkar, V. The diagnosis of deep vein thrombosis using the ^{125}I fibrinogen test. *Archives of Surgery*, 104: 152-159, February, 1972.

36. Kniseley, R. M. The bone marrow. In Wagner, Henry N. *Principles of Nuclear Medicine*. Philadelphia: W. B. Saunders Co., 1968, pp. 404-412.

37. Koplowitz, J. M. *et al.* Measurement of thyroid function. In Blahd, William H. *Nuclear Medicine*, 2nd ed. New York: McGraw-Hill Book Co., 1971, pp. 175-228.

38. Kriss, J. P. et al. Radioisotopic angiocardiography. *Radiologic Clinics of North America*, 9: 369-383, December, 1971.

39. Kuhl, D. E. *et al.* The brain scan in Sturge-Weber Syndrome. *Radiology*, 103: 621-626, June, 1972.

40. Laughlin, J. S. *et al.* The cyclotron: Source of short-lived radionuclides and positron emitters for medicine. In Lawrence, John H. (ed.). *Recent Advances in Nuclear Medicine.* New York: Grune & Stratton, 1971, pp. 39-62.

41. Laughlin, J. S. The cyclotron and cancer. *Ca — A Cancer Journal for Clinicians*, 21: 334-340, September-October, 1971.

42. LeMay, M. J. and New, P. E. Pneumoencephalography and cisternography in the diagnosis of occult normal pressure hydrocephalus. *Radiology*, 96: 347-358, August, 1970.

43. Lyman, James D. and Loeb, Benjamin, Sl (eds.). *Nuclear Terms.* Washington, D. C.: Division of Technical Information, U.S. Atomic Division, 1964, pp. 1-35 (*verbatim*).

44. Mitsuma, T. *et al.* Radioimmunoassay of triiodothyronine in unextracted human serum. *Journal of Clinical Endocrinology and Metabolism*, 33: 364-367, October, 1971.

45. National Bureau of Standards No. 48. *Control and Removal of Radioactive Contamination in Laboratories.* Washington, D.C.

46. National Council on Radiation and Measurements. Report No. 36. *Precautions in the Management of Patients Who Have Received Therapeutic Amounts of Radionuclides.* Washington, D.C.

47. New, P. F. J. and Weiner, M. A. The radiological investigation of hydrocephalus. *Radiologic Clinics of North America*, 9: 117-140, April, 1971.

48. Nordyke, R. A. Radioactive chlormerodrin kidney uptake test. In Blahd, William H. *Nuclear Medicine*, 2nd ed. New York: McGraw-Hill Book Co., 1971, pp. 395-396.

49. Powell, M. R. Clinical applications of the scintillation camera. In Blahd, William H. *Nuclear Medicine*, 2nd ed. New York: McGraw-Hill Book Co., 1971, pp. 533-573.

50. Powell, M. R. and Weiss, J. M. Radioisotopic kidney studies. In Smith, Donald R. *General Urology*, 7th ed. Los Altos, California: Lange Medical Publications, 1972, pp. 85-113.

51. Quimby, Edith H., Feitelberg, Sergei and Gross, William. *Radioactive Nuclides in Medicine and Biology*, 3rd ed. Philadelphia: Lea & Febiger, 1970, pp. 7-16.

52. Quinn, J. L. Radionuclidic imaging procedures in the diagnosis of cancer — *Ca — A Cancer Journal for Clinicians*, 21: 292-301, September-October, 1971.

53. Richards, A. G. *et al.* Unexpected renal scanning during placental scanning with ^{113m}In. *Radiology*, 104: 611-614, September, 1972.

54. Saenger, E. L. *et al.* The safe tracer dose in medical investigation. In Lawrence, John H. (ed.). *Recent Advances in Nuclear Medicine.* New York: Grune & Stratten. 1971, pp. 139-165.

55. Schall, G. L. and Quinn, J. L. Brain scanning. In Blahd, William H. *Nuclear Medicine*, 2nd ed. New York: McGraw-Hill Book Co., 1971, pp. 236-277.

56. Schilling. R. F. Diagnosis of pernicious anemia and other vitamin B_{12} malabsorption syndromes with radioactive vitamin B_{12} In Blahd, William H. *Nuclear Medicine*, 2nd ed. New York: McGraw-Hill Book Co., 1971, pp. 444-447.

57. Sterling, K. *et al.* T-3 thyrotoxicosis due to elevated serum triiodothyronine levels. *Journal of American Medical Association*, 213: 571-575, July 27, 1970.

58. Tauxe, W. N. Renal clearance techniques. In Blahd, William H. *Nuclear Medicine*, 2nd ed. New York: McGraw-Hill Book Co., 1971, pp. 396-415.

59. Thoma, George E., M.D. *Glossary of Terms in Nuclear Medicine.* St. Louis University School of Medicine.

60. Thoma, G. E. Diagnostic procedures for the estimation of thyroid function. *Southern Medical Journal*, 53: 410, April, 1960.

61. Thompson, R. W. The diagnostic value of brain scanning in intracranial lymphomas. *Radiology*, 102: 111-116, January, 1972.

62. Turner, D. A. *et al.* The use of ^{67}Ga scanning in the staging of Hodgkin's disease. *Radiology*, 103: 97-101, June, 1972.

63. Ultman, J. E. The management of lymphoma. *Ca — A Cancer Journal for Clinicians.* 21: 342-359, November-December, 1971.

64. Wagner, H. N. and Mishkin, F. The liver. In Wagner, Henry N. *Principles of Nuclear Medicine.* Philadelphia: W. B. Saunders Co., 1968, pp. 599-620.

65. Wagner, H. N. Technical details of common procedures. In Wagner, Henry N. *Principles of Nuclear Medicine.* Philadelphia: W. B. Saunders Co., 1968, pp. 833-858.

66. _____. Radioactive tracers and the circulation. *Circulation*, 45: 8-10.

67. Wahner, H. W. *et al.* Interpretation of serum triiodothyronine levels measured by the Sterling technique. *New England Journal of Medicine*, 284: 225-230, February 4, 1971.

68. Weinstein, I. M. Measurement of bone marrow. In Blahd, William H. *Nuclear Medicine*, 2nd ed. New York: McGraw-Hill Book Co., 1971, p. 439.

69. Weinstein, I. M. Measurement of iron metabolism and erythropoiesis. In Blahd, William H. *Nuclear Medicine*, 2nd ed. New York: McGraw-Hill Book Co., 1971, pp. 416-439.

70. Winter, C. C. Radioisotope diagnostic tests in urology. In Campbell, Meredith F. and Harrison, Hartwell J. *Urology*, 3rd ed. Philadelphia: W. B. Saunders Co., 1970, pp. 295-312.

Index

Amastia, 24
Amaurosis fugax, 246
Ambivalence, 68
Amblyopia, 246
  ex anopsia, 246
Ameba, 268
Amebic dysentery, 271, 278
Amenorrhea, 194
Ametropia, 246
Amnesia, 68
Amniocentesis, 208, 217
Amniography, 208
Amnion, 207
Amniotic fluid, 207
  analyses, 212
Ampulla, 194
  See uterine tubes, 195
Amputation, 35
  below knee, 49
  forearm, 47
Amputation neuroma. See neuroma, 54
Amputation of
  aural deformity, 260
  ear, 264
Amylase, 155
Amyloidosis, 112
  primary systemic, 112
  secondary parenchymatous, 112
Amylolytic, 155
Amyotrophic lateral sclerosis, 57
ANA, 27, 280
Ana, 271
Anaclitic, 68
Anacusis, 261
Anaerobes, 268
Analeptics, 299
Anal fistula. See fistula in ano, 148
Analgesia, 63, 299
Analgesics, 299
Analysis, 64
Anaphylaxis, 273
Anaplasia, 291
Anasarca, 88
Anastomosis, 146
  aortic coarctation, 91
  blood vessels, 91
ANC, 27
Anemia, 108
  aplastic, 110
  blood loss, 108
  congenital pancytopenia. See
    Faconi syndrome, 110
  Cooley's anemia. See thalassemia
    major, 110
  erythroblastosis fetalis. See
    hemolytic anemia of newborn, 110
  hereditary spherocytosis, 110
  iron deficiency, 108
  megaloblastic, 108
  pernicious, 108
  sickle cell, 108
  spherocytic. See hereditary
    spherocytosis, 110
  thalassemia, 110
Anencephalia, 57
  anencephalus, 57
Anes., 302
Anesthesia, 12, 63
  general, 299
  local, 299
Anesthesiologist, 299
Anesthesiology, 299
Anesthetic, 299
Anesthetic agents
  nonvolatile, 304

  volatile, 304
Anesthetist, 299
Aneurysm, 79
  aorta, 90
  dissecting, 90
  fusiform, 90
  heart, 79
  sacculated, 90
ANF, 27
Anger camera, 318
Angiectasis, 3
Angiitis, angitis, 7
Anginal syndrome, 88
Angina pectoris. See anginal
  syndrome, 88
Angio, 89
Angiocardiography, 93
  rapid biplane, 93
Angiocardiography, selective
  coronary arteriography, 93
  internal mammary arteriography, 93
  retrograde aortography, 94
  right ventricular angiography, 94
Successive angiocardiograms, 94
Angioedema, 20
Angiography, 312
Angioma, 295
Angioneurotic edema. See
  angioedema, 20
Angiorrhexis, 4
Angiosarcoma, 295
Angiospasm, 92
Angiotomy, 7
ANHA, 285
Animal inoculation, 277
Anisocytosis, 6, 113
Anisometr., 251
Anisometropia, 246
Ankyle, 36
Ankyloglossia, 141
Ankylosing spondylitis, 48
Ankylosis, 37
  artificial, 39
Anode. See electrotherapy, 307
Anomalies, congenital, 79
Anorchism, 177
Anorexia, 147
Anosmia, 125
Anovulation, 196
Anoxemia, 133
Anoxia, 133
ANS, 72
Anteflexion, 2
Antenatal, 12
Antepartum, 12
Anterior, 17
Anthracosis, 131
Antianxiety agents, 68
Antibody labeling with fluorescein, 280
Anti-D antibody injection, 208
Antidepressants, 68
Antigen, 120, 207, 268
Antiglobulin reaction, 212
Antipsychotic agents, 68
Antipyretic, 12
Antisepsis, 12
Antiseptic, 268
Antistreptolysin-O titer, 94
Antitoxin, 12, 268
Antrectomy,
  mucosal, 161
Antrotomy, 5, 127
Antrum, 126
Antrum of Highmore. See maxillary
  sinus, 127

Antrum window operation, 137
Anular, 23
Anulus fibrosus. See intervertebral
  disc, 37
Anuria, 171
Anus, 147
Anxiety neurosis. See neurosis, 65
AOA, 285
AOC, 310
Aorta, 89
Aortic
  anastomosis, 101
  arch syndrome, 90
  bifurcation occlusion syndrome, 286
  coarctation, 101
  sinuses, 79
  stenosis, 90
  stenosis and insufficiency, 101
Aortocoronary artery bypass, 84, 100
Aortography, 93
  abdominal, 93
  thoracic, 93
Aortoiliac
  disease, 90
  endarterectomy, 101
  occlusions, 286
  thrombosis, 286
AP, 46, 136
APA, 72
APC, 280
Apex of lung, 129
Apgar score, 210
Aphagia, 143
Aphasia, 63
  motor, 63
  sensory, 63
APHA, 27
Aphonia, 128
Aphthous stomatitis, 141
Aplasia
  bronchus, 129
  lung, 131
Apnea, 12, 133
Apoplexy, 312. See cerebrovascular
  accident, 59
Aponeurosis, 42
Appendectomy, 3, 149, 160
Appendicitis, 148
Appendix, 147
  vermiformis, 147
Apraxia, 285
APRL, 310
APTA, 310
Aqueous humor, 251
Arachnodactyly. See Marfan's
  syndrome, 274
Arachnoid, 57
ARC, 27
Archimedes principle, 308
Arcus, 283
  senilis, 242, 284
ARD, 136, 280
Areola, 24
Argentaffinoma. See carcinoid, 291
Argyll-Robertson pupil, 246
ARRS, 329
ARRT, 329
Arterial spiders, 154
Arteriolar nephrosclerosis, 167
Arteriosclerosis, 4, 90
  arteriolosclerosis, 90
  atherosclerosis, 90
  Mönckeberg's medial calcific
    sclerosis, 90
Arteriosclerosis obliterans, 90

Arteritis
  cranial, 283
  giant cell, 283
  of the aged, 283
Artery, 89
Arthralgia, 7, 40
Arthritis, 7, 37
  atrophic, 37
  gouty, 37
  infectious, 37
  hypertrophic, 7
  Marie Strümpell, 37
  traumatic, 37
Arthroclasia, 39
Arthrodesis, 5, 39
Arthrology, 7
Arthroplasty, 5
Arthrodynia. See arthralgia, 40
Arthrography, 44
Arthrolysis, 39
Arthron, 36
Arthropathy, 38
Arthroplasties of hip, 39
  Charnley, 39, 48
  Colonna, 40, 48
  Moore and Thompson, 40, 48
  Vitallium mold, 40, 48
Arthroplasties of knee, 40
  Geomedic, 40
  MacIntosh, 40
  MGH, 40
Arthroplasty, 39
Arthroplasty of
  temperomandibular joint, 40
Arthrotomy, 40
Articulation, 37
  cartilaginous, 37
  diarthrodial, 37
  fibrous, 37
  synovial, 37
as, 263
Asbestosis, 131
Aschheim-Zondek, 211
Aschoff bodies, 89
Ascites, 152
ASCP, 122
ASD, 8
ASHD, 98
ASO, 98
Aspergillosis, 271
Aspermia, 229
Asphyxia neonatorum, 209
Aspirin tolerance test, 117
Asplenia, 116
Association neurons, 53
ASS, 46
Asthenia, 12, 283
Astigm., 251
Astigmatism, 246
Astro, 291
Astrocytoma. See primary brain
  tumor, 59
Asystole, 89
Ataractics, 68
Ataraxics, 299
Ataxia, 63
Atelectasis, 3, 131
  neonatorum, 3, 209
Athelia, 24
Atherosclerosis, 90
Atherosclerotic
  aortoiliac occlusion, 101
  heart disease, 100
  occlusive disease, 286
  vascular disease, 286

aortoiliac, 286
  femoropopliteal, 286
  renal, 286
Athetosis. See dyskinesia, 64
Athlete's foot. See epidermophytosis, 21
Atom, 315
  electrons, 315
  neutrons, 315
  protons, 315
Atomic weight, 315
Atony of bladder, 173
Atopic skin disorders, 20
ATP, 235, 310
Atresia, 12, of
  anus. See imperforate anus, 209
  choanae, 125
  esophagus, 143
  external auditory meatus, 258
  hymen, 199
  vagina, 189
  vulva, 189
Atria. See cavities of heart, 78
Atrial
  arrhythmias, 81
  fibrillation, 81
  flutter, 81
  septal defect, 79
Atrioseptostomy by balloon catheter.
  See Rashkind operation, 84
Atriotomy, 100
Atrioventricular block, 82, 100
  first degree, 82
  second degree, 82
  third degree, 82
Atrioventricular
  bundle, 78
  nodal arrhythmias, 81
  nodal rhythm, 81
Atrophy and degeneration of retina, 243
ATS, 137
Attitude, obstetric, 206
Audiometric test, 262
Audiometry, 262
  electrodermal, 262
  electroencephalic, 262
  impedance, 262
  speech, 262
Auditio, 256
Auditory agnosia, 261
Auditory tube, 256
Augmentation mammaplasty, 25, 29
Aura, 63
Aural barotrauma. See aerotitis
  media, 258
Aural
  discharge, 261
  furunculosis, 262
  polyp, 258
  vertigo, 56
Auricle, 256
Auscultation, 137
Austin Moore or Fred Thompson
  arthroplasty, 48
Autism, 68
Auto, 271
Autoagglutinin. See agglutinin, 119
Autoantibodies, 273
Autofluoroscope, 318
Autogenous graft, 287
Autograft, 274
Autografting of bone. See bone
  grafting, 35
Autohemolysins, 273
Autoimmune diseases, 273
Autoimmunization, 273

Autologous marrow infusion, 292
Automatic bladder, 175
Automation, 86
Autonomous bladder, 175
Autonomy, 291
Autoradiograph. See
  radioautograph, 318
Autosomal chromosome. See
  chromosome, 227
Autosome, 227
Autosplenectomy, 116
Autotransplantation. See bone
  grafting, 35
AV, 98
Avascular necrosis of bone, 31
Avertin, 304
Avulsion of endolymphatic
  labyrinth, 265
Axon, axone, 53
Ayre's surface cell biopsy, 197
AZ, 215
Azotemia, 171

— B —

Ba, 158
Babinski reflex, 71
Bacillary dysentery, 270, 277
Bacillus, 268
Background radiation, 315
Bacterio, 268
Balanitis, 177
Balano, 176
Baldy-Webster suspension, 194
Ballism. See dyskinesia, 64
Ballistocardiography, 97
Ballottement, 206
Banding of pulmonary artery, 99
Bandl's ring, 206
Barbiturate serum concentration, 71
Barium enema, 154
Barium swallow in cardiovascular
  disorders, 94
Barotitis media. See aerotitis
  media, 258
Barr test of nuclear sex. See buccal
  smear test, 234
Bartholin's
  abscess, 199
  adenitis, 189
  retention cysts, 189
Bartholin's glands. See vestibular
  glands, 189, 199
bas, 121
Basal
  anesthesia, 299
  body temperature, 203
  cell carcinoma, 21, 159, 293
  metabolism, 231
Base of lung, 129
Basis, 299
Basset operation, 199
BBB, 98
BBT, 215
BC, 263
BCG, 136
BDAC, 72
BE, 46, 310
Bedsonia virus, 276
Behavior of tumor, 291
BEI, 235
Bell's palsy, 54
Bence-Jones protein, 45
Benign, 291

Cerebellum, 56
Cerebral, 7
  angiography, 69
  aneurysm, 59
  arteriovenous malformation, 59
  atherosclerosis, 59
  concussion, 59
  cortex, 56
  embolism, 59
  hemisphere, 312
  hemorrhage, 209
  localization, 56
  palsy, 59
  thrombosis, 59
Cerebral aqueduct. See ventricles, 57
Cerebrospinal, 7
  otorrhea, 63
  rhinorrhea, 64
Cerebrovascular accident, 59, 312
Cerebrum, 56
Cerumen, 256
  gland adenoma, 258
Cervical, 7
  canal, 192
  mediastinotomy, 134
  region, 17
  rib, 31, 91
  segment, 312
Cervicectomy, 7, 194
Cervicitis, 193
Cervicovesical, 7
Cervix, 190
Cervix of uterus, 192
  cervical canal, 192
  external os. See ostium, 192
Cesarean hysterectomy, 205
Cesarean section, 205, 216
  classical, 205
  low uterine segment, 205
  vaginal hysterectomy, 205
CF, 121
CFT, 280
Chadwick's sign, 206
Chalasis, 283
Chalazion, 247
Chambers of eye, 240
  anterior, 240
  posterior, 240
Charnley low-friction arthroplasty, 48
c.gl., 251
C_2H_4, 302
C_3H_6, 302
$CHCl_3$, 302
C_2HCl_3, 302
C_2H_5Cl, 302
CHD, 98
CHF, 98
Cheilitis, chilitis, 7, 141
Cheiloplasty, 7, 142
Cheilos, 141
Cheilosis, chilosis, 7, 141
Cheilostomatoplasty, 142
Chemical analysis of CSF. See exam.
  of CSF, 70
Chemosis, 248
Cheyne-Stokes respiration, 133
Chickenpox, 269, 275
Chief salivary glands, 142
Chiromegaly, 7
Chiropody, 7
Chirospasm, 6
Chloasma, 23
Chloride salts, 234
Chloroform, 304
Choana, 125

Choked disk. See papilledema, 244
Cholangi, 149
Cholangiography, 155
  operative, 155
Cholangitis, 7, 152
Chole, 149
Cholecyst, 7, 149
Cholecystectomy, 153, 162
Cholecystitis, 152
Cholecystogram, 7
Cholecystography, 155
Cholecystostomy, 153
Choledoch, 149
Choledochoduodenostomy, 153
Choledocholithotomy, 153
Choledochoplasty, 153
Cholelithiasis, 3, 152
Cholelithotomy, 5
Cholemia. See hepatic coma, 151
Cholesteatoma, 258
Cholesterol, 158, 233, 234
  esters, 158
Chondrectomy, 8, 40
Chondritis, 38
Chondroblastoma, 38
Chondrocalcinosis, 38
Chondrofibroma, 8
Chondroma, 8, 38, 294
Chondromalacia of patella, 49
Chondroplasty, 40
Chondros, 36, 127
Chondrosarcoma, 38, 294
Chorea. See dyskinesia, 64
  Huntington's, 60
  Sydenham's, 60
Choriocarcinoma, 204, 294
Choroid, 240
Choroidal hemorrhage, 242
Chorion, 207
Christmas disease, 111
Chroma, 227
Chromatin, 227
Chromosomal aberration, 227
  acquired, 227
  congenital, 227
  monosomy, 227
  trisomy, 227
Chromosome, 227
Chronaxie, 310
Chronic
  airway obstruction, 129
  brain syndrome, 285
  congestive splenomegaly, 116
  granulomatous disease, 112
Chvostek's sign, 210
Cicatrix of skin, 23
Cicatrization, 23
Cilia, 247
Ciliary body, 240
Ciliary zonule, 240
Cineangiocardiography, 94
Cinecholedochography, 155
Cineradiography, 155, of
  urinary tract, 179
Cineroentgenography. See
  cineradiography, 155
Cingulumotomy, 62
Circinate degeneration, 243
Circulation time, 94
Circulatory arrest, 303
Circumcision, 177
Circumstantiality, 68
Cirrho, 149
Cirrhosis of liver, 151
CIS, 198

Cisternal puncture, 70
Claudication, 43, 92
  lower extremity, 92
  upper extremity, 92
Cleft lip, 141
Cleft palate, 141
Clinitest, 180
Clipping of frenum linguae, 142, 210
Clitorectomy, 199
Clitoris, 189
Clonic spasm, 44
Clostridium
  botulinum, 277
  perfringens, 277
Closure of
  bronchopleural fistula, 129
  vesicovaginal fistula, 199
Clot formation (nuclear) studies, 322
  fibrinogen uptake ^{125}I or ^{131}I, 322
Clotlysis, 117
Clot retraction, 117, 119
Clotting time. See coagulation
  time, 117, 119
cm, 122
CM, 263, 330
CMV, 275
Coagulant, 117
Coagulation time, 117, 119
Coagulum, 117
Coarctation of aorta, 90, 98
Coats of arteries
  tunica externa, 89
  tunica media, 89
  tunica intima, 89
Coats of eye
  cornea, 240
  retina, 240
  uvea, 240
COC, 310
CO_2, 235, 302
CO_2 capacity, 232
Coccidioides immitis, 278
Coccidioidomycosis, 271, 278
Coccus, 268
Cochlea, 256
Codman's exercises, 309
COH, 158
Cold agglutinin. See agglutinin, 119
Cold anoxic arrest, 87
Cold conization of uterine
  cervix, 193
Cold knife cone biopsy of uterine
  cervix. See cold conization, 193
Cold punch transurethral resection of
  vesical neck, 174
Cold quartz, 308
Colic, 149
Colitis, 148
  ischemic, 148
  mucous, 148
  ulcerative, 148
Colla, 274
Collagen, 274
  diseases, 274
Collapse surgery, 133
Collection of cerebrospinal fluid, 70
Collecting tubule, 167
Colon, 147
Colonnar capsular arthroplasty, 48
Colonfiberoscopy, 153
Colonoscopy, 153
Colon resection, 149
Color blindness, 246
Colostomy, 5, 149, 161
Colostrum, 206

340

Cyanosis, 133
Cyclic vomiting, 147
Cyclo, 240
Cyclodialysis, 245, 252
Cyclodiathermy, 245
Cyclopropane, 304
Cyclothymic, 68
Cyclothymic personality. See
  personality disorder, 66
Cyclotron, 316
cyl, 251
Cyst, 8
Cystadenocarcinoma, 293
  pseudomucinous, 293
  serous, 293
Cystadenoma, 293
  pseudomucinous, 293
  serous, 293
Cystadenoma of ovary, 195
Cystectomy, 174
Cystic
  degeneration of macula, 243
  disease of breast, 24
  disease of lungs, 131, 138
  duct, 151
  fibrosis of pancreas, 152
Cystine stones, 180
Cystitis, 173
Cysto, 172, 182
Cystocele, 3
Cyst of
  iris, 253
  ovary, 195
Cystogram, 178
Cystographic placentography, 210
Cystography, 8
Cystolithotomy, 174
Cystometrogram, 176
Cystometry, 176
  air, 176
Cystoplasty, 174, 184
Cystorrhaphy, 174, 184
Cystoscope, 8
Cystoscopy, 5, 174, 184
  ultraviolet, 175
Cystostomy, 5, 174, 184
Cyto, 107, 227
Cytogenetics, 227
Cytologic studies of cervix
  Papanicolaou, 197
  Ayre, 197
  Gravlee, 197
Cytology, 8
  spinal fluid, 70
Cytomegalic inclusion disease, 269, 275
Cytomegalovirus, 275
  infections, 269
  perfusion syndrome, 82
  posttransfusion syndrome, 269, 275
Cytotoxicity, 273
CZI, 235

— D —

D₁, 46
D₂, 46
Dacryadenitis, 8
Dacryo-, 247
Dacryoaden-, 247
Dacryoadenectomy, 248, 253
Dacryoadenitis, 248
Dacryocele, 8
Dacryocyst, 8

Dacryocystectomy, 248
Dacryocystitis, 248
Dacryocystography,
  distention, 248
Dacryocystorhinostomy, 248, 253
Dacryocystotomy, 253
Dactylitis, 8
Dactylogram, 8
Dactylomegaly, 8
Dactylospasm, 6
Dark adaptation, 250
Darkfield illumination, 280
D&C, 198
DC, 310
DCR, 72
Debilitated, 99
Debility, 122
Decalcification, 36
Decay, radioactive, 316
Decompression
  brain, 62, 73
  endolymphatic sac, 261
  spinal cord, 62
Decontamination, 316
Decubitus ulcer, 21
Dedifferentiation, 291
Deferens, 176
Defibrillator, 87
Deflection of septum, 125
Degenerative arthritis, 48
Deglutition, 143
Dehiscence of
  graafian follicle, 195
  wound, 195
Dehiscere, 194
Delirium, 68
Delusions of
  grandeur, 68
  persecution, 68
  reference, 68
Dema, 221
Dement, 64
Dementia, 69
Dendrite, 53
Dendron. See dendrite, 53
Denial, 69
Dense, 315
Density, 135
Dent, 141
Dental caries, 141
Depersonalization, 69
Depigmentation, 23
Depression, 285
Derm., 27
Derma, dermis, 20
Dermabrasion, 23
Dermabrasion and excision of
  furrowed brows, 284
  perioral wrinkles, 284
Dermal, 8
Dermatitis, 8, 21
  contact, 21
  exfoliative, 21
  external ear, 258
  medicamentosa, 21
  venenata, 21
Dermatographism, 23
Dermatomyositis, 274
Dermatosis, 4
Dermographia, 23
Dermoid, 240
Dermopathy, 8
Descensus uteri. See prolapse, 193
Descriptive psychiatry, 64
Desensitization, 26

Destructive coxopathy, 38
Detachment of cartilage, 40
Detachment of retina, 243
Determination of calcium in urine
  and feces, 45
Detrusor urinae muscle, 173
Dextroposition of aorta, 79
Diabetes insipidus, 225
Diabetes mellitus, 225
Diabetic retinopathy, 243
Dialysis, 176
  peritoneal, 176
  prophylactic, 176
Diaphragm, 42
Diaphragmatic hernia. See hiatus
  hernia, 43
Diaphysis, 31
Diarrhea, 149
Diarthrodial joint. See synovial joint, 37
Diastase, 155
Diastole, 89
Diastolic augmentation procedure, 87
Diathermy, 308
Dicrotic pulse, 92
Didymos, 176
Diencephalon, 56
Dietl crisis, 171
Differential leukocyte count, 107, 109
Differentiation, 291
Digital autofluoroscope. See
  autofluoroscope, 318
Digital, 92
  blanching, 92
Dilatation and curettage, 194
Dilatation of
  aorta, 90
  cervix, 206
  esophagus, 143
  larynx, 128
Diopter, 250
Diplegia, 64
Diplococcus pneumoniae, 249, 262,
  264, 276
Diploë, 31
Diplopia, 246
Direct
  contact, 268
  current defibrillation, 87
  immunofluorescent staining, 280
  revascularization, 100
  smears and cultures of middle ear
    secretions, 262
  vision cardiac surgery for
    tetralogy of Fallot, 85
Disciform macular degeneration, 243
Discission of lens, 245
Discography, 70
Discoid, 23
Discrete, 23, 135
Dislocation, 38
  ossicles, 259
  patella, 49
Displacement, 69
Displacements of uterus, 193
  anteflexion, 193
  retroflexion, 193
  retroversion, 193
  prolapse, 193
Disruptive trauma of joint, 37
Dissecting aneurysm of thoracic
  aorta, 101
Disseminated lupus
  erythematosus, 273, 274
Disseminated sclerosis. See multiple
  sclerosis, 61

Heterograft. See xenograft, 274
HEW, 137
Hg, 98
5-HIAA, 158, 232
Hiatal hernia, 145
Hiatus hernia, 43, 145
  recurrent, 160
Hiccough, 133
Hiccup. See hiccough, 133
H-ICDA, 27
High femoral osteotomy, 48
Hilus of
  lung, 131
  renal pelvis, 167
Hip flexion contracture, 49
Hip fracture, 33, 48
  femoral neck, 48
  intertrochanteric, 48
Hirschsprung's disease. See congenital
  megacolon, 148
Hirsutism, 224
Histo, 268
Histocompatibility, 273
Histological
  derivation, 293, 294, 295, 296
Histoplasma capsulatum, 278
Histoplasmosis, 131, 271, 278
Histos, 271
Hives. See urticaria, 21
HLR, 98
HM, 251
Hodgkin's disease, 115, 122
Hofmeister technique, 146
Homograft. See allograft, 274
Homografting. See bone grafting, 35
Homotransplantation. See
  bonegrafting, 35
Hordeolum
  external, 247
  internal, 247
Horizontal, 17
Hormone, 221
Hormones of adenohypophysis, 221, 222
  adenocorticotrophic, 221, 222
  diabetogenic, 222
  follicle stimulating, 221, 222
  interstitial cell-stimulating, 222
  luteinizing, 222
  prolactin, 221
  somatotrophic, 222
  thyrotrophic, 222
Howard test, 181
HP, 46
HPL, 215
HPO, 198
HP Soc., 329
HS, hs, 158
HSG, 215
Ht, 121
HUD, 285
Huebner-Todaro hypothesis, 297
Human placental lactogen, 211
Hunner's ulcer, 173
Huntington's chorea. See chorea, 60
HVD, 98
Hyaline membrane disease. See
  idiopathic respiratory distress, 209
Hydatidiform mole, 204
Hydramnios. See polyhydramnios, 205
Hydro, 307
Hydrocele, 3
  tunica vaginalis, 177
  spermatic cord, 177
Hydrocephalus, 60, 209
  adult, 60

ex vacuo. See adult, 60
  infantile, 60
  nonobstructive, 60
  obstructive, 60
  posttraumatic, 61
17-hydrocorticosteroids, 230
Hydrogen ion concentration, 180
Hydronephrosis, 169, 182, 183
Hydrophobia. See rabies, 270
Hydropneumothorax, 134
Hydrops of gallbladder, 152
Hydrosalpinx, 195
Hydrotherapy, 308
Hydroureter, 172
Hymen, 189
  atresia of, 199
Hymenectomy, 199
Hymenotomy, 199
Hypaque, 178
Hyperacidity, 14
Hyperadrenalism, 14
Hyperaeration, 133
Hyperalimentation, 154
Hyperbaric oxygenation, 88
Hyperbaroxia. See hyperbaric
  oxygenation, 88
Hyperbilirubinemia, 217
  neonatal, 209
Hypercalcemic syndrome, 223
Hypercarbia, 121
Hyperchloremia, 226
Hyperchlorhydria, 147
Hypercholesterolemia, 226, 233, 234
Hyperchylomicronemia, 226, 234
Hyperemesis gravidarum, 14, 204
Hyperemia, 14, 248
Hyperesthesia, 64
Hyperglycemia, 3, 226
Hyperglyceridemia, 233, 234
Hyperglycosemia, 3
Hyperinsulinism due to islet cell
  tumor, 223
Hyperkalemia, 226
Hyperkinesia, 44, 224
Hyperlipemia, 233, 234
Hyperlipidemia, 161
Hyperlipoproteinemia, 226
Hypermastia, 24
Hypermetropia, 246
Hypernatremia, 226
Hyperopia. See hypermetropia, 246
Hyperparathyroidism, 223, 236
Hyperpigmentation, 23
Hyperpituitarism, 74
Hyperplasia, 292
  breast, 24
Hyperpnea, 133
Hyperpyrexia, 14
Hyperresonance, 137
Hypersensitivity, 268
  delayed, 268
  immediate, 268
  subacute delayed, 268
Hypersplenic syndrome, 116
Hypersplenism, 116
Hypertension, 14, 90
Hypertensive
  encephalopathy, 61
  retinopathy, 243
  vascular disease, 90
Hypertensive disorders of
  pregnancy, 204
  eclampsia, 204
  preeclampsia, 204
Hyperthyroidism, 223, 330

Hypertriglyceridemia, 226
Hypertrophic pyloric stenosis,
  congenital, 145
Hypertrophy, 14
  conchae, 137
  kidney, 169
  prostate, benign, 177
  right ventricle, 79
  tonsils, 143
Hyperuricemia, 226
Hyperuropiresia, 175
Hyperventilation, 133, 299
  syndrome, 133
Hyphemia, 246
Hypno, 301
Hypnosis, 67
Hypocarbia, 121
Hypochlorhydria, 147
Hypochondriac region, 14, 16
Hypodermic injection, 14
Hypogastric region, 16
Hypoglycemia, 14
Hypolipoproteinemia, 226
Hypomastia, 24, 229
Hypometabolism, 303
Hyponatremia, 226
Hypoparathyroidism, 223
Hypophysis, 221
Hypoplasia of
  breast, 24
  epiglottis, 127
Hypopyon, 242
Hypothalamus. See brain stem, 56
Hypothermia, 100
  induced, 302, 303
Hypothyroidism, 223, 235
Hypotonia, 44
Hypoxia, 133, 299
Hysterectomy, 194
  Cesarean, 205
  subtotal, 194
  supracervical, 194
  vaginal, 194, 205
  Wertheim's, radical, 194, 200
Hysteria, 9, 190
Hysterical deafness, 260
Hysterical neurosis, 65
  conversion type, 65
Hysteropexy, 5
Hysterorrhexis, 4. See rupture of
  uterus, 205
Hysterosalpingography, 210

—I—

I, 330
IASD, 98
IC, 27, 330
ICDA, 27
ICF, 235
ICM, 215
ICN, 27
ICRP, 329
ICSH, 235
ICT, 72
Icterus, 154
Ictotest, 180
ICU, 182
Identification, 69
Idio, 227
Idiogram, 229
Idiopathic respiratory distress, 209
IDK, 46
IF, 235

Mental
deficiency, 65
health, 65
mechanism, 69
retardation, 65
mEq/1, 122
Mesencephalon, 57
Mesocolon, 147
Metabole, 225
Metabolic
acidosis, 225
alkalosis, 225
stone disease, 226
Metabolite, 234
Metaphase, 229
Metastases to bone, 45
Metastasis formation, 292
Metastasize, 292
Metastatic
adenopathy, 159
tumor, 58
Metathalamus. See brain stem, 56
Meter, 307
Methohexital, 304
Methoxyflurane, 304
Metra, 190
Metritis, 10
Metrorrhagia, 10, 194
Metrorrhexis, 10
See rupture of uterus, 205
Mev, MeV, 330
MFT, 312
mg, mgm, 122
MH, 27, 198
MPH, 329
MI, 98
Microcephalus, 61
Microcurie (nuclear), 317, 329
Microcytosis, 115
Microneurosurgery, 62
of pituitary gland, 224
Hardy's approach, 224
Rand's approach, 224
Microorganism, 268
Microphages. See phagocytes, 108
Microsurgery of ear, 260
Micturition, 175
Midbrain. See mesencephalon, 57
Middle
cerebral artery, 312
ear, 256
ear effusion, 259
Miles' operation. See abdomino-
perineal resection, 161
Milia (pl.), 23
milium (sing.), 23
Milieu therapy, 67
Millicurie (nuclear), 317, 329
min, 122
Minimal erythematous dose, 309
Minnesota Multiphasic Personality
Inventory, 71
Miotics, 252
Mitos, 227
Mitosis, 229
Mitral
commissurotomy, 84
insufficiency, 101
stenosis, 101
valve, 78
valvoplasty, 101
Mix. Astig., 251
ml, 122
MLD, 329
mm, 122

mm^3, 122
mm Hg, 98
MMPI, 72
MN system, 120
Modified Gilliam procedure. See
suspension of uterus, 194, 200
Modified Hibbs arthrodesis, 48
Molds, 268
Mole. See nevus, 21
mon, 122
Mönckeberg's medial calcific
sclerosis, 90
Mondini's deafness, 260
Mongolism. See Down's syndrome, 209
Monilia. See Candida albicans, 278
Moniliasis. See candidiasis, 141
Moniliform, 23
Monitoring, 317
Mono, 227
Monocular blindness, 246
Monocytes, 108
Monospot. See spot test, 279
Morbid obesity, 161
Moro's reflex, 210
Motor aphasia, 63
MPC, 329
MPL, 329
MS, 72, 98
MSH, 235
MSL, 46, 137
MSRPP, 72
mμ, 215
Mucopurulent discharge, 178
Mucosal antrectomy, 146
Mucoviscidosis, 217
See cystic fibrosis, 152
Multi, 203
Multiform, 24
Multipara, 203
Multiple detrusor myotomy, 174
Multiple
myeloma, 45, 112, 294
polyposis, 148
rib resection. See extrapleural
thoracoplasty, 133, 138
sclerosis, 61
Mumps, 270, 275
Mural lesions
adventitial, 287
medial, 287
Murmur, 89
Muscle
insertion, 43
origin, 43
Muscle contraction
concentric, 309
eccentric, 309
isokinetic, 309
isometric, 309
isotonic, 309
Muscle relaxants, 303
Muscular
dystrophy, 43
rheumatism. See fibrositis, 38
Mustard operation, 84
Mutant, 227
Mutation, 229
Myasthenia gravis, 43, 236
Myco, 268
Mycobacterium
leprae, 277
tuberculosis, 277
Mycology, 268, 271
Mycosis, 271
Myelencephalon. See medulla

oblongata, 57
Myelin sheath, 53
Myelitis, 10, 61
Myelo, 56
Myelocele, 3
Myelogenous, 10
Myelography, 70
Myeloma
multiple, 33
solitary, 33
Myelopathy, 4
Myelopoiesis, 108
Myeloproliferative, 108
disorders, 112
Myelos, 31
Myelosarcoma, 10
Myelosclerosis, 112
Myitis, 10
Myo, 42
Myocardial
infarction, acute, 83
ischemia, 100
revascularization, 84
sinusoids, 78
Myocardial disease
primary:
myocarditis, 83
myocardosis, 83
secondary:
with noninfectious systemic
diseases, 83
Myocardium, 10, 78
Myolysis, 6
Myoma, 43
Myomectomy, 4, 194
abdominal, 194
vaginal, 194
Myometrium, 92
Myop, 251
Myopathy, 4
Myopia, 246
Myoplasty, 43
Myorrhaphy, 43
Myosarcoma, 43
Myositis, 10, 43
Myotasis, 43
Myotomies, 49
Myringa, 256
Myringitis, 258
Myringotomy, 261, 264
Myringoplasty, 261, 264
Myxedema, 223, 235
Myxoma of right atrium, 100
Myxovirus, 275

— N —

N, 317, 329, 330
NaCl, 235
NAMH, 72
Nanocurie, 329
NARC, 72
Narcoanalysis, 67
Narcose, 299
Naris, pl. nares, 125
Nasal meatus, 125
Nasolacrimal duct, 247
Nasopharyngeal cancer, 125
Nasopharyngitis, 125
Nasopharynx, 225
Natural childbirth, 203
Read's method, 203
psychoprophylactic, 203
Natus, 208

Paresis, 64
Paresthesia, 64, 287
Paries, 134
Parietal pleura, 134
Pario, 203
Parkinson's disease. See paralysis
    agitans, 61, 74
Paronychia, 21
Parotid, 142
    gland. See salivary glands, 142
    tumor, 160
Parotidectomy, 160
Parotitis, 15, 142
    infectious. See mumps, 270, 275
Paroxysmal
    atrial tachycardia, 81
    digital cyanosis, 92
    hyptertension, 224
    pain, 56
Parrot fever, 270
Parturient, 203
Pasteurella tularensis, 277
PAT, 98
Patellectomy, 49
Patelloplasty, 49
Patency, 287
Patent ductus arteriosus, 79
Path, 198
Pathogenic, 6, 269
PBI, 231, 235
PC, pc, 158
Pco$_2$, 120
    arterial, 120
    venous, 120
PCT, 122
PCV, 122
PDA, 98
PDR, 302
Peau d'orange, 25
Pedal circulation, 92
Pediculosis, 21
PEG, 72
Pel-Ebstein type of fever, 116
Pelvic
    exenteration, 194, 293
    inflammatory disease, 195
    inlet. See pelvic brim, 204
    outlet, 204
Pelvimetry, 210
Pelvis, 31, 203, 204
    false, 204
    true, 204
Pemphigus, 21, 27
    vulgaris, 27
Pemphix, 20
Penia, 107
Penis, 176
Pent., 302
Penthrane, 304
Pentothal, 304
Perceptual motor testing, 310
Percussion, 137
Percutaneous
    cordotomy, 62, 74
    needle biopsy, 132
    splenoportography, 93
    transfemoral catheterization of
        coronary arteries, 96
Perforated viscus, 148
Perforation of tympanic membrane, 258
Perfusion in
    intracardiac surgery, 88
    treatment of cancer, 293
Perfusion scan. See lung
    scanning, 320

Periapical abscess, 141
Periarteritis nodosa, 274
Periarthritis. See fibrositis, 38
Periarticular fibrositis. See
    fibrositis, 38
Peribronchial, 135
Pericardial tamponade. See cardiac
    tamponade, 82
Pericardiectomy, 85, 100
Pericardiolysis, 100
Pericarditis, 15, 83
    constrictive, 83
    purulent, 83
Pericardium, 15, 78
Perichondritis, 127
    of auricle, 258
Perimetritis, 15, 193
Perimetrium, 15
Perimetry, 250
Perineorrhaphy, 216
Perineum, 189
Periodontal disease, 141
Periosteum, 15, 31
Periostitis, 15
Peripheral, 17
    arterial insufficiency of
        extremities, 90
    iridotomy, 245
    nerve, 281
    vascular disease, 91
Peripheral pulses
    femoral, 287
    pedal, 287
    popliteal, 287
Peritoneal lavage, 176
Peritoneoscopy, 153
Peritoneum, 149, 151
Peritonsillar abscess, 143
Personality disorder, 66
    alcohol addiction, 66
    cyclothymic p., 66
    drug dependence, 66
    inadequate p., 66
    schizoid p., 66
Persuasion, 67
Pes, ped, 31, 36
Petechiae, 23
Petrissage, 308
Petrositis, 260
PFT, 312
PGH, 235
PH, 27
pH, 121, 182
    arterial pH, 121
    venous pH, 121
Phage, 107
Phagocytes, 108
Phakos, 240
Phantom limb pain, 36
Pharyngeal tonsil, 143
Pharyngitis, 143
    febrile, 269, 275
Pharyngoconjunctival fever, 269
Pharyngotympanic tube. See
    auditory tube, 256
Pharynx, 143
Phenotype, 229, 234
Phenylalanine, 213
Phenylketonuria, 226
    detection, 213
Phenolsulfonphthalein, 181
Phimosis, 177
Phleb, 89
Phlebitis, 91
Phlebosclerosis, 91

Phlebotomy, 92
Phleborrhaphy, 92
Phlegmasia alba dolens, 205
Phobia, 69
Phocomelia, 209
Phono, 127
Phonocardiography, 7, 97
    intracardiac, 97
Phoresis, 271, 307
Phosphate and carbonate stones, 180
Phospholipid-P, 233
Photo, 307
Photocoagulation, laser, 245
    argon laser beam, 245
    krypton, laser, 245
    ruby laser, 245
    xenon laser, 245
Photocoagulation, ocular, 245
Photon, 317
Photophobia, 246
Photoscan. See scan, 318
Phototherapy for neonate, 213
Phragm, 42
Phren, 64, 134
Phrenicotripsy, 5
Phylaxis, 271
Physiatrist, 307
Physical, 307
    agents, 307
    medicine, 307
    therapist, 307
    therapy, 307
    therapy assistant, 307
Physical dependence, 73
Physio, 307
Physis, 31, 221
PI, 27
Pia mater, 57
Pica, 207
Pick's disease, 285
Picocurie, 329
Picornavirus, 275
    coxsackie A, 275
    coxsackie B, 275
    ECHO, 275
PID, 198
Pigment, 20
    forming tissue, 296
Pigmentum, 20
Piles. See hemorrhoids, 148
Pilonidal cyst, 148
    excision of, 149
    exteriorization, 149
    marsupialization, 149
Pilus, pili, 20
Pinna. See auricle, 256
PIT, 329
Pituita, 221
Pituitary
    gland. See hypophysis, 221
    tumor, 59, 74
PL, 251
Placenta, 203, 204
    ablatio, 205
    abruptio, 205
    previa, 205, 216
Placental scanning, 321
Placentography, 210
    cystographic, 210
    intravenous, 210
Plakia, 291
Planigrams. See laminograms, 25, 135
Planta, 31
Planus, 36

RMT, 215
ROA, 215
Roentgenogram, 25
Roentgenography, 25
Roentgenologist, 25
Roentgen rays, 25
ROM, 312
Romberg
  sign, 71
  test, 263
Roots of spinal nerves, 54
  dorsal, 54
  ventral, 54
ROP, 215
Rorschach personality test, 71
ROT, 215
Rouleaux formation, 115
RPCF, 280
RPF, 182
RPR, 280
RR, 98
RSA, 215
RScA, 215
RScP, 215
RSNA, 329
RSP, 215
RTA, 182
Rubella (pregnancy), 213.
  See German measles, 269
  virus, 276
Rubeola. See measles, 270, 276
  virus, 276
Rubin test. See tubal insufflation, 212
Ruga, 145
Rupture of
  aneurysm, 91
  bladder, 184
  quadriceps tendon, 49
  tuboovarian abscess, 195
  tympanic membrane, 258
  uterus, 205
RV, 98
RVH, 98
R wave, 97
Rx, 27

— S —

S, 46
SA, 98
Sabin-Feldman dye test, 278
SACH, 46, 312
Sacral region, 17
Sagittal, 17
SAL, 263
Saline abortion, 206
Salivary gland virus disease. See
  cytomegalic inclusion disease, 269
Salivation. See ptyalism, 142
Salmonella
  paratyphi, 277
  typhi, 277
Salmonella infection, 270
Salmonellosis. See salmonella
  infection, 270
Salpingectomy, 196, 200
Salpingitis, 195
  of eustachian tube, 259
Salpingo, 194, 256
Salpingolysis, 196
Salpingo-oophorectomy, 196, 200
Salpingoplasty. See tuboplasty, 196

Saphenofemoral junction, 287
Saphenous vein, 287
Saprophyte, 269
Sarco, 291
Sarcoma, 4, 292
  of breast, 24
Sarcomas
  angiosarcoma, 295
  chondrosarcoma, 38, 294
  Ewing's sarcoma, 33, 294
  fibrosarcoma, 294
  hemangiosarcoma, 295
  lymphangiosarcoma, 295
  lymphosarcoma, 115, 295
  meningosarcoma, 295
  neurofibrosarcoma, 295
  osteogenic sarcoma, 35, 294
  osteosarcoma, 294
  reticulum cell sarcoma, 295
SAT, 72
Saucerization, 47
SB, 72
SBE, 98
SC, 302
Scabies, 21
Scalene anticus syndrome, 91
Scaler, 318
Scan, 318
  photoscan, 318
  scintillation scan, 318
Scanning, 319
  speech, 64
Scanogram, 44
Scanography, 44
Scars of cornea, 242
  leukoma, 242
  macula, 242
  nebula, 242
Schiller test, 198
Schilling's hemogram, 107, 109
Schisis, 240
Schizo, 4
Schizoid personality. See personality
  disorder, 66
Schizophrenia, 66
  catatonic, 66
  hebephrenic, 67
  latent, 67
  paranoid, 67
Sciatic neuritis, 54
Sciatica. See sciatic neuritis, 54
Scintilla, 315
Scintillation
  camera. See Anger camera, 318
  counter, 319, 330
  scan. See scan, 318
Scintiphotography, 319
Scirrhous, 291, 292
Sclera, sclero, 240, 274
Scleral buckling operation, 246, 252
Sclerectomy, 252
Scleritis, 242
Scleroderma, 274
Scolios, 36
Scoliosis, 38
Scope, 128
Scotoma, 246
Scotometry, 250
Scout film, 155
Scrotum, 176
SD, 46
Sebaceous glands, 20
Seborrheal, 24
  seborrheic, 24
Sebum, 20

Secretory
  otitis media, 259
  tubule, 167
Secundines, 204
SED, 312
Sedation, 299
Segment, 301
Segmental resection of lung, 133, 138
Selective
  intra-arterial infusion of
    vasopressor, 154
  segmental bronchography, 136
SEM, 263
Semen, 176
Semicircular canals, 15
Semicoma, 15
Semilunar valves, 15, 78
Seminiferous tubule dysgenesis. See
  Klinefelter's syndrome, 229
Senescence, 283
Senile
  dementia. See psychoses with organic
    brain syndrome, 66
  macular degeneration, 284
  osteoporosis, 284
  pruritus, 284
  purpura, 284
  sebaceous adenomas, 284
  tremor, 284
Senile psychoses, 285
  delirium and confusion, 285
  dementia, 285
  depression and agitation, 285
  paranoia, 285
  presbyophrenia, 285
  Wernicke's syndrome. See
    presbyophrenia, 285
Senilis, 283
Senility, 283
Senium, 283
Senopia. See gerontopia, 284
Sensitivity, 269
Sensitivity studies, 136
Sensory
  aphasia, 63
  deprivation, 69
Septectomy, 125, 137
Septic shock, 196
Septum, 125
  deflection of, 125
  nasal, 125
Sequestration, 35
Sequestrectomy, 36, 47
Sequestrum, 35
Serous otitis media, 259, 264
  with hemotympanum, 259
Serpiginous, 24
Serum, 108
  acid phosphatase, 182
  albumin, 157
  alkaline phosphatase, 157
  bilirubin, 157
  calcium, 44
  carotene level, 156
  cholinesterase, 158
  diastase, 156
  globulin, 157
  iron, 121
  leucine aminopeptidase, 156
  lipase, 156
  phenylalanine, 213
  phosphorus, 44
  protein-bound fucose level, 198
  proteins, total, 157
  uric acid, 45